AF676803

Subarachnoid Hemorrhage

NEUROLOGICAL DISEASE AND THERAPY

Series Editor

WILLIAM C. KOLLER

Department of Neurology
University of Kansas Medical Center
Kansas City, Kansas

1. Handbook of Parkinson's Disease, *edited by William C. Koller*
2. Medical Therapy of Acute Stroke, *edited by Mark Fisher*
3. Familial Alzheimer's Disease: Molecular Genetics and Clinical Perspectives, *edited by Gary D. Miner, Ralph W. Richter, John P. Blass, Jimmie L. Valentine, and Linda A. Winters-Miner*
4. Alzheimer's Disease: Treatment and Long-Term Management, *edited by Jeffrey L. Cummings and Bruce L. Miller*
5. Therapy of Parkinson's Disease, *edited by William C. Koller and George Paulson*
6. Handbook of Sleep Disorders, *edited by Michael J. Thorpy*
7. Epilepsy and Sudden Death, *edited by Claire M. Lathers and Paul L. Schraeder*
8. Handbook of Multiple Sclerosis, *edited by Stuart D. Cook*
9. Memory Disorders: Research and Clinical Practice, *edited by Takehiko Yanagihara and Ronald C. Petersen*
10. The Medical Treatment of Epilepsy, *edited by Stanley R. Resor, Jr., and Henn Kutt*
11. Cognitive Disorders: Pathophysiology and Treatment, *edited by Leon J. Thal, Walter H. Moos, and Elkan R. Gamzu*
12. Handbook of Amyotrophic Lateral Sclerosis, *edited by Richard Alan Smith*
13. Handbook of Parkinson's Disease: Second Edition, Revised and Expanded, *edited by William C. Koller*
14. Handbook of Pediatric Epilepsy, *edited by Jerome V. Murphy and Fereydoun Dehkharghani*
15. Handbook of Tourette's Syndrome and Related Tic and Behavioral Disorders, *edited by Roger Kurlan*
16. Handbook of Cerebellar Diseases, *edited by Richard Lechtenberg*
17. Handbook of Cerebrovascular Diseases, *edited by Harold P. Adams, Jr.*
18. Parkinsonian Syndromes, *edited by Matthew B. Stern and William C. Koller*
19. Handbook of Head and Spine Trauma, *edited by Jonathan Greenberg*
20. Brain Tumors: A Comprehensive Text, *edited by Robert A. Morantz and John W. Walsh*

21. Monoamine Oxidase Inhibitors in Neurological Diseases, *edited by Abraham Lieberman, C. Warren Olanow, Moussa B. H. Youdim, and Keith Tipton*
22. Handbook of Dementing Illnesses, *edited by John C. Morris*
23. Handbook of Myasthenia Gravis and Myasthenic Syndromes, *edited by Robert P. Lisak*
24. Handbook of Neurorehabilitation, *edited by David C. Good and James R. Couch, Jr.*
25. Therapy with Botulinum Toxin, *edited by Joseph Jankovic and Mark Hallett*
26. Principles of Neurotoxicology, *edited by Louis W. Chang*
27. Handbook of Neurovirology, *edited by Robert R. McKendall and William G. Stroop*
28. Handbook of Neuro-Urology, *edited by David N. Rushton*
29. Handbook of Neuroepidemiology, *edited by Philip B. Gorelick and Milton Alter*
30. Handbook of Tremor Disorders, *edited by Leslie J. Findley and William C. Koller*
31. Neuro-Ophthalmological Disorders: Diagnostic Work-Up and Management, *edited by Ronald J. Tusa and Steven A. Newman*
32. Handbook of Olfaction and Gustation, *edited by Richard L. Doty*
33. Handbook of Neurological Speech and Language Dis-orders, *edited by Howard S. Kirshner*
34. Therapy of Parkinson's Disease: Second Edition, Revised and Expanded, *edited by William C. Koller and George Paulson*
35. Evaluation and Management of Gait Disorders, *edited by Barney S. Spivack*
36. Handbook of Neurotoxicology, *edited by Louis W. Chang and Robert S. Dyer*
37. Neurological Complications of Cancer, *edited by Ronald G. Wiley*
38. Handbook of Autonomic Nervous System Dysfunction, *edited by Amos D. Korczyn*
39. Handbook of Dystonia, *edited by Joseph King Ching Tsui and Donald B. Calne*
40. Etiology of Parkinson's Disease, *edited by Jonas H. Ellenberg, William C. Koller, and J. William Langston*
41. Practical Neurology of the Elderly, *edited by Jacob I. Sage and Margery H. Mark*
42. Handbook of Muscle Disease, *edited by Russell J. M. Lane*
43. Handbook of Multiple Sclerosis: Second Edition, Revised and Expanded, *edited by Stuart D. Cook*
44. Central Nervous System Infectious Diseases and Therapy, *edited by Karen L. Roos*
45. Subarachnoid Hemorrhage: Clinical Management, *edited by Takehiko Yanagihara, David G. Piepgras, and John L. D. Atkinson*

Additional Volumes in Preparation

Neurology Practical Guidelines, *edited by Richard Lechtenberg and Henry Schutta*

Subarachnoid Hemorrhage

Medical and Surgical Management

edited by
Takehiko Yanagihara
David G. Piepgras
John L. D. Atkinson
Mayo Clinic
Rochester, Minnesota

MARCEL DEKKER, INC. NEW YORK • BASEL • HONG KONG

ISBN 0-8247-9519-9

The publisher offers discounts on this book when ordered in bulk quantities. For more information, write to Special Sales/Professional Marketing at the address below.

This book is printed on acid-free paper.

Copyright © 1998 by MARCEL DEKKER, INC. All Rights Reserved.

Neither this book nor any part may be reproduced or transmitted in any form or by any means, electronic or mechanical, including photocopying, microfilming, and recording, or by any information storage and retrieval system, without permission in writing from the publisher.

MARCEL DEKKER, INC.
270 Madison Avenue, New York, New York 10016
http://www.dekker.com

Current printing (last digit):
10 9 8 7 6 5 4 3 2 1

PRINTED IN THE UNITED STATES OF AMERICA

Preface

Subarachnoid hemorrhage is one of the most devastating of neurological disorders, with a catastrophic outcome in many instances. It represents up to 10% of all strokes worldwide. Although several causes of subarachnoid hemorrhage are well known, head injury is the single most common cause. The major structural causes include intracranial aneurysms and vascular malformations. While there have been a fair number of monographs on intracranial aneurysms, particularly with emphasis on the surgical aspects, monographs dealing with subarachnoid hemorrhage from structural lesions are rare. Those dealing comprehensively with the epidemiological, neurological, neurosurgical, neuroradiological, radiosurgical, and rehabilitation aspects of subarachnoid hemorrhage are even rarer, even though the management of these patients with subarachnoid hemorrhage does require a comprehensive team approach by physicians having expertise in many different subspecialties.

In spite of a general decline in the mortality following cerebral infarction and intracerebral hemorrhage in the past 30 to 40 years, there has been no such decline in the mortality rate following subarachnoid hemorrhage in many parts of the world, including the United States and Japan. Many patients still die before reaching hospitals or before implementation of life-saving or salvage measures. There have been clear advances in the management of patients with subarachnoid hemorrhage over the past few decades, past experiences accumulated by our predecessors have aided in decision making for surgical intervention, as have advances in imaging technology and surgical techniques and the development of interventional neuroradiology. As a result more patients who would have been considered inoperable in the past are able to undergo surgical or interventional radiological procedures, with permanent cure as the goal. In addition, recent advances in stereotactic radiosurgery have changed management decisions regarding arteriovenous malformations. The management of patients with vasospasm, based on accumulating knowledge of pathophysiology and new information on neuropharmacology, has improved and is in constant evolution. Even those patients with mental and cognitive impairments following subarachnoid hemorrhage and sequelae have been identified more promptly and have been treated with appropriate rehabilitation to facilitate convalescence before returning to society.

While these advances have no doubt improved the quality of care we can provide to patients following subarachnoid hemorrhage, there is still a wealth of diverse information coming from physicians who treat them. Difficulty maybe encountered in gathering broad-based up-to-date information despite the fact that the multidisciplinary approach does require comprehensive knowledge and mutual understanding of the various subspecialized fields. The present volume was thus planned as two components: First, to have those specialized in different disciplines review recent advances in their own fields, and second, to comprehensively present the major subfields pertaining to the clinical aspects of neurological disorders causing subarachnoid hemorrhage, particularly intracranial aneurysms and vascular malformations. It is likely that some of our readers would prefer reading individual chapters separately according to their needs, but other readers may wish to have a more comprehensive review or to have a reference book. We therefore designed each chapter as an independent entity so that our readers can use individual chapters as the source of specific information, but we also designed this volume to be used as a reference book for any issues related to subarachnoid hemorrhage. We did not include subarachnoid hemorrhage secondary to head injury primarily because of current clinical uncertainty as to its contribution to outcome. However, any future publication on subarachnoid hemorrhage may need coverage of this topic, which is currently in rapid evolution.

Each chapter was written by the staff and former trainees in the Departments of Neurology, Neurologic Surgery, Diagnostic Radiology, Physical Medicine and Rehabilitation, and Health Science Research of the Mayo Clinic. At the Mayo Clinic, we practice the multidisciplinary team approach and have constantly incorporated the above-mentioned technological advances over the past 30 to 40 years for care of patients with subarachnoid hemorrhage from the acute stage to the chronic convalescence period. During this period, Dr. Thoralf M. Sundt, former Chair of the Department of Neurologic Surgery at the Mayo Clinic, played a pivotal role in advancing technology and improving care of patients with subarachnoid hemorrhage. To his contemporaries, he was a colleague with consummate skill, a keen mind, and great discipline and drive. To his patients, he was a compassionate surgeon. To his students currently practicing neurosurgery, he was an excellent teacher and role model. To his memory, we the editors and authors, dedicate this volume.

We are grateful to Mr. Paul Dolgert, former Executive Editor, and Ms. Sandra Beberman, Assistant Vice President of Marcel Dekker, Inc., for providing us with this opportunity, and to Ms. Lia Pelosi, Production Editor, for her excellent editorial assistance.

Takehiko Yanagihara
David G. Piepgras
John L. D. Atkinson

Contents

Contributors

John L. D. Atkinson, M.D., F.A.C.S. Assistant Professor, Department of Neurological Surgery, Mayo Clinic, Rochester, Minnesota

Jeffrey R. Basford, M.D. Associate Professor and Consultant, Department of Physical Medicine and Rehabilitation, Mayo Clinic and Mayo Foundation, Rochester, Minnesota

Bradley F. Boeve, M.D. Senior Associate Consultant and Instructor, Department of Neurology, Mayo Clinic and Mayo Foundation, Rochester, Minnesota

Robert D. Brown, Jr., M.D. Consultant, Department of Neurology, Division of Cerebrovascular Disease, Mayo Clinic, Rochester, Minnesota

Robert J. Coffey, M.D. Associate Professor, Department of Neurological Surgery, Mayo Clinic, Rochester, Minnesota

Nicolee C. Fode, R.N., M.S. Associate and Instructor, Department of Neurosurgery, Mayo Clinic, Rochester, Minnesota

J. R. Fulgham, M.D. Consultant, Department of Neurology, Mayo Clinic, Rochester, Minnesota

Timothy J. Ingall, M.B., B.S., Ph.D., F.R.A.C.P. Assistant Professor, Department of Neurology, Mayo Clinic Scottsdale, Scottsdale, Arizona

Phyo Kim, M.D., Ph.D. Associate Professor, Department of Neurosurgery, Dokkyo University School of Medicine, Tochighi, Japan

Bob Lefsrud, M.D. Department of Diagnostic Radiology, May Clinic, Rochester, Minnesota

Irene Meissner, M.D., F.R.C.P.(C) Associate Professor and Consultant, Department of Neurology, Mayo Clinic, Rochester, Minnesota

Fredric B. Meyer, M.D. Professor, Department of Neurosurgery, Mayo Clinic, Rochester, Minnesota

Gary M. Miller, M.D. Assistant Professor, Department of Diagnostic Radiology, Mayo Clinic, Rochester, Minnesota

Michael K. Morgan, M.D., B.S., F.R.A.C.S. Associate Professor, Department of Surgery, University of Sydney, Sydney, New South Wales, Australia

Akio Morita, M.D. Assistant Professor, Department of Neurosurgery, George Washington University, Washington, D.C.

Vittorio M. Morreale, M.D. Doctor, Department of Neurological Surgery, Mayo Clinic, Rochester, Minnesota

Douglas A. Nichols, M.D. Consultant, Department of Diagnostic Radiology, Mayo Clinic, Rochester, Minnesota

Ronald C. Petersen, M.D., Ph.D. Professor, Department of Neurology, Mayo Clinic and Mayo Medical School, Rochester, Minnesota

George W. Petty, M.D. Associate Professor and Consultant, Department of Neurology, Mayo Clinic and Mayo Medical School, Rochester, Minnesota

David G. Piepgras, M.D. Professor and Chairman, Department of Neurological Surgery, Mayo Clinic, Rochester, Minnesota

Michael R. Puumala, M.D. Department of Neurosurgery, Mayo Clinic, Rochester, Minnesota

Gabriel J. E. Rinkel, M.D. Department of Neurology, University of Utrecht, The Netherlands

Thoralf M. Sundt, Jr., M.D.† Department of Neurological Surgery, Mayo Clinic, Rochester, Minnesota

Jack P. Whisnant, M.D. Emeritus Professor, Department of Neurology, Mayo Clinic, Rochester, Minnesota

David O. Wiebers, M.D. Professor and Chair, Division of Cerebrovascular Diseases, Mayo Clinic, Rochester, Minnesota

Eelco F. M. Wijdicks, M.D., Ph.D., F.A.C.P. Professor, Department of Neurology, Mayo Clinic, Rochester, Minnesota

Takehiko Yanagihara, M.D.* Professor and Chairman, Department of Neurology, Mayo Clinic, Rochester, Minnesota

---

†Deceased.

**Current affiliation*: Osaka University Medical School, Osaka, Japan.

1

Subarachnoid Hemorrhage: An Overview

Takehiko Yanagihara,* David G. Piepgras, and John L. D. Atkinson
Mayo Clinic, Rochester, Minnesota

I. INTRODUCTION

The mortality rate due to cerebrovascular disease has declined steadily in the United States and Europe and precipitously in Japan in the past 30 years. The most notable decline has occurred among patients with intracerebral hemorrhage and to a lesser degree among those with cerebral infarction. For these patients, control of hypertension may have played a role, and risk factors for intracerebral hemorrhage and cerebral infarction have been well defined. However, the mortality from subarachnoid hemorrhage (SAH) has not declined in either the United States or Japan, and these sudden tragic events are still encountered in daily medical practice. Hence, identification of risk factors, improvement in medical and surgical management, and concentrated effort in rehabilitation are still necessary.

The most common cause of SAH is head injury, however, this subject will not be addressed in this text. Subarachnoid hemorrhage caused by structural lesions are most commonly ruptured intracranial aneurysms and intracranial vascular malformations. In addition, SAH can be caused by hematologic disorders without any detectable structural causes. While SAH is the common denominator, the diagnostic and therapeutic approaches are somewhat different among these disorders. Even when a structural cause of SAH has been identified, surgical treatment may not be feasible because of the general and/or neuro-

---

**Current affiliation*: Osaka University Medical School, Osaka, Japan.

logical conditions of the patients and the size and/or location of the responsible aneurysms, or vascular malformations. One of the most serious complications of SAH remains vasospasm, which may lead to serious focal neurological deficits or cognitive impairment despite successful obliteration of the hemorrhagic source. While we have witnessed technical advances in interventional radiology to relieve vasospasm and have tried various pharmacological agents for prevention and amelioration of vasospasm, further development of efficacious therapeutic agents is needed. In spite of the best available medical and surgical management, a significant percentage of patients with SAH still experience serious sequelae of cognitive and/or focal neurologic deficits as a result of the primary hemorrhage or secondary complications. For these patients, intensive and sometimes prolonged rehabilitation efforts are necessary to optimize neurologic recovery.

With these problems in mind, this volume was designed to review experimental SAH models currently utilized, and review the current multispecialty clinical practice in the diagnosis and management of SAH and sequelae.

II. SUBARACHNOID HEMORRHAGE, VASOSPASM, AND PHARMACOLOGICAL MODIFICATION OF VASOSPASM IN ANIMAL MODELS

Experimental studies of SAH have focused on two major events during acute and chronic stages following SAH. Immediately after rupture of an aneurysm, an increase in intracranial pressure, decrease in cerebral blood flow, and induction of cerebral ischemia often causes a high mortality. This acute condition has been reproduced in many experimental models. The main focus of animal experimentation related to SAH, however, is delayed ischemia caused by prolonged constriction of cerebral arteries, commonly known as vasospasm, which typically begins 4 to 6 days following SAH and lasts for 2 to 3 weeks in human patients. This temporal profile is believed to represent vasoconstriction caused by cellular damage to smooth muscle, possibly damage to endothelium, and subsequent subendothelial proliferation. Another significant characteristic of this condition is a refractoriness to various pharmacological agents, indicating the presence of a mechanism different from physiologic vasoconstriction. In animal models, it is therefore crucial that the characteristic temporal profile and pharmacologic refractoriness be reproduced. In primates, it is possible to produce an accurate temporal profile of acute and chronic vasospasm either by placement of a blood clot over the surface of the brain or intracisternal administration of blood. The subsequent vasospasm reduced luminal diameter and cerebral blood flow by loss of endothelium-dependent relaxation with histological alterations such as endothelial damage, subendothelial proliferation, corrugation of internal elastic lamina, and myonecrosis. However, despite excellent human clinical correlation, there are reasons to limit the use of primates in any animal experimentation, and other animal models have been developed. While acute pathophysiological changes can be produced in rats, which is one of the most commonly utilized species for animal research, chronic vasospasm is short lived and mild. Other experimental models include dog, cat, and rabbit. Although those models are less suitable than primate models, they have been utilized successfully to investigate certain aspects involving the pathophysiology of SAH and pharmacologic manipulations.

Despite many attempts to pharmacologically alter chronic vasospasm, there has been no major breakthrough thus far. Based on existing hypotheses for the pathophysiology of vasospasm, various pharmacological agents have been tried both experimentally and clinically. Neurotransmitter receptor agonists and antagonists have been utilized, however, adrenergic agonists and antagonists have not provided a definitive answer, and serotonin antagonists have not shown positive effects for treatment of chronic vasospasm. Calcium channel blockers have been tried since the early 1980s and have shown some efficacy on chronic vasospasm. Nimodipine has been the most successful of these for the prevention of vasospasm induced ischemic deficits; however, vasospasm itself, as visualized by angiogram, remains unchanged. While traditional vasodilating agents, phosphodiesterase inhibitors, and nitrovasodilators have not been effective when given intravenously, they can be transiently effective when given intraarterially, and papaverine is now in clinical use among interventional radiologists. Suppression of inflammatory prostaglandins, leukotrienes, and free-radial formation have met with some success in animal models. Methylprednisolone, ibuprofen, and tirilazad belong to this group of agents. A recent multicenter clinical trial of tirilazad, which appeared very promising, has met with limited success. A newer approach has been the intrathecal administration of agents with different pharmacologic function such as serine proteases and tissue plasminogen activators.

While we do not have a definitive answer for the management of chronic vasospasm, there are promising future approaches. Unraveling the mechanism of chronic vasospasm will eventually occur and then pharmacologic intervention will play a major role in its prevention.

III. CLINICAL MANIFESTATION OF SUBARACHNOID HEMORRHAGE

A. Epidemiology of Subarachnoid Hemorrhage

Population-based epidemiologic studies are essential in tracing the incidence and prevalence of many diseases and SAH is not an exception. Hospital-based statistics may be biased due to referral patterns and by exclusion of patients who die before coming to the hospital; therefore, accurate accrual of information within the general population is vital. Over the past 40 years there have been at least 56 surveys on SAH from all over the world. However, many of these studies have had methodologic problems included in analyses, and comparison of the remaining studies is difficult because of methodologic differences. Despite these limitations, these studies suggest SAH may represent 5 to 10% of all strokes and the age-adjusted standardized incidence rate ranged from 4.8 to 15.1 per 100,000 per year. In Rochester, Minnesota, the incidence rate has remained stable between 1945 and 1984 at 11.8 per 100,000 per year. Of interest is that the incidence increases with age and is higher in women in most countries. Subarachnoid hemorrhage remains a life threatening disease and more than 10% of patients die before hospital arrival, and the fatality rate within the first 3 months reaches 40% or more. However, encouraging new information suggests a slight decline in the annual mortality rate in many parts of the world.

B. Clinical Characteristics of Neurological Disorders Causing Subarachnoid Hemorrhage

Subarachnoid hemorrhage is one of the most devastating of all cerebrovascular disorders. Intracranial aneurysms and arteriovenous malformations (AVMs) are the two leading structural disorders causing SAH, yet clinical manifestations and prognosis are considerably different. Subarachnoid hemorrhage secondary to intracranial aneurysms occurs in 10 to 16 per 100,000 persons per year, but rupture of aneurysms occurs more often with increasing age and is said to reach 40 per 100,000 per year for ages greater than 75 years. A large-scale prospective study is currently underway in the Unites States, however retrospective studies suggest that aneurysms 1 cm or greater in diameter are at increased risk to rupture.

Clinical manifestations of intracranial aneurysms consist of generalized symptoms ranging from headache to loss of consciousness and focal manifestations due to a local mass effect of the aneurysm, space-occupying hematoma, or subsequent vasospasm. The location and size of the aneurysm and the extent of focal or diffuse SAH dictate the clinical patient parameters. In order to assess the clinical condition of the patient and determine the need for surgical intervention, several clinical grading scales have been advocated. The World Federation of Neurological Surgeons has proposed a universally accepted grading scale based on the Glascow coma scale score and focal neurologic deficit. Natural history suggests rebleeding occurs in 30 to 40% of patients within the first 6 months unless the aneurysm is repaired. Vasospasm occurs in 20 to 40% of patients with ruptured intracranial aneurysms and has increasingly severe neurologic consequences directly related to the size and location of the clot.

Intracranial arteriovenous malformation is the second most common structural cause of nontraumatic SAH accounting for approximately 10% of cases. While AVMs are the most common, other types of vascular malformations including cavernous hemangiomas and dural arteriovenous fistulae can also cause SAH. Although patients with intracranial AVMs do experience SAH, it is important to realize that they actually suffer intracerebral and intraventricular hemorrhage more often than SAH alone. Clinical manifestations encompass not only those associated with intracranial hemorrhage such as severe headaches and loss of consciousness, but also seizures, migraine-like symptoms, and progressive neurologic deficits. The risk of intracranial hemorrhage among patients without prior history of bleeding approximates 2 to 4% per year and this risk persists over time. The risk of rebleeding is even higher, at least temporarily, reaching 6% during the first year after the initial hemorrhage. Subarachnoid hemorrhage is seen in patients with dural arteriovenous fistula. Unlike other vascular malformations, this is an acquired disease related to intracranial sinus thrombosis. Subarachnoid hemorrhage from spinal AVMs comprises less than 1% of all cases of SAH and is suggested by focal or regional spinal or suboccipital symptoms.

Subarachnoid hemorrhage but without an identifiable source after vigorous investigations occurs in perhaps 20% of all SAH patients. Among them, idiopathic perimesencephalic hemorrhage is a distinct variant. This condition is said to make up as high as 10% of all patients with SAH and consists of hemorrhage confined to the perimesencephalic cisterns on cranial computerized tomography (CT) scan, a normal angiogram, and good prognosis.

C. Behavioral Disorders Following Ruptured Intracranial Aneurysms and Surgical Treatment

Cognitive and behavioral disorders are common after SAH. Some neurobehavioral impairments may become permanent and hamper daily professional and social activities. Among them, amnesia, confabulation, and apathy are well known. Amnesia usually is associated with a ruptured aneurysm of the anterior communicating artery and typically occurs as part of the symptom complex of amnesia, confabulation, and personality change. Neuroradiological and autopsy studies have revealed damage to the basal forebrain of these patients. The most frequently encountered personality changes are apathy and fatigue.

IV. NONINVASIVE LABORATORY PROCEDURES FOR DIAGNOSIS OF SUBARACHNOID HEMORRHAGE, INTRACRANIAL ANEURYSMS, VASCULAR MALFORMATIONS, AND VASOSPASMS

Since the advent of CT in the early 1970s, the diagnosis of SAH has increased in accuracy and has obviated the need for diagnostic lumbar puncture in many instances. The advent of magnetic resonance imaging (MRI) in the early 1980s has expanded the opportunity to identify the source of SAH without conventional cerebral angiography. Furthermore, recent advances in diagnostic ultrasound procedures, particularly Transcranial Doppler Ultrasonography (TCD), has augmented the detection of vasospasm. However, there are certain advantages and disadvantages in these diagnostic procedures.

Despite the superiority of MRI in general, CT scan remains the modality of choice to diagnose SAH. The sensitivity in detecting even small amounts of hemorrhage is close to 100% within the first 24 to 48 hours of hemorrhage, and may still be as high as 40% 3 to 4 weeks after large hemorrhages. Even so, a negative CT examination does not necessarily rule out the possibility of SAH and lumbar puncture revealing hemorrhage or xanthochromia can be diagnostic in these situations. The appearance of blood on MRI is quite variable depending on the time after extravasation, oxidation state of red blood cell iron, and pulse sequences as well as field strength of the magnet. Despite these factors, MRI may improve in the future for detection of SAH if the examination time is shortened and new pulse sequences are developed. One such possibility is a recently introduced pulse sequence called fluid attenuated inversion recovery (FLAIR).

The appearance of intracranial aneurysms on MRI may also be variable depending on pulse sequences, the extent of intraluminal thrombosis, and the condition of the surrounding tissues. Although it is commonly accepted that an aneurysm larger then 5.0 mm in diameter can be detected with the current MRI technique, aneurysms smaller than 3.0 mm are not readily visualized due to limitation of the spatial resolution. A powerful diagnostic tool in identifying both symptomatic and asymptomatic vascular malformations, MRI is often capable of differentiating AVMs, capillary malformations, cavernous angiomas, and venous malformation by their characteristic appearances. Angiographically occult lesions such as partially or completely thrombosed vascular malformations can also be detected by MRI. Although both CT imaging and MRI can disclose dural arteriovenous fistulae by visualizing dilated veins and sinuses, MRI provides better anatomic resolution. Magnetic resonance (MR) angiography may be useful in this area, particularly with phase contrast MR angiography, which can demonstrate the direction of blood flow. For detection of spinal AVMs, MRI is considered to be superior to CT myelography and has become the screening modality of choice because of its ability in detecting both parenchymal and vascular changes. However, selective spinal angiography is still necessary in many instances for appropriate management of such patients.

TCD can strongly suggest the presence of vasospasm following SAH by detecting an increase in the mean velocity of cerebral blood flow, provided adequate insonation can be achieved through the skull. The sensitivity of this type of instrument is in the range of mid 80% with the M-1 segment of the middle cerebral artery and the basilar artery, and the specificity for detection of vasospasm in the presence of SAH is in the range of 89 to 100% in the anterior circulation and 82 to 88% in the posterior circulation. Devices for TCD are lightweight, portable, and ideally suited to application at bedside, and the procedure can be repeated easily, thus contributing to detection of vasospasm and decision making for medical, surgical, or interventional treatment.

V. MEDICAL MANAGEMENT OF PATIENTS WITH SUBARACHNOID HEMORRHAGE

The goal of medical management of patients with SAH is to prevent rebleeding and secondary deterioration and to treat medical complications associated with SAH. The best way to prevent rebleeding is repair of the structural source of hemorrhage. However, the general and neurological condition of the patient, and the type, location, and size of the underlying pathology may prevent surgical or neuroradiologic intervention. After SAH, hyponatremia may occur as cerebral salt-wasting syndrome, where both hyponatremia and hypovolemia occur simultaneously. Failure to recognize this syndrome may lead to neurologic deterioration and may accelerate delayed ischemic events. Hydrocephalus has been observed in up to 20% of patients following SAH. Removal of cerebrospinal fluid by lumbar puncture or external ventricular drainage may become necessary in select cases in the acute phase, and ventriculoperitoneal shunting may be necessary in refractory cases.

Clinical vasospasm occurs in 20 to 30% of patients following aneurysmal SAH. The resulting delayed ischemic neurologic deficits may be devastating. Maintenance of normal blood pressure and vascular volume may reduce ischemic effects and nimodipine may lessen clinical ischemic events. Once vasospasm occurs, the treatment is concentrated on maintaining adequate cerebral blood flow. Adequate cerebral blood flow can be indirectly ensured by augmenting cerebral perfusion pressure, which is the difference between mean arterial blood pressure and intracranial pressure. This therapy should aim at maintaining cerebral perfusion by increasing vascular volume and elevation of blood pressure and decreasing any elevated intracranial pressure. Obviously, obliteration of the source of hemorrhage allows more aggressive medical treatment. If neurologic deterioration progresses despite maximal medical therapy, angiographic infusion of papaverine or transluminal angioplasty may play an important role.

VI. SURGICAL MANAGEMENT OF PATIENTS WITH SUBARACHNOID HEMORRHAGE

The outcome of SAH caused by ruptured intracranial aneurysms remains relatively bleak. Even with surgical intervention in good grade patients, only about 50% of patients achieve favorable outcomes after 3 months. There are several important factors that determine surgical intervention. Patients in good clinical grades are generally operated early within 3 to 4 days of hemorrhage despite an increase in the degree of surgical difficulty. However, this is offset by eliminating the source of a repeat hemorrhage and its attendant markedly increased morbidity and mortality. Surgical techniques for repair of intracranial aneurysms have improved greatly thanks to many pioneer neurosurgeons in the past, particularly after introduction of the operating microscope and subsequent development of microsurgical techniques. The shape, size and, location of some aneurysms make them a high surgical risk. Under these circumstances, other techniques such as repair under cardiopulmonary bypass or augmenting neuroradiologic or cerebrovascular bypass procedures may be necessary. High-risk aneurysms are perhaps best treated by centers with experience in the management of these often treacherous lesions.

The surgical intervention for intracranial AVMs differs from intracranial aneurysms. The intracerebral location, size, and vascular pattern dictate the need for surgical intervention as well as intracerebral hematoma and anticipated quality of survival. Surgical procedures may be sufficient by themselves, or augmented with neuroradiologic embolization of part or most of the lesion, or even partial staged ablation with radiosurgery and subsequent surgery years later. Surgical complications for AVMs may be different from those of aneurysmal surgery. Among them, normal perfusion pressure breakthrough, obstructive venous hypertension, and postoperative hemorrhage are major concerns. Normal perfusion pressure breakthrough, an unexpected degree of global postoperative brain swelling, is a controversial issue. There is no well-accepted theory, and it may occur in 3 to 5% of patients, particularly with large AVMs. Strict control of blood pressure offers the best treatment. Obstructive venous hypertension occurs in perhaps 5% of patients postoperatively as the result of venous stasis in the remaining postoperative venous drainage system. Postoperative hemorrhage from residual AVMs occurs in 3 to 5% of patients. This can be prevented by immediate reoperation when residual AVMs are discovered by postoperative cerebral angiography. Parenchymal AVMs in the spinal cord pose different problems with the surgical mortality of 2 to 5%, clinical deterioration of 14 to 20%, and incomplete resection of up to 40%.

VII. ROLE OF INTERVENTIONAL NEURORADIOLOGY AND STEREOTACTIC RADIOSURGERY FOR TREATMENT OF INTRACRANIAL ANEURYSMS AND VASCULAR MALFORMATIONS

Stereotactic radiosurgery has gained solid ground in the past several years for treatment of AVMs, particularly after introduction of the cobalt-60 unit. Other instruments include the linear-accelerator-based system and the charged-particle unit. The advantages of stereotactic radiosurgery are the ability to treat deep-seated AVMs and a short convalescent period. However, the size of AVMs amenable to stereotactic radiosurgery are limited to a range of about 33 cm^3 and it takes 2 years or longer before the nidus completely obliterates. The success rate is over 90% and radiosurgery will remain a significant treatment for management of intracranial AVMs; however, expertise is required to minimize delayed radiation injury to surrounding neural structures.

There are three major roles for interventional neuroradiology in the management of intracranial aneurysms and AVMs. The first is endovascular treatment of intracranial aneurysms. Selective obliteration of saccular aneurysms or occlusion of the parent artery is used for fusiform aneurysms or wide-necked aneurysms involving the cavernous or paraclinoid segment of the internal carotid artery. For selective aneurysmal obliteration, detachable balloons were initially used and failed, but the development of detachable platinum coils has advanced the technology in this field because of their flexibility and their capability for electrothrombosis. It is now possible to carry out this procedure within a few hours after rupture of the aneurysm. However, long term efficacy remains to be proven. The second is endovascular treatment of vasospasm by balloon angioplasty after failure of medical management. It is rare that vasospasm recurs once an artery has been dilated, and this procedure can be combined with intra-arterial administration of vasodilating agents. However, there is a limit in the caliber of the arteries where balloon angioplasty can be performed effectively and safely, and there is a risk of aneurysmal rerupture if balloon angioplasty is performed prior to aneurysmal obliteration. The third is endovascular treatment of AVMs. The most common indication is preoperative embolization and devascularization of AVMs to make surgical intervention easier, but other indications include treatment of steal phenomenon occurring around large AVMs and reduction of the size prior to radiosurgery. Attempts to cure AVMs without surgical resection or radiosurgery by using permanent embolic agents are being utilized, and *n*-butyl cyanoacrylate is rapidly emerging as the embolization agent of choice worldwide.

VIII. REHABILITATION OF PATIENTS FOLLOWING SUBARACHNOID HEMORRHAGE

Cognitive and neurologic deficits may occur following SAH. While 60 to 75% of patients who survive SAH may be functionally independent, many of them may suffer subtle cognitive and emotional deficits. There are two major aspects of SAH that are relevant to rehabilitation. The first is the generalized effect of SAH that may result in confusion, lethargy, agitation, emotional lability, and impaired judgement during the early recovery period. The second aspect is associated with vasospasm and development of focal neurological deficits. Rehabilitation during the acute period is directed to general care with orientation and stimulation and gradual shift toward individual deficits in the chronic period. Physicians specialized in rehabilitation are responsible for organizing individual rehabilitation efforts and they deal with general medical and behavioral problems, where input from behavioral neurologists is important. The role of physiotherapists ranges from prevention of contracture to eventual ambulation, while the role of occupational therapists ranges from cognitive stimulation to eventual home evaluation. In addition, psychological assessment and counseling, speech therapy, recreational therapy and social services play crucial roles in the chronic period. While many patients are transferred to a rehabilitation unit for inpatient rehabilitation where they have daily contact with experienced rehabilitation nurses, it should be kept in mind that the patients who will have the full benefit of a rehabilitation unit are those who have deficits but are motivated to regain independence and have social and family support. While many patients manage to return home, it has been shown repeatedly that patients with "good" clinical outcomes report excessive problems with fatigue, anxiety, lack of concentration, and other mood as well as behavioral disturbances. Thus, careful follow-up after discharge from a hospital or a rehabilitation unit is very important for maximal recovery of patients following SAH.

IX. SUMMARY

Subarachnoid hemorrhage is one of the most devastating of neurologic disorders. The incidence and prevalence has remained stable for decades and despite an exponential improvement in technical and medical management, the morbidity and mortality remain dismal. Current management goals include identification by radiologic screening and, in select cases, preventive obliteration of structural lesions before devastating hemorrhage can occur. Laboratory efforts and clinical studies will further advance treatment and, combined with early detection of potential hemorrhagic sources, will improve our future management in the next generations.

2
Animal Models of Subarachnoid Hemorrhage and Vasospasm

Phyo Kim
Dokkyo University School of Medicine, Tochighi, Japan

I. INTRODUCTION

Animal models of subarachnoid hemorrhage (SAH) have been devised and utilized to study disturbance of perfusion and pathological changes in the brain, as well as to study delayed alterations occurring in the cerebral arteries known as chronic vasospasm. Experimental studies are performed with a focus on either acute or delayed events following subarachnoid hemorrhage. Alterations occurring immediately after rupture of aneurysms, such as an increase in intracranial pressure (ICP), a decrease in cerebral blood flow (CBF), and ischemia of the brain are often very severe in clinical situations and are the reasons for high mortality in the acute period. In fact, a large percentage of patients expire before reaching regional medical institutions [1,2].

Delayed ischemia caused by prolonged constriction of the cerebral arteries occurring in the chronic phase remains a major complication of subarachnoid hemorrhage. The chronic vasospasm and resultant ischemia are superimposed on the course of recovery from the initial insult and often after surgical repair of aneurysms. The arterial spasm develops and persists with a characteristic time course: it starts typically four to six days following the hemorrhage and lasts for two or three weeks [3]. Numerous experimental studies have been performed to elucidate pathogenesis of the chronic spasm and to develop an effective treatment. However, despite the volume of such efforts, an integrative view of the mechanism has yet to be delineated.

To reproduce pathological conditions of subarachnoid hemorrhage and chronic vasospasm in animals, various experimental models have been devised. Rats, rabbits, cats, dogs, pigs, sheep, monkeys, and baboons have been used for this purpose. A variety of techniques have been applied in these animals to induce subarachnoid hemorrhage.

II. CHARACTERISTICS OF THE CLINICAL CONDITION OF CHRONIC VASOSPASM

Following subarachnoid hemorrhage, cerebral arteries undergo sustained constriction. The vasoconstriction evolves in a characteristic time course with a delayed onset of several days after the hemorrhage and lasting for a few weeks, and therefore is often referred to as chronic vasospasm [3]. The constriction and decrease in cerebral blood flow may cause focal ischemia and neurological deficits, which can result in a permanent infarction. The degree of constriction is correlated with the amount and volume of the subarachnoid clot that covers the cerebral vascular tree throughout the cistern.

During chronic vasospasm, the cerebral arteries respond poorly to conventional pharmacological treatments. Ordinary systemic doses of vasodilator agents, such as phosphodiesterase inhibitors and calcium channel blockers, do not reverse or prevent the constriction, although efficacy of the latter in dilating collateral channels and improving the clinical outcome has been demonstrated. With the advent of interventional angiography and improvement of intravascular techniques, selective catheterization and local injection into the spastic segment became feasible. Intra-arterial delivery of vasodilator agents can achieve high local concentrations and cause positive responses, but usually the effect is not long lasting.

The unique temporal profile of cerebral vasospasm as well as the refractoriness to pharmacological treatments indicate that the vasoconstriction is not caused by physiological mechanisms of smooth muscle contractions, such as those elicited by interaction of agonist with receptor. Rather it probably represents constriction due to degeneration or cellular damage of the smooth muscle resulting from interaction with the clot [4,5]. Proliferation of the noncontractile components [6] in the arterial wall may also contribute to the increased rigidity [7,8]. Morphological alterations of the arterial wall, such as damage to the endothelium, subendothelial proliferation, and necrosis of smooth muscle have been described in clinical specimens [6,9,10,11,12]. However these findings have been contradicted by reports of failure to observe such changes [13,14]. The reason for the discrepancy is not certain, but may be due partially to inadequately fixed clinical specimens that are difficult to obtain in a fresh state.

III. PREREQUISITES FOR THE ANIMAL MODELS OF CHRONIC CEREBRAL VASOSPASM

When studying pathophysiology of cerebral arterial spasm in animal models, it is crucial that the arterial constrictions caused by the experimental SAH possess characteristics comparable to clinical cerebral vasospasm. These features include the temporal profile of the sustained contraction with delayed onset and refractoriness to vasodilatory agents.

Focal neurological deficits due to a decrease in CBF and ischemia are not usually reproduced in nonprimate models due to relatively abundant collateral circulation. For example, following blood injections into the cisterna magna in dogs, intense chronic vasoconstriction can be induced in the basilar artery perfusing the brainstem, but focal neurological deficits are not observed. When studying alterations in cerebral blood flow and ischemia, it is essential to use appropriate models where these changes are known to occur.

Morphological alterations of the cerebral arterial wall during chronic vasospasm have been described under both clinical and experimental conditions. However, a great amount of controversy exists as to its significance. In experimental models, histological findings such as damage to the endothelium, subendothelial proliferation, necrosis of the smooth muscle and inflammatory reactions in the adventitia have been described [15,16,17,18], but there are reports of the absence of those changes in identical animal models [14,19a,20,21]. In the canine model of vasospasm, where the characteristic time course and pharmacological refractoriness are analogous to the clinical situation, significance of pathological alterations have been controversial: reports of findings such as smooth muscle necrosis and endothelial damage have been contradicted by negative observations [14,19a,20,21]. In our own experience with this model, frank necrosis of smooth muscle was not characteristic in the spastic arteries, although alterations such as condensation and shrinkage of the cytoplasm of the smooth muscle cells were frequently observed [5]. Generally, pathological changes are not remarkable in small animal models [22,23].

In view of these controversies, studies need to be conducted that consider the variability in histological findings in these models and rigorously define baseline alterations in the preparations obtained by the specific method and protocol in each laboratory.

IV. SPECIES VARIABILITY

The use of small rodent models has great advantages in terms of supply and maintenance and these models are suitable for studying the acute alterations in CBF and ICP following hemorrhage [23,24,25,26,27,28,29,30,31]. Arterial spasm has been reproducible angiographically in rats; however, the time course is not quite analogous to that in humans, having a short duration and little delay [32,33].

The pathophysiology of vasospasm has been studied in rats, especially regarding the possible involvement of neural mechanisms [34]. However, alterations in the pharmacological responsiveness of arteries are studied more often in larger animal models such as in dogs and monkeys due to the size of the vasculature. Nonetheless, with increasing concerns about the ethical aspects in the use of experimental animals in general, small rodent models gradually replace the use of larger animals.

Anatomical characteristics of each species—the size of the brain and the cerebral arteries—influence their suitability for the study of different aspects of vasospasm following subarachnoid hemorrhage. Complexity of contour of the cisterns determines wash-out of the clot by cerebrospinal fluid (CSF). This factor influences persistence of the clot, encasement of the arteries, and thus generation of vasospasm. In monkeys, a single placement of clot in the sylvian cistern suffices to produce spasm in their middle cerebral arteries [18]. By contrast, repetitive blood injections are required for reliable clot formation in the prepontine cistern surrounding the basilar arteries in dogs [35,36] or rabbits [37,38].

Abundance of collateral circulation would prevent development of delayed ischemic deficits, another important factor to characterize models. The injection of blood into the cisterna magna in canine or rabbit models reliably reproduces severe vasoconstriction in the basilar artery; however, the animals develop signs of meningeal irritation and do not usually develop neurologic deficits. This is presumably due to abundance in the collateral circulation and a relative tolerance of the brainstem against ischemia in these animals. Delayed ischemic deficits are observed in monkeys, albeit infrequently, as the result of vasospasm of the middle cerebral arteries after placement of blood clot in the sylvian fissure [18]. Recognizing variability in these characteristics between different species is the critical factor when planning studies of delayed events after subarachnoid hemorrhage.

V. METHODS OF INDUCTION OF SAH

Several methods have been used to induce SAH in experimental animals. To ensure reproducible induction of vasospasm, it is necessary to produce formation of a firm clot surrounding the cerebral artery. Principles of the methods typically employed for induction of hemorrhage are as follows:

1. Injection of blood into the cerebral cistern with puncture or an implanted catheter,

2. Disruption of a cerebral artery and bleeding into the cistern, and
3. Craniotomy and placement of a blood clot in apposition of the cerebral arteries.

Each of the methods has advantages and disadvantages.

Injection can deliver a constant amount of blood in the cistern and is technically simple and less invasive. Typically the cisterna magna is punctured percutaneously with a spinal needle [39]. Alternatively the chiasmatic cistern is punctured with a needle advanced through the orbita to instill blood on the circle of Willis [40]. Injection can be done by a small catheter implanted in the subarachnoid space, however one concern regarding this method is that inflammatory reaction of the arachnoid tissue may occur, possibly causing adhesive arachnoiditis and fibrosis surrounding the artery. We have observed instances of chronic arachnoiditis causing severe vasospasm in the basilar arteries in dogs. The injection/instillation method does not cause direct injury to the arterial wall and does not evoke vascular mechanisms of hemostasis such as interaction with platelets and acute contraction of smooth muscles. Increase in intracranial pressure is moderate as compared to the clinical situation or the condition in the extravasation models where the cerebral artery is ruptured and arterial blood pressure is released into the intracranial cavity. Despite these limitations, instillation of a sufficient amount of blood, especially with multiple injections, allows formation of durable clot and induces vasospasm reliably with a temporal profile analogous to the clinical phenomenon.

Tearing the artery and causing extravasation in the cistern is another standard method of induction of hemorrhage [41,42]. Typically it is done during craniotomy by placing a needle or suture, piercing the cerebral artery, and withdrawing after closure. The ensuing events include blood extravasation and clot formation in the surrounding subarachnoid space and acute constriction of the artery. The extravasation occurs with the arterial blood pressure and if the puncture is effective, the subarachnoid hemorrhage tends to be intense, distributing the clot distally along the arterial tree and causing a rise in the intracranial pressure. The method reproduces the complex conditions of vascular injury with hemorrhage that occur in the actual clinical situation. A drawback to this technique is that the volume of blood extravasated is not controlled, and it is difficult to maintain a constant condition of interaction between the blood clot and the cerebral artery. High mortality of the animals, if the bleeding is intense and protracted, is another disadvantage of this method.

Placement of blood clot over the surface of the cerebral arteries after craniotomy has been done as a method of induction of SAH in monkeys [18]. The advantage of the method is the ability to place the clot in a relatively large volume in direct apposition with the cerebral artery. Vasospasm of the middle cerebral artery in monkeys induced by this method can cause ischemia of the brain perfused by the arterial tree. The ischemic change is reportedly unilateral and symptoms of motor deficit appear. An additional advantage of the method is that the cerebral arteries of the contralateral hemisphere can be utilized as the normal control. The disadvantage of the model is that it requires the full operative procedure of craniotomy and suitable facilities. Absence of direct injury to the arterial wall or disruption is another factor to consider if the study is aimed at the pathogenetic mechanism of vasospasm.

An appropriate method of induction of subarachnoid hemorrhage has to be selected for the specific purpose of the project and the focus of the pathological events to be studied in the experiment.

VI. SPECIFIC MODELS

Models of subarachnoid hemorrhage using various species of animal have been described in the past. Those include models of dogs, cats, monkeys, rabbits, rats, pigs, and goats. Methods that have been employed in each species and characteristics of these models are as follows.

A. Canine Models

In dogs, to reproduce the condition of subarachnoid hemorrhage, methods such as percutaneous injection into the cisterna magna [43,44,45,46,15,35], instillation into the chiasmatic cistern with a surgical approach through the orbita [40,48,19a,20], and disruption of the cerebral arteries after placement of a needle piercing through the arteries [49,50,51] have been employed.

Injection of autogenous blood into the cisterna magna [52,39,44] causes prolonged constriction of the basilar artery. To enhance the intensity and the duration of vasoconstriction, double injection with an interval of 2 days has been used by Varsos et al. According to their report [35], the basilar artery spasm after repeated injection of autologous venous blood was resistant to treatments with vasodilators such as phosphodiesterase inhibitor and calcium channel blocker. It was also reported that histological changes such as myonecrosis and edematous changes of the endothelium take place.

For details of the surgical techniques, the reader is referred to the original articles. Usually dogs are anesthetized by intravenous thiopental or pentobarbital. After intubation, artificial ventilation is started, and if necessary, the animal can be maintained on gaseous anesthesia. Angiograms can be performed in dogs either by using a Seldinger technique with a catheter inserted in the femoral artery or by direct catheterization of the vertebral artery. In the latter case, the right vertebral artery is exposed through an incision medial to the sternocleidomastoid muscle extending to the upper margin of the clavicle. The origin of the vertebral artery is found by following the subclavian artery proximally, in the region lateral to the right carotid artery sheath. The vertebral artery is ligated close to its takeoff from the subclavian artery and cannulated for contrast injection. With a selective catheterization by the Seldinger technique, it is possible to inject dyes into the basilar artery or the internal carotid artery. During angiogram, arterial blood gases are monitored to safeguard against a fluctuation in the values of pCO_2. In case of blood injection into the cisterna magna, the foramen magnum is punctured, 4–5 mL of cerebrospinal fluid is withdrawn and 7–10 mL of autologous venous blood is injected. The head is kept 30 degrees down for at least 15 minutes to ensure placement of the blood in the prepontine cistern surrounding the basilar artery. The injection is repeated in 48 hours. The double injection ensures formation of the clot encasing the basilar artery and interaction between the clot and the artery, resulting in spasm with increased severity and prolonged duration lasting several days to 2 weeks. The temporal profile of the vasoconstriction is comparable to the clinical situation; a moderate spasm is seen in 3 days after the initial injection, it reaches its maximum around the seventh day, and returns to normal configuration in two to three weeks [53]. The reliable reproduction of vasospasm made the "double hemorrhage" cisternal injection model the most thoroughly studied experimental model.

Alterations in the functional, biochemical, and morphological aspects of the cerebral artery have been reported in the spastic canine basilar artery. Changes in pharmacological responsiveness in the basilar artery were studied in isolated preparations as well as in situ through clival exposure. Increased contractility to serotonin and norepinephrine [19], decreased sensitivity to serotonin, norepinephrine, and potassium [50], impaired relaxation to aminophylline and papaverine [35], loss of endothelial-dependent relaxations [54,55,56], and impairment in relaxations to calcium channel blockers [35,57] have been reported. A decrease in production of cyclic guanosine monophosphate (GMP), which is the key substance for vasodilatation [58] was observed along with a decrease in the content of high-energy phosphates [4] in the canine spastic arteries [59]. Impairment in the regulation and homeostasis of intracellular calcium was demonstrated in the preparations [5]. Other features, such as alteration of the mechanical properties and decrease in distensibility/compliance of the arterial wall [7,60] have been demonstrated in this model as well.

Histological findings of necrosis of the smooth muscle, subendothelial proliferation, inflammatory reactions of the adventitia, detachment and vacuolization of the endothelium have also been reported [15,17]. However, as discussed earlier, these reports have been contradicted by reports of absence of myonecrosis, subendothelial proliferation, and endothelial damage in this model [14,19a,20]. In our own experience, patterns of damage to the smooth muscle cells, alterations such as shrinkage and condensation of the cytoplasm, are reliably observed, but frank necrosis of muscle is not characteristic in the spastic arteries. The canine model has been criticized for the variability in the histological observations; however, in fact, findings in the clinical conditions are equally controversial.

The chronic vasospasm of the basilar artery does not cause neurological deficits in dogs; focal signs ascribed to infarction of the brain stem such as motor weakness, cerebellar signs, cranial nerve palsy are not observed. The animals with successful instillation and clot formation show signs of meningeal irritation, such as nuchal rigidity, irritability, and hypersensitivity when touched in the head or neck region. The absence of the delayed ischemic deficit is the limitation of the model.

Injection into chiasmatic cisterns through the orbita has been tried and used in dogs to induce chronic vasospasm in the arteries of the circle of Willis [48,51]. Disruption or tearing of the artery by withdrawing a needle previously placed through the wall or by retracting a ligature tied around the artery has produced vasospasm in the delayed phase [50,41]. However the disruption method is not frequently used in recent investigations for pathogenesis and experimental therapy probably due to the difficulty in controlling the extent of hemorrhage.

B. Primate Models

Methods of inducing subarachnoid hemorrhage used in primates include percutaneous puncture and injection of autologous blood into the cisterna magna [61], and surgical exposure of the chiasmatic cistern and needle instillation of blood [62,63]. In combination with craniotomy, placement of blood clot [64], puncture of the cerebral arteries [65,66,67,42,60], and avulsion by withdrawal of a needle inserted in the arterial wall [68] have been used.

Extensive studies have been done by the group of Weir et al. on a monkey craniotomy model [64,18]. The advantage of the model is that delayed neurological deficits can be reproduced since the clot placed over the sylvian cistern causes vasospasm in the branches of the middle cerebral artery and thus can produce focal infarcts in the fronto-parietal cortex. Since the clot is formed over the surface of the cerebrum (as opposed to brainstem in the canine model) CT scan can be used effectively to delineate the distribution of clots. Another advantage is that because of the symmetrical nature of the middle cerebral arteries, the contralateral arteries can be used as the normal control in the studies. Disadvantages of the model are the cost of procurement and maintenance of the monkeys, variability in the supply, as well as the requirement of complete craniotomy with appropriate anesthetic techniques.

Time course of the vasospasm in monkey SAH models, either by clot placement/craniotomy [18] or by needle or catheter injection of blood into the cistern [69,64a], are comparable to that of clinical spasm. Echlin described in detail the constriction of the cerebral arteries immediately after the injection of blood into the prepontine or premedullary cistern through a catheter, followed by a second phase of constriction at 24 to 72 hours [69]. Espinosa reported that the maximum point of vasoconstriction was obtained at 7 days after the SAH and returned to near-normal caliber in about 14 days [18]. Histological studies reported substantial alterations such as endothelial damages, subendothelial proliferation, corrugation of internal elastica lamina, and myonecrosis [70,64]. Development of delayed ischemia was observed in the craniotomy/clot placement model, albeit the incidence was low [18]. Acquired in the acute phase of vasospasm following rupture of the vessels, CBF studies indicate decreased flow corresponding to the onset of the acute spasm, along with increase in ICP and decrease in CO_2 reactivity [65,67]. Recent studies of CBF in the chronic phase by Handa et al. demonstrated a reduction in CBF secondary to vasospasm and decreased capacity of autoregulation during the phase of chronic spasm [71]. A pharmacological study reported loss of endothelium-dependent relaxations [55].

C. Feline Models

In cats, experimental hemorrhage has been made by injection of blood percutaneously [72,73,22] or via an implanted catheter [74,75] into the foramen magnum, as well as by operative exposure of the prepontine cistern by removing a part of the clivus [76]. Rupture of the middle cerebral artery via craniotomy or via transorbital approach has been employed in cats [77]. Mayberg et al. reported absence of histological changes in the feline basilar artery during vasospasm induced by injection of blood into the cisterna magna [22].

D. Rabbit Models

Alterations of pharmacological responsiveness and histological changes of the arterial wall have been studied in rabbit models. Methods of transorbital injection [78] or craniotomy/arterial rupture [79] have been employed as well as cisternal injection by percutaneous puncture [80,81,38,47,54] or by injection through exposed dura [37]. The cisternal injection causes vasospasm of the basilar artery in a delayed and prolonged fashion. Angiographical vasospasm reaches maximum in 4 to 6 days and returns to normal caliber over 10 days to 2 weeks [37,38,78,81]. Histological changes of myonecrosis and damage of the endothelium have been observed on the third day following single cisternal injection [80]. However, myonecrosis was absent in the same model [54], as well as after repeated injections into the cisternal magna [47]. Symptoms such as lethargy, decreased food intake, paresis of the hind limbs, gait disturbance [81] have been reported but whether they represent brain-stem ischemia is not certain. Otsuji et al. observed infarction in the cerebral cortex, the hippocampus, and in the brainstem after ligation of the bilateral carotid arteries and cisternal blood injection [82].

Angiograms have been performed in rabbits by methods such as surgical exposure of the brachial artery and direct catheterization [38], retrograde catheterization of the carotid artery and injection at the aortic arch [81,82], and femoral artery puncture and catheterization into the aortic arch [80].

E. Rat Models

Subarachnoid hemorrhage has been made in rats by various methods, such as transclival exposure of the basilar artery and needle puncture followed by withdrawal [83,28,32], rupturing the internal carotid artery by traction of a suture placed intraluminally [24,31], injection into the cisterna magna [84,27], cisternal injection via an implanted catheter [29,30,33], cortical blood injection via a needle inserted through a bone wax sealing a burr hole on the convexity [26], and injection into the basal cistern surrounding the Willisian circle [85].

Vasospasm in the rat is generally short-lived; it is observed on the second day, and the vessel caliber returns to normal within 3–4 days. The angiographic narrowing in this phase is very mild [32,33]. Biphasic time course has been observed following cisterna magna injection [86,33] with the early phase spasm observed for the initial 10–15 minutes and delayed spasm at 2 days, which is very mild as compared to chronic vasospasm produced in other species. The temporal profile is significantly different from that observed in larger animal models or in humans. Measurement of the caliber of the basilar arteries has been done either by direct visualization with clival exposure [32] or by angiography using a catheter inserted in the axillary artery [33].

Histological changes observed in the rat spastic arteries include myonecrosis in the peri-intimal portion of the medial layer and infiltration of phagocytotic cells in the adventitia, which were most remarkable at 48 hours after SAH [27]. However absence of such arteriopathy in the basilar artery, on days 3, 7 and 14, was reported [28]. Swift and Solomon also failed to observe histological changes of smooth muscle necrosis and intimal proliferation in the cisternal injection model at 72 hours following SAH [23]. Veelken et al., in their carotid artery rupture model, reported histological findings of cerebral ischemia in the hippocampus [31]. Neurological changes such as lethargy and worsening of limb motor function have been reported [83] following basilar artery puncture and subarachnoid hemorrhage, but the significance of these symptoms as focal ischemic deficit resulting from chronic vasospasm is not certain.

Alterations of the physiological parameters in the acute phase have been extensively studied in the rat model. Increase in intracranial pressure and decrease in CBF have been observed in the cisternal injection model as well as vessel rupture model [24,25,27,30,31]. Electrocardiographic alterations and bradycardia have been observed as well [85]. A study has shown that the temporal profile of the CBF changes in the second phase does not correspond with the angiographic course of the spasm [29]. In a cisternal injection model, sham operation of injection of artificial CSF caused comparable reduction in CBF as in the SAH group, which returned to normal in 24 hours in both groups [23].

F. Miscellaneous Models

Other species used for SAH model include pigs and goats.

Takemae et al. injected autologous arterial blood into the prepontine cistern of pigs via an indwelling catheter twice with an interval of two days, resulting in vasospasm observed angiographically at day 4. They reported histological changes in the arterial wall such as myonecrosis and intimal proliferation at day 7 to day 14 [87].

Alabadi et al. made SAH in goats by injection of blood into the basal cistern via a catheter implanted through a parieto-temporal burr hole. Increase in cerebrovascular resistance and decrease in CBF was observed on the third day after SAH. Decreased responsiveness to the calcium channel blocker nicardipine as well as increased responsiveness to endothelin-1 was demonstrated in the middle cerebral artery in vivo as well as in vitro [88].

VII. SUMMARY

The temporal profile of delayed onset and prolonged duration, as well as its refractoriness to conventional pharmacological treatments, are the hallmarks of cerebral arterial spasm following subarachnoid hemorrhage. These characteristics suggest that the vasoconstriction is not caused by ordinary smooth muscle contraction but is elicited as the result of damage to the smooth muscle, and in fact this notion is supported by recent experimental studies. When studying pathophysiology of cerebral vasospasm in animal models, it is crucial that the characteristic time course and refractoriness are reproduced. Morphological changes of the artery, such as damage of the endothelium, subendothelial proliferation, and necrosis of the smooth muscle have been described in clinical specimens and in the experimental models, but there is no unanimous agreement on their true significance.

In the canine model, especially in the double-injection model, the temporal profile of the spasm in the basilar artery as well as its resistance to pharmacological agents are comparable to the clinical condition. Alterations of the pharmacological, biochemical, and mechanical properties of the cerebral artery, as well as derangement in the smooth muscle regulatory mechanism were well documented in the model. Histological changes such as endothelial damage and smooth muscle necrosis have been described, but contradicted by negative reports. Focal neurologic deficits are not observed in the basilar artery spasm models despite severe arterial constriction, presumably due to abundance in the collateral circulation.

In the primate models of subarachnoid hemorrhage, both acute and chronic arterial spasm can be induced after injection of autologous blood or instillation of blood clot, with concomitant reduction in CBF. Delayed ischemic deficit has been reported after placement of the clot over a hemisphere. Histological studies done in these models described damage to endothelium and the smooth muscle.

In the rabbit model, a temporal profile of vasospasm analogous to the clinical condition was reported, with its maximum at day 4 and resolution over 2 weeks. Histological change of the artery was observed but absence of such changes have been also reported in the same model.

In the rat, a variety of techniques have been employed to induce subarachnoid hemorrhage. Chronic spasm in these models is short and less intense, typically reaching maximum on the second day. Earlier spasm is seen for the initial 10 to 15 minutes. Regarding histological changes, both positive and negative reports have been documented. Alterations in ICP, CBF, have been also described in the acute phase in the model.

REFERENCES

1. Aho K, Fogekholm R. Incidence and early prognosis of stroke in Espoo–Kauniainen Area, Finland, in 1972. *Stroke* 1974; 5:258–261.
2. Sundt TM, Whisnant JP. Subarachnoid hemorrhage from intracranial aneurysms. Surgical management and natural history of disease. *N Engl J Med* 1978; 299:116–122.
3. Saito I, Ueda Y, Sano K. Significance of vasospasm in the treatment of ruptured intracranial aneurysms. J Neurosurg 1977; 47:412–429.
4. Kim P, Jones JD, Sundt TM Jr. Decrease of high–energy phosphates in the spastic cerebral arteries after subarachnoid hemorrhage. *J Neurosurg* 1992; 76:991–996.
5. Kim P, Yoshimoto Y, Iino M, Sasaki T, Kirino T, Nonomura Y. Impaired calcium regulation of smooth muscle during chronic vasospasm following subarachnoid hemorrhage. *J Cereb Blood Flow Metab* 1996; 16:334–341.
6. Smith RR, Clower BR, Grotendorst GM, Yabuno N, Cruse JM. Arterial wall changes in early human vasospasm. *Neurosurgery* 1985; 16:171–176.
7. Kim P, Sundt TM Jr, Vanhoutte PM. Alteration of mechanical properties in canine basilar arteries after subarachnoid hemorrhage. *J Neurosurg* 1989; 71:430–436.
8. Bevan JA, Bevan RD, Frazee JG. Functional arterial changes in chronic cerebrovasospasm in monkeys: An in vitro assessment of the contribution to arterial narrowing. *Stroke* 1987; 18:472–481.

9. Yamashima T, Kida S, Yamamoto S. An electron microscopic study of cerebral vasospasm with resultant myonecrosis in cases of SAH, meningitis and trans–sylvian surgery. *J Neurol* 1986; 233:348–357.
10. Crompton MR. The pathogenesis of cerebral infarction following the rupture of cerebral berry aneurysms. *Brain* 1964; 87:491–510.
11. Hughes JT, Schianchi PM. Cerebral artery spasm. A histological study at necropsy of the blood vessels in cases of subarachnoid hemorrhage. *J Neurosurg* 1978; 48:515–525.
12. Mizukami M, Kim H, Araki G, Mihara H, Yoshida Y. Is angiographic spasm real spasm? *Acta Neurochirurgica* 1976; 34:247–259.
13. Conway LW, McDonald LW. Structural changes of the intradural arteries following subarachnoid hemorrhage. *J Neurosurg* 1972; 37:715–723.
14. Eldevik OP, Kristiansen K, Torvik A. Subarachnoid hemorrhage and cerebrovascular spasm. Morphological study of intracranial arteries based on animal experiments and human autopsies. *J Neurosurg* 1981; 55:869–876.
15. Liszczak TM, Varsos VG, Black PM, Kistler JP, Zervas NT. Cerebral arterial constriction after experimental subarachnoid hemorrhage is associated with blood components within the arterial wall. *J. Neurosurg* 1983; 58:18–26.
16. Clower BR, Hining JL, Smith RR. Pathological changes in the cerebral artery after subarachnoid hemorrhage. In: Wilkins RH, (ed). Cerebral Arterial Spasm. Baltimore, London: Williams & Wilkins, 1980, pp 124–131.
17. Tanabe Y, Sakata K, Yamada H, Itoh T, Takada M. Cerebral vasospasm and ultrastructural changes in cerebral arterial wall. An experimental study. *J Neurosurg* 1978; 49:229–238.
18. Espinosa F, Weir B, Overton T, Costar W, Grace M, Boisvert D. A randomized placebo–controlled double–blind trial of nimodipine after SAH in monkeys. Part 1: Clinical and radiological findings. *J Neurosurg* 1984; 60:1167–1175.
19. Pickard JD, Perry S. Spectrum of altered reactivity of isolated cerebral arteries following subarachnoid hemorrhage: response to potassium, pH, noradrenaline, 5–hydroxytryptamine, and sodium loading. *J Cereb Blood Flow Metab* 1984; 4:599–609.
19a. Pickard JD, Graham DI, Matear E, Macpherson P, Tamura A, Fitch W. Ultrastructure of cerebral arteries following experimental SAH. *J Neurol Neurosurg Psychiatry* 1985; 48:256–262.
20. Tani E, Yamagata S, Ito Y. Intercellular granules and vesicles in prolonged cerebral vasospasm. *J Neurosurg* 1978; 48:179–189.
21. Yamashima T, Yamamoto S. Cerebral arterial pathology in experimental subarachnoid hemorrhage. *J Neurosurg* 1983; 58:843–850.
22. Mayberg MR, Houser OW, Sundt TM Jr. Ultrastructural changes in feline arterial endothelium following SAH. *J Neurosurg* 1978; 48:49–57.
23. Swift DM, Solomon RA. Subarachnoid hemorrhage fails to produce vasculopathy or chronic blood flow changes in rats. *Stroke* 1988; 19:878–882.
24. Bedersen JB, Germano IM, Guarino L. Cortical blood flow and cerebral perfusion pressure in a new non-craniotomy model of subarachnoid hemorrhage in the rat. *Stroke* 1995; 26:1086–1092.
25. Doczi T. The pathogenetic and prognostic significance of blood–brain barrier dam-

age at the acute stage of aneurysmal subarachnoid hemorrhage. Clinical and experimental studies. *Act Neurochir Wien* 1985; 776:110–132.

26. Doczi T, Joo F, Adam G, Bozoky B, Szerdahelyi P. Blood–brain barrier damage during the acute stage of subarachnoid hemorrhage, as exemplified by a new animal model. *Neurosurgery* 1986; 18:733–739.
27. Jackowski A, Crockard A, Burnstock G, Russell RR, Krastek F. The time course of intracranial pathophysiological changes following experimental subarachnoid hemorrhage in the rat. *J Cereb Blood Flow Metab* 1990; 10:835–849.
28. Kader A, Krauss WE, Onesti ST, Elliott P, Solomon RA. Chronic cerebral blood flow changes following experimental subarachnoid hemorrhage in the rat. *Stroke* 1990; 21:577–581.
29. Rasmussen G, Hauerberg J, Waldemar G, Gjerris F, Juhler M. Cerebral blood flow autoregulation in experimental subarachnoid hemorrhage in rat. *Acta Neurochir (Wien)* 1992; 119:128–133.
30. Solomon RA, Antunes L, Chen RY, Bland L, Chien S. Decrease in cerebral blood flow in rats after experimental subarachnoid hemorrhage. A new animal model. *Stroke* 1985; 16:58–64.
31. Veelken JA, Laing RJC, Jakubowski J. The Sheffield model of subarachnoid hemorrhage in rats. *Stroke* 1995; 26:1279–1284.
32. Barry KJ, Gogjian MA, Stein BM. Small animal model for investigation of subarachnoid hemorrhage and cerebral vasospasm. *Stroke* 1979; 10:538–541.
33. Delgado TJ, Brismar J, Svendgaard NA. Subarachnoid haemorrhage in the rat: angiography and fluorescence microscopical evaluation of the major cerebral arteries. *Stroke* 1985; 16:595–602.
34. Svendgaard NA, Delgado-Zygmunt TJ, Shiokawa Y. Involvement of trigeminal afferents in cerebral vasospasm in monkey. In: Findlay JM (ed). Cerebral Vasospasm, Developments in Neurology vol 8. Amsterdam: Elsevier, 1993; 235–238.
35. Varsos VG, Liszczak TM, Han DH, Kistler JP, Vielma J, Black PMcL, Heros RC, Aervas NT. Delayed cerebral vasospasm is not reversible by aminophylline, nifedipine or papaverine in a "two-hemorrhage" canine model. *J Neurosurg* 1983; 58:11–17.
36. Zabramski JM, Spetzler RF, Bonstelle C. Chronic cerebral vasospasm: Effect of volume and timing of hemorrhage in a canine model. *Neurosurgery* 1986; 18:1–6.
37. Spallone A, Pastore FS. Cerebral vasospasm in a double–injection model in rabbit. *Surg Neurol* 1989; 32:408–417.
38. Baker KF, Zervas NT, Pile-Spellman J, Vacanti FX, Miller D. Angiographic evidence of basilar artery constriction in the rabbit: a new model of vasospasm. *Surg Neurol* 1987; 27:107–112.
39. Landau B, Ransohoff J. Prolonged cerebral vasospasm in experimental subarachnoid hemorrhage. *Neurology (Minneapolis)* 1968; 18:1056–65.
40. Lougheed WM, Tom M. A method of introducing blood into the subarachnoid space in the region of the circle of Willis in dogs. *Canad J Surg* 1961; 4:329–337.
41. Brawley BW, Strandness DE Jr., Kelly WA. The biphasic response of cerebral vasospasm in experimental subarachnoid hemorrhage. *J Neurosurg* 1968; 28:1–8.
42. Simeone FA, Ryan KG, Cotter JR. Prolonged experimental cerebral vasospasm. *J Neurosurg* 1968; 29:357–366.

43. Allen GS, Gold LHA, Chou SN, French LA. Cerebral arterial spasm. Part 3: In vivo intracisternal production of spasm by serotonin and blood and its reversal by phenoxybenzamine. *J Neurosurg* 1974; 40:451–458.
44. Kuwayama A, Zervas NT, Belson R, Shintani A, Pickren K. A model for experimental cerebral arterial spasm. *Stroke* 1972; 3:49–56.
45. Sasaki T, Wakai S, Asano T, Takakura K, Sano K. Prevention of cerebral vasospasm after SAH with a thromboxane synthetase inhibitor, OKY–1581. *J Neurosurg* 1982; 57:74–82.
46. Chyatte D, Rusch N, Sundt TM. Prevention of chronic experimental cerebral vasospasm with ibuprofen and high–dose methylprednisolone. *J Neurosurg* 1983; 59:925–932.
47. Liszczak TM, Black P McL, Tzouras A, Foley L, Zarvas NT. Morphological change of the basilar artery, ventricles and choroid plexus after experimental SAH. *J Neurosurg* 1984; 61:486–493.
48. McQueen JD, Jeanes LD. Influence of hypothermia on intracranial hypertension. *J Neurosurg* 1962; 19:277–288.
49. Nagai H, Suzuki Y, Sugiura M, Noda H. Experimental cerebral vasospasm. Part 1: Factors contributing to early spasm. *J Neurosurg* 1974; 41:285–292.
50. Toda N, Ozaki T, Ohta T. Cerebrovascular sensitivity to vasoconstricting agents induced by subarachnoid hemorrhage and vasospasm in dogs. *J Neurosurg* 1977; 46:296–303.
51. Wilkins RH, Levitt P. Intracranial arterial spasm in the dog. A chronic experimental model. *J Neurosurg* 1970; 33:260–269.
52. Chow RWB, Newton TH, Smith MC, Adams JE. Cerebral vasospasm induced by subarachnoid blood and serotonin. An angiographic study. *Invest Radiol* 1968; 3:402–407.
53. Yoshimoto Y, Kim P, Sasaki T, Takakura K. Temporal profile and significance of metabolic failure and trophic changes in the canine cerebral arteries during chronic vasospasm after subarachnoid hemorrhage. *J Neurosurg* 1993; 78:807–813.
54. Nakagomi T, Kassel NF, Sasaki T, Fujiwara S, Lehman RM, Johshita H, Nazar GB, Torner JC. Effect of subarachnoid hemorrhage on endothelium–dependent vasodilatation. *J Neurosurg* 1987; 66:915–923.
55. Kanamaru K, Weir BKA, Findlay JM, Krueger CA, Cook DA. Pharamcological studies on relaxation of spastic primate cerebral arteries. *J Neurosurg* 1989; 71:909–915.
56. Kim P, Sundt TM Jr, Vanhoutte PM. Alterations in endothelium–dependent responsiveness of the canine basilar artery after subarachnoid hemorrhage. *J Neurosurg* 1988; 69:239–246.
57. Matsui T, Kaizu H, Itoh S, Asano T. The role of active smooth–muscle contraction in the occurrence of chronic vasospasm in the canine two–hemorrhage model. *J Neurosurg* 1994; 80:276–282.
58. Furchgott RF, Vanhoutte PM. Endothelium–derived relaxing and contracting factors. *FASEB J* 1989; 3:2007–2018.
59. Kim P, Schimi V, Sundt TM Jr, Vanhoutte PM. Reduced production of cyclic GMP explains the loss of endothelium-dependent relations in the canine basilar artery after subarachnoid hemorrhage.

60. Bevan RD, Bevan JA, Frazee JG. Diltiazem protects against functional change in chronic cerebrovasospasm in monkeys. *Stroke* 1988; 19:73–79.
61. Sahlin C, Brismar J, Delgado T, Owman C, Salford LG, Svendgaard NA. Cerebrovascular and metabolic changes during the delayed vasospasm following experimental subarachnoid hemorrhage in baboons, and treatment with a calcium antagonist. *Brain Res* 1987; 403:313–332.
62. Boisvert DPJ, Pickard JD, Graham DI, Fitch W. Delayed effects of subarachnoid haemorrhage on cerebral metabolism and the cerebrovascular response to hyperemia in the primate. *J Neurol Neurosurg Psychiatry* 1979; 42:892–898.
63. Pelofsky S, Jacobson ED, Fisher R. Effects of prostaglandin E1 on experimental cerebral vasospasm. *J Neurosurg* 1972; 36:634–639.
64. Espinosa F, Weir B, Shnitka T, Overton T, Boisvert D. A randomized placebo–controlled double–blind trial of nimodipine after SAH in monkeys. Part 2: Pathological findings. *J Neurosurg* 1984; 60:1176–1185.
64a. Espinosa F, Weir B, Boisvert D, Overton T, Costor W. Chronic cerebral vasospasm after large subarachnoid hemorrhage in monkeys. *J Neurosurg* 1982; 57:224–232.
65. Fein JM, Boulos R. Local cerebral blood flow in experimental middle cerebral artery vasospasm. *J Neurosurg* 1973; 39:337–347.
66. Roy VC, Sundt TM Jr, Murphey F. Experimental subarachnoid hemorrhage: A study for spasm with the production of aneurysms. *Stroke* 1970; 1:248–252.
67. Kamiya K, Kuyama H, Symon L. An experimental study of the acute stage of subarachnoid hemorrhage. *J Neurosurg* 1983; 59:917–924.
68. Frazee JG, Giannotta SL, Stern WE. Intravenous nitroglycerin for the treatment of chronic cerebral vasoconstriction in the primate. *J Neurosurg* 1981; 55:865–868.
69. Echlin FA. Experimental vasospasm, acute and chronic, due to blood in the subarachnoid space. *J Neurosurg* 1971; 35:646–656.
70. Fein JM, Flor WJ, Cohan SL, Parkhurst J. Sequential changes of vascular ultrastructure in experimental cerebral vasospasm. Myonecrosis of subarachnoid arteries. *J Neurosurg* 1974; 41:49–58.
71. Handa Y, Kubota T, Tsuchida A, Kaneko M, Caner H, Kobayashi H, Kubota T. Effect of systemic hypotension on cerebral energy metabolism during chronic cerebral vasospasm in primates. *J Neurosurg* 1993; 78:112–119.
72. Ohmoto T, Yoshioka K, Shibata K, Morooka H, Matsumoto Y, Nishimoto A. Cerebral vasospasm following subarachnoid hemorrhage: Experimental and clinical studies. *Neurol Med Chir (Tokyo)* 1979; 19:73–81.
73. Waters A, Harder DR. Altered membrane properties of cerebral vascular muscle following subarachnoid hemorrhage: An electrophysiological study. *Stroke* 1985; 16:990–997.
74. Lobato RD, Marin J, Salaies M, Burgios J, Rivilla F, Garcia AG. Effect of experimental subarachnoid hemorrhage on the adrenergic innervation of cerebral arteries. *J Neurosurg* 1980; 53:477–479.
75. Peterson EW, Cardoso ER. The blood brain barrier following experimental subarachnoid hemorrhage. Part 1: Response to insult caused by arterial hypertension. *J Neurosurg* 1983; 58:338–344.
76. Duff TA, Scott G, Feilbach JA. Ultrastructural evidence of arterial denervation following experimental subarachnoid hemorrhage. *J Neurosurg* 1986; 64:292–297.

77. Hayakawa T, Waltz AG. Experimental, subarachnoid hemorrhage from a middle cerebral artery. Neurologic deficits, intracranial pressure, blood pressure and pulse rate. *Stroke* 1977; 8:421–426.
78. Owman C, Edvinsson L, Olin T, Sahlin C, Svendgaard NA. Pathophysiology of cerebral vasospasm: Transmitter changes in perivascular sympathetic nerves and increased pial artery sensitivity to norepinephrine and serotonin. In: Price TR, Nelson E, (eds). Cerebrovascular Disease. New York: Raven Press, 1979; 295–305.
79. Logathetis J, Karacostas D, Karoutas G, Artemis N, Mansouri A, Mironas I. A new model of subarachnoid hemorrhage in experimental animals with the purpose to examine cerebral vasospasm. *Exp Neurol* 1983; 81:257–278.
80. Chan RC, Durity FA, Thompson GB, Nugent RA, Kendall M. The role of the prostacyclin–thromboxane system in cerebral vasospasm following induced subarachnoid hemorrhage in the rabbit. *J Neurosurg* 1984; 61:1120–1128.
81. Endo S, Branson PJ, Alksne JF. Experimental model of symptomatic vasospasm in rabbits. *Stroke* 1988; 19:1420–1425.
82. Otsuji T, Endo S, Hirashima Y, Nishijima M, Takaku A. An experimental model of symptomatic vasospasm induced by oxyhemoglobin in rabbits. *Stroke* 1994; 25:657–662.
83. Barth KNM, Onesti ST, Kraus WE, Kader A, Solomon RA. Transclival basilar artery puncture followed by middle cerebral artery occlusion in the Rat: A new model for delayed cerebral ischemia after subarachnoid hemorrhage. In: Sano K, Takakura K, Kassell NF, Sasaki T, (eds). Cerebral Vasospasm. Tokyo: University of Tokyo Press, 1990, pp 207–210.
84. D'Avella D, Germano A, Santoro G, Costa G, Zuccarello M, Caputi AP, Hayes RL, Tomasello F. Effect of experimental hemorrhage on CSF eicosanoids in the rat. *J Neurotrauma* 1990; 7:121–129.
85. Lacy PS, Earle AM. A small model for electrocardiographic abnormalities observed after an experimental subarachnoid hemorrhage. *Stroke* 1983; 14:371–377.
86. Svendgaard NA, Brismar J, Delgado TJ, Diemer NH. The effect on the development of cerebral vasospasm in the rat of lesioning of the peripheral and central catecholamine systems. *Neurol Res* 1985; 7:30–34.
87. Takemae T, Branso PJ, Alksne JF. Intimal proliferation of cerebral arteries after subarachnoid blood injection in pigs. *J Neurosurg* 1984; 61:494–500.
88. Alabadi JA, Salom JB, Torregrosa G, Miranda FJ, Jover T, Alborch E. Changes in the cerebrovascular effects of endothelin–1 and nicardipine after experimental subarachnoid hemorrhage. *Neurosurgery* 1993; 33:707–715.

3
Pharmacological Modifications of Experimental Vasospasm

Phyo Kim
Dokkyo University School of Medicine, Tochighi, Japan

I. INTRODUCTION

An undisputed pharmacological management protocol for cerebral arterial spasm remains to be developed. This vasospasm develops with a characteristic time course in a delayed fashion following subarachnoid hemorrhage (SAH), with a typical onset of several days after ictus and a duration of days to weeks. The vasoconstriction is the chief cause of cerebral ischemia, neurological deficits, and mortality in the late phase following recovery from the initial insult of hypoperfusion at the time of the arterial bleeding. Treatments using various classes of vasodilators have not been reproducibly effective. The unique temporal profile and the refractoriness to conventional treatments are the hallmark of cerebral vasospasm and it remains a major cause of neurological deterioration. Based on various hypotheses with respect to the pathogenesis of the vasospasm, numerous pharmacological trials have been performed on experimental models of subarachnoid hemorrhage. Underlying each hypothesis are findings in the alterations of cellular functions and biochemical pathways in the vasculature of the spastic cerebral arteries. Such observations made in the experimental models of subarachnoid hemorrhage include production of vasoconstrictive substances such as catecholamines and prostaglandins in the subarachnoid space, release of neural transmitters from vasomotor nerve endings, free radical formation by the clot and membrane lipid peroxidation in the smooth muscle, dysfunction of the NO-cyclic GMP pathway, alterations in the Ca^{2+} regulation and in the contractile mechanisms of the smooth muscle, growth factor production and proliferative arteriopathic changes, and immunological/inflammatory reactions.

Agents used in experimental therapeutic trials include drugs that can be practically applicable in vivo as well as those applicable only in vitro. Numerous agents have been tried on the isolated cerebral arteries in an organ bath, which is used as a preliminary screening bench test. In this chapter, results of the pharmacological therapeutic trials performed in vivo on subarachnoid hemorrhage models—the experiments performed on the intact animal models—are reviewed with special attention to the pharmacokinetic and pharmacodynamic viewpoints.

II. THERAPEUTIC TRIALS USING ADRENERGIC AGONISTS AND ANTAGONISTS

A. Alpha-Adrenergic Blockers

Fraser et al. [1] demonstrated in a clival exposure model in rhesus monkeys that the acute spasm produced by topical application of blood was reversed by phenoxybenzamine (10^{-5} to 10^{-3} *M*). Pharmacological depletion of noradrenergic stores (topical application of tyramine 10^{-5} to 10^{-3} *M* or bretylium 10^{-5} *M*) prior to exposure to the blood dilated the basilar artery but did not prevent development of the acute spasm.

Flamm et al. [2], in a cat clival exposure model, observed that parenteral phenoxybenzamine (i.v., 6 to 12 mg/kg), given 120 minutes prior to the transclival application of blood, prevented development of acute vasospasm. Topical application of phentolamine, a competitive α-adrenergic blocker, and phenoxybenzamine dilated the basilar artery after blood injection, but the duration of the effect of the former was short.

Smigiel and Sundt [3] tried topical application of phentolamine (10^{-3} *M*) and phenoxybenzamine (10^{-4} *M*) in a cat clival exposure model. The acute vasospasm induced by application of autologous blood was not reversed by the alpha blockers but the duration of the vasoconstriction was reduced (JNS 1974).

White et al. [4] reported that the intracisternal injection of the α-adrenergic antagonist, phenoxybenzamine (10^{-2} *M*, 15 minutes or 24 hours after SAH) was not effective in reversal of the acute vasospasm. Preventive protocol with the drug (intravenous, 12 mg/kg) given 2 hours prior to the cisternal injection of blood was not effective either.

Ishibashi et al. [5] reported prazosin, a peripheral α_1-adrenergic antagonist, was effective in prevention of acute vasospasm, when given via NG tube (0.5 mg/kg) prior to induction of acute spasm by application of oxyhemoglobin. When given after application of oxyhemoglobin, prazosin caused only partial reversal of the vasospasm.

By contrast Allen et al. [6] reported that cisternal injection of phenoxybenzamine (10^{-2} *M*) reversed the acute vasospasm observed 30 to 60 minutes after cisternal blood injection in dogs.

In a recent study Matsui et al. [7] examined the effects of transclival topical application of phentolamine (10^{-6} *M*), atropine (10^{-6} *M*), methysergide (serotonin antagonist, 10^{-6} *M*), and diphenhydramine (H1 histamine antagonist, 3×10^{-6} *M*) on the chronic vasospasm observed on day 7 in the double hemorrhage canine model. The mixed solution was ineffective in dilatation of the constricted basilar artery.

B. Beta-Adrenergic Stimulants

Isoproterenol (3μ g/kg/min, intravenous) in combination with a phosphodiesterase inhibitor aminophylline (3 mg/kg/min) was tried in cat and monkey models and was effective in reversing the acute vasospasm after induction of subarachnoid hemorrhage by topical application or cisternal injection of autologous blood [8]. Smigiel and Sundt [3] tried topical application of isoproterenol (10^{-4} *M*) in a cat clival exposure model. The acute vasospasm in the basilar artery was not reversed but the duration of the spasm was shortened. Sundt et al. [3] tried a combination of isoproterenol and lidocaine hydrochloride in humans. The rationale for the protocol was observation of vasodilatory effect of β-adrenergic agonists in the isolated cerebral arteries and the latter drug's suppressive effect on arrhythmia, which is possibly caused by isoproterenol. They found the protocol to be effective in improving the ischemic neurological deficits resulting from the chronic vasospasm.

C. Beta-Adrenergic Blockers

Edvinsson et al. [10] studied the effect of propranolol in a cat model where SAH was induced by rupture of the basilar artery. The Beta blocker was reportedly effective in prevention of acute vasospasm.

D. Summary

The adrenergic receptor manipulation was found to have some effect in the situation of acute vasospasm. Definitive effect on chronic vasospasm has not been observed in the experimental models.

III. PHOSPHODIESTERASE INHIBITORS AND NITROVASODILATORS: MODIFICATION OF NITRIC-OXIDE–CYCLIC GMP PATHWAYS

Dilatation of the spastic cerebral arteries with vasodilatory drugs, such as phosphodiesterase inhibitors and nitrovasodilators, has been attempted in animal models of chronic vasospasm. Recent progress in the biochemical pharmacology delineated that these traditional classes of vasodilators acts on the NO-cyclic GMP pathway, which is the pivotal mechanism of vasodilatation. The mechanism is shared by relaxations mediated by the endothelium in response to various physiological agonists. Impairment of the mechanism has been demonstrated in experimental models of subarachnoid hemorrhage/chronic vasospasm [11–16]. The phosphodiesterase inhibitors suppress hydrolysis of cyclic nucleotides and thus causes cumulation of cyclic GMP, which is the key substance in mediating relaxation in the smooth muscle. Nitrovasodilators increase activity of guanylate cyclase and increase the amount of cyclic GMP in the smooth muscle.

A. Phosphodiesterase Inhibitors

Aminophylline (3 mg/kg/min) was tried in combination with a beta stimulant, isoproterenol, in cat and monkey models and was effective in ameliorating the acute vasospasm after induction of subarachnoid hemorrhage by topical application or cisternal injection of autologous blood [8].

Papaverine induced temporary relief of the chronic vasospasm in a monkey model. After induction of subarachnoid hemorrhage in rhesus monkeys (autologous arterial blood injection into the basal cistern), infusion of papaverine (0.03% solution, 20 mL infused over 2 hours) into the subarachnoid space ameliorated chronic vasospasm observed on day 6–8, albeit duration of the effect was short [17].

In another study using a canine model (induction of SAH by perforation of the posterior communicating artery, [18]), papaverine (vertebral artery injection, 4mg/kg) and isoxsuprine (beta-adrenergic agonist, intraarterial, 0.5 mg/kg) were effective both on the early (15 minutes after SAH) and late vasospasm (24 hours after SAH), although the duration of the effect on the delayed phase was short. By contrast, receptor specific antagonists such as alpha or beta adrenergic blockers, concurrently tried in their study, had little effect on the late vasospasm.

In a double injection canine model, chronic vasospasm (observed 96 hours after two injections of autologous blood into the cisterna magna) was not reversible by papaverine (2 mg/kg bolus intravenous injection) or aminophylline (10 mg/kg/hr, intravenous infusion) (Varsos et al., [19]). The refractoriness was interpreted as the characteristics of the canine model shared with the clinical conditions.

In a rabbit model (blood injected into the cisterna magna), the degree of chronic vasospasm, as assessed with postmortem morphometry, was reduced with an intraarterial injection of a mixture of papaverine (10^{-4} *M*), sodium nitroprusside (2×10^{-4} *M*) plus adenosine (10^{-5} *M*) [20].

However, in another study using a similar rabbit model in which a long-lasting spasm of the basilar artery was observed over a period of nine days, papaverine (vertebral artery injection, 2 mg/kg) reversed angiographic narrowing in the first 3 days after hemorrhage but not in the chronic phase from day 5 to 9 [21,22]. In their study, refractoriness to papaverine in vivo was positively correlated with decreased vessel wall distensibility measured in vitro. The data suggested that the initial cause of arterial narrowing is mediated by activation of physiologic contraction, whereas in the later phase the sustained constriction is associated with abnormal tone and probably with tissue damage and structural changes.

In an attempt to evaluate the role of active smooth-muscle contraction in chronic vasospasm, the effect of papaverine was studied in the canine two-hemorrhage model, along with efficacy of a calcium channel blocker, nicardipine, and a protein kinase C inhibitor, H-7 [23]. The agents dilated the cerebral artery in the chronic vasospasm. However, the dilation induced by papaverine progressively decreased from day 2 to day 7.

In the clinical condition of chronic vasospasm, superselective intraarterial injection of papaverine (0.2% solution) was shown to be effective in dilating the spastic arteries [24]. Recently the treatment has been widely used in clinical practice; however, the duration of the effect is often limited. Frequent recurrence of spasm after injection is seen, but successive treatment is possible and often effective [25]. It seems that the vasodilator agent is effective on the portion of the constriction caused by activation of physiological contractile mechanisms, but not on the pathological contraction that takes place in the damaged smooth muscle.

The successful clinical experience signifies the importance of pharmacokinetic consideration. Introduction of superselective catheterization into the cerebral arteries enables the attainment of much higher local concentrations of the agents than by the conventional method of administration. Consideration of the distribution of therapeutic agent and accomplishment of effective local concentrations is mandatory prior to evaluation of the efficacy of the agent.

B. Nitrovasodilators

Kistler et al. [26] tried nitroglycerin in the canine cisternal injection model of subarachnoid hemorrhage. On angiographical spasm observed 48 hours after the induction of subarachnoid hemorrhage, intravenous administration of nitroglycerin (bolus 300 μ g/kg, followed by infusion of 100 μ g/min for 2 hours, resulting in 5–13% decrease in blood pressure) was effective and caused 39% increase in the diameter. However the effect lasted less than 60 minutes after discontinuation of the infusion. In a primate model of chronic vasospasm, in which subarachnoid hemorrhage was produced by withdrawal of a needle transfixed in the carotid artery, intravenous infusion of nitroglycerin (0.7 to 1.25 μ g/kg/hr, causing decrease in the blood pressure 5–10%) caused a modest dilatation of the arterial constriction observed on day 5 following hemorrhage [27].

Sodium nitroprusside has been tried in the canine model in the form of intraarterial as well as intravenous injection. Hirsh in 1980 [28] reported that intraarterial infusion of the nitrovasodilator (380 μ g/min, vertebral artery catheterization) reversed the acute vasospasm in dogs induced by cisternal injection of blood. Heros [29] demonstrated in a canine model (single cisternal injection) that intravenous infusion of sodium nitroprusside (1–25 μ g/kg/hr) was effective in reversing the acute (90 minutes after SAH) and chronic phase (24 and 48 hours after SAH) of vasospasm.

C. Inhibitors of Endothelial Production of NO

Release of nitric oxide from endothelium in response to various pharmacological and physiological stimuli and the subsequent production of cyclic GMP in the smooth muscle play crucial roles in mediating vasodilatation. Alterations in the function of the pathway, such as loss of endothelial relaxations [1,12,16,30] and impaired production of cyclic GMP in the smooth muscle [14,31] have been demonstrated in experimental models of chronic vasospasm. Modifications of the endothelial pathway have been tried in an attempt to treat chronic vasospasm.

Kajita et al. [32], in a double hemorrhage canine model, tried intrathecal L-arginine (a substrate for the formation of nitric oxide), NG-monomethyl-L-arginine (L-NMMA, an analog of L-arginine that inhibits the formation of nitric oxide from L-arginine), and superoxide dismutase, which protects nitric oxide from oxidation by the superoxide anion. In normal dogs, intracisternal bolus injection of L-arginine (1, 10, or 100 μmol) produced a dose-dependent dilatation of the basilar artery, whereas L-NMMA produced constriction. During chronic vasospasm (days 4 and 7 after SAH), L-arginine produced transient vasodilation, whereas L-NMMA produced no significant vasoconstriction. Intracisternal injection of super oxide dismutase (SOD) enhanced the duration of the effect of L-arginine on the chronic vasospasm. The data suggest the NO-cyclic GMP pathway was impaired after subarachnoid hemorrhage, which could be supplemented by administration of L-arginine.

D. Summary

The two traditional classes of vasodilatory agents, phosphodiesterase inhibitors and the nitrovasodilators, directly act on the intracellular NO-cyclic GMP pathway. The impairment of the pathway has been reproducibly demonstrated in the experimental models of subarachnoid hemorrhage. When combined with an appropriate method of drug delivery, which achieves sufficient concentration over a prolonged period without side effect, these classes of agent can be an effective tool.

IV. CALCIUM CHANNEL BLOCKERS

A. Effects on the Acute Phase of Vasospasm

In 1982, nimodipine was tried in a cat model of subarachnoid hemorrhage, and a positive effect on the acute phase of vasospasm was reported [33]. Intravenous administration (0.1 mg/kg) 20–30 min after SAH (cisternal injection of autologous blood) resulted in a complete disappearance of acute spasm in the pial arteries.

In another study on the acute phase of cerebral vasospasm in a cat model (clival window experiment), verapamil (0.1 mg/kg, topical application) effectively reversed the acute spasm 30 minutes after induction by human platelet-rich plasma aggregated with ADP. The effect lasted for about 60 minutes [34].

B. Efficacy of Effect on the Chronic Phase of Vasospasm

A study of the effect of a preventive protocol on chronic vasospasm was performed in a primate model [35], in which subarachnoid hemorrhage was induced by withdrawal of a needle transfixed in the internal carotid artery. Administration of diltiazem, given orally 25 mg/kg twice per day for two days prior to induction of subarachnoid hemorrhage and for five days afterwards, was effective in prevention of both angiographical spasm and "neurological symptoms" such as hyperreflexia and hypotonia.

Intraarterial injection of four different calcium channel blockers—diltiazem, cinnarizine, verapamil, and nifedipine—was tried in a dog model of subarachnoid hemorrhage and the effects of the agents were compared [36]. Injection of the calcium channel blockers (1 mL of 10^{-6} or 10^{-7} M solution into the vertebral artery) reversed the vasospasm observed 24 hours after subarachnoid hemorrhage. The effect lasted at least 30 minutes.

Bevan et al. reported that the oral administration of diltiazem (25 mg/kg twice daily, started 2 days prior to induction of SAH) in a monkey model prevented chronic vasospasm and the development of associated changes in the stiffness of the arterial wall as well as impairment in the arterial contractility [37].

Tadie et al. [38] studied the effect of oral administration of nimodipine (5 mg/kg per day) as a prevention started immediately after SAH prior to development of vasospasm, or as a postictal treatment started on day 2, in their canine model where subarachnoid hemorrhage was produced by clot placement via craniotomy and cisternal injection. The preventive protocol was effective in reducing the severity of vasospasm both on the cortical arteries as well as on the basilar artery, whereas the treatment protocol was mainly effective on the cortical arteries on day 5 but the effect was not significant on vasospasm of the basilar artery.

Alterations in the mitochondrial respiration in the rat brain following subarachnoid hemorrhage and a protective effect of nimodipine were reported. [39]. Subarachnoid hemorrhage, induced by injection of autologous arterial blood (0.35 mL) into the cisterna magna, significantly affected respiratory parameters of nonsynaptic mitochondria isolated from the brain 1 hour after the hemorrhage. Respiratory control ratio was changed during the acute phase of vasospasm. Intravenous administration of nimodipine (2 μgrams/kg/min for 30 minutes) started immediately after the hemorrhage significantly ameliorated the mitochondrial respiratory parameters.

C. Failure of Effect on the Chronic Vasospasm

These reports showing positive effects of the calcium channel blockers have been contradicted by a number of reports of negative findings.

Varsos et al. [19] observed that the vasospasm seen 96 hours following subarachnoid hemorrhage in their double injection canine model (cisternal injection) was not reversible by nifedipine (1 mg/kg, i.v. infusion over 30 minutes). In a primate model of chronic vasospasm (induced by clot placement over the cerebral arteries, the maximum intensity on day 7), nimodipine (via nasogastric tube, 1 mg/kg every 8 hours, from 20 hours after the SAH until day 14) did not have an ameliorating effect [40]. Histological changes of the arterial wall such as endothelial swelling, subendothelial proliferation, corrugation of the elastic lamina, and myonecrosis were not prevented by the treatment either [41]. Nosko et al. [42] tried nimodipine treatment in the same model with increased dosage (3, 6, 12 mg/kg every 8 hours, from 20 hours after the SAH until day 14 via nasogastric tube) but the protocols also failed to alter the incidence or intensity of vasospasm.

Efficacy of nimodipine treatment on the alterations of contractility in the spastic cerebral arteries was studied by the same group [43]. Treatment with nimodipine (via nasogastric tube, 3, 6, 12 mg/kg every 8 hours, from 20 hours after the subarachnoid hemorrhage until day 14) did not prevent decrease in the maximal contractilities in response to norepinephrine, serotonin, and KCl seen in the spastic cerebral arteries. Sahlin et al. [44] studied the effect of nimodipine on chronic vasospasm in a baboon model of subarachnoid hemorrhage (triple cisternal injection of autologous blood in the course of 4 days). The vasoconstriction of the cerebral arteries along with reduction in cerebral blood flow and impairment in CO_2 responses and autoregulation were all confirmed in the chronic phase. Nimodipine (i.v. infusion, 0.5μ g/kg/min over 45 minutes) increased cerebral blood flow before experimental subarachnoid hemorrhage but no such effect was observed after the hemorrhage.

The effect of nimodipine infusion was studied in a rat model [45]. Subarachnoid hemorrhage was induced in rats by injection of autologous blood into the cisterna magna. On day 8, presence of vasospasm was confirmed by corrosion casts examination showing grooving and vertical relief. Nimodipine infused on day 8 (45 μg/kg/hour, i.v.) failed to ameliorate the chronic vasospasm. Elevated extracellular calcium and potassium concentrations observed in the SAH group were not altered by the treatment either.

In the canine model of subarachnoid hemorrhage, single cisternal administration of nimodipine (10^{-3} M, 4 mL) reversed vasospasm in the acute (30 minutes after hemorrhage) and chronic phases (1–4 days following single blood injection or 3–6 days after double hemorrhage) effectively, but the duration of the effect lasted only several hours [46]. Intravenous or sublingual administration of nimodipine was not effective in reversal of chronic vasospasm.

The effect of nicardipine on chronic vasospasm in a canine model was examined by Sakaki et al. [47]. Dilation responses to nicardipine (intracisternal injection 3.0 mL solution containing 0.25 mg) were observed at 48 hours after subarachnoid hemorrhage, but were markedly reduced at 7 and 14 days after hemorrhage.

A significant decline in the responsiveness to diltiazem (10^{-7} and 10^{-6} M) following subarachnoid hemorrhage was observed in a cat basilar artery [48]. Contraction of the vessels in response to noradrenaline and adrenaline during the course of subarachnoid hemorrhage was reduced. In fact, impairment in the calcium regulation of the smooth muscle in the spastic arterial wall has been demonstrated in the canine model [49]. Membrane calcium permeability was increased and the shift was only partially reversed by a calcium channel blocker, diltiazem.

Efficacy of nicardipine to increase CBF was diminished during chronic vasospasm in a goat model [50]. Subarachnoid hemorrhage was induced by injection of autologous blood into the basal cistern. Increase in CBF in response to intraarterial infusion of nicardipine (3μ g/min) was significantly diminished on day 3 after the subarachnoid hemorrhage. The ability of the calcium blocker to inhibit endothelin-1-induced CBF reductions was significantly less in the subarachnoid hemorrhage group than in the control group.

Matsui et al. [22] studied the effects of nicardipine, H-7 (protein kinase C inhibitor), and papaverine in the two-hemorrhage canine model. The drugs applied via a transclival window reversed the chronic vasospasm. When the vasodilatory effect of each agent was compared, the effect of nicardipine or papaverine progressively decreased from day 2 to day 7, whereas that induced by H-7 increased.

D. Trials of Novel Ca Channel Blockers

A few new calcium-blocking compounds with different properties have been tried on experimental chronic vasospasm. "Intracellular calcium antagonists," HA1004 (*N*-(2-guanidinoethyl)-5-isoquinolinesulfonamide), and HA 1077 (1-(5-isoquinolinesulfonyl) homopiperazine) were tried on the delayed cerebral vasospasm in a canine model of subarachnoid hemorrhage [51]. Contraction induced by a calcium ionophore, A23187, was antagonized by the HA compounds (10^{-5} *M*) but not by the conventional calcium entry blockers, nicardipine, diltiazem, and verapamil (10^{-5} *M*). The data indicate the HA compounds act on the intracellular mechanism. The angiographical spasm observed on day 7 was dilated by HA 1004 and 1077 (3 and 10 mg/kg, i.v.). Intracisternal administration (6 mg) completely reversed the chronic vasospasm.

The prophylactic potential of HA1077 on chronic cerebral vasospasm was reported in a study done in a two-hemorrhage canine model [52]. Intravenous infusion of HA1077 (3 mg/kg over 30 min twice daily [day 1–day 7) after the first intracisternal injection of 5 mL autologous blood significantly prevented the occurrence of chronic cerebral vasospasm. Bolus intravenous administration of HA1077 (0.1 and 0.3 mg/kg) increased cerebral blood flow.

The effect of a "cerebrovascular-selective" calcium channel blocker clentiazem (8-chlorodiltiazem), a derivative of a diltiazem with an enhanced cerebrovascular selectivity, was studied in a rabbit model [20]. Subarachnoid hemorrhage was induced by multiple injections of blood into the prepontine cisterns. Clentiazem (5 mg/kg, administered 4 times daily from 24 hours before subarachnoid hemorrhage), reduced the angiographic vasospasm seen on days 2, 5, and 9. Spasm in the untreated rabbits was resistant to papaverine, whereas spasm in the clentiazem-treated animals was responsive to papaverine.

E. Summary

The earlier studies reported efficacy of nimodipine or verapamil on the acute vasospasm, as well as beneficial effects of nimodipine and diltiazem in prevention and treatment of the chronic vasospasm. These were followed by a number of studies in chronic spasm models reporting inadequate efficacy on the vasoconstriction. Decreased responsiveness to conventional Ca blockers in the course of chronic vasospasm were demonstrated. However, protective effects on the cerebral blood flow and parenchymal mitochondrial parameters were reported, presumably due to improvement in the collateral flow and microcirculation. A few novel classes of Ca blockers have been tried and the results were encouraging in experimental chronic vasospasm.

V. INHIBITION OF PROSTAGLANDIN PATHWAY, SUPPRESSION OF FREE-RADICAL FORMATION AND LIPID PEROXIDATION

Findings of release of vasoconstricting prostaglandins in the cerebrospinal fluid and reduced synthesis of prostacyclin have led into the hypothesis that the vasoconstrictor prostanoids increase in the subarachnoid space and the imbalance between the vasoconstrictor and vasodilator prostanoids mediate cerebral vasospasm. Therapeutic trials were performed to evaluate the effect of suppression of the prostaglandin pathway using steroids or nonsteroid anti-inflammatory drugs. Specific blockers of the receptor–agonist interaction in the pathway were also tried in the experimental subarachnoid hemorrhage.

A. Inhibitors of Prostaglandin Synthesis-Anti-Inflammatory Agents

White et al. [53] performed a study to assess the effect of nonsteroidal anti-inflammatory agents: piroxicam, meclofenamate, ibuprofen, and aspirin. They used the canine cisternal injection model and the drugs were given intravenously 30 minutes before and 3 hours after the blood injection. The treatment significantly reduced occurrence of vasospasm at 24 hours after subarachnoid hemorrhage. They observed the drug with a longer half-life, piroxicam, was more efficacious than meclofenamate, ibuprofen, or aspirin. By contrast, a vasodilator prostanoid, prostacyclin, infused via the vertebral artery failed to affect the vasospasm at 24 hours after the subarachnoid hemorrhage.

Preventive administration of anti-inflammatory agents during the developmental phase of vasospasm was tried by Chyatte et al. [54]. Intravenous administration of the anti-inflammatory agent ibuprofen (12.5 mg/kg every 8 hours, started from the first day after subarachnoid hemorrhage until day 7) or methylprednisolone (30 mg/kg every 8 hours) was effective in preventing angiographic vasospasm observed on day 7.

A study performed by Yamakawa et al. [55] confirmed the efficacy of methylprednisolone (i.v., 10 mg/kg, every 12 hours) in the canine model, and in addition, found that the treatment suppressed the increase in platelet aggregation observed from days 4 to 7 after subarachnoid hemorrhage. They also demonstrated that high-dose methylprednisolone treatment had a nonspecific vasodilatory effect on the basilar artery and has beneficial effects in restoring impairment in autoregulation of CBF following subarachnoid hemorrhage.

The role of intrinsic arachidonate metabolites released from the erythrocyte breakdown products and inhibition by anti-inflammatory agents were demonstrated by Okamoto et al. [56]. Contraction of the canine basilar artery in response to ghost-free hemolysate from dog erythrocytes was attenuated by treatment with either aspirin or polyphloretin phosphate, a prostaglandin antagonist. Mesenteric arteries were contracted only slightly by high concentrations of hemolysate. A superfusion study showed release of a prostaglandin-like substance by the hemolysate application. They showed that hemolysate contracts basilar arteries mainly through prostaglandins synthesize in and released from the vascular wall.

B. Suppression of Free-Radical Formation and Lipid Peroxidation

Free-radical formation and lipid peroxidation of the membrane fatty acids provokes prostaglandin release and has been proposed as a mechanism that may play a significant role in the pathogenesis of cerebral vasospasm along with neuronal damage. Gaetani et al. [57] studied the effects of 21-aminosteroid tirilazad mesylate (U74006F), which is an inhibitor of iron-dependent lipid peroxidation, or high-dose methylprednisolone on the ex-vivo synthesis of eicosanoids in brain slices of rats. Production in the brain slices of prostaglandin D_2 and 6-keto F_1 alpha (a stable metabolite of prostacyclin) were significantly higher at 48 hours after subarachnoid hemorrhage; prostaglandin E_2 release was significantly enhanced at 6 hours after SAH. Release of a lipoxygenase metabolite, leukotriene C_4, was enhanced at 1, 6, and 48 hours after subarachnoid hemorrhage. Treatment regimens with U74006F or high-dose methylprednisolone significantly reduced the ex-vivo synthesis of prostaglandin D_2, prostaglandin E_2, and leukotriene C_4 at 1, 6, and 48 hours after subarachnoid hemorrhage.

Kanamaru et al. [58] studied effects of U74006F on lipid peroxidation in subarachnoid clot in a cynomolgous monkey model. Intravenous administration (0.3 or 1.0 mg/kg, every 8 hours for 6 days) significantly suppressed development of vasospasm measured at the 7th day after the subarachnoid hemorrhage and reduced the levels of malondialdehyde, the by-product of lipid peroxidation, in the clot. Preventive effects of U74006F on chronic cerebral vasospasm were confirmed in the double hemorrhage canine model by Matsui and Asano [59]. An intravenous administration of U74006F (0.5, 1.5, and 3.0 mg/kg, repeated every 8 hours) was effective in preventing development of vasospasm.

Another compound, U88999E, a tropolone derivative, which possesses properties as an inhibitor of lipid peroxidation and also as a calcium antagonist, caused relaxation of the rabbit basilar artery precontracted with KCl, UTP, or endothelin-1 [60]. In the rabbit model of subarachnoid hemorrhage, vasospasm observed on day 2 was suppressed by intravenous administration (1.0 to 3.0 mg/kg, every 8 hours, starting 8 hours prior to SAH) of U88999E.

The possibility of treatment/prevention using deferoxamine, an iron-chelating agent, was investigated by Harada and Mayberg [61]. In a rabbit femoral artery spasm model, where whole blood application causes chronic vasoconstriction, a preventive effect by topical application of the agent was reported.

One well-documented source of free radicals is the reaction catalyzed by xanthine oxidase (XO). The pathway of purine catabolism is activated as the nucleotides contained in the clot undergo degradation, and the end product of the enzyme is uric acid. In the double hemorrhage canine model, the cerebrospinal fluid (CSF) level of uric acid was in fact increased on day 7, signifying concomitant production of superoxide radicals in the subarachnoid space. A specific inhibitor of xanthine oxidase, allopurinal, in a regimen of 25 mg/kg, i.v., every 6 hours, completely suppressed the pathway and the level of uric acid, but the angiographic vasospasm as well as the elevation of the CSF prostaglandin on day 7 after SAH were not affected by the treatment [62,63].

C. Suppression of the Thromboxane System

Chan et al. [64] studied the therapeutic effect of prostacyclin and suppression of the thromboxane system in cerebral vasospasm in the rabbit cisternal injection model. Exogenous prostacyclin and carbacyclin decreased chronic vasospasm observed on day 3, but failed to improve cerebral perfusion. Chronic spasm was absent in the group treated with a selective thromboxane A_2 (TXA_2) synthetase inhibitor, sodium(E)-3-[4-(3-pyridylmethyl)phenyl]-2-methyl-2-propenoate (OKY-1581), or linoleic acid. The latter is a precursor of eicosapentaenoic acid, which is transformed into trienoic prostanoids such as thromboxane A_3 and prostaglandin I_3 and thus suppresses TXA_2 production. The compound TXA_3 does not possess proaggregatory activity and eicosapentaenoic acid thus reduces platelet aggregation and TXA_2 production. Cerebral blood flow measurements on the 4th posthemorrhage day using the xenon-133 technique revealed significantly higher values in the groups treated with linoleic acid or

OKY-1581. The inhibitor TXA_2 is not only formed during platelet aggregation but also induces platelet aggregation.

The OKY agents were also tried in the canine model [65]. They studied effects of OKY-1581 and OKY-046 ((E)-3-[4-(1-imidazolylmethyl) phenyl]-2-propenoic acid hydrochloride monohydrate, an inhibitor of TXA_2 synthetase) on the chronic vasospasm in the canine cisternal injection model. Vasospasm observed angiographically on day 5 was not reversed by intravenous infusion (50μ g/kg/min for 1 or 2 hours), in spite of the efficacy of the regimen in suppression of platelet aggregation in the systemic venous blood.

Yokota et al. [66] studied the effect of OKY-046 on intracerebral production of prostaglandins in a double hemorrhage canine model. Intravenous infusion of OKY-046 had little effect on angiographic vasospasm but increased CBF. During delayed vasospasm, the cortical levels of prostaglandin $F_{2\alpha}$ ($PGF_{2\alpha}$) were significantly decreased, whereas the plasma levels of $PGF_{2\alpha}$ and TXB_2 sampled in the transverse sinus were increased. The intravenous infusion of OKY-046 reversed the changes; the drug induced an increase in the levels of cortical PGF_2, an increase in the plasma 6-keto-$PGF_{1\alpha}$ (the stable metabolite of prostacyclin), and a decrease in the plasma TXB_2 in the transverse sinus. The increased plasma $PGF_{2\alpha}$ and TXB_2 levels during delayed vasospasm may reflect enhancement of intravascular coagulation, and the decreased cortical levels of $PGF_{2\alpha}$ may reflect a decrease in CBF.

Kondo et al. [67] studied effects of ONO-3708, an antagonist of the thromboxane A_2/prostaglandin endoperoxide receptor, on blood vessels. The antagonist ONO-3708 inhibited contractions induced by thromboxane A_2, prostaglandin H_2, 11,9-epoxymethano-prostaglandin H_2 (U-46619), or $PGF_{2\alpha}$ without affecting the contractions induced by angiotensin II, serotonin, or norepinephrine. In a concentration of 1 to 100 n*M*, the drug acted as a competitive inhibitor of the contractile responses of the canine basilar artery to 9,11-epithio-11,12-methano-thromboxane A_2, U-46619, and $PGF_{2\alpha}$, and as a noncompetitive inhibitor of the contractile responses to 15-hydroperoxy-eicosatetraenoic acid (15-HPETE). Infusion of ONO-3708 (10 and 30 μgrams/kg per min, i.v.) prevented cerebral vasospasm in the canine subarachnoid hemorrhage model.

D. Others: A Leukotriene Antagonist and a Vasodilator Prostanoid

For suppression of the vasoconstrictive effect of lipoxygenase products, ONO-1078, a novel leukotriene antagonist (i.v., once a day for 7 days, started immediately after SAH) was tried in a double hemorrhage canine model [68]. The levels of leukotriene C_4 in the cerebrospinal fluid were increased after subarachnoid hemorrhage. The treatment effectively suppressed the increase and partially prevented the chronic vasospasm observed on day 7.

A vasodilator prostanoid, prostaglandin E_1, was tried in humans. Lipoprostaglandin E_1 has a longer half life than PGE_1, which is mainly degraded in the lung. Treatment of patients after clipping in the acute phase after subarachnoid hemorrhage with lipo-PGE_1 (15 μ g, intravenously every 8 hours for two weeks) reportedly yielded a better outcome as compared to the nontreated group [69].

E. Summary

Efficacy of steroids and nonsteroidal anti-inflammatory agents has been repeatedly demonstrated in the experimental chronic cerebral arterial spasm. Suppression of free radical formations and lipid peroxidation by novel compounds yielded positive preventive effects on the chronic spasm in the canine and the primate models. However complete suppression of superoxide production mediated by an archetypal radical-producing enzyme, xanthine oxidase, did not result in reducing the development of vasospasm. Beneficial effects with inhibitors of thromboxane synthetase, eicosapentaenoic acid, leukotriene antagonist, and vasodilator prostaglandin were reported.

VI. SUPPRESSION OF RELEASE AND ACTION OF SEROTONIN

Zervas et al. [70] observed that dogs treated with reserpine (0.1 mg/kg for 2 days) did not develop vasospasm, which would be observed at 30 minutes and 2 days after cisternal injection of blood taken from nontreated animals. Reserpine (intramuscularly, 0.1 mg/kg, given for 2 days prior to SAH) or kanamycin (per os, 100 mg/kg/day, given for 14 to 28 days prior to SAH), which reduce the platelet serotonin contents, prevented experimental vasospasm observed in rhesus monkeys after subarachnoid hemorrhage induced by puncture of the middle cerebral artery [71].

Boullin et al. [72] observed that the intracisternal injection of a serotonin antagonist, alpha-amino N-2-chlorphenoxypropyl-acetamidine HCL monohydrate (BW501C67, Wellcome Laboratories) did not reverse the acute spasm induced by cisternal blood injection in baboons, although the agent at the same concentration was effective in suppressing the vasoconstriction caused by serotonin injected into the cistern. The agent was also effective in suppression of serotonin-induced platelet aggregation in vitro. The data suggested that serotonin played little role in the genesis of acute spasm after subarachnoid hemorrhage.

Boisvert et al. [73] found that the acute spasm (up to 3 hours) and alteration of CBF observed after autologous blood injection into the cistern in the cynomolgus monkeys was unaffected by a serotonin-blocking agent cyproheptadine (i.v., 1.0 mg/kg). Concurrently, intracisternal injection of serotonin at a concentration normally present in monkey serum (5×10^{-6} M), which is sufficient to cause contraction of cerebral artery in vitro, had little effect in vivo. The result suggested that serotonin had little contribution to the genesis of the acute vasospasm.

Noseworthy et al. [74] studied the effect of treatment with reserpine and kanamycin in a monkey model where platelet-enriched blood was injected in the chiasmatic cistern. Treatment with reserpine (0.0013 mg/kg, i.m.) and kanamycin (50 mg/kg, p.o.) administered 3 hour after SAH and daily thereafter to day 7, did not reduce the incidence or severity of the chronic vasospasm, in spite of the efficacy of the protocol in suppression of the systemic levels of serotonin.

A. Summary

As stated by Zervas in a commentary [74], treatment with reserpine and kanamycin, which reduces storage of serotonin, is meaningful only if given prior to hemorrhage, and administration of the agents after subarachnoid hemorrhage has little effect on the events occuring in the clot extravasated in the subarachnoid space. Specific serotonin antagonists, despite concentrations sufficient to block serotonin-induced spasm, also failed to ameliorate acute vasospasm induced by injection of blood.

VII. SUPPRESSION OF SYNTHESIS OR EFFECT OF ENDOTHELIN

Endothelin (ET) is a potent vasoconstrictor peptide isolated from cultured endothelial cells. Contribution of the substance in the pathogenesis of chronic vasospasm is not firmly established. There are conflicting reports of increase in cerebrospinal fluid ET levels and histological findings such as in-situ hybridization demonstrating expression of the peptide in the endothelium or subendothelial layers of the spastic cerebral arteries [75]. Endothelin was present in both plasma and cerebrospinal fluid after subarachnoid hemorrhage, but did not correlate with the intensity of vasospasm [75]. In a study done in the double-hemorrhage canine model of chronic vasospasm, levels of immunoreactive ET in plasma and cerebrospinal fluid were not affected by development of vasospasm [76]. At the present time, the best evidence suggesting contribution of the substance to vasospasm are results from the prevention/treatment of vasospasm in animal models.

A. Inhibitors of Endothelin Production

The active form of endothelin, endothelin-1 (ET-1), is converted from big endothelin-1. The conversion is inhibited by phosphoramidon, which is a metalloproteinase inhibitor. In the canine double-hemorrhage model of chronic vasospasm, intrathecal administration of phosphoramidon (2μ mol/4 mL saline, on day 0 and 2 prior to the cisternal blood injections) inhibited the increase in the CSF endothelin level and chronic vasospasm observed on day 7 after subarachnoid hemorrhage [77]. However, in two other studies using the same canine model, phosphoramidon failed to prevent the development of vasospasm [75,76] (2×10^{-4} *M*, daily cisternal injection). Agents to block production of endothelin by inhibition of RNA and DNA synthesis, such as actinomycin D, were effective in preventing the development of vasospasm in the dog model [75].

B. Blockade of Action of Endothelin

Contribution of ET_A and ET_B receptor activation was investigated in a rabbit double-hemorrhage model. An endothelin ETA receptor antagonist, BQ610 (1μ *M*; homo piperidinyl-CO-Leu-D-Trp(CHO)-D-Trp-OH), and an endothelin ET_A/ET_B receptor antagonist, PD145065 (1μ *M*; Ac-D-Bhg-L-Leu-L-Asp-L-Ile-L-Ile-L-Trp), topically applied via a cranial window, relaxed the vasospastic basilar artery on day 6 after subarachnoid hemorrhage in situ [78].

In a rat cisternal injection model, a selective antagonist of the ETA receptor, BQ-123, (cyclo[Dtrp, Dasp, pro-D-ValLeu], cisternal injection) was effective in preventing decrease in CBF observed at 60 minutes and 120 minutes following subarachnoid hemorrhage [79]. Whether the reduction in CBF in that phase represents the phenomenon analogous to chronic vasospasm is not certain. The alteration may be secondary to acute vasospasm or due to cerebral swelling.

In the double-hemorrhage canine model, daily intracisternal injections of BQ-123 (10^{-4} *M*) failed to prevent chronic vasospasm [76]. The drug, at a lower concentration (10^{-5} *M*) selectively inhibited contractions by ET-1 (10^{-11}-3×10^{-8} *M*) of the isolated canine basilar arteries. The negative result with the regimen, despite the efficacy in blocking the action of endothelin in vitro, presents evidence against a role of ET-1 in mediating chronic vasospasm.

An ET_A receptor antagonist, FR139317 (intracisternal administration, 0.1 mg/1 mL saline, given on day 0, 2, and 4) partially prevented the vasoconstriction of the basilar artery measured at day 7 in the double-hemorrhage canine model (62% in the control group versus 76% in the treated group). Interestingly, cisternal injection of the drug did not dilate the normal basilar artery [80].

Another antagonist to the ET_A receptor, BQ-485, was reportedly effective in the double-hemorrhage canine model. Systemic continuous administration of 120 mg/day of the agent inhibited the narrowing of canine basilar artery on day 7 following experimental subarachnoid hemorrhage [81].

A nonpeptide ET_A receptor antagonist, SB 209670, (intracisternal continuous injection via osmotic minipump for 7 days, 360 $\pm$ 10 μgrams/day), partially prevented vasospasm in the canine model on day 7 [82]. The antagonist SB 209670 caused inhibition of contraction of the canine basilar and anterior spinal arteries by ET. An IT_B-selective agonist, sarafotoxin 6c, did not contract these posterior cerebral vessels. The antagonist SB 209670 also produced a concentration-dependent inhibition ($IC_{50} = 1$ nmol/L) of the mitogenic response induced by ET-1 in the culture of vascular smooth muscle.

C. Summary

Trials of blockage of production or action of endothelin yielded at best conflicting results in the canine model. Efficacy of the agents in other established animal models of chronic vasospasm remains to be examined.

VIII. MODIFICATION OF VASOMOTOR NERVE AND NEUROTRANSMITTER FUNCTIONS

Contribution of autonomic nerve dysfunction in the pathogenesis of chronic vasospasm has been studied extensively in rat models, where the onset and duration of the delayed vasospasm is relatively short. Participation of substance P, calatonin gene related peptide (CGRP), serotonergic, adrenergic, and dopaminergic pathways have been studied.

Chemical destruction of the central serotonergic and dopaminergic pathways prior to the cisternal blood injection failed to affect the vasospasm observed on day 2 in the rat model of subarachnoid hemorrhage [83].

An antagonist to arginine vasopressin (AVP) was tried in the Sprague-Dawley rat model [84]. The acute vasospasm was observed maximally 10 minutes after induction of subarachnoid hemorrhage and late vasospasm 2 days after the hemorrhage. In Brattleboro rats, which are deficient in arginine vasopressin, the acute vasospasm was not observed although the late vasospasm developed in an intensity comparable to that seen in Sprague-Dawley rats. Cisternal injection of arginine vasopressin induced acute vasospasm in the Sprague-Dawley rats. Intravenous vasopressin antagonist, or intracisternal vasopressin antiserum, when administered prior to the subarachnoid hemorrhage, prevented the acute vasospasm but not the late spasm. The data suggest that an increased release of AVP may contribute to the acute vasospasm.

Capsaicin, an agent that causes depletion of substance P, or spantide, a substance P antagonist, prevented the acute (10 minutes after SAH) and chronic (day 2 after SAH) vasospasm observed in the rat model, when injected intracisternally prior to induction of SAH []85. Cisternal injection of either agent 2 hours after the subarachnoid hemorrhage prevented development of chronic spasm as well.

Therapeutic potential of calcitonin gene-related peptide (CGRP) was investigated in the rabbit model of subarachnoid hemorrhage [86]. Infusion of CGRP (either intracisternally or intravenously, 100 ng/kg/min, 2 hours), on the second day after induction of subarachnoid hemorrhage, dilated the spastic basilar artery significantly. Intravenous infusion of CGRP caused significant hypotension.

Shiokawa et al., [87] studied the involvement of cerebrovascular sensory nerves in the development of the vasospasm. In a squirrel–monkey model, a unilateral surgical section of the trigeminal nerve at the postganglionic (Gasserian) level—but not at the preganglionic level—constricted ipsilateral cerebral arteries. Intrathecal injection of antibody to substance P, a sensory neurotransmitter in the trigeminal system, prevented chronic vasospasm after subarachnoid hemorrhage and the decrease in CBF. Antibody to CGRP reduced the baseline diameter but did not affect development of chronic vasospasm.

A. Summary

The significance of the participation of the perivascular autonomic nervous system has been mostly studied in the small animal models. It remains to be established in the larger animal models or in human cases.

IX. IMMUNOSUPPRESSANTS

It has been postulated that the immunological reactions taking place against extravasated blood might play a role in the development of chronic vasospasm after subarachnoid hemorrhage, and therefore the chronic spasm is refractory to conventional pharmacological treatments. The hypothesis was in part supported by the findings of the presence of inflammatory cells in the perivascular subarachnoid space. Agents to suppress immunological responses have been tried on experimental vasospasm.

An immunosuppressant treatment with cyclosporine A was tried in a double-hemorrhage canine model [88]. A prophylactic protocol with the agent 6 mg/kg/day and adjunctive low-dose steroid reportedly prevented occurrence of severe chronic vasospasm.

The effect of cyclosporine was also studied in a monkey craniotomy-clot placement model [89]. Cyclosporine (5 mg/kg/day) was administered intramuscularly for 7 days starting immediately after the induction of SAH. Angiographical spasm was partially prevented by the treatment, but no effect was seen on the deposition of IgG in the arterial wall of the cerebral artery.

Another immunosuppressant, FK-506, was tried in the double-hemorrhage canine model to assess the role of cell-mediated immune reactions. Despite suppression of lymphocytic infiltration in the arterial wall, FK-506 alone or in combination with steroid failed to prevent chronic vasospasm or pathological changes observed in the arterial wall [90].

Nishizawa et al. [91] studied the efficacy of FK-506 (0.15 or 0.3 mg/kg/day, intramuscular injection started 6 hours after subarachnoid hemorrhage and continued through day 7) on the development of chronic vasospasm in the canine model. They found no significant effect despite achievement of a therapeutic concentration of the drug. Levels of the third factor of complement (C3) and the activity of complement inducing 50% hemolysis of sheep erythrocytes (CH_{50}) in serum were not affected by the treatment. There were no changes in the levels between day 1 and day 7 in the untreated group as well.

A. Summary

Conflicting results were reported with cyclosporine and FK506 in canine or primate models. The positive effect of cyclosporine was not necessarily associated with findings of effective suppression of immunological reaction. The compound FK-506 was ineffective despite effective suppression of lymphocytic infiltration in the vascular wall. In one study, the complement levels did not vary in the course of development of chronic vasospasm, suggesting that the activation of the system is not contributing to chronic vasospasm.

X. MISCELLANEOUS TREATMENTS

A. Protease Inhibitors

Ito in 1980 [92] observed in a dog model of subarachnoid hemorrhage (chiasmatic cistern injection of blood) that intravenous administration of the combination of gabexate mesilate (nonpeptide proteinase inhibitor FOY, Ono Pharmaceuticals Inc., 3.3–13.3 mg/kg, intravenous injection) and diphenhydramine (H_1 receptor antagonist, 2 mg/kg intravenous injection) ameliorated vasospasm observed on day 3 to 5. Topical application of haptoglobin, which forms a stable compound with hemoglobin stoichiometrically, was effective in reversal of the spasm when applied after removal of the peri-arterial clot by exposing the artery [92].

Yanamoto et al. [93] studied the effect of a protease inhibitor, FUT-175, in a rabbit model. The maximal vasospasm was seen on day 2 after a single injection of blood into the cisterna magna, and the serine protease inhibitor FUT-175 (intravenous injection, 3 doses of 1, 2, or 3 mg) inhibited development of this spasm.

B. Angiotensin-Converting Enzyme Inhibitors

An angiotensin-converting enzyme inhibitor, teprotide, was tried in a dog model of chronic vasospasm 3 days after subarachnoid hemorrhage [94]. Effective release of vasospasm was observed 30 to 90 minutes following injection of the drug. Andrews et al. [95] examined the effect of teproside on the acute phase of vasospasm 30 minutes after cisternal injection of blood in dogs and observed effective reversal of the acute vasospasm.

C. Potassium Channel Openers

A novel class of vasodilator, potassium channel opener, has been tried in the double-hemorrhage canine models. Intravenous infusion of nicorandil (10 μ g/kg/min for 6 hours on day 3 and for 3 hours twice per day on day 4, 5, and 6) ameliorated the chronic vasospasm [96].

D. Protein Kinase C Inhibitors

In the chronic spasm of the double-hemorrhage model, transclival topical application of the protein kinase C inhibitors staurosporine (10^{-8}–10^{-7} *M*) and H-7 compound (10^{-5} *M*) dilated the spastic basilar artery [7].

E. Analogues of Nucleotide

Dibutyryl-3',5'-adenosine monophosphate (dibutyryl cyclic AMP) when applied topically (10 mg/2 mL) via a Rickham reservoir inserted in the cistern, reversed the acute spasm in macaque rhesus monkeys after injection of blood. The drug penetrates the membrane of the smooth muscles and acts as an analog of cyclic AMP, which causes relaxation [97].

F. Heparin and Antithrombin III

A preventive effect of heparin on the pathological changes in the cerebral arteries has been reported in the rat model of subarachnoid hemorrhage. Intracisternal injection of heparin one hour after injection of autologous blood reportedly decreased the proliferative histological changes [98].

Irrigation/infusion of the cistern with saline containing antithrombin III (2-hour intracisternal infusion of 100 IU on day 3) resulted in amelioration of the basilar artery constriction [99] in the rabbit subarachnoid blood injection model. Antithrombin III (10 IU/mL) induced relaxation in the rabbit basilar arteries in vitro as well.

In a cat model, in which subarachnoid hemorrhage was induced by puncture of the middle cerebral artery, the proliferative changes seen in the arterial wall were suppressed by administration of heparin (75 mg/kg subcutaneous injection every 6 hours, started 7 days prior to the hemorrhage and continued through day 16) ([100].

G. Magnesium

The effect of topical (n=30) and intravenous (n=20) magnesium sulfate on the spastic artery on day 3 in the rat cisternal injection model was evaluated by Ram et al. [101]. Intravenous magnesium sulfate dilated the spastic basilar artery. Magnesium sulfate given topically via clival exposure dilated the basilar artery of the control and the subarachnoid hemorrhage groups. All rats receiving intravenous magnesium sulfate reached therapeutic plasma levels of the ion. Hemodynamic effects were mild and immediately reversible upon cessation of magnesium sulfate administration.

H. Chlorpromazine

Possibility of treatment with chlorpromazine was examined in a cat model of cerebral vasospasm [102]. Acute vasospasm induced by rupturing the branches of the basilar artery via transclival approach and by electrical, mechanical, and pharmacological stimulation, was reversed by topical application of chlorpromazine (10^{-7}–10^{-4} *M*). The phenothiazine agent has a direct inhibitory effect on the smooth muscle by inhibition of calmodulin, as well as an effect to antagonize the alpha adrenergic action.

In a canine model of chronic vasospasm (double cisternal injection), infusion of chlorpromazine solution (10^{-6}–10^{-5} *M*) was effective in reversal of the vasospasm observed on day 7, without causing major alterations in the EEG or neurological status [103].

I. Intrathecal Clot Lysis

Lysis of the clot using fibrinolytic substances such as urokinase or recombinant tissue plasminogen activator (rt-PA) have been demonstrated to be efficacious in reducing the incidence and severity of chronic vasospasm in primate and canine models. Cisternal injection of rt-PA via the Ommaya reservoir (0.5 mg in 0.5 mL saline, every 8 hours × 3 started 24 hours after hemorrhage) or slow-release gel (1.25 mg) was effective in lysis of the subarachnoid clot in the monkey craniotomy-clot placement model and prevention of the development of vasospasm as observed on the angiograms taken 7 days after hemorrhage [104,105] The intrathecal injection of the thrombolytic agent (0.75 mg) was effective when injected within 24 or 48 hours of subarachnoid hemorrhage but was not effective when injected after 72 hours in the model [106].

A bolus intrathecal injection of urokinase (200,000 IU) was as effective in lysing the subarachnoid clot in the primate model as rt-PA (2 mg) given via an Ommaya reservoir [107]. When the lysing agents were given in a reduced dose (100,000 IU or 1 mg), substantial clot remained.

Single intracisternal bolus injection of the agent (25 μg) 48 hours after the first and 6 hours after the second injection of blood into the cisternal magna in dogs was effective in prevention of the chronic vasospasm [108]. Intrathecal application of recombinant tissue plasminogen activator (2 mg) resulted in an almost total restoration of CSF absorption after experimental SAH [109] in a cat model. After a cisternal blood injection, CSF outflow resistance was found to be elevated, in parallel to the amount of blood injected. The elevation was reversed after intrathecal injection of tissue plasminogen activator (2 mg), indicating effective clot lysis in the subarachnoid space.

In a cat transorbital cisternal injection model, tissue plasminogen activator (25 μg) injected within 10 minutes of subarachnoid hemorrhage inhibited intimal platelet accumulation as demonstrated using indium-111 labeled platelets. Injection at 60 minutes after hemorrhage did not inhibit platelet accumulation, although the extent of subarachnoid clot was reduced [110].

In a recent large-scale clinical study, which was a multicentered, randomized, placebo-controlled trial conducted with one hundred patients, efficacy of a single injection with rt-PA (1 mg/mL, 10 mL) into the basal cistern immediately following aneurysm clipping was examined [111]. The overall incidence of angiographic vasospasm measured between the seventh and eleventh day was similar between the placebo and the rt-PA groups. A trend toward a lesser degree of vasospasm was found in the rt-PA group, and when a comparison was made in the subgroup of patients with thick subarachnoid clots, there was a significant risk reduction of severe vasospasm [111].

XI. CONCLUSION

Various classes of pharmacological agents have been tried on the cerebral vasospasm following experimental subarachnoid hemorrhage in animal models. Therapeutic trials have been made on the acute cerebral vasospasm occurring shortly after the induction of hemorrhage, as well as on the chronic vasospasm that develops over several days afterwards and that lasts for 2 to 3 weeks.

In the pharmacological trials performed on acute spasm, the contraction of the cerebral artery is reversed by vasodilatory agents acting directly on the smooth muscle, such as calcium channel blockers, phosphodiesterase inhibitors, and nitrovasodilators. The responsiveness to the vasodilators suggests that the acute spasm is caused by activation of a physiological mechanism in the smooth muscle.

Chronic vasospasm and resultant ischemic brain damage are the chief cause of mortality and morbidity after recovery from the initial insult of subarachnoid hemorrhage, and it is for this condition that therapeutic measures are being sought. It has been reproducibly demonstrated in experimental vasospasm that the cerebral artery during chronic vasospasm becomes less responsive to different vasodilators such as phosphodiesterase inhibitors, nitrovasodilators, and calcium channel blockers. In fact, the mechanism of the NO-cyclic GMP pathway, which plays a pivotal role for relaxations of smooth muscle and is the target of modification by nitrovasodilators and phosphodiesterase inhibitors, becomes impaired in the cerebral arteries during chronic vasospasm. These changes are associated with findings of cellular damage to smooth muscles. The diminished responsiveness to vasodilators is a hallmark of chronic vasospasm, and an important factor to be considered when designing pharmacological treatment. Pharmacological agents should be chosen with a consideration to the pharmacodynamics that circumvent the degenerative alterations occuring in the smooth muscle cells.

Experimental and clinical findings are suggesting that the smooth muscles of the spastic arterial wall are not completely or homogeneously affected, but the cellular damage takes place in a mosaic fashion, sparing a population of smooth muscle cells that are less affected and maintain relative responsiveness to dilating agents. Conventional dilators acting directly on the smooth muscle can be effective on the cell population if the local concentration of the agent is sustained above the therapeutic range for a sufficient duration. Positive results with the superselective intraarterial administration of papaverine or calcium channel blockers for clinical chronic vasospasm—albeit the effect may not be long lasting—indicate that the pathological constriction can be reversed if the dilators are presented in an adequate condition of distribution. Negative results of therapeutic trials should be interpreted carefully with attention to whether the problems lie in the pharmacodynamics, the mechanism of action of the drug, or in the distribution. If the latter is the cause of failure, enhancement in drug delivery, if achieved without causing adverse effects, can possibly yield improved results.

In contrast to the efforts to dilate the vessels once constricted, another rational strategy is to prevent the development of cellular damage that leads to constriction. Pharmacological inhibition of free-radical generation, lipid peroxidation, prostaglandin synthesis, and protease inhibitors have been tried. Adequate pharmacokinetic design is crucial for successful treatment with this approach, since the treatment has to cover the period of development of delayed vasospasm with a sufficient concentration of the agents.

Removal of blood clots in the subarachnoid space using lytic agents such as urokinase or tissue plasminogen activators has been recently tried experimentally and clinically. Oxyhemoglobin itself is a potent vasoconstrictor in vitro and in situ and has been demonstrated to generate free radicals, to cause cell damage in cultured smooth muscle, to release prostaglandins, and to scavenge nitric oxide, the relaxing factor. Encasement of the vascular wall with a clot containing oxyhemoglobin is probably one of the most important factors in the genesis of delayed vasoconstriction. Lysis of the hematoma and removal by irrigation, if effectively achieved in the intact cranium and in the entire subarachnoid space, can remove the interactions between the clot and the arterial wall.

A pragmatic approach to improving the efficacy of pharmacological treatments is to enhance the pharmacokinetic factor. Enhanced drug delivery and distribution, with the local concentration sustained in an effective therapeutic range over an extended period of time, would improve the responsiveness of the artery to the preexisting classes of vasodilators.

Concurrently, with the advancements in the understanding of the nature of the pathological vasoconstriction that it is not simply due to the activation of the normal contractile mechanisms but involves cell damage process, pharmacological interventions with novel pharmacodynamic schemes will be devised in the future to prevent the development of chronic vasospasm.

REFERENCES

1. Fraser RAR, Stein BM, Barrett RE, Pool JL. Noradrenergic mediation of experimental cerebrovascular spasm. *Stroke* 1970; 1:356–362.
2. Flamm ES, Yasargil MG, Ransohoff J Jr. Alteration of experimental cerebral vasospasm by adrenergic blockade. *J Neurosurg* 1972; 37:294–301.
3. Smigiel MR Jr, Sundt TM Jr. The comparative effectiveness of alpha–blockade and beta–stimulation in modifying experimental basilar arterial spasm. *J Neurosurg* 1974; 41:300–305.
4. White RP, Hagen AA, Robertson JT. Effect of nonsteroid anti-inflammatory drugs on subarachnoid hemorrhage in dogs. *J Neurosurg* 1979; 51: 164–171.
5. Ishibashi Y, Konda R, Yoshimoto T, Suzuki J. The effect of prazosin hydrochloride on cerebral vasospasm. An experimental study. *Noushinkei-Geka* 1984; 12:133–139.
6. Allen GS, Gold LHA, Chou SN, French LA. Cerebral arterial spasm. Part 3: In vivo intracisternal production of spasm by serotonin and blood and its reversal by phenoxybenzamine. *J Neurosurg* 1974; 40:451–457.
7. Matsui T, Takuwa Y, Johshita H, Yamashita K, Asano T. Possible role of protein kinase C–dependent smooth muscle contraction in the pathogenesis of chronic cerebral vasospasm. *J Cereb Blood Flow Metab* 1991; 11: 143–149.
8. Flamm ES, Kim J, Lin J, Ransohoff J. Phosphodiesterase inhibitors and cerebral vasospasm. *Arch Neurol* 1975; 32:569–571.
9. Sundt TM Jr, Onofrio BM, Merideth J. Treatment of cerebral vasospasm from subarachnoid hemorrhage with isoproterenol anmd lidocaine hydrochloride. *J Neurosurg* 1973; 38:557–560.
10. Edvinsson L, Hardebo JE, Mackenzie ET, Stewart M. Dual action of serotonin on pial arterioles in situ and the effect of propranolol on the response. *Blood Vessels* 1975; 14:366–371.
11. Nakagomi T, Kassel NF, Sasaki T, Fujiwara S, Lehman RM, Johshita H, Nazar GB, Torner JC. Effect of subarachnoid hemorrhage on endothelium–dependent vasodilatation. *J Neurosurg* 1987; 66:915–923.
12. Kim P, Sundt TM Jr, Vanhoutte PM. Alterations in endothelium–dependent responsiveness of the canine basilar artery after subarachnoid hemorrhage. *J Neurosurg* 1988; 69:239–246.
13. Kim P, Lorenz RR, Sundt TM Jr, Vanhoutte PM. Release of endothelium–derived relaxing factor after subarachnoid hemorrhage. *J Neurosurg* 1989; 70:108–114.
14. Kim P, Schini V, Sundt TM Jr, Vanhoutte PM. Reduced production of cyclic GMP explains the loss of endothelium–dependent relaxations in the canine basilar artery after subarachnoid hemorrhage. *Circ Res* 1992; 70:248–256.
15. Kim P, Jones JD, Sundt TM Jr. Decrease of high–energy phosphates in the spastic cerebral arteries after subarachnoid hemorrhage. *J Neurosurg* 1992; 76:991–996.
16. Kanamaru K, Weir BKA, Findlay JM, Krueger CA, Cook DA. Pharmacological studies on relaxation of spastic primate cerebral arteries. *J Neurosurg* 1989; 71:909–915.

17. Ogata M, Marshall BM, Lougheed WM. Observations n the effects of intrathecal papaverine in experimental vasospasm. *J Neurosurg* 1973; 38:20–25.
18. Noda S. Experimental subarachnoid hemorrhage in dogs—effect of various drugs and sympathectomy on cerebral arterial spasm (author's transl). *No Shinkei Geka* 1975; 3: 747–755.
19. Varsos VG, Liszczak TM, Han DH, Kistler JP, Vielma J, Black PM, Heros RC, Zervas NT. Delayed cerebral vasospasm is not reversed by aminophylline, nifedipine, or papaverine in a "two-hemorrhage" canine model. *J Neurosurg* 1983; 58:11–17.
20. Nakagomi T, Kassell NF, Hongo K, Sasaki T. Pharmacological reversibility of experimental cerebral vasospasm. *Neurosurgery* 1990; 27: 582–586.
21. Vorkapic P, Bevan JA, Bevan RD. Clentiazem protects against chronic cerebral vasospasm in rabbit basilar artery. *Stroke* 1991; 22: 1409–1413.
22. Vorkapic P, Bevan JA, Bevan RD. Two indices of functional damage of the artery wall parallel the time course of irreversible narrowing in experimental vasospasm in the rabbit. *Blood Vessels* 1991; 28: 179–182.
23. Matsui T, Kaizu H, Itoh S, Asano T. The role of active smooth–muscle contraction in the occurrence of chronic vasospasm in the canine two–hemorrhage model. *J Neurosurg* 1994; 80: 276–282.
24. Kaku Y, Yonekawa Y, Tsukahara T, Kakezawa K. Superselective intra–arterial infusion of papaverine for the treatment of cerebral vasospasm after subarachnoid hemorrhage. *J Neurosurg* 1992; 77:842–847.
25. Clouston JE, Numaguchi Y, Zoarski GH, Aldrich EF, Simard JM, Zitnay KM. Intraarterial papaverine infusion for cerebral vasospasm after subarachnoid hemorrhage. *AJNR Am J Neuroradiol* 1995; 16:27–38.
26. Kistler JP, Lees RS, Candia G, Zervas NT, Crowell RM, Ojemann RG. Intravenous nitroglycerine in experimental cerebral vasospasm. A preliminary report. *Stroke* 1979; 10:26–29.
27. Frazee JG, Giannotta SL, Stern WE. Intravenous nitroglycerin for the treatment of chronic cerebral vasoconstriction in the primate. *J Neurosurg* 1981; 55:865–868.
28. Hirsh LF. Intra–arterial nitroprusside treatment of acute experimental vasospasm. *Stroke* 1980; 11:601–605.
29. Heros RC, Zervas NT, Lavyne MH, Pickren KS. Reversal of experimental cerebral vasospasm by intravenous nitroprusside therapy. *Surg Neurol* 1976; 6:227–229.
30. Suzuki Y, Kajita Y, Oyama H, Tanazawa T, Takayasu M, Shibuya M, Sugita K. Dysfunction of nitric oxide in the spastic basilar arteries after subarachnoid hemorrhage. *J Auton Nerv Syst* 1994; 49 Suppl: S83–87.
31. Edwards DH, Byrne JV, Griffith TM. The effect of chronic subarachnoid hemorrhage on basal endothelium–derived relaxing factor activity in intrathecal cerebral arteries. *J Neurosurg* 1992; 76:830–837.
32. Kajita Y, Suzuki Y, Oyama H, Tanazawa T, Takayasu M, Shibuya M, Sugita K. Combined effect of L–arginine and superoxide dismutase on the spastic basilar artery after subarachnoid hemorrhage in dogs. *J Neurosurg* 1994; 80: 476–483.
33. Tanaka K, Gotoh F, Muramatsu F, Fukuuchi Y, Okayasu H, Suzuki N, Kobari M. Effect of nimodipine, a calcium antagonist, on cerebral vasospasm after subarachnoid hemorrhage in cats. *Arzneimittelforschung* 1982; 32(12): 1529–1534.

34. Leblanc R, Feindel W, Yamamoto LY, Milton JG, Frojmovic MM, Hodge CP. The effects of calcium antagonism on the epicerebral circulation in early vasospasm. *Stroke* 1984; 15:1017–1020.
35. Frazee JG, Bevan JA, Bevan RD, Jones KR. Effect of diltiazem on experimental chronic cerebral vasospasm in the monkey. *J Neurosurg* 1985; 62:912–917.
36. Takagi T, Fukuoka H, Kamiya K, Nagai H, Hotta K. Effect of diltiazem on experimental vasospasm in comparison with effects of cinnarizine, verapamil and nifedipine. *Noushinkei geka* 1983; 11:605–611.
37. Bevan RD, Bevan JA, Frazee JG. Diltiazem protects against functional changes in chronic cerebrovasospasm in monkeys. Stroke 1988. 19:73–79.
38. Tadie M. Effect of nimodipine on vasospasm of cortical arteries. Experimental study. *Neurochirurgie* 1992; 38(3): 134–137.
39. Rodriguez-y-Baena R, Gaetani P, Silvani V, Spanu G, Marzatico F. Effect of nimodipine on mitochondrial respiration in different rat brain areas after subarachnoid haemorrhage. *Acta Neurochir Suppl Wien* 1988; 43: 177–181.
40. Espinosa F, Weir B, Overton T, Castor W, Grace M, Boivert D. A randomized placebo controlled trial of nimodipine after subarachnoid hemorrhage in monkeys: Part 1. Clinical and radiological findings. *J Neurosurg* 1984; 60:1167–1175.
41. Espinosa F, Weir B, Shnitka T, Overton T, Boivert D. A randomized placebo controlled trial of nimodipine after subarachnoid hemorrhage in monkeys: Part 2. Pathological findings. *J Neurosurg* 1984; 60:1176–1185.
42. Nosko M, Weir B, Krueger C, Cook D, Norris S, Overton T, Boisvert D. Nimodipine and chronic vasospasm in monkeys: Part 1. Clinical and radiological findings. *Neurosurgery* 1985; 16:129–136.
43. Krueger C, Weir B, Nosko M, Cook D, Norris S. Nimodipine and chronic vasospasm in monkeys: Part 2. Pharmacological studies of vessels in spasm. *Neurosurgery* 1985; 16: 137–140.
44. Sahlin C, Brismar J, Delgado T, Owman C, Salford LG, Svendgaard NA. Cerebrovascular and metabolic changes during the delayed vasospasm following experimental subarachnoid hemorrhage in baboons, and treatment with a calcium antagonist. *Brain Res* 1987; 403:313–332.
45. Rickels E, Zumkeller M. Vasospasm after experimentally induced subarachnoid haemorrhage and treatment with nimodipine. *Neurochirurgia Stuttg* 1992; 35: 99–102.
46. Gioia AE, White RP, Bakhtian B, Robertson JT. Evaluation of the efficacy of intrathecal nimodipine in canine models of chronic cerebral vasospasm. *J Neurosurg* 1985; 62:721–728.
47. Sakaki S, Ohue S, Kohno K, Takeda S. Impairment of vascular reactivity and changes in intracellular calcium and calmodulin levels of smooth muscle cells in canine basilar arteries after subarachnoid hemorrhage. *Neurosurgery* 1989; 25: 753–761.
48. Yoshida K, Nakamura S, Umezawa T, Nakano M, Tsubokawa T. Effect of diltiazem and thromboxane A2 synthetase inhibitor (OKY–046) on vessels following experimental subarachnoid hemorrhage. *Surg Neurol* 1990; 34: 309–317.
49. Kim P, Yoshimoto Y, Iino M, Sasaki T, Kirino T, Nonomura Y. Impaired calcium

regulation of smooth muscle during chronic vasospasm following subarachnoid hemorrhage. *J Cereb Blood Flow and Met* 1996; 16:334–341.

50. Alabadi JA, Salom JB, Torregrosa G, Miranda FJ, Jover T, Alborch E. Changes in the cerebrovascular effects of endothelin–1 and nicardipine after experimental subarachnoid hemorrhage. *Neurosurgery* 1993 Oct; 33(4): 707–714.
51. Takayasu M, Suzuki Y, Shibuya M, Asano T, Kanamori M, Okada T, Kageyama N, Hidaka H. The effects of HA compound calcium antagonists on delayed cerebral vasospasm in dogs. *J Neurosurg* 1986; 65: 80–85.
52. Satoh S, Suzuki Y, Harada T, Ikegaki I, Asano T, Shibuya M, Sugita K, Hidaka H. Possible prophylactic potential of HA1077, a Ca2+ channel antagonist and vasodilator, on chronic cerebral vasospasm. *Eur J Pharmacol* 1992; 220: 243–248.
53. White RP, Robertson JT. Comparison of piroxicam, meclofenamate, ibuprofen, aspirin, and prostacyclin efficacy in a chronic model of cerebral vasospasm. *Neurosurgery* 1983; 12: 40–46.
54. Chyatte D, Rusch N, Sundt TM Jr. Prevention of chronic experimental vasospasm with ibuprofen and high–dose methylprednisolone. *J Neurosurg* 1983; 59:925–932.
55. Yamakawa K, Sasaki T, Tsubaki S, Nakagomi T, Saito I, Takakura K. Effect of high-dose methylprednisolone on vasospasm after subarachnoid hemorrhage. *Neurol Med Chir Tokyo* 1991; 31: 24–31.
56. Okamoto S, Handa H, Toda N. Role of intrinsic arachidonate metabolites in the vascular action of erythrocyte breakdown products. *J Neurosurg* 1984; 61: 1120–1128.
57. Gaetani P, Marzatico F, Lombardi D, Adinolfi D, Rodriguez-y-Baena R. Effect of high–dose methylprednisolone and U74006F on eicosanoid synthesis after subarachnoid hemorrhage in rats. *Stroke* 1991; 22: 215–220.
58. Kanamaru K, Weir BK, Simpson I, Witbeck T, Grace M. Effect of 21–aminosteroid U–74006F on lipid peroxidation in subarachnoid clot. *J Neurosurg* 1991; 74: 454–59.
59. Matsui T, Asano T. Effects of new 21–aminosteroid tirilazad mesylate (U74006F) on chronic cerebral vasospasm in a "two-hemorrhage" model of beagle dogs. *Neurosurgery* 1994; 34: 1035–1039.
60. Takahashi S, Kassell NF, Toshima M, Dougherty DA, Foley PL, Lee KS. Effect of U88999E on experimental cerebral vasospasm in rabbits. *Neurosurgery* 1993; 32: 281–288.
61. Harada T, Mayberg MR. Inhibition of delayed arterial narrowing by the iron–chelating agent deferoxamine. J *Neurosurg* 1992; 77: 763–767.
62. Kim P, Yaksh TL, Burnett PC, Blum MR, Sundt TM Jr. Cerebrospinal fluid levels of uric acid in dogs and the effect of allopurinol. *Brain Res* a987; 402: 87–92.
63. Kim P, Yaksh TL, Romero JC, Sundt TM Jr. Production of uric acid in cerebrospinal fluid after subarachnoid hemorrhage in dogs. Investigation of the possible role of xanthine–oxidase in chronic vasospasm. *Neurosurgery* 1987; 21: 39–44.
64. Chan RC, Durity FA, Thompson GB, Nugent RA, Kendall M. The role of the prostacyclin–thromboxane system in cerebral vasospasm following induced subarachnoid hemorrhage in the rabbit. *J Neurosurg* 1984 61: 1120–1128.

65. Fukumori T, Tani E, Maeda Y, Sukenaga A. Effect of selective inhibitor of thromboxane A2 syntetase on experimental cerebral vasospasm. *Stroke* 1984; 15:306–311.
66. Yokota M, Tani E, Fukumori T, Maeda Y, Yamaura I. Effects of subarachnoid hemorrhage and a thromboxane A2 synthetase inhibitor on intracranial prostaglandins. *Surg Neurol* 1991; 35: 345–349.
67. Kondo K, Seo R, Omawari N, Imawaka H, Wakitani K, Kira H, Okegawa T, Kawasaki A. Effects of ONO–3708, an antagonist of the thromboxane A2/prostaglandin endoperoxide receptor, on blood vessels. *Eur J Pharmacol* 1989; 168: 193–200.
68 Kobayashi H, Ide H, Handa Y, Aradachi H, Arai Y, Kubota T. Effect of leukotriene antagonist on experimental delayed cerebral vasospasm. *Neurosurgery* 1992; 31: 550–556.
69. Korosue K, Kondoh T, Ishikawa A, Suzuki H, Nagao T, Tamaki N, Matsumoto S. Lipo prostaglandin E1 administration in the acute stage following subarachnoid hemorrhage. *No Shinkei Geka* 1988; 16(5 Suppl): 509–515.
70. Zervas NT, Kuwayama A, Rosoff CB, Salzman EW. Cerebral arterial spasm. Modification by inhibition of platelet function. *Arch Neurol* 1973; 28:400–404.
71. Zervas NT, Hori H, Rosoff CB. Experimental inhibition of serotonin by antibiotic: prevention of cerebral vasospasm. *J Neurosurg* 1974; 41:59–62.
72. Boullin DJ, Du Boulay GH, Rogers AT. Aetiology of cerebral arterial spasm following subarachnoid haemorrhage: evidence against a major involvement of 5–hydroxytryptamine in the production of acute spasm. *Br J Clin Pharmacol* 1978; 6:203–215.
73. Boisvert DPJ, Weir BKA, Overton TR, Reiffenstein RJ, Grace MGA. Cerebrovascular responses to subarachnoid blood and serotonin in the monkey. *J Neurosurg* 1979; 50:441–448.
74. Noseworthy TW, Weir B, Boisvert D, Espinosa F, Overton T, Marshal ML. Effect of reserpine–kanamycin treatment on chronic vasospasm after platelet–enriched subarachnoid hemorrhage in primates. *Neurosurgery* 1984; 14:193–197.
75. Shigeno T, Mima T, Yanagisawa M, Saito A, Fujimori A, Shiba R, Goto K, Kimura S, Yamashita K, Yamasaki Y, et al. Possible role of endothelin in the pathogenesis of cerebral vasospasm. *J Cardiovasc Pharmacol* 1991; 17 (Suppl 7): S480–483.
76. Cosentino F, McMahon EG, Carter JS, Katusic ZS. Effect of endothelinA–receptor antagonist BQ–123 and phosphoramidon on cerebral vasospasm. *J Cardiovasc Pharmacol* 1993; 22 (Suppl 8): S332–33.
77. Matsumura Y, Ikegawa R, Suzuki Y, Takaoka M, Uchida T, Kido H, Shinyama H, Hayashi K, Watanabe M, Morimoto S. Phosphoramidon prevents cerebral vasospasm following subarachnoid hemorrhage in dogs: the relationship to endothelin–1 levels in the cerebrospinal fluid. *Life Sci* 1991; 49: 841–848.
78. Zuccarello M, Lewis AI, Rapoport RM. Endothelin ETA and ETB receptors in subarachnoid hemorrhage–induced cerebral vasospasm. *Eur J Pharmacol* 1994; 259: R1–2.
79. Clozel M, Watanabe H. BQ–123, a peptidic endothelin ETA receptor antagonist, prevents the early cerebral vasospasm following subarachnoid hemorrhage after intracisternal but not intravenous injection. *Life Sci* 1993; 52: 825–834.
80. Nirei H, Hamada K, Shoubo M, Sogabe K, Notsu Y, Ono T. An endothelin ETA

receptor antagonist, FR139317, ameliorates cerebral vasospasm in dogs. Life–Sci. 1993; 52(23): 1869–1874.

81. Itoh S, Sasaki T, Ide K, Ishikawa K, Nishikibe M, Yano M. A novel endothelin ETA receptor antagonist, BQ–485, and its preventive effect on experimental cerebral vasospasm in dogs. *Biochem Biophys Res Commun* 1993; 195: 969–975.
82. Willette RN, Zhang H, Mitchell MP, Sauermelch CF, Ohlstein EH, Sulpizio AC. Nonpeptide endothelin antagonist. Cerebrovascular characterization and effects on delayed cerebral vasospasm. *Stroke* 1994; 25: 2450–2456.
83. Svendgaard NA, Brismar J, Delgado TJ, Rosengren E, Stenevi U. Subarachnoid haemorrhage in the rat: effect on the development of cerebral vasospasm of lesions in the central serotoninergic and dopaminergic systems. *Stroke* 1986; 17: 86–90.
84. Delgado TJ, Arbab MA, Warberg J, Svendgaard NA. The role of vasopressin in acute cerebral vasospasm. Effect on spasm of a vasopressin antagonist or vasopressin antiserum. *J Neurosurg* 1988; 68: 266–273.
85. Delgado-Zygmunt TJ, Arbab MA, Edvinsson L, Jansen I, Svendgaard NA. Prevention of cerebral vasospasm in the rat by depletion or inhibition of substance P in conducting vessels. J *Neurosurg* 1990; 72: 917–925.
86. Toshima M, Kassell NF, Tanaka Y, Dougherty DA. Effect of intracisternal and intravenous calcitonin gene–related peptide on experimental cerebral vasospasm in rabbits. *Acta Neurochir Wien* 1992; 119: 134–138.
87. Shiokawa Y, Svendgaard NA. Cerebrovascular sensory innervation involved in the development of cerebral vasospasm following a subarachnoid hemorrhage. *J Auton Nerv Syst* 1994; 49 Suppl: S167–170.
88. Peterson JW, Nishizawa S, Hackett JD, Bun T, Teramura A, Zervas NT. Cyclosporine A reduces cerebral vasospasm after subarachnoid hemorrhage in dogs. *Stroke* 1990; 21: 133–137.
89. Handa Y, Hayashi M, Takeuchi H, Kobayashi H, Kawano H, Kabuto M. Effect of cyclosporine on the development of cerebral vasospasm in a primate model. Neurosurgery 1991; 28: 380–386.
90. Mori T, Nagata K, Ishida T, Sasaki T, Nirei H, Hamada K, Ohami H, Kirino T. FK–506: a new immunosuppressive agent, failed to reduce cerebral vasospasm after experimental subarachnoid hemorrhage. *J Vet Med Sci* 1993; 55: 581–586.
91. Nishizawa S, Peterson JW, Shimoyama I, Iwasaki K, Uemura K. Therapeutic effect of a new immunosuppressant, FK–506, on vasospasm after subarachnoid hemorrhage. *Neurosurgery* 1993; 32: 986–992.
92. Ito M. Experimental vasospasm. Significance of oxyhemoglobin, fibrin degradation products and breakdown products of white ghost in the pathogenesis of cerebra; vasospasm. Treatment of vasospasm with gabexate mesilate and diphenhydramine. *Neurol Med Chir (Tokyo)* 1980; 20:225–236.
93. Yanamoto H, Kikuchi H, Okamoto S, Nozaki K. Preventive effect of synthetic serine protease inhibitor, FUT–175, on cerebral vasospasm in rabbits. *Neurosurgery* 1992; 30: 351–357.
94. Gavras H, Andrews P, Papadakis N. Reversal of experimental delayed cerebral vasospasm by angiotensin–converting enzyme inhibition. *J Neurosurg* 1981; 55: 884–888.

95. Andrews P, Papadakis N, Gavras H. Reversal of experimental acute cerebral vasospasm by angiotensin converting enzyme inhibition. *Stroke* 1982 13: 480–483.
96. Matsui T, Nagafuji T, Tsutsumi K, Uchida H, Miyauchi T, Asano T. The effect of Nicorandil on chronic cerebral vasospasm. *Acta Neurochir Wien* 1994; 126: 165–169.
97. Peterson EW, Searle R, Mandy FF, Leblanc R. The reversal of experimental vasospasm by dibutyryl–3',5'–adenosine monophosphate. *J Neurosurg* 1973; 39: 730–734.
98. Tekkok IH, Tekkok S, Ozcan OE, Erbengi T, Erbengi A. Preventive effect of intracisternal heparin for proliferative angiopathy after experimental subarachnoid haemorrhage in rats. *Acta Neurochir Wien* 1994; 127: 112–117.
99. Vollmer DG, Hongo K, Kassell NF, Ogawa H, Tsukahara T, Lehman RM. Effect of intracisternal antithrombin III on subarachnoid hemorrhage–induced arterial narrowing. *J Neurosurg* 1989; 70: 599–604.
100. Kapp JP, Clower BR, Azar FM, et al. Heparin reduces proliferative angiopathy following subarachnoid hemorrhage in cats. *J Neurosurg* 1985; 62:570–575.
101. Ram Z, Sadeh M, Shacked I, Sahar A, Hadani M. Magnesium sulfate reverses experimental delayed cerebral vasospasm after subarachnoid hemorrhage in rats. *Stroke* 1991; 22: 922–927.
102. Blaumanis OR, Grady PA. Experimental cerebral vasospasm: resolution by chlorpromazine. *Surg Neurol* 1982; 17:263–268.
103. Nakano M, Tani E, Fukumori T, Yokota M. Effects of chlorpromazine on experimental delayed cerebral vasospasm. *J Neurosurg* 1984; 61:857–863.
104. Findlay JM, Weir BK, Steinke D, Tanabe T, Gordon P, Grace M. Effect of intrathecal thrombolytic therapy on subarachnoid clot and chronic vasospasm in primate model of SAH. *J Neurosurg* 1988; 69:723–35.
105. Findlay JM, Weir BK, Gordon P, Grace M, Baughman R. Safety and efficacy of intrathecal thrombolytic therapy in a primate model of cerebral vasospasm. *Neurosurgery* 1989; 24:491–498.
106. Findlay JM, Weir BK, Kanamaru K, Grace M, Baughman R. The effect of timing of intrathecal fibrinolytic therapy on cerebral vasospasm in a primate model of subarachnoid hemorrhage. *Neurosurgery* 1990; 26:201–206.
107. Hariton GB, Findlay JM, Weir BKA, Kasuya H, Grace MGA, Mielke BW. Comparison of intrathecal administration of urokinase and tissue plasminogen activator on subarachnoid clot and chronic vasospasm in a primate model. *Neurosurgery* 1993; 33:691–697.
108. Seifert V, Eisert WG, Stolke D, Goets C. Efficacy of single intracisternal bolus injection of recombinant tissue plasminogen activator to prevent delayed cerebral vasospasm after experimental subarachnoid hemorrhage. *Neurosurg* 1989; 25:590–598.
109. Brinker T, Seifert V, Stolke D. Effect of intrathecal fibrinolysis on cerebrospinal fluid absorption after experimental subarachnoid hemorrhage. *J Neurosurg* 1991; 74: 789–793.
110. Yamamoto Y, Clower BR, Haining JL, Smith RR. Effect of tissue plasminogen activator on intimal platelet accumulation in cerebral arteries after subarachnoid hemorrhage in cats. *Stroke* 1991; 22: 780–784.

111. Findlay JM, Kassell NF, Weir BK, Haley EC, Kongable G, Germanson T, Truskowski L, Alves WM, Holness RO, Knuckey NW, Yonas H, Steinberg GK, West M, Winn HR, Ferguson G. A randomized trial of intraoperative, intracisternal tissue plasminogen activator for the prevention of vasospasm. *Neurosurgery* 1995; 37:168–176.

4
Epidemiology of Subarachnoid Hemorrhage

Timothy J. Ingall
Mayo Clinic Scottsdale, Scottsdale, Arizona

Jack P. Whisnant
Mayo Clinic, Rochester, Minnesota

I. INTRODUCTION

In the last forty years there have been at least 56 studies of subarachnoid hemorrhage (SAH) that have reported on the various epidemiologic aspects of subarachnoid hemorrhage including incidence rates, case fatality rates, and mortality [1–56]. These are studies of primary SAH that include SAH due to aneurysmal rupture, rupture of arteriovenous malformations, and SAH of unknown cause. Reports have come from many different countries including the United States [1–7], England [8–10], Finland [11–19], New Zealand [20–22], Faroe Islands [23], Australia [24–26] Canada [27], Sweden [28–33], Denmark [34,35], Greenland [36], Iceland [37], Estonia [38], Norway [39], Rhodesia [40], Libya [41], Italy [42–44], Japan [45–51], China [52], France [52], the Netherlands [54], Poland [55], and Saudia Arabia [56] (Table 1). However, because these studies used significantly different methods, comparison of results is difficult.

Many of these studies have significant methodologic problems that limit the interpretation of their data. Of the criteria for an ideal stroke incidence study listed by Malmgren et al. [57], there are three criteria that are frequently not satisfied: first-ever stroke only, representative population, and complete case ascertainment. Many of the studies either included both first and recurrent cases of SAH [4,15,17,27,29,34,50,54,55] or did not specify that only first-ever SAHs were in-

Table 1 Epidemiological Studies of Subarachnoid Hemorrhage

United States of America	Finland	Denmark	Japan
Rochester, MN [1,2]	Helsinki [11]	Frederiksberg [34,35]	Shibata [45]
Framingham, MA [3,7]	Middle Finland [12,18]	Greenland [36]	Hisayama [46]
South Alabama, AB [4]	Espoo-Kauniainen [13,17]	Iceland [37]	Akita [47]
North Manhattan, NY [5]	Kuopio [14]	Estonia	Hiroshima and Nagasaki [48]
Cincinnati, OH [6]	Countrywide cohort study [15]	Tartu [38]	Izumo City [49,51]
England	Three community study [16]	Norway	Okinawa [50]
Carlisle [8]	South and Middle Finland [19]	Oslo [39]	China
Oxfordshire [9]	New Zealand	Rhodesia [40]	Beijing [52]
Surrey [10]	Auckland [20,22]	Libya	France
Sweden	National study [21]	Benghazi [41]	Dijon [53]
Söderhamn [28]	Faroe Islands [23]	Italy	Netherlands
Göteberg [29,32]	Australia	Florence [42]	Tilburg [54]
Enkoping-Habo [30]	Perth [24,25]	The Valle d'Aosta [43]	Poland
Malmo [31]	Melbourne [26]	Reggio Emilia [44]	Poznan District [55]
North Sweden [33]	Canada		Saudi Arabia [56]
	Quebec [27]		

cluded in the analyses [10,22,26,36,37,39,40,47,48]. Other studies did not study the whole population, limiting the study to either a cohort or specific age groups [3,4,7,10,16,26–30,32,33,40–42,45,46,51,52,55,56]. Incomplete case ascertainment, or incomplete information regarding accuracy of case ascertainment, is a methodologic problem present in many of the studies [5,19,21,26,36,39–41,47,49,53,56]. Some studies surveyed all hospitals in the community, but did not use death-certificate surveillance or cases from the coroner or medical examiner as part of their screening procedure for case ascertainment [5,21,26,36,39–41,47,49,53,56]. In Rochester, Minnesota, in the period 1975–1984, 12% of cases of SAH died before receiving medical attention [2]. In Middle Finland from 1980 to 1987, 13% of cases of SAH died before receiving medical attention [18]. Thus, studies that do not monitor death certificates or cases from the coroner or medical examiner will have incomplete case ascertainment because they do not include cases without medical attention prior to death.

Another issue to consider in assessing these studies is whether standard diagnostic criteria have been used. All of the studies used accepted clinical criteria in diagnosing SAH. However, the diagnostic tests available for SAH have varied over the forty years of SAH epidemiologic reports studied here. Cerebrospinal fluid (CSF) analysis has been available throughout the period but computerized tomographic (CT) scanning has only been generally available over the last 15 to 20 years. CT scanning increases the certainty of stroke subtype diagnosis. In particular, it helps to differentiate between SAH and intracerebral hemorrhage with secondary subarachnoid extension. In the 1988 Greater Cincinnati Study, 20 out of 268 cerebral hemorrhage cases had intracerebral hemorrhage (ICH) and SAH concurrently, with the CT scan differentiating the underlying etiology [Broderick—personal communication]. In Middle Finland in the period 1976–1978, no patients diagnosed with SAH had a CT scan, while in the period 1980–1987, 51% of patients with a diagnosis of SAH had CT scans performed. The SAH incidence rate per 100,000 population per year, age- and sex-adjusted to the 1980 Finnish population, was 20.1 and 16.4 respectively for these two periods. Other data from Espoo-Kauniainen and the South and Middle Finland regions covered the time periods from 1972–1973 to 1989–1991 [19]. This study also spans a period from when CT scans were not available through the late 1980s, when CT scans were available. The age-specific annual SAH incidence, adjusted to the 1970 Finnish population, was 22.7 in the period 1972–1973, 13.1 in the period 1978–1980, and 8.4 in the period 1989–1991. The incidence of cerebral hemorrhage increased from 12.9 in the period 1978–1980 to 20.2 in the period 1989–1991. The data from these studies raises the possibility that the introduction of CT scanning in Finland could have led to an artifactual decline in the SAH incidence rate by allowing for a more accurate differentiation between SAH and parenchymal intracerebral hemorrhage with secondary subarachnoid extension. Thus, the utilization of CT scanning is a factor that should be considered when comparing studies from time periods that differ in the availability of CT scanning to diagnose SAH.

There are 17 published reports that met the stroke incidence study criteria of Malmgren et al [57]. The study from Frederiksberg, Denmark [35] satisfied the study criteria, but had only 2 cases of SAH during the observation period from 1989 to 1990, which limited the ability to interpret the data. Data from that study will not be included in further analysis. The other 16 reports were from Rochester, Minnesota [1,2] and Cincinnati, Ohio [6], in the United States; Carlisle [8] and Oxfordshire [9] in England; Helsinki [11], Middle Finland [12,18], Espoo-Kauniainen [13], and Kuopio [14] in Finland; Auckland, New Zealand [20]; the Faroe Islands [23]; Perth, Australia [24,25]; Malmo, Sweden [31]; and the Valle d'Aosta, Italy [43]. Further discussion of incidence rates, case fatality rates, and mortality rates will be limited to these 16 studies.

II. INCIDENCE RATES

All rates quoted are per 100,000 population per year.

Most population-based studies have shown that SAH represents about 5 to 10% of all strokes [2,8,9,13,20,24,25,43] (Table 2). The only exceptions to this are SAH in the Valle d'Aosta in Italy [43] and the Espoo-Kauniainen area of Finland [13], where SAH represents 2.4% and 13% of all strokes respectively.

Comparison of crude incidence rates (Table 3) from the different popula-

Table 2 Subarachnoid Hemorrhage as a Percentage of All Strokes

Study	Percentage (%)
Rochester, Minnesota, USA	
1945–1954[a]	5.2
1955–1964[a]	6.9
1965–1974[a]	8.7
1975–1984 [2]	7.7
1945–1984[a]	7.2
Carlisle, England, 1955–1961 [8]	7.6
Oxfordshire, England, 1981–1986 [9]	5.0
Espoo-Kauniainen, Finland, 1978–1980 [13]	13.0
Auckland, New Zealand, 1981–1983 [20]	6.8
Perth, Australia	
1986 [24]	4.5
1989–1990 [25]	4.0
The Valle d'Aosta, Italy, 1989 [43]	2.4

[a] Unpublished observations.

Table 3 Crude Incidence Rates of Subarachnoid Hemorrhage

Study	Period of observation	Average yearly population	Crude incidence rates (per 100,000 population per year)		
			Men	Women	Total
Rochester, Minnesota[a]	1945–1985	43,935	7.3	12.6	10.2
Cincinnati, Ohio, USA [6]	1988–White	1,086,462	—	—	5.7
	1988–Black	171,718	—	—	10.5
Carlisle, England [8]	1955–1961	71,101	—	—	10.6
Oxfordshire, England [9]	1981–1986	105,476	4.2	11.5	7.8
Helsinki, Finland [11]	1954–1961	439,751	15.0	16.4	15.7
Middle Finland [12]	1976–1978	241,000	19.2	19.6	19.4
Kuopio, Finland [14]	1978–1980	95,420	17	13	15
Auckland, New Zealand [20]	1981–1983	829,454	10.6	17.8	14.3
Faroe Islands [23]	1962–1975	38,524	—	—	7.4
Perth, Australia [24,25]	1986 [24]	134,690	—	—	6.2
	1989–1990 [25]	138,708	7.7	9.6	8.6
Malmo, Sweden [31]	1989	232,448	5.4	6.6	6.0
The Valle d'Aosta, Italy [43]	1989	114,325	5.3	5.2	5.2

[a] Unpublished observations.

tions is difficult because of the potential for significant differences in age and sex distributions among the populations. Standardized incidence rates (SIRs) allow for comparison between studies. For this chapter, where studies provided age-specific incidence rates, an age-adjusted total SIR was calculated. For studies where age- and sex-specific incidence rates were supplied, the following SIRs were calculated: age-adjusted for men and women separately, age-adjusted total, and age- and sex-adjusted total. The United States white population in 1980 was used as the reference population. All SIRs are quoted as per 100,000 population per year.

A. Geographic Differences in Incidence Rates

There were 9 studies [2,6,8,9,11,20,23,25,31] where age-adjusted SIRs could be calculated (Table 4). The lowest age-adjusted total SIR was 4.8 for Malmo, Sweden, and the highest was 15.1 for Helsinki, Finland. The age-adjusted total SIRs for the other studies were 7.9 for Oxfordshire, England; 8.5 for Perth, Australia; 8.7 for the Faroe Islands; 9.5 for Carlisle, England; 11.8 for Rochester, Minnesota; and 12.3 for Auckland, New Zealand. The crude total incidence

Table 4 Standardized Incidence Rates of Subarachnoid Hemorrhage[a]

	Age-adjusted			Age- and sex-adjusted
Population	Men	Women	Total	Total
Rochester, Minnesota (1945–1984)	8.3	14.7	11.8	11.6
Carlisle, England (1955–1961)	—	—	9.5	—
Oxfordshire, England (1981–1986)	4.0	11.9	7.9	8.0
Helsinki, Finland (1954–1961)	14.6	15.4	15.1	15.0
Auckland, New Zealand (1981–1983)	8.1	16.3	12.3	11.6
Faroe Islands (1962–1975)	—	—	8.7	—
Perth, Australia (1989–1990)	7.7	9.2	8.5	8.4
Malmo, Sweden (1989)	—	—	4.8	—
Cincinnati, Ohio, USA (1988)—White	—	—	—	6
—Black	—	—	—	12

[a] All rates standardized to 1980 U.S. white population.

rates vary over a slightly wider range from 5.2 for the Valle d'Aosta [43] to 19.4 for Middle Finland [12] (Table 3). The SAH incidence rate in Finland is higher than other countries, with crude incidence rates varying from 14.0 in Espoo-Kauniainen [13] to 19.4 in Middle Finland [12]. Although the exact reasons for the higher Finnish SAH incidence rates are unclear it may be related to higher incidence rates for men in Finland compared to other countries, or the rates may be artifactually high (see later discussions on sex-specific SAH incidence rates and the temporal decline in SAH incidence rates). Excluding Finland and the Faroe Islands, which represents a study in a distinctly separate population, age-adjusted total SIRs in other populations span a fairly narrow range between 4.8 (Malmo, Sweden) and 12.3 (Auckland, New Zealand). This is not surprising considering that the populations involved in the studies from Rochester, Minnesota; Carlisle and Oxfordshire in England; Malmo, Sweden; and Auckland, New Zealand, are predominantly white European in origin. Although many studies of SAH have been reported from Japan, none of these has been done in a population where the whole population has been studied, so no total population incidence rates are available for comparison.

B. Temporal Trends in Incidence Rates

Few data are available regarding the temporal trends of SAH incidence. The only fully population-based, long-term data come from Rochester, Minnesota, where information is available for the 40-year period 1945–1984 [2]. In contrast to the well-documented decrease in the incidence of other types of stroke during the same period [58], there has been essentially no change in the incidence of SAH in Rochester, Minnesota over these 40 years. The age-adjusted total incidence rates (age-adjusted to 1960 U.S. white population) for SAH in the four 10-year periods, 1945–1954, 1955–1964, 1965–1974, and 1975–1984 were 9.5, 12.0, 12.1, and 10.2, respectively [2]. The population-based study in Söderhamn, Sweden [28], only included patients 16 years old and older so the total incidence rates are not comparable directly to other studies. However, there was little variation between the crude total incidence rates between two different time periods. The crude total SAH incidence rate in 1975–1978 was 13 per 100,000 population per year compared to 11 in the period 1983–1986. Two other age-limited studies from Sweden, Göteberg (15–65 years of age) [32] and Northern Sweden (35–74 years of age) [33], covered time periods from 1971–1987 and 1985–1991 respectively. No significant temporal trends were observed in the incidence of SAH in any age or sex group.

The only studies showing a possible temporal decline in the incidence of SAH come from Finland. In Middle Finland [18], the incidence of SAH, age- and sex-adjusted to the 1980 Finnish population, was 20.1 in the period 1976–1978 compared to 16.4 in the period 1980–1987. Other data from Espoo-Kauniainen and the South and Middle Finland regions covered time periods from 1972–1973 and 1978–1980 (Espoo-Kauniainen) and 1989–1991 (South and Middle Finland) [19]. The age-specific annual SAH incidence, adjusted to the 1970 Finnish population, was 22.7 in the period 1972–1973, 13.1 in the period 1978–1980, and 8.4 in the period 1989–1991. As discussed previously, the introduction of CT scanning in Finland in the 1980s may have allowed for a more accurate differentiation between SAH and parenchymal intracerebral hemorrhage with secondary subarachnoid extension. Therefore, the observed changes in SAH incidence in the Finnish studies may be artifactual. However, CT scanning was not routinely available in Rochester, Minnesota, until the late 1970s, and no significant change was seen in the incidence of SAH between the periods 1945–1974 and 1975–1984 [2]. Thus, the Finnish data may reflect a true temporal decline in the incidence of SAH. Overall, however, the incidence of SAH appears to have been stable over time. This is in contrast to the incidence rates of cerebral infarction and cerebral hemorrhage, which have declined over the last 30 years [58]. It is not clear why there is a difference in the temporal trends of the incidence of different types of stroke. One possible reason could be that there are different risk factors for the different types of stroke. Successful treatment of only some of the risk factors could lead to a differential effect on stroke subtype incidence rates.

C. Age- and Sex-Related Incidence Rates

The incidence of SAH increases with age. In Rochester, Minnesota, the age-specific SAH incidence rates due to all causes in the period 1945–1984 increased with age until age 70 and then decreased slightly (unpublished observation). These rates increased from 1.1 in the less than 30 years age group to 35.1 in the 60 to 69 years age group. The rate then decreased slightly over the next two age groups with rates of 32.0 in the 70 to 79 year age group, and 28.5 in the 80 years and older age group. This may reflect variability due to relatively few persons over the age of 70 years in Rochester, Minnesota. Other population-based studies also show a similar increase with age in the incidence of SAH [6,8,9,11,12,20,23,25,31,51] with the rates either plateauing or decreasing after the age of 59 years [8], 64 years [23], 69 years [11], 74 years [20], or 85 years [9,25]. The studies from Cincinnati, Ohio [6], Middle Finland [12], and Malmo, Sweden [31] showed a continual increase with age over all the age groups. In Japan, the studies from Shibata [45] and Izumo City [51] are the only population-based studies with adequate case ascertainment but are limited to the population 20 years and older. In both studies, the age-specific SAH incidence rates increased with age, but declined in the oldest age groups.

Over the 40-year period 1945–1984, the age-adjusted SIRs for men and women in Rochester Minnesota, show that the incidence of SAH is greater in women than men (14.7 for women and 8.3 for men) (Table 4). This difference between age-adjusted SIRs for women and men is also seen in Auckland, New Zealand (16.3 for women, 8.1 for men) and Oxfordshire, England (11.9 for women and 4.0 for men). In Perth, Australia, however, there is little difference in the age-adjusted SIRs between men and women (9.2 for women, 7.7 for men). The only other study where age-adjusted SIRs for men and women are available is the Helsinki, Finland, study where there is little difference between men and women (15.4 for women, 14.6 for men). Of the other population-based studies, 3 from Finland reported crude incidence rates for men and women [12,13,14] (Table 3). The rates in these studies showed either little difference between the sexes [12] or rates for men slightly lower than women [13,14]. Why the pattern of SAH incidence among the sexes is different in Finland is unclear. As discussed previously, the unexplained higher SAH incidence rates for men in Finland may be a significant factor in the higher total SAH incidence rates observed in that country. In Malmo, Sweden [31], there was little difference in the SAH incidence rates between men and women (7 for women, 5 for men). In Shibata, Japan [45], the SAH incidence rates were markedly greater for men in some age groups. The age- and sex-specific rates were no different for men and women in the 20 to 29 year, 30 to 39 year, 70 to 79 year, and the 80 years and over age groups. In the 40 to 49 year, 50 to 59 year, and 60 to 69 year age groups the rates for men and women were 42 and 5, 51 and 28, and 93 and 28 respectively. Like the Finnish studies, the reasons behind this observation are unknown. The studies from other countries where comparative data are available show a consistently higher incidence of SAH in women compared to men [2,9,20]. Overall, the majority of studies reported significantly higher SAH incidence rates for women. The reasons behind this sex difference are unknown.

D. Racial Differences in Incidence Rates

There are only two studies that have compared the SAH incidence rates of different races from within the same study population. In Cincinnati, Ohio, USA [6], the SAH incidence rates, age- and sex-adjusted to the 1980 U.S. population, were 12 for the black population and 6 for the white population. Marks et al. [22] studied the incidence of SAH in the Auckland, New Zealand, population. The crude incidence rates were 25.7 for the Maori (Polynesian) population, and 14.3 for the European population. However, the interpretation of the data from the New Zealand study was limited because there was no death certificate surveillance, and it was not stated whether recurrent cases were excluded from the study. Nonetheless, the data from these studies suggest that there may be significant racial differences in the incidence of SAH. However, a more systematic study is needed to determine whether racial differences in the incidence of SAH do exist.

III. SURVIVAL FOLLOWING SAH

There is a high early mortality from SAH. In Rochester, Minnesota, in the period 1975–1984, 12% of the cases died before receiving medical attention [2]. In Middle Finland from 1980 to 1987, 13% of cases of SAH died before receiving medical attention [18]. Although not all studies have reported case fatality rates (CFR) at similar times after the onset of SAH, the majority of CFRs within the first 3 months are greater than 40% (Table 5). The exceptions are CFRs of 21% (30 days) for Malmo, Sweden [31], 33% (28 days) for Perth, Australia [25], and 38% (2 months) for the Faroe Islands [23]. Other CFRs reported within the first 3 months after the onset of the SAH [2,6,9,11,12,13,18,20,24] vary from 40% at 21 days in Helsinki, Finland [11], to 58% at 30 days for Rochester, Minnesota, 1945–1974 [2]. Most of the mortality due to SAH occurs within the first 30 days. Mortality at one year differs little from 30-day mortality, ranging from 45% in Espoo-Kauniainen, Finland [13], to 57% in Auckland, New Zealand [20].

Only two studies have addressed specifically the issue of temporal trends in SAH mortality [2,21]. In Rochester, Minnesota, for the period 1945–1984, the age-adjusted average annual mortality rates per 100,000 population (adjusted to 1960 U.S. white population) were 6.3 for 1945–1954, 6.8 for 1955–1964, 6.6 for 1965–1974, and 4.3 for 1975–1984. Over the first 30 years of observation (1945–1974) the average annual mortality rates varied between 6.3 and 6.8 per 100,000 per year. For the last 10 years (1975–1984) the rate decreased to 4.3. The relatively small number of patients in the study makes it difficult to assess the statistical significance of this observation. However, a similar decrease was also noted in the recent mortality rates for U.S. white males

Table 5 Subarachnoid Hemorrhage Case Fatality Rates

Study	Period	7 Days	21 Days	28 Days	30 Days	2 Months	3 Months	6 Months	1 Year	3 Years	5 Years
Rochester, Minnesota, USA [2]	1945–74	—	—	—	58%	—	—	—	—	—	—
	1975–84	—	—	—	43%	—	—	—	—	—	47%
Cincinnati, OH, USA [6]—White	1988	—	—	—	44%	—	—	—	—	—	—
—Black	1988	—	—	—	50%	—	—	—	—	—	—
Oxfordshire, England [9]	1981–86	—	—	—	46%	—	—	—	48%	—	—
Helsinki, Finland [11]	1954–61	—	40%	—	—	—	—	—	—	—	—
Middle Finland [12,18]	1976–78	—	59%	—	—	—	49%	—	—	49%	—
	1980–87	—	62%	—	—	—	—	—	—	52%	—
Espoo-Kauniainen, Finland [13]	1978–80	—	—	—	—	—	45%	—	45%	—	—
Auckland, New Zealand [20]	1981–83	43%	—	—	—	—	—	57%	57%	—	—
Faroe Islands [23]	1962–75	—	—	—	—	38%	—	—	—	—	53%
Perth, Australia [24,25]	1986	—	—	57%	—	—	—	—	—	—	—
	1989–90	—	—	33%	—	—	—	—	—	—	—
Malmo, Sweden [31]	1989	—	—	—	21%	—	—	29%	—	—	—

and females in the same time period [2]. Bonita et al. [21] have reported a similar decline in SAH mortality rates in the New Zealand population for the period 1959 to 1979. They age adjusted the crude annual mortality rates for males and females to the 1951 New Zealand population. Annual mortality rates for males remained relatively stable at about 10.6 until 1972 and then declined to 8.7 in 1979. Annual mortality rates for females showed a gradual increase reaching a peak of 17.5 around 1969 and then declined to 14.2 in 1979.

Several factors could contribute to the observed decrease in SAH mortality rates. A lower mortality would result from a decrease in the incidence of SAH. However, as described previously, available evidence shows that the incidence rate of SAH has changed little over the last 40 years. Even if the incidence rate had decreased slightly it would not explain fully the observed decrease in mortality rate. Lower mortality rates could result from improved case fatality rates. In Rochester, Minnesota, case fatality rates for aneurysmal or presumed aneurysmal SAH decreased from 57% in 1945–1974 to 42% in 1975–1984 [2], although this difference was not statistically significant ($p = 0.10$). Due to small numbers of patients it was unclear whether changes in medical treatment, changes in surgical treatment, both or neither contributed to the change in case fatality rates. Thus, the exact reasons behind the decrease in mortality rates for SAH have yet to be determined.

IV. REFERRAL BIAS IN ASSESSING THE NATURAL HISTORY OF SAH

Studying the natural history of SAH involves collecting data on the frequency, distribution, and prognosis associated with SAH. However, most of the information on the natural history of SAH comes from studies performed at large referral-based medical centers. Each center has its own selection bias for patient referral based on the distance of the referral, the condition of the patient, the particular interests of the physicians in the referral center, and other variables that may affect the outcome reported for such patients. This in turn may affect what is reported as the natural history of the disease [59].

In a unique study, Whisnant et al. [60] compared the characteristics of 49 patients with aneurysmal SAH from the Rochester, Minnesota community with those of 328 referral patients in the same medical care setting (i.e., the Mayo Clinic) to assess the effect of referral bias on survival. The community patients were seen in the period 1975–1984, while the referral patients were seen in the period 1980–1984. A number of significant differences were found between the two groups. Using the Hunt and Hess clinical grading scale, there were relatively more patients in the better clinical grades 1 through 3 in the referral group than in the community group (78.3% versus 59.2, $p = 0.0002$).

Survival for the referral group was significantly better than that of the community group. Survival at 30 days after onset of SAH was 83% in the referral group and 59% in the community group. The survival at 5 years for the referral and community group was 63% and 53%, respectively. The referral patients had better survival than the community patients because the referral patients did not include patients who died before the opportunity for referral and because less severely ill patients were referred preferentially. The fact that referral factors affect the reported natural history of SAH will need to be considered when interpreting the effects of different treatment options on outcome from SAH.

V. SUMMARY

The epidemiology of subarachnoid hemorrhage has been investigated in at least 23 countries. SAH represents between 5 to 10% of all strokes. Comparison of age-adjusted SAH standardized incidence rates from 7 countries showed that SAH incidence rates per 100,000 population per year ranged from 4.8 (Malmo, Sweden) to 15.1 (Helsinki, Finland). However, it is possible that the Finnish rates may be artifactually high since there was evidence that SAH incidence rates had declined after the introduction of CT scanning, which would allow for better differentiation between SAH and parenchymal intracerebral hemorrhage with secondary subarachnoid extension. SAH incidence rates have not changed over time, which is in contrast to the incidence rates of cerebral infarction and cerebral hemorrhage, which have declined over the last 30 years. The incidence of SAH increases with age, except in the oldest age groups where the incidence appears to decline. Subarachnoid hemorrhage is more common in women, except in Finland where, for reasons that are unclear, SAH occurs equally in men and women. Limited information on racial differences in SAH incidence rates suggests that it is more common in American blacks than whites and may be more common in New Zealand Maoris compared to New Zealanders of European origin.

There is a high early mortality from SAH with approximately 12% of patients dying before receiving medical attention. The majority of studies have reported a 30-day case fatality rate of more than 40%. Limited data was available regarding long-term trends in SAH mortality. Studies from New Zealand and Rochester, Minnesota, USA, have shown a decreasing trend in SAH mortality over time. It was not clear whether this was due to better treatment of SAH or a decline in SAH incidence rates.

REFERENCES

1. Phillips LH, Whisnant JP, O'Fallon WM, Sundt TM, Jr. The unchanging pattern of subarachnoid hemorrhage in a community. *Neurology* 1980; 30:1034–1040.

2. Ingall TJ, Whisnant JP, Wiebers DO, O'Fallon WM. Has there been a decline in subarachnoid hemorrhage mortality? *Stroke* 1989; 20:718–724.
3. Sacco RL, Wolf PA, Bharucha NE, Meeks SL, Kannel WB, Charette LJ, McNamara PM, Palmer EP, D'Agostino R. Subarachnoid and intracerebral hemorrhage: Natural history, prognosis, and precursive factors in the Framingham Study. *Neurology* 1984; 34:847–854.
4. Gross CR, Kase CS, Mohr JP, Cunningham SC, Baker WE. Stroke in South Alabama: Incidence and diagnostic features—a population based study. *Stroke* 1984; 15:249–255.
5. Sacco RL, Hauser WA, Mohr JP. Hospitalized stroke in blacks and Hispanics in Northern Manhattan. *Stroke* 1991; 22:1491–1496.
6. Broderick JP, Brott T, Tomsick T, Huster A, Miller R. The risk of subarachnoid and intracerebral hemorrhages in blacks as compared to whites. *New England Journal of Medicine* 1992; 326:733–736.
7. Wolf PA, D'Agostino RB, O'Neal MA, Sytkowski P, Kase CS, Belanger AJ, Jannel WB. Secular trends in stroke incidence and mortality. The Framingham Study. *Stroke* 1992; 23:1551–1555.
8. Brewis M, Poskanzer DC, Rolland C, Miller H. Neurological disease in an English city. *Acta Neurologica Scandinavica* 1966; 42(Suppl 24):1–89.
9. Bamford J, Sandercock P, Dennis M, Burn J, Warlow C. A prospective study of acute cerebrovascular disease in the community: the Oxfordshire Community Stroke Project—1981–1986. 2. Incidence, case fatality rates and overall outcome at one year of cerebral infarction, primary intracerebral and subarachnoid hemorrhage. *Journal of Neurology, Neurosurgery and Psychiatry* 1990; 53:16–22.
10. Crawford MD, Sarner M. Ruptured intracranial aneurysm. Community Study. *Lancet* 1965; 2:1254–1257.
11. Pakarinen S. Incidence, aetiology, and prognosis of primary subarachnoid hemorrhage. A study based on 589 cases diagnosed in a defined urban population during a defined period. *Acta Neurologica Scandinavica* 1967; 43(Suppl 29):1–128.
12. Fogelholm R. Subarachnoid hemorrhage in Middle–Finland: Incidence, early prognosis and indications for neurosurgical treatment. *Stroke* 1981; 12:296–301.
13. Kotila M. Declining incidence and mortality of stroke? *Stroke* 1984; 15:255–259.
14. Sivenius J, Heinonen OP, Pyörälä K, Salonen J, Riekkinen P. The incidence of stroke in the Kuopia area of East Finland. *Stroke* 1985; 16:188–192.
15. Reunanen A, Aho K, Aromaa A, Knekt P. Incidence of stroke in a Finnish prospective population study. *Stroke* 1986; 17:675–681.
16. Sarti C, Tuomilehto J, Salomaa V, Sivenius J, Kaarsalo E, Narva EV, Salmi K, Torppa J. Epidemiology of subarachnoid hemorrhage in Finland from 1983 to 1985. *Stroke* 1991; 22:848–853.
17. Aho K, Fogelholm R. Incidence and early prognosis of stroke in Espoo–Kauniainen area, Finland, in 1972. *Stroke* 1974; 5:658–661.
18. Fogelholm R, Hernesniemi, Vapalahti M. Impact of early surgery on outcome after aneurysmal subarachnoid hemorrhage. A population based study. *Stroke* 1993; 24:1649–1654.
19. Numminen H, Kaste M, Kotila M, Waltimo O. Incidence of stroke in Finland: three population based studies form 1972 to 1989. Epidemiology and Prevention of

Stroke, Satellite Symposium to 3rd European Stroke Conference, Umeå, Sweden, May 29–31, 1994; (unpublished data).
20. Bonita R, Thomson S. Subarachnoid hemorrhage: Epidemiology, diagnosis, management, and outcome. *Stroke* 1985; 16:591–594.
21. Bonita R, Beaglehole R, North JDK. Subarachnoid hemorrhage in New Zealand: An epidemiological study. *Stroke* 1983; 14:342–347.
22. Marks PV, Hope JKA, Cluroe AD, Furneaux CE. Racial differences between Maori and European New Zealanders in aneurysmal subarachnoid hemorrhage. *British Journal of Neurosurgery* 1993; 7:175–182.
23. Joensen P. Subarachnoid hemorrhage in an isolated population. Incidence on the Faroes during the period 1962–1975. *Stroke* 1984; 15:438–440.
24. Ward G, Jamrozik K, Stewart-Wynne E. Incidence and outcome of cerebrovascular disease in Perth, Western Australia. *Stroke* 1988; 19:1501–1506.
25. Anderson CS, Jamrozik KD, Burvill PW, Chakera TMH, Johnson GA, Stewart-Wynne EG. Determining the incidence of different subtypes of stroke: results from the Perth Community Stroke Study, 1989–1990. *Medical Journal of Australia* 1993; 158:85–89.
26. Christie D. Some aspects of the natural history of subarachnoid haemorrhage. *Aust NZJ Med* 1981; 11:24–27.
27. Mayo NE, Goldberg MS, Levy AR, Danys I, Korner-Bitensky N. Changing rates of stroke in the province of Quebec, Canada: 1981–1988. *Stroke* 1991; 22:590–595.
28. Terént A. Increasing incidence of stroke among Swedish women. *Stroke* 1988; 19:598–603.
29. Harmsen P, Berglund G, Larsson O, Tibblin G, Wilhelmsen L. Stroke registration in Göteborg, Sweden, 1970–1975. *Acta Med Scand* 1979; 206:337–344.
30. Åsberg KH, Parrow A. Event, incidence, and fatality rates of cerebrovascular diseases in Enköping-Håbo, Sweden, 1986–1988. *Scandinavian Journal of the Society of Medicine* 1991; 19:134–139.
31. Jerntorp P, Berglund G. Stroke registry in Malmö, Sweden. *Stroke* 1992; 23:357–361.
32. Harmsen P, Tsipogianni A, Wilhelmsen L. Stroke incidence rates were unchanged, while fatality rates declined, during 1971–1987 in Göteborg, Sweden. *Stroke* 1992; 23:1410–1415.
33. Stegmayr B, Asplund K, Wester PO. Trends in the incidence, case–fatality rate, and severity of stroke in Northern Sweden, 1985–1991. *Stroke* 1994; 25:1738–1745.
34. Hansen BS, Marquardsen J. Incidence of stroke in Frederiksberg, Denmark. *Stroke* 1977; 8:663–665.
35. Jørgensen HS, Plesner A-M, Hübbe P, Larsen K. Marked increase of stroke incidence in men between 1972 and 1992 in Frederiksberg, Denmark. *Stroke* 1992; 23:1701–1704.
36. Kristensen MO. Increased incidence of bleeding intracranial aneurysms in Greenlandic eskimos. *Acta Neurochirurgica* 1983; 67:37–43.
37. Gudmundsson G. Primary subarachnoid hemorrhage in Iceland. *Stroke* 1973; 4:764–767.
38. Zupping R, Roose M. Epidemiology of cerebrovascular disease in Tartu, Estonia, USSR, 1970 through 1973. *Stroke* 1976; 7:187–190.

39. Kristiansen K. A clinical and radiologic evaluation of spontaneous subarachnoid hemorrhage. *Acta Radiologica* 1956; 46:326–32.
40. Levy LF, Rachman I, Castle WM. Spontaneous primary subarachnoid haemorrhage in Rhodesian Africans. *Afr J Med Sci* 1973; 4:77–86.
41. Radhakrishnan K, Ashok PP, Sridharan R, Mousa ME. Stroke in the young: Incidence and pattern in Benghazi, Libya. *Acta Neurol Scand* 1986; 73:434–438.
42. Nencini P, Inzitari D, Baruffi MC, Fratiglioni L, Gagliardi R, Benvenuti L, Buccheri AM, Cecchi L, Passigli A, Rosselli A, Amaducci L. Incidence of stroke in young adults in Florence, Italy. *Stroke* 1988; 19:977–981.
43. D'Alessandro G, Di Giovanni M, Roveyaz L, Iannizzi L, Campagnoni MP, Blanc S, Bottacchi E. Incidence and prognosis of stroke in the Valle d'Aosta, Italy. First–year results of a community–based study. *Stroke* 1992; 23:1712–1715.
44. Guidetti D, Baratti M, Zucco R, Greco G, Terenziani S, Vescovini E, Sabadini R, Bondavalli M, Masini L, Salvarani C, Solimé F. Incidence of stroke in young adults in the Reggio Emilia area, Northern Italy. *Neuromepidemiology* 1993;12:82–87.
45. Tanaka H, Ueda Y, Date C, Baba T, Yamashita H, Hayashi M, Shoji H, Owada K, Baba K-I, Shibuya M, Kon T, Detels R. Incidence of stroke in Shibata, Japan: 1976–1978. *Stroke* 1981; 12:460–466.
46. Kiyohara Y, Ueda K, Hasuo Y, Wada J, Kawano H, Kato I, Sinkawa A, Ohmura T, Iwamoto H, Omae T, Fujishima M. Incidence and prognosis of subarachnoid hemorrhage in a Japanese rural community. *Stroke* 1989; 20:1150–1155.
47. Suzuki K, Kutsuzawa T, Takita K, Ito M, Sakamoto T, Hirayama A, Ito T, Ishida T, Ooishi H, Kawakami K, Hirota K, Ogasawara T, Yoshida J, Tamura T, Hattori S, Iwabuchi S, Karouji Y, Waga T, Oosato Y, Yazaki K, Saito T, Oouchi T, Kojima S. Clinicoepidemiologic study of stroke in Akita, Japan. *Stroke* 1987; 18:402–406.
48. Lin CH, Shimizu Y, Kato H, Robertson TL, Furonaka H, Kodama K, Fukunaga Y. Cerebrovascular diseases in a fixed population of Hiroshima and Nagasaki, with special reference to relationship between type and risk factors. *Stroke* 1984; 15:653–660.
49. Inagawa T, Ishikawa S, Aoki H, Takahashi M, Yoshimoto H. Aneurysmal subarachnoid hemorrhage in Izumo City and Shimane Prefecture of Japan. Incidence. *Stroke* 1988; 19:170–175.
50. Kinjo K, Kimura Y, Shinzato Y, Tomori M, Komine Y, Kawazoe N, Takashita S, Fukiyama K, COSMO Group. An epidemiologic analysis of cardiovascular diseases in Okinawa, Japan. *Hypertension Research* 1992; 15:111–119.
51. Inagawa T, Tokuda Y, Ohbayashi N, Takaya M, Moritake K. Study of aneurysmal subarachnoid hemorrhage in Izumo City, Japan. *Stroke* 1995; 26:761–766.
52. Chen D, Román GC, Wu G, Wu Z, Yao C, Zhang M, Hirsch RP. Stroke in China (Sino–MONICA–Beijing Study) 1984–1986. *Neuroepidemiology* 1992; 11:15–23.
53. Giroud M, Milan C, Beuriat P, Gras P, Essayagh E, Arveux P, Dumas R. Incidence and survival rates during a two–year period of intracerebral and subarachnoid haemorrhages, cortical infarcts, lacunes and transient ischaemic attacks. The Stroke Registry of Dijon: 1985–1989. *International Journal of Epidemiology* 1991; 20:892–899.
54. Herman B, Leyten ACM, van Luijk JH, Frenken CWGM, Op de Coul AAW, Schulte BPM. Epidemiology of stroke in Tilburg, The Netherlands. The population-based

stroke incidence register: 2. Incidence, initial clinical picture and medical care, and three week case fatality. *Stroke* 1982; 13:629–634.
55. Wender M, Lenart-Jankowska D, Pruchnik D, Kowal P. Epidemiology of stroke in the Poznan District of Poland. *Stroke* 1990; 21:390–393.
56. Nogueira GJ. Spontaneous subarachnoid haemorrhage and ruptured aneurysms in the Middle East. A myth revisited. *Acta Neurochirgica (Wien)* 1992; 114:20–25.
57. Malmgren R, Warlow C, Bamford J, Sandercock P. Geographical and secular trends in stroke incidence. *Lancet* 1986; 2:1196–1200.
58. Whisnant JP. The decline of stroke. *Stroke* 1984; 15:160–168.
59. Melton LJ III. Selection bias in the referral of patients and the natural history of surgical conditions (editorial). *Mayo Clin Proc* 1985; 60:880–885.
60. Whisnant JP, Sacco SE, O'Fallon WM, Fode NC, Sundt TM Jr. Referral bias in aneurysmal subarachnoid hemorrhage. *J Neurosurg* 1993; 78:726–732.

5
Intracranial Aneurysms

Vittorio M. Morreale and Irene Meissner
Mayo Clinic, Rochester, Minnesota

I. FREQUENCY AND DISTRIBUTION OF ANEURYSMS

The average annual incidence of aneurysms is 12.2/100,000 in females and 7.6/100,000 in males, making the female-to-male ratio about 1.6:1–1.7:1. Intracranial aneurysms are common in the general population. Contrary to popular belief, aneurysms are likely not congenital, but appear to develop with increasing age [200]. Aneurysms usually occur between the 4th and 7th decades of life with a mean age of onset of 58 years. The age specific incidence rises with age and reaches up to 40/100,000 for ages greater than 75 years. Adult aneurysms most frequently involve the anterior circulation [77,137,145,175]. From autopsy studies, the incidence of aneurysms ranges from 0.8% [77] to 5% [70]. In 84% of patients, the aneurysms are multiple [77]. About 400,000 people in the United States have an aneurysm of considerable size and each year there are about 25,000 new cases of ruptured intracranial aneurysms [70]. The epidemiologic data regarding aneurysms that occur in children is different. In children under 18 years of age, aneurysms occur more frequently in males than in females, with a prevelence of 3:1. The posterior circulation is most frequently involved [58,111]. Children under the age of 15 account for about 1% of aneurysm cases and children under 20 account for about 3% of cases [138]. With regard to ruptured aneurysms, the ratio of whites to blacks is 1.6:1 [129].

II. INCIDENCE OF BLEEDING

The overall incidence of bleeding aneurysms is 10/100,000 to 16/100,000 [137,198]. In one study [82], 142 patients with a total of 181 aneurysms were followed for at least 10 years. The research found that the average annual rupture rate was 1.4%. Fifty percent of these ruptures were fatal. The cumulative rupture rate was 10% at 10 years, 26% at 20 years, and 32% at 30 years. They also found that rupture was more likely in aneurysms greater than 10 mm in diameter. In patients with multiple aneurysms, the risk of rupture was inversely proportional to age. Other studies have shown the annual risk of rupture to be 2 to 3% [205].

Wiebers, et al. have reported 2 long-term natural history studies [202,203] for patients with unruptured intracranial aneurysms involving a total of 130 patients with 161 unruptured intracranial aneurysms. Over a mean followup interval of 8.3 years, 15 of 130 patients had intracranial hemorrhage. Of the 102 aneurysms less than 1 cm in diameter, none ruptured during the followup period, whereas of the 51 aneurysms 1 cm or greater in diameter, 15 eventually ruptured. Five of the 15 ruptures ocurred within 3 months of the diagnosis of intracranial aneurysms and 14 of the 15 ruptures were fatal. A multivariate discriminate analysis assessed the relationship of several independent variables to aneurysmal rupture. The only single variable of unquestionable significance for predicting aneurysmal rupture was aneurysmal size. However, with only 36 aneurysms in the 6 to 9 mm category and only 10 in th 8 to 9 mm category, considerable doubt remained about using 10 mm as the critical size below which the risk of rupture would be negligable. Furthermore, many studies did not uniformly correct for angiographic magnification and therefore cannot be accurately interpreted with regard to critical size of rupture.

III. THE IMPACT OF SUBARACHNOID HEMORRHAGE ON PUBLIC HEALTH

Thirty to fifty percent of patients who have had a major rupture of an intracranial aneurysm die or are severely impaired [21,70,196]. In a study of patients with angiographically negative subarachnoid hemorrhage (SAH) a 5% mortality and a 7% rebleed rate was demonstrated. Forty percent described persistent headache and fatigue, 29% had dementia, 5% had severe and persistent objective neurologic symptoms, and 84% returned to normal functioning capacity [45]. Subarachnoid hemorrhage accounts for 10% of all strokes [69] and is responsible for 8% of sudden death due to stroke [144]. The estimated lifetime cost for annual cases of patients hospitalized with unruptured aneuysms is $522,500,000 compared with $1,755,600,000 for patients with aneurysmal SAH [200].

IV. ETIOLOGY AND PUTATIVE RISK FACTORS

The etiology of intracranial aneurysms is unclear, with many theories available based on speculation, observation, and experimentation. The congenital theory and the acquired/degenerative theory are most popular. The congenital theory states that there is an underlying pathology involving blood vessel walls that predisposes them to pressure effects of hypertension and jet streaming due to blood flow. This theory is supported by the clinical evidence that certain disease states are more prone to aneurysm formation such as seen in collagen deficiency states such as patients with type III collagen deficiency [134,148], and defective collagen formation conditions including coarctation of the aorta, polycystic kidney disease, and Marfan's syndrome. Also, aneurysms occur in children even though associated diseases such as Marfan's may not present until adulthood [111]. Aneurysms are also seen in patients with anomalies of the circle of Willis such as reduplication of the anterior communicating artery and asymmetries of the posterior communicating artery and anterior cerebral artery stem [32]. Patients with arteriovenous malformations commonly have associated aneurysms and their cerebral blood vessels have been found to have defects that predispose to aneurysm formation [32]. There is also evidence for a genetic linkage [133]. The degenerative theory is supported by the evidence of aneurysms being associated with conditions that are not directly involved with connective tissue disorders such as hypertension and athersclerosis [6,32]. Also, as mentioned earlier, aneurysms most commonly present at an older age (40–70 years) consistent with a degenerative process [175]. Other associated exogenous factors that may predispose to aneurysm formation and rupture include cigarette smoking [22], oral contraceptive use [143], alcohol [74], and age [114].

There are a number of diseases in which the incidence of SAH is higher than the average population. Hypertension is the most commonly associated medical disorder, but it is probably a contributing factor for aneurysm formation rather than a primary cause since there are more males afflicted with hypertension than there are females [145]. Aneurysms are commonly seen in association with arteriovenous anomalies. High blood flow in association with a presumed blood vessel abnormality may contribute to aneurysm formation. There is an association between autosomal dominant polycystic kidney disease (ADPKD) and berry aneurysms of the circle of Willis [30,201]. One study demonstrated that 64% of patients with ADPKD had rupture of an intracerebral aneurysm before the patients were 50 [167]. Intracranial aneurysms are also seen in diseases that produce defects in the walls of blood vessels such as Ehlers–Danlos syndrome, Marfan's syndrome [174], and pseudoxanthoma elasticum [70]. There are a variety of conditions associated with intracranial aneurysms including coarctation or hypoplasia of the aorta [70,168], neurosarcoidosis [19], Churg–Strauss syndrome with necrotizing vasculitis of the choroid plexus [29], orgasmic cephalgia [106], and fibromuscular dysplasia [70]. Subarachnoid hemorrhage can occur in up to 30% of patients with systemic lupus erythematosus. These patients may be predisposed to aneurysm formation as a result of focal trasmural angiitis [44,186]. A rare disorder, Familial Idiopathic Nonarteriosclerotic Cerebral Calcification (FINCC), consists of intracranial aneurysms and symmetrical cerebral calcifications and extraneural involvement including cirrhosis and pulmonary emphysema [84]. Multiple intracranial aneurysms have also been seen in association with cardiac myxomas [34]. In addition, SAH may occur as a presenting complication of many brain tumors such as malignant gliomas, vascular tumors, and pituitary adenomas with malignant degeneration [59,139,157]. The tumor location is not predictive of the likelihood of SAH [59]. Common symptoms include headache, nuchal rigidity, dysesthesias, neck pain, fever and diplopia, and common signs are coma, fixed pupils, hyperreflexia, Babinski's sign, restlessness, emesis, respiratory difficulty, seizures, hemiplegia, and nuchal rigidity [59].

V. PATHOPHYSIOLOGY

Microscopic examination of aneurysms reveals the primary defect to occur in the medial wall and the internal elastic lamina of the blood vessel [131,175]. Pressure, caused by either jet force at a bifurcation or hypertension, results in ballooning out at the area of relative weakness. The media is thinned out and the muscular component is replaced with fibrotic tissue and calcification [131]. The wall of the aneurysm is composed of intima with or without an intact endothelium, the thinned out media, and the adventitia. In degenerative aneurysms, atherosclerosis may be the cause. Atherosclerosis commonly affects the parent blood vessel of the aneurysm. The atherosclerotic disease process weakens the vessel by damage to the intima and medial layers resulting in dissection of the vessel wall [32].

VI. CLINICAL FEATURES

A. Location

Aneurysms are most commonly seen at bifurcations. The description of the distribution of aneurysms within the cerebral vasculature varies by author (Table 1). According to Sundt, anterior cerebral artery (ACA) and internal carotid

Table 1 Location of Intracranial Aneurysms

	Fox (%) [55]	Makenzie (%) [108]	Nehls (%) [124]
ICA	37	31.5	14.5
ACA-AComm	30.7	33.5	14.5
ICA-PComm	13.4		22
MCA	13.4	29	21.5
BA	8.9	6	3.5

artery (ICA) aneurysms occur in equal frequency and account for 60–70% of aneurysms; middle cerebral artery (MCA) aneurysms account for 15–30%; and 15–20% are posterior [177]. Twenty percent of aneurysms are multiple. Fifteen to twenty percent of aneurysms may be localized according to the presenting signs and symptoms, to be described below [105].

B. Signs and Symptoms

Patients with SAH may present with a wide variety of signs and symptoms that may confound the diagnosis. Because of the likelihood of serious neurologic and life-threatening sequelae, it is imperative that the common and rare manifestations of SAH are not overlooked. In fact, since headache is the most common presenting symptom, it is not surprising that SAH is often mistaken for migraine headache in the emergency room [80,162,135]. Another frequent misdiagnosis is transient ischemic attack (TIA) [80,181]. Some of the most common emergency room presentations of SAH are headache (74%), nausea or vomiting (77%), loss of consciousness (53%), altered consciousness (64%), and nuchal rigidity (35%) [54]. Some have reported headache to be a presenting feature in as many as 90% of patients diagnosed with SAH [135]. Cranial nerve palsies are very commonly associated with intracerebral aneurysms. The most commonly affected cranial nerve (CN) is CN III but CN IV, V, VI as well as the lower cranial nerves may also be involved [13,91,97,152,173,105]. Weakness and paraplegia ipsilateral to a ruptured aneurysm are usually signs of a large hemorrhage with mass effect or ischemia [48,88]. Rarely, the weakness may be ipsilateral, secondary to hematoma or ischemia affecting the secondary motor area of Reil [96]. Other symptoms include periorbital pain, transient blindness secondary to ischemia of the retina and optic nerve [36,160,182], tinnitus [126], paresthesias of the extremities [176], peduncular hallucinosis [63], transient global amnesia [164], deafness [7], and photophobia [196]. Seizures [65,199], vitreous hemorrhages (Terson's syndrome) [47], retinal hemorrhages [46], abnormal tongue protrusion and abnormal movement affecting the eyes [75], dizziness [105], and sudden death [92] may also be seen.

C. The Warning or Sentinel Bleed

The warning headache is the headache that occurs up to weeks before the major aneurysmal rupture. It corresponds to what is called the "sentinel bleed." It is unique in character and is described by many patients as the "worst headache of my life." It is often referred to as a "thunderclap" headache. Indeed, the nature and frequency of association of the headache with SAH makes it almost pathognomonic of SAH and it may be the symptom bringing patients to the emergency room. It is usually acute in onset, severe, and occasionally radiates to the neck. When reported, the most common signs and symptoms of the sentinel bleed are headache, nausea, vomitting, dizziness, disturbance of consciousness, and transient motor deficits [16,169]; that is, nonspecific signs and symptoms that may be confused for other illnesses.

Table 2 lists the incidence of warning signs and symptoms corresponding to the sentinel bleed, which is variable depending on the reporting group, ranging from 20% to 60%.

The etiology of the premontory or sentinel headache has been elucidated by postmortem pathological studies [11] that suggest that the warning hemorrhage comes from a small tear in the aneurysm wall. The tear becomes plugged by intraluminal, well-organized thrombus. The aneurysm is surrounded by layers of fresh thrombus displaying lines of Zahn [11]. It is postulated that localized pain is caused by SA blood stimulating the vessels of the circle of Willis, which are innervated by cranial nerves V, IX, and X and spinal nerves C1–C3 [135]. Generalized headache is probably due to meningeal inflammation and when hydrocephalus develops, increased intracranial pressure [55,135]. In general, the site of the headache is not absolutely specific for the location of the bleeding aneurysm [135]. It has been reported that the location or laterality of the headache may help pinpoint the location of the bleeding aneurysm up to 85% of the time [16]. For example, the headache associated with posterior inferior cerebellar artery (PICA) aneurysm rupture is usually occipital and is accompanied by neck pain, ICA-PComm aneurysms usually produce ipsilateral and retroorbital pain, and AComm and MCA aneurysms often produce bifrontal pain [135,208]. The symptoms of intraparenchymal hemorrhages are usually due to mass effect and in contrast to SAH, intraparenchymal hemorrhages in and of themselves do not usually produce pain unless they are associated with significant mass effect or rupture into the subarachnoid space.

Table 2 Incidence of Warning Signs and Symptoms

Author	Incidence of promontory signs/symptoms (%)
Bassi et al. [16]	20.3
Waga [192]	58.8
Leblanc [102]	39
Fisher [49]	20
Duffy [40]	28
Lyrer [107]	40
Shapiro [169]	40
Calvert [26]	37.5
Average	35

The average time interval between the sentinel bleed and rupture is 14 days [83]. However, this interval can vary depending on the location of the aneurysm. For anterior cerebral and anterior communicating artery aneurysms the average interval is 16.9 days, for middle cerebral artery aneurysms it is 6 days, and for intradural internal carotid artery aneurysms it is 7.3 days [192].

D. Diagnosis/Diagnostic Tests

Twenty-three percent of patients admitted to the hospital have a delay in diagnosis of subarachnoid hemorrhage of 4–7 days. Common misdiagnoses include systemic illnesses, migraine, and hypertensive encephalopathy. In 2% of these patients, rebleeding occurs before the correct diagnosis is made [1]. Traditionally, lumbar puncture (LP) has been considered a reliable and relatively safe diagnostic test [140]. One looks for xanthrochromia, a yellowish discoloration in the cerebrospinal fluid (CSF) caused by pigments released by lysed red blood cells (RBC) [189]. Xanthrochromia can develop within a few hours to twelve hours after SAH [189]. In some cases, the diagnosis of SAH is confounded by a "traumatic tap" in which blood from the epidural plexus of veins is torn with the spinal needle while procuring a CSF specimen. In order to distinguish fresh blood from SA blood, the specimen is centrifuged and the supernatant is examined for xanthrochromia by visual inspection or, preferably, by spectrophotometry [189]. In certain circumstances an LP may not be desirable and even hazardous such as in a patient with an intracranial hematoma and mass effect where the removal of CSF may result in brain herniation [189]. One study demonstrated that 7 out of 55 SAH patients deteriorated after LP, presumably due to intracranial hematoma [41]. The amount of blood found on LP does not correlate with outcome. In contrast, there is a good correlation between the amount of blood on presenting computerized tomography (CT) and patient outcome. In fact, CT may be better at predicting outcome than clinical grading [8] and CT has almost replaced LP as the diagnostic test of choice. Not only does CT show subarachnoid blood, it also shows the amount and location of blood and other complicating conditions such as hematoma, hydrocephalus, mass effect, intraventricular hemorrhage, and edema [147,209,189]. The CT technique is also superior to LP for diagnosing rebleed [189]. Furthermore, CT has been shown to diagnose aneurysm as a cause for SAH 76% of the time [209]. The amount and location of blood on the CT scan correlates well with the severity of symptoms and with prognosing the location of vasospasm [147]. In some studies, CSF lactate has been shown to correlate well with the patient's clinical status [171]. Whereas magnetic resonance imaging (MRI) has not been of value in diagnosing acute subarachnoid blood, it has been shown to be at least as effective as CT in localizing and identifying the cause of SAH. In addition, MRI often shows the actual aneurysm and has even demonstrated a double lumen in dissecting aneurysms [78]. Current postoperative imaging has higher resolution with MRI than CT because clips cause more interference artifacts on CT than on MRI [79]. The more recent use of nonparamagnetic clips allows for the increasing use of MRI scanning for follow-up purposes. Angiography is still considered the gold standard test for identifying intracerebral aneurysms and is able to demonstrate an aneurysm in 60–80% of cases [194]. The combined diagnostic accuracy of all tests is estimated at 85% [54].

E. Complications of SAH

The complications of subarachnoid hemorrhage may be divided into immediate and delayed effects. Immediate complications occur secondary to the direct effect of the hemorrhage. Mortality from these complications is usually within the first 48 hours and is caused by an acute rise in intracranial pressure (ICP) secondary to uncontrolled arterial bleeding, intracranial hematoma formation, and the subsequent impedance of cerebral circulation due to decreased cerebral perfusion pressure (CPP). This is shown by the formula, CPP = MAP − ICP, where MAP is the mean arterial pressure. Delayed effects usually start after about 72 hours and are usually the result of rebleeding, ischemia and infarction due to vasospasm, and hydrocephalus [178]. Sarachnoid hemorrhage also poses a threat to a variety of organ systems, as discussed below.

1. Rebleeding

Rebleeding is not an uncommon complication [196]. It may occur in 15% to 22% of patients after the initial bleed [21,72]. During the first 2 weeks, the risk of rebleeding is about 2.1%/day [158], and the cumulative two-week rebleed rate is 19% [89]. The risk of rebleeding is about 30–40% within the first 6 months after the initial hemorrhage [70]. The risk of rebleed is maximal at about day 7–10 [105]. Patients with a lower clinical (lesser deficits) grade on admission have a lower risk of bleeding than those with a higher grade (greater deficits) [158]. Of patients who survive the initial major hemorrhage, 25–35% will die from a subsequent hemorrhage if left untreated [70]. A prospective study [72] showed a high mortality rate among patients who rebled, with an 18% survival at 3 months following initial SAH. This study also showed that even though the risk of rebleeding cannot be inferred from the initial clinical presentation, the most common symptom associated with rebleed consisted of loss of consciousness (LOC) in 90% and headache in 33%.

2. Cerebral Ischemia

The mechanism of cerebal ischemia in SAH may be on the basis of mass effect from a hematoma, mass effect from the aneurysm itself, vasospasm, or from intraluminal thrombus formation at the base of an aneurysm with subsequent embolization. The CT technique can document infarcts and atrophy long after the SAH has resolved [71]. There is no clear correlation between the initial symptoms of ischemia and the location of the aneurysm [98]. The average length of time from aneurysmal rupture to the onset of ischemic symptoms is 8 days. Cerebral ischemia is characterized by focal neurologic signs, disturbances of consciousness, cognitive changes, hemiparesis, and mutism in the context of documented absence of hydrocephalus on CT [71,98]. Patients who exibit disturbances of consciousness early following SAH (within 1 week) tend to have a worse prognosis [98].

3. Hydrocephalus

The presentation of hydrocephalus in SAH consists of those signs and symptoms that are usually caused by increased intracranial pressure such as mental status changes, changes in level of consciousness, dizziness, headache, and visual disturbances, to name a few. Communicating hydrocephalus and noncommunicating hydrocephalus is seen very commonly in SAH [151,35,180]. According to different authors, the incidence of hydrocephalus with SAH varies from 1% to 63% [55,113]. The incidence of hydrocephalus has been shown to correlate with the clinical grade of presentation: low grades, 3–5% and high grades, 21–42% [113]. There is a relative increased likelihood of hydrocephalus in patients with anterior communicating artery aneurysms [170]. Many patients will require ventricular shunting, usually with good results [149]. The onset of hydrocephalus after the initial SAH occurs as acute within 3 days, subacute within 4–9 days, or chronic after 10 days [55]. There are many proposed etiologies for the development of hydrocephalus. These include ventricular casting by blood [130], abnormal uptake of CSF (shown to occur in up to 70% of patients) [197], loculation of blood in cisterns, RBCs in arachnoidal tissue such as Liliequist's membrane, blood causing sluggish flow over cortical surfaces, and RBCs blocking the resorption of CSF by arachnoid granulations [55].

4. Elevated ICP

Elevated intracranial pressure may be seen in SAH. This may be caused by cerebral edema, hematoma, hydrocephalus, and vasodilation. Increased ICP may cause ischemia secondary to vasospasm [55] or decreased cerebral perfusion secondary to a decreased cerebral perfusion pressure.

5. Seizures

Seizures have been noted in up to 26% of patients with subarachnoid hemorrhage [65,86]. In fact, intracerebral aneurysm is often the undiagnosed etiology of unexplained epilepsy [86,167]. Seizures are most commonly associated with either ruptured or unruptured aneurysms of the middle cerebral artery [53,65]. Intracerebral hematoma as a result of MCA aneurysm predisposes to seizures [65]. Complex partial seizures are seen with giant aneurysms of the MCA with or without SAH, presumably due to mass effect or ischemia of the MCA territory [199].

6. Motor Deficits

Weakness contralateral to an aneurysmal SAH is often seen [48]. It is presumably caused by vasospasm, mass effect from hematoma, or may be seen after partial seizures. Generalized weakness may also be caused by hydrocephalus and increased intracranial pressure. Ipsilateral motor weakness may be caused by compression from a hematoma on the secondary motor area of Reil [96].

7. Cranial Nerves

The oculomotor nerve is the most commonly affected cranial nerve in SAH. It is affected in 30–87% of ICA-PComm aneurysms [141,105], in unruptured aneurysms of the basilar artery, and in uncal herniation secondary to hematoma and edema. Partial CN III palsies are seen in 50% of unruptured ICA and 50% of unruptured distal basilar aneurysms [14]. Mydriasis and paralysis of ocular motility are frequent presenting signs of intracranial aneurysms, with diplopia as a frequent presenting symptom [13,91,97,141,152]. The abducens nerve is the second most commonly affected cranial nerve and it also presents with diplopia [101,122]. The caudal cranial nerves can also be affected. They usually present with dysphagia and throat pain [85]. To a lesser degree, cranial nerves IV, V1 and V2 are also affected.

8. Transient Ischemic Attacks (TIAs)

TIAs have been seen as a presenting sign of SAH. Associated mechanisms include secondary ischemic vasoconstriction from SAH related vasospasm and ischemia by mass effect from the aneurysm itself The intra-aneurysmal thrombus may also provide a source of embolus in unruptured aneurysms [52], explaining the appearance of small infarcts in the distal territory of the parent vessel of an aneurysm.

9. Ophthalmologic Signs and Symptoms

Visual disturbances range from unilateral field loss [36] to transient blindness secondary to ischemia of the retina and optic nerve [182]. Fundoscopic examination may reveal retinal hemorrhages [46] and vitreous hemorrhages (Terson's syndrome) [47]. One form of vision deterioration is caused by optochiasmal arachnoiditis, which improves with steroid therapy [110,153]. Retroorbital pain is frequently seen as a lateralizing feature of the headache of SAH and occasionally SAH presents with eye pain. A proposed mechanism is the transmission of pain along sensory nerves on CN III [100].

10. Cardiovascular Complications

The cardiovascular effects of SAH are common and multiple. Changes in electrocardiogram (ECG) are the most frequent cardiovascular effects of SAH. In some instances, chest pain may even be the presenting symptom of SAH [15]. In fact, in one study arrhythmias were seen 100% of the time [55]. A large variety of rhythm changes may be seen in patients with SAH [112], most of which are transient. Prolonged Q-T interval, T-wave inversion, and prominent U-waves are strongly associated with SAH [55]. Other ECG abnormalities include nonspecific ST-T changes, sinus tachycardia, ventricular premature complexes, and sick sinus symdrome [93,207]. Some of the ECG changes may also occur during vasospasm [55]. The etiology of the rhythm disturbances may be a large catecholamine release concomitant with the SAH, catecholamine discharge secondary to increased ICP, electrolyte disturbances, pH abnormality secondary to respiratory disturbances, hemodynamic factors, or underlying coronary artery disease [55,207]. It has been postulated that coronary artery vasospasm may accompany SAH [185]. Changes in ECG were studied at the time of surgery and it was found that manipulating the circle of Willis precipitated arrhythmias [62]. One study showed that 41% of patients with SAH had elevated creatine phosphokinase MB isoenzyme (CB-MB), of these 71% had ECG changes consistent with cardiac injury [90]. In another study, 59.6% of patients showed laboratory evidence of ischemic changes [109]. In some instances, there are ECG changes and symptoms suggestive of myocardial infarction (MI) without evidence for myocardial damage [123]. Subarachnoid hemorrage can present as cardiopulmonary arrest [92]. Seventeen percent of patients were found to have a loss of consciousness associated with a cardiorespiratory disorder brought on by SAH [73]. In a prospective study of patients less than 70 years old with spontaneous SAH and without prior history of cardiac disease, 91% had cardiac arrhythmias and 41% had serious cardiac arrhythmias consisting of torsades de pointe, V-flutter, and V-fib. Thus, continuous ECG monitoring is recommended [4]. Hypertension is also seen in SAH [181]. This may be different from the hypertension caused by increased ICP and may be related to an alteration in catecholamine metabolism as described above.

11. Pulmonary Complications

Pulmonary complications occur as pulmonary edema or respiratory insufficiency and are often seen in patients presenting moribund or deceased to the hospital [92]. They are often associated with ECG changes [123] and cerebral edema and may be caused by a large sympathetic discharge secondary to increased ICP [55]. Aneurysm location is not a predisposing factor [55]. In one study of 254 patients with SAH, 15% required assisted ventillation [73].

12. Mental Status

The spectrum of disturbances in the level of consciousness ranges from agitation or transient LOC to coma. There is a direct correlation between the amount of SA blood and the level of consciousness on presentation. The severity of disturbance of consciousness depends on many factors including the degree of vasospasm, hydrocephalus, fluid and electrolyte abnormalities, and the location of the aneurysm if present, causing ischemic effects [55].

The data suggest that the clinical features at presentation are not predictive of cognitive outcome [191]. Overall, the degree of impairment with respect to standardized psychometric testing that a patient has after a good surgical outcome correlated with the patient's age [104]. No significant correlation was seen between the source of bleeding, sex, age, interval between SAH and admission, level of consciousness, cognitive function, Hunt and Hess grading, and Glascow coma score on long-term social prognosis. There appeared to be a positive correlation between the neurological, cognitive, and activities of daily living (ADL) deficit that persists and the decline of social and familial function. Less than 50% of patients who were employed premorbidly were employed 12 months post SAH [127].

Memory disorders are commonly seen [120]. Thirty-one percent of patients' families note memory deficits but only 6% of patients are aware of these. Objective testing showed that verbal memory deficits gradually improved to normal but nonverbal memory deficits were significant in 47% of patients tested at 12 months. Twenty-seven to seventy-six percent of patients had moderately impaired visuospatial deficits at 12 months [128]. The clinical grade at discharge was shown to be the best predictor of permanent cognitive impairment. The presumed mechanism for cognitive deficits is widespread, diffuse cortical damage secondary to toxic effects of subarachnoid blood or transient ischemia secondary to increased intracranial pressure or brief intracranial circulatory arrest after SAH. Transient global amnesia has been seen with SAH and is presumed to be caused by diffuse cerebral arterial spasm [164]. Depression is also observed following SAH. In one study, 70% of patients were found to have major depression following SAH, 10% committed suicide, and only 10% fully recovered [136].

13. Electrolytes

Electrolyte disturbances of the serum and CSF commonly accompany SAH. Electrolyte abnormalities include hyponatremia in 16% [119] and hypokalemia and hypocalcemia in serum and CSF [191]. The syndrome of inappropriate antidiuretic hormone secretion (SIADH) may be the cause of hyponatremia. The hyponatremia that develops often correlates to the patient's clinical condition, which may also reflect other intracranial pathology [206]. It has been shown that elevated levels of atrial natriuretic hormone after SAH are followed by salt wasting and volume depletion [204].

14. Endocrine Abnormalities

Endocrine abnormalities have been seen particularly in association with aneurysms of the anterior cerebral artery and its branches. Presumably these are related to ischemia of the hypothalamus. A small percentage of patients have presented with pituitary apoplexy and SAH, which is usually due to bleeding from a pituitary adenoma having undergone malignant transformation [193]. In about 9.3% of patients after SAH, SIADH is seen, and 10% of patients with AComm aneurysms develop SIADH [37]. This phenomenon usually develops approximately 7 days after SAH.

15. Aseptic Meningitis

The presentation of SAH can mimic an inflammatory asceptic meningitis. The onset is usually within 4–24 hours of the hemorrhage. It consists of the usual signs and symptoms of meningitis: fever, positive Kernig's sign, irritability, confusion, lethargy, delerium, photophobia, hyperacusis, and hyperventillation secondary to acidic pH [55].

16. Subdural Hematoma

Subdural hematomas are not uncommon. They may be caused by tearing of the arachnoid membrane with bleeding directly into the subdural space or the aneurysm may have eroded through the arachnoid prior to rupture [55]. In one study, it was found that subdural hematomas were uniformly fatal if left untreated for greater than 4 hours [155].

17. Gastrointestinal Complications

As in severe brain injury patients, SAH can be complicated by gastrointestinal hemorrhage, which is seen in up to 12% of patients with SAH. It is commonly associated with aneurysms of the anterior cerebral artery or anterior communicating artery [55]. Nausea and vomiting are seen in up to 55% of patients, especially in those with hydrocephalus and increased ICP [55].

18. Deafness

Bilateral deafness has been reported as a complication of basilar artery rupture [7]. Mass effect from an aneurysm in the CPA can affect CN VII as well.

19. Myelopathy

Spinal arachnoiditis following intracranial SAH may present as thoracic myelopathy [9].

F. Clinical Manifestations of Aneurysms by Location

Aneurysms often cause site-specific signs and symptoms. The following is a breakdown of signs and symptoms associated with anuerysms according to their location. These phenomena include symptoms and signs of rupture, as well as those in unruptured aneurysms on the basis of cranial nerve palsies, mass effect and compression, and ischemia in the territory of—or distal to—the parent vessel.

1. Internal Carotid Artery (ICA)

Petrous pyramid ICA aneurysms may affect cranial nerves 7 and 8 causing facial weakness, tinnitus, vertigo, dizziness, and hearing loss. With medial enlargement of the aneurysm, the trigeminal nerve may become affected and the patient can develop a cavernous sinus syndrome. Ruptured aneurysms may bleed out through the eustachian tube causing epistaxis [55]. Paraclinoid ICA aneurysms usually present with an oculomotor nerve palsy and nonfocal hemispheric signs. There may be a localizing headache [55]. In addition to nonlocalizing signs and symptoms of SAH, there may be an ipsilateral localizing headache and contralateral focal cerebral signs with carotid artery-ophthalmic artery aneurysms. Visual disturbances may be caused, in particular by large aneurysms secondary to compression of the optic apparatus [55]. Twenty-nine percent of patients with ruptured aneurysms experience preoperative visual abnormalities, usually with the onset of bleeding. In 35% of patients with unruptured aneurysms the visual loss is slowly progressive [99]. Nasal field loss may be present [36]. Anterior choroidal artery aneurysms usually present with general signs of SAH plus CN III palsy with or without contralateral hemiplegia.

One may see Abbie's syndrome consisting of contralateral motor and sensory loss and a homonymous hemianopsia. Pain may be localized behind the ipsilateral eye or forehead [55]. Carotid bifurcation aneurysms may be associated with hemiplegia, related hemispheric localizing signs, and a localizing ipsilateral frontal headache [55].

2. Anterior-Cerebral–Anterior-Communicating Arteries (ACA–AComm)

Anterior communicating artery aneurysms and SAH secondary to these aneurysms present with a variety of signs and symptoms. The mechanism is likely to be ischemia or pressure on adjacent structures, including the hypothalamus.

In addition, aneurysms in this location may cause bilateral anterior cerebral artery insufficiency with ensuing mental status changes. These include emotional lability, personality changes, psychomotor retardation, intellectual retardation, memory deficits, confusion, Korsakoff's confabulatory-amnestic syndromes, impaired concentration, and akinetic mutism [55]. There may be unilateral or bilateral vision abnormalities [160]. On ophthalmologic examination, retinal, subhyaloid and vitreous hemorrhages, and papilledema can be seen. Headache is usually bifrontal and retroorbital. Contralateral hemiplegia affecting the arm greater than the leg may be present. Other signs include Babinski signs, decerebrate posturing, dysphasia, diabetes mellitus, electrolyte disturbances, and disturbances of micturition and defecation. In addition, bilateral CN VI palsies may be seen [122]. The signs and symptoms of anterior cerebral artery aneurysms are similar to those seen with ICA bifurcation and AComm aneurysms. In addition, syndromes of neglect may occur [60]. There may also be disturbances in micturition secondary to ischemia of the septal and preoptic regions of the telencephalon and rostral part of the hypothalamus [5], mental deficits secondary to frontal lobe disturbances, pyramidal tract signs including leg weakness [55], and visual disturbances [105].

3. Internal-Carotid–Posterior-Communicating Arteries (ICA–PComm)

Carotid artery-posterior communicating artery aneurysms commonly produce symptoms prior to major rupture [55]. They present with general signs of SAH including CN III palsy [173]. In addition, there may be focal hemispheric signs causing contralateral hemiparesis and pain localized to the ipsilateral orbit or forehead [55]. Orbital pain with or without CN III palsy [100,105] and numbness and/or paresthesias of V1 and V2 have also been reported [105]. Cranial nerves IV and VI may also be affected [105].

4. Middle Cerebral Artery (MCA)

In addition to the general features relating to aneurysmal rupture, there are other symptoms attributable to ischemia in the vascular territory of the MCA. These include contralateral hemiplegia (the arm more affected than the leg) [96,105], motor, receptive or global aphasia in dominant hemisphere aneurysms, homonymous hemianopsia, and cortical sensory deficits [55,105]. Seizures in association with intracerebral aneurysms and SAH are most commonly seen with MCA aneurysms. Postulated seizure mechanisms include ischemia to the temporal lobe or direct pressure from a hematoma or a giant aneurysm [105]. Symptoms of SAH are lateralizing in 50% of cases [55].

5. Basilar Artery

Symptoms from vertobrobasilar artery aneurysms are generally caused by mass effect and ischemia. For example, compression of CN V, VI, and VII may result in trigeminal neuralgia, diplopia, and hemifacial spasm. Compression of the aqueduct of Sylvius may lead to hydrocephalus. Commonly, ischemia may affect the brainstem, cerebellum, and occipital lobes [55]. Thrombosis in branching vessels may lead to infarction causing permanent neurologic deficit, coma, or death [42,142].

Fox [55] divides the deficits caused by aneurysms of the basilar artery into upper and lower basilar artery syndromes. Upper basilar artery aneurysms may cause a unilateral or bilateral CN III palsy, Parinaud's syndrome secondary to pretectal ischemia, vertical or rotatory nystagmus, and internuclear ophthalmoplegia secondary to ischemia of the medial longitudinal fasciculus. With aneurysm rupture, homonymous hemianopsia or cortical blindness secondary to ischemia in the distribution of the posterior cerebral artery (PCA) or the lateral geniculate body may occur. Ischemia to the various structures causes specific symptomatology: ischemia of the cerebral peduncles may cause hemiplegia, quadriplegia, or alternating hemiplegia; ischemia of the medial lemniscus and red nucleus can cause Benedikt's syndrome consisting of contralateral hemianesthesia and dystonias; a peduncle and CN III nucleus causes Weber's syndrome with ipsilateral CN III palsy and contralateral hemiplegia; corticobulbar pathways cause pseudobulbar palsy with an inability to control swallowing, talking, and facial movement. If the sympathetic pathways are involved, the patient may develop Horner's syndrome. Damage to the reticular formation may present as coma. Also seen is superior cerebellar artery syndrome consisting of ipsilateral cerebellar signs; Horner's syndrome; contralateral loss of pain, temperature, and touch; partial or complete deafness; mask-like facies; and dysarthria. Aneurysms of the lower basilar artery, in addition to having the general features of SAH, show signs of ischemia to the pons and medulla. Classic but rare signs of basilar artery rupture include sudden coma, flaccid quadriplegia, fixed and dilated or mid-position pupils, absent respiration, and no response to stimulation. Such patients appear brain dead but they may improve with resucitation. Rupture of basilar artery aneurysms has been shown to be associated with deafness due to blood extending into Rosenthal's canal and fluid channels of the modiolus [7]. Hemorrhage is seen in the interpeduncular cistern. Posterior cerebral artery aneurysms cause ischemia to the occipital lobes resulting in homonymous hemianopsia [55,146]. There may also be a CN III palsy and occasionally a CN IV palsy. Coma may be seen [146]. Posterior choroidal artery aneurysms here can cause contralateral hemiparesis along with the general signs of SAH [55]. Superior cerebellar artery aneurysms may manifest with the superior cerebellar artery syndrome as described above. Other signs may include ocular bobbing and trigeminal neuralgia [55]. In anterior inferior cerebellar artery aneurysm, symptoms may be caused with or without SAH. Mass effect, commonly on CN 7 or 8, may cause facial paresis, tic, loss of taste to anterior ⅔ of tongue, hearing loss, tinnitus, rushing sounds, vertigo, nausea, vomitting, and horizontal nystagmus [55].

6. Vertebral Artery and Branches

Posterior inferior cerebellar artery aneurysms are most common and can cause paraplegia [88]. Common signs are those of SAH and dysphagia, dysarthria, Meniere's hemifacial spasm, and hemiatrophy of the tongue. With rupture of a vertebral artery, one sees brainstem findings, loss of touch and vibratory sense, loss of pain and temperature response, leg dysesthesias, coma, and respiratory depression [55].

7. Giant Aneurysms

Generally, these lesions produce symptoms on the basis of mass effect and ischemia to specific structures in addition to symptoms and signs of SAH specific to the location of the aneurysm.

G. Mycotic Aneurysms

1. Incidence

Mycotic aneurysms are found to occur in 1–3% of all patients with infective endocarditis (IE) [117]. In one study, fifty-seven percent of patients with mycotic aneuysms and infective endocarditis suffered SAH [161]. Other studies showed that 10% of patients with IE had SAH, 17–40% had an infarct and 6% had meningitis [64,81]. Twenty to forty percent of all patients with infective bacterial endocarditis will describe neurologic symptoms. In 60% of these patients, the neurologic complaint was either the chief complaint or a major presenting symptom [81,117]. There appears to be no difference in the frequency of neurologic symptoms between patients with or without aneuysms, which suggests that most neurologic symptoms are due to emboli from infected valvular vegetations [161]. In some instances SAH is the presenting sign of infective endocarditis [154]. The mortality rate from rupture of mycotic aneurysms is as high as 50%. This is 1.6 times higher than the overall population of patients with infective bacterial endocarditis. All ages are affected. In one study the ages ranged from 11 to 82. Patients at higher risk are those with rheumatic heart disease, congenital heart disease, and parental drug abuse [25]. Mycotic aneurysms occur earlier but less frequently in acute endocarditis and more often but later in subacute endocarditis [103]. Late aneurysms have been reported to appear 3 months to 2 years after surgical excision of an aneurysm in a different location or after effective treatment of IE [25,156].

2. Clinical Presentation

Osler's triad of symptoms of patients presenting with IE are fever, heart murmur, and stroke [132]. Other presenting features of infective bacterial endocarditis (IBE) include petechiae, thrombocytopenia, splenomegaly, hematuria, Roth spots, arthritis, clubbing and splinter hemorrhages. Warning signs of mycotic aneurysms are not unlike those of other intracerebral aneurysms. These include headache, nuchal rigidity, and neurologic problems such as coma, altered consciousness, hemiparesis, and dilated pupils [117]. Other major neurologic symptoms associated with mycotic cerebral aneurysms include toxic encephalopathy, meningitis, organic headache, mononeurities, convulsions, and visual impairment. A TIA precedes a major stroke in 27%. Major emboli account for 50% of neurologic complications and embolization often precedes the diagnosis of mycotic aneurysm [27,103,121]. Mycotic aneurysms as complications of infective endocarditis also occur at the abdominal aorta, sinus of valsalva, ligated ductus arteriosus, and superior mesenteric, splenic, coronary, and pulmonary arteries [154].

3. Pathology

It is thought that infected emboli from cardiac vegetations seed the intracranial circulation with pathogens. Usually, aneurysms are located at vessel bifurcations. The MCA is the most frequently affected vessel and is involved 4 times as often than either the ACA or PCA [20,118]. Several proposed mechanisms for the formation of aneurysms exist. Molinari's experiments showed that infection begins in the adventitia layer. Bacteria then pass through the vasa vasorum and extend medially, weakening the blood vessel wall and causing it to dilate [116]. Another described mechanism involves septic emboli as the cause of inflammatory destruction of blood vessel walls beginning at the endothelial layer [20]. It is also suggested that congenital aneurysms may become infected [20,121]. Another proposed etiology is an immune-mediated attack of blood vessels causing either aneurysm or blood vessel rupture [188].

4. Diagnosis

The diagnosis of mycotic aneurysm requires a history of infective bacterial endocarditis: rarely is a mycotic aneurysm seen in the absence of IBE; examination, positive laboratory studies; and usually angiographic evidence of an aneurysm. The physical examination may reveal signs of infective endocarditis as described above. In addition, there may be heart murmurs on auscultation. Blood cultures are positive 93% of the time. Streptococcus species and staphylococcus aureus are the most common pathogens and rarely gram negative organisms like *E. coli* are involved. The erythrocyte sedimentation rate is generally greater than 40 mm/hr. and the CSF may be abnormal. In one study, the CSF was normal in 30%, purulent in 28% (polymorphonuclear cells, decreased glucose, increase protein), aseptic in 25%, and hemorrhagic in 13% [150]. There may be a mildly elevated protein (80–180 mg/mL), RBCs or xanthrochromia (especially in patients with meningitis), and an elevated WBC up to 1,600/mL mostly consisting of lymphocytes and polymorphonuclear cells. The EEG may show focal abnormalities with focal lesions such as cerebral hemorrhage, infarct, or abscess, or it may show a diffuse abnormality in patients with toxic encephalopathy [81]. The echocardiogram usually demonstrates vegetations.

5. Complications

In addition to SAH, complications from mycotic aneurysms include abscess formation, meningitis, and meningoencephalitis [103]. Abscess formation depends on the level and duration of bacteremia, virulence of the infecting organism, and occurrence of preceeding septic emboli [103]. Microabscesses are usually found at autopsy. They are often too small to be detected by MRI or CT. The antibiotics used to treat the IBE and mycotic aneurysm will also treat the microabscesses. Larger abscesses present with headache, increased ICP, and focal neurologic signs. These require surgical drainage [103]. Patients with meningoencephalitis present with headache, stiff neck, confusion, and "toxic encephalopathy" [103]. Seizures can result from emboli, antibiotic therapy (e.g., penicillin) or from infarction [150]. Intracranial hemorrhage occurs in about 5%. When the infecting organism is staphylococcus, hemorrhage usually occurs early and is lobar [66].

6. Treatment

Aneurysms can either disappear, as documented by serial angiography or they can grow. Ruptured mycotic aneurysms carry a very high risk of mortality. Thus, followup with frequent serial angiograms is recommended [57]. Antibiotic therapy specific to the sensitivity of the organism is used. If cultures are negative, empiric broad spectrum coverage is used including vancomycin and gentamicin [117]. Enlargement of the aneurysm after a full course of antibiotic therapy, peripheral location, ease of surgical resection, and single aneurysm are all potential indications for surgical resection [18,20]. Morowetz et al. have developed treatment guidelines for patients with mycotic aneurysm [118]. They recommend 4-vessel angiography in all patients with bacterial endocarditis who develop a neurological deficit, presumably secondary to embolization. Antibiotic therapy should be instituted as soon as blood cultures are obtained and a diagnosis is made and should be continued for 4 to 6 weeks regardless of any decision for surgical intervention. Underlying cardiac disorders, including the need for valvular surgery must be addressed as well. Intracerebral hemorrhage should be operated on if it produces significant mass effect. Unruptured mycotic aneurysms should be followed with serial angiograms at 6 weeks, 3 months, 6 months, and 1 year after the diagnosis of mycotic aneurysm is made and antibiotics are started; some authors recommend more frequent angiography. Frazee et al. [57] recommend angiograms at 7–10 day intervals. Finally, CT should be performed on all patients with IBE who develop neurologic symptoms [56].

H. Symptomatology of Vasospasm

1. Incidence

Vasospasm is a common and often severe complication of SAH. It occurs in 20–40% of patients with intracranial aneurysms [61,196,172], and is the cause of delayed ischemia [178]. The etiology for vasospasm is somehow related to breakdown products of subarachnoid blood, but the exact mechanism has not yet been clearly elucidated. There is a strong association between the amount of subarachnoid blood seen at surgery and the degree of vasospasm that develops postoperatively [183]. It has been suggested that volume depletion may be a contributing factor in the development of vasospasm as 85% of patients who develop hyponatremia develop vasospasm [69,119]. There is no association between the presenting clinical grade and the degree of vasospasm that develops but in general, patients who present with a lower clinical grade are at a low risk [172]. There is an association between poor clinical grade on admission, the amount of blood on CT, and the occurrence of vasospasm [13]. Focal collections of blood on the admission CT is the best predictor of vasospasm. If subarachnoid (SA) blood is not detected on CT, vasospasm is unlikely. If subarachnoid blood collections are layered 1 mm or more in fissures or cisterns, spasm is usually severe. There is an almost exact correlation between the location of SA blood and the distribution of vessels that go into spasm [50]. Usually the degree of spasm is worse for the vessel on which the aneurysm is located [55]. The vessels most commonly affected are the ACA and MCA [2,50].

2. Symptoms

Nearly all patients who experience vasospasm will have some kind of ischemic deficit [51]. Delayed onset of new or progressive neurologic decline usually suggests vasospasm. Symptoms and signs include headache; vomiting; focal neurologic signs such as hemiparesis; blood pressure elevation; mental status changes such as excitement, confusion, increased drowsiness, and irritability; coma; respiratory irregularity; and decerebrate posturing. Vasospasm of the anterior cerebral arteries may be manifest in abulia [51]. Eighty-four percent of patients with severe vasospasm had delayed hemiplegia and 100% of patients with hemiplegia had angiographic evidence of severe vasospasm. Vasospasm may lead to infarction if left untreated [55]. The temporal profile of vasospasm is as follows. It usually begins on day 3 post SAH [51]. The earliest signs are related to the vessel in spasm. At day 6–8, the severity of neurologic symptoms is worst, corresponding to severe evidence of vasospasm on objective testing. By day 12, the reversible symptoms of vasospasm resolve leaving the patient with residual defects of infarction [13,51,55,195]. Patients with vasospasm may develop fever, hypertension, tachycardia, and leukocytosis [13]. If fever develops it may peak at 37–38 °C or develop on approximately day 5, last for about one week, and peak at 38–39 °C [159]. Increased intracranial pressure is seen in patients with diffuse vasospasm. Fifty percent of patients will show clinical evidence of vasospasm. This is followed by a rise in ICP, which is associated with ischemic brain swelling or infarction [67]. Typically, initially increased ICP may be seen without angiographic evidence of vasospasm. This is followed by a fall in ICP concomitant with the onset of vasospasm. Changes in the ECG may accompany vasospasm [55].

I. Clinical Grading Systems

Numerous grading systems have been developed to facilitate determining treatment outcomes relative to defined groupings of clinical status. The first widely used system was that of Botterell [23]. This was an easy to apply, five-category system that defined operative risk based on neurological function and level of consciousness: grade 1 patients may or may not have signs of SAH, are conscious, and have no neurologic deficit; grade 2 patients are drowsy and do not have significant neurological deficit; grade 3 patients are drowsy and have a neurologic deficit; grade 4 patients have a major neurologic deficit and are deteriorating or are older patients with less severe neurologic deficit; grade 5 patients are moribund, essentially dying, and have extensor rigidity. Nishioka [125] and Hunt and Hess [76] modified the Botterell system. They essentially eliminated Botterell's group 4 and subdivided Botterell's group 1 into 2 separate groups: patients who are basically asymptomatic and patients who have minimal symptoms and minimal neurologic deficit. See Table 3. The Hunt and Hess grade 2 differs from the Nishioka grade 2 in its inclusion of patients with a focal neurologic deficit. According to Hunt and Hess, good correlation is observed between presenting clinical grade and patient outcome. According to Sundt [177], the Botterell system simplifies data analysis but it fails to relate improvement in patients clinical status with resolution of meningeal symptoms. Sundt used a modified Botterell classification based on 4 grades: grade 1 includes those patients with or without headache, alert, and no major neurologic deficit; grade 2 includes patients with severe headache, meningeal signs, altered consciousness, and focal deficit; grade 3 includes patients with a major alteration of consciousness and a major focal deficit; and grade 4 includes patients who are comatose, with or without lateralizing signs. There have been other suggestions for grading systems arising out of failure to consistently obtain good correlation between clinical grade and prognosis. In one system, the grading is

Table 3 The Hunt and Hess and Nishioka Subarachnoid Hemorrhage Grading Scales

Grade	Hunt and Hess[a] [76]	Nishioka [125]
I	Asymptomatic, or minimal headache and slight nuchal rigidity	Symptom-free: completely recovered from last hemorrhage
II	Moderate to severe headache, nuchal rigidity, no neurologic deficit except cranial nerve palsy	Headache, alert and responsive, no major neurologic deficit
III	Drowsiness, confusion, or mild focal deficit	Either a) lethargic, headache, nuchal rigidity, no hemispheric defect; or b) alert, recovered from effects of SAH, hemispheric defect
IV	Stupor, hemiparesis, possible decerebrate rigidity or vegetative disturbances	Either a) obtunded, no major deficit; or b) lethargic, poorly responsive, hemispheric defect
V	Coma, decerebrate, moribund	Moribund, decerebrate or unresponsive

[a] Systemic diseases such as hypertension, diabetes, arteriosclerosis, chronic pulmonary disease, and severe vasospasm on angiogram result in placement of patient in next less favorable category.

based on the presence or absence of vomitting and the duration of unconsciousness at the time of initial bleed [165]. Good correlation was demonstrated between clinical severity and patient outcome in this system. Another author showed that there is a good correlation between "wakefulness" on admission and prognosis [24].

Table 4 WFNS[a] Subarachnoid Hemorrhage Grading Scale

WFNS[a] Grade	GCS Score	Motor deficit
I	15	Absent
II	14–13	Absent
III	14–13	Present
IV	12–7	Present or absent
V	6–3	Present or absent

[a] WFNS = World Federation of Neurological Surgeons, GCS = Glascow Coma Scale.

The World Federation of Neurological Surgeons (WFNS) Committee on a Universal Subarachnoid Hemorrhage Grading Scale worked for 6 years to devise a universally acceptable grading scale that could be used to standardize clinical groupings of patients to evaluate treatment effects, identify changes in patient status, and predict patient prognoses, and which would be easy to apply. There are 5 grades based on level of consciousness and degree of major neurological deficit. This system also incorporates the Glascow Coma Scale [179], as shown in Table 4.

REFERENCES

1. Adams HP Jr, Jergenson DD, Kassell NF, Sahs AL. Pitfalls in the recognition of subarachnoid hemorrhage. *JAMA* 1980; 244(8):794–796.
2. Adams HP Jr, Kassell NF, Torner JC, Haley EC Jr. Predicting cerebral ischemia after aneurysmal subarachnoid hemorrhage: influences of clinical condition, CT results, and antifibrinolytic therapy. A report of the Cooperative Aneurysm Study. *Neurology* 1987; 37(10):1586–1591.
3. Alksne JF, Lovings ET. The role of the arachnoid villus in the removal of red blood cells from the subarachnoid space. An electron microscopic study. *J Neurosurg* 1972; 36:192–200.
4. Andreoli A, di Pasquale G, Pinelli G, Grazi P, Tognetti F, Testa C. Subarachnoid hemorrhage: frequency and severity of cardiac arrhythmias. A survey of 70 cases studied in the acute phase. *Stroke* 1987; 18(3):558–564.
5. Andrew J, Nathan PW, Spanos NC. Disturbances of micturition and defecation due to aneurysms of anterior communicating or cerebral arteries. *Journal of Neurosurgery* 1966; 24(1):1–10.
6. Andrews RJ, Spiegel PK. Intracranial aneurysms. Age, sex, blood pressure, and multiplicity in an unselected series of patients. *Journal of Neurosurgery* 1979; 51(1):27–32.
7. Arnold W, Vosteen KH. [Sudden deafness as a consequence of rupture of a basilar artery aneurysm (author's transl)] Akute Ertaubung als Folge der Ruptureines Basilarisaneurysma *HNO* 1977; 25(4):127–130 (Published in German).
8. Auer LM, Schneider GH, Auer T. Computerized tomography and prognosis in early aneurysm surgery. *J Neurosurg* 1986; 65(2):217–221.
9. Augustijn P, Vanneste J, Davies G. Chronic spinal arachnoiditis following intracranial subarachnoid haemorrhage. *Clin Neurol Neurosurg* 1989; 91(4):347–350.
10. Austin DC. A review of intracranial aneurysms. *Henry Ford Hosp Med Bull* 1964; 12:251–271.
11. Ball MJ. Pathogenesis of the "sentinel headache" preceding berry aneurysm rupture. *Can Med Assoc J* 1975; 112(1):78–79.
12. Balla JI, Morley JB. Oculomotor nerve paralysis. *Med J Aust* 1967; 1(15):755–758.
13. Barker FG 2d, Heros RC. Clinical aspects of vasospasm. *Neurosurg Clin N Am* 1990; 1(2):277–288.
14. Bartleson JD, Trautmann JC, Sundt TM Jr. Minimal oculomotor nerve paresis sec-

ondary to unruptured intracranial aneurysm. *Arch Neurol* 1986; 43(10):1015–1020.

15. Barton CW. Subarachnoid hemorrhage presenting as acute chest pain: a variant of le coup de poignard. *Ann Emerg Med* 1988; 17(9):977–978.
16. Bassi P, Bandera R, Loiero M, Tognoni G, Mangoni A. Warning signs in subarachnoid hemorrhage: a cooperative study. *Acta Neurol Scand* 1991; 84(4):277–281.
17. Berek K, Kiechl S, Willeit J, Birbamer G, Vogl G, Schmutzhard E. Subarachnoid hemorrhage as presenting feature of isolated neurosarcoidosis. *Clin Investig* 1993; 71(1):54–56.
18. Bingham WF. Treatment of mycotic intracranial aneurysms. *Journal of Neurosurgery* 1977; 46(4)428–437.
19. Bohm E, Hugosson R. Experiences of surgical treatment of 400 consecutive rutured cerebral arterial aneurysms. *ACTA Neurochir* 1978; 40:33–43.
20. Bohmfalk GL, Story JL, Wissinger JP, Brown WE Jr. Bacterial intracranial aneurysm. *Journal of Neurosurgery* 1978; 48(3):369–382.
21. Bolander HG, Kourtopoulos H, West KA. Retrospective analysis of 162 consecutive cases of ruptured intracranial aneurysms. Total mortality and early surgery. *Acta Neurochir (Wien)* 1984; 70(1–2):31–41.
22. Bonita R. Cigarette smoking, hypertension and the risk of subarachnoid hemorrhage: a population–based case–control study. *Stroke* 1986; 17(5):831–835.
23. Botterell EH, Lougheed WM, Scott JW, Vanderwater SL. Hypothermia, and interruption of carotid or carotid and vertebral circulation, in the surgical management of intracranial aneurysms. *J Neurosurg* 1956; 13:1–42.
24. Brismar J, Sundbarg G. Subarachnoid hemorrhage of unknown origin: prognosis and prognostic factors. *J Neurosurg* 1985; 63(3):349–354.
25. Brust JC, Dickinson PC, Hughes JE, Holtzman RN. The diagnosis and treatment of cerebral mycotic aneurysms *Ann Neurol* 1990; 28(3):364 See comments in: *Ann Neurol* 1990; 27(3):238–246.
26. Calvert JM. Premonitory signs and symptoms of subarachnoid hemorrhage. *Med J Aust* 1966; 1:651–657.
27. Cantu RC, LeMay M, Wilkinson HA. The importance of repeated angiography in the treatment of mycotic–embolic intracranial aneurysms. *Journal of Neurosurgery* 1966; 25(2):189–193.
28. Alajouanine T, Castaigne P, Lhermitte F et al. Cerebral arteritis of bacterial endocarditis: its late complications. *JAMA* 170:1858–1959 and Cerebral arteritis in Osler's disease: its late complications. Sem Hop Paris 35: 1160–1165, 1959 (Fre).
29. Chang Y, Kargas SA, Goates JJ, Horoupian DS. Intraventricular and subarachnoid hemorrhage resulting from necrotizing vasculitis of the choroid plexus in a patient with Churg–Strauss syndrome. *Clin Neuropathol* 1993; 12(2):84–87.
30. Chapman AB, Rubinstein D, Hughes R, Stears JC, Earnest MP, Johnson AM, Gabow PA, Kaehny WD. Intracranial aneurysms in autosomal dominant polycystic kidney disease [see comments]. *New England Journal of Medicine* 1992; 327(13):916–920.
31. Clarke E, Walton JN. Subdural hematoma complicating intracranial aneurysm and angioma. *Brain* 1953; 76:378–404.
32. Crompton MR. The pathogenesis of cerebral aneurysms. *Brain* 1966; 89:797–814.

33. Dalessio DJ. The cerebral circulation and the headache of subarachnoid hemorrhage. In: Wolffs Headache and Other Head Pain. 3rd ed. New York: Oxford University Press, 1972; 189–212.
34. Damasio H, Seabra-Gomes R, da Silva JP, Damasio AR, Antunes JL. Multiple cerebral aneurysms and cardiac myxoma. *Arch Neurol* 1975; 32(4):269–270.
35. Danilewicz B, Zwolinska G, Jedlinska M. [Hydrocephalus following subarachnoid hemorrhage] Wodoglowie po krwotokach podpajeczynowkowych. *Neurol Neurochir Pol* 1987; 21(2):130–133.
36. Day AL. Aneurysms of the ophthalmic segment. A clinical and anatomical analysis. *J Neurosurg* 1990; 72(5):677–691.
37. Doczi T, Bende J, Huszka E, Kiss J. Syndrome of inappropriate secretion of antidiuretic hormone after subarachnoid hemorrhage. *Neurosurgery* 1981; 9(4):394–397.
38. Dott NM. Intracranial aneurysms: cerebral arterio–radiography: surgical treatment. *Edinburgh Med J* 1933; 40:219–234.
39. Drake CG, Hunt WE, Kassel N, Pertuiset B, Sano K, Teasdale G, DeVilliers JC. Report of World Federation of Neurological Surgeons Committee on a Universal Subarachnoid Hemorrhage Grading Scale. *J Neurosurg* 1988; 68:985–986.
40. Duffy GP. The "warning leak" in spontaneous subarachnoid haemorrhage. *Med J Aust* 1983; 1(11):514–516.
41. Duffy GP. Lumbar puncture in spontaneous subarachnoid hemorrhage. *British Medical Journal Clinical Research* 1982; 285(6349):1163–1164.
42. Echiverri HC, Rubino FA, Gupta SR, Gujrati M. Fusiform aneurysm of the vertebrobasilar arterial system. *Stroke* 1989; 20(12):1741–1747.
43. Eguchi T, Nakagomi T, Teraoka A. Treatment of bilateral mycotic intracavernous carotid aneurysms. Case report. *Journal of Neurosurgery* 1982; 56(3):443–447.
44. Ellis SG, Verity MA. Central nervous system involvement in systemic lupus erythematosus: a review of neuropathologic findings in 57 cases, 1955–1977. *Seminars in Arthritis and Rheumatism* 1979; 8(3):212–221.
45. Eskesen V, Sorensen EB, Rosenorn J, Schmidt K. The prognosis in subarachnoid hemorrhage of unknown etiology. *J Neurosurg* 1984; 61(6):1029–1031.
46. Fahmy JA. Symptoms and signs of intracranial aneurysms with particular reference to retinal haemorrhage. *Acta Ophthalmol (Copenh)* 1972; 50(2):129–136.
47. Fahmy JA. Vitreous haemorrhage in subarachnoid haemorrhage—Terson's syndrome. Report of a case with macular degeneration as a complication. *Acta Ophthalmol (Copenh)* 1972; 50(2):137–143.
48. Ferrante L, Acqui M, Mastronardi L, Celli P, Lunardi P, Fortuna A. Posterior inferior cerebellar artery (PICA) aneurysm presenting with SAH and contralateral crural monoparesis: a case report. *Surg Neurol* 1992; 38(1):43–45.
49. Fisher CM. Headache in acute cerebrovascular disease. Vinken PJ, Bruyn GW (eds). Headache and Cranial Neuralgias. Vol 5. NY: John and Sons, 1968: 124–156.
50. Fisher CM, Kistler JP, Davis JM. Relation of cerebral vasospasm to subarachnoid hemorrhage visualized by computerized tomographic scanning. *Neurosurgery* 1980; 6(1):1–9.
51. Fisher CM, Roberson GH, Ojemann RG. Cerebral vasospasm with ruptured saccular aneurysm—the clinical manifestations. *Neurosurgery* 1977; 1(3):245–248.

52. Fisher M, Davidson RI, Marcus EM. Transient focal cerebral ischemia as a presenting manifestation of unruptured cerebral aneurysms. *Ann Neurol* 1980; 8(4):367–372.
53. Fitz CR, Harwood-Nash DC. Early venous filling and controlled hyperventilation in cerebral angiography. *Acta Radiol Suppl (Stockh)* 1976; 347:77–81.
54. Fontanarosa PB. Recognition of subarachnoid hemorrhage [see comments] *Ann Emerg Med* 1989; 18(11):1199–1205.
55. Fox JL. Intracranial Aneurysms. Vol 1. New York: Springer-Verlag, 1983.
56. Frazee JG, Cahan LD. Treatment of mycotic aneurysms. *J Neurosurg* 1981; 54:566.
57. Frazee JG, Cahan LD, Winter J. Bacterial intracranial aneurysms. *Journal of Neurosurgery* 1980; 53(5):633–641.
58. Gerosa M, Licata C, Fiore DL, Iraci G. Intracranial aneurysms of childhood. *Childs Brain* 1980; 6(6):295–302.
59. Glass B, Abbott KH. Subarachnoid hemorrhage consequent to intracranial tumors. *Arch Neurol Psychiat* 1955; 73:369–379.
60. Goldenberg G. Neglect in a patient with partial callosal disconnection. *Neuropsychologia* 1986; 24(3):397–403.
61. Gotoh O, Tamura A, Nihei H, Manaka S, Tsujita Y, Oka H, Sano K. [Vasospasm and its outcome after early surgery for ruptured cerebral aneurysms: changing pattern of its incidence and outcome during this 9-year period] *No Shinkei Geka* 1993; 21(4):299–304 (Published in Japanese).
62. Hammer WJ, Luessenhop AJ, Weintraub AM. Observations on the electrocardiographic changes associated with subarachnoid hemorrhage with special reference to their genesis. *Am J Med* 1975; 59(3):427–433.
63. Harada Y, Ishimitsu H, Miyata I, Honda C, Nishimoto K. Peduncular hallucinosis associated with ruptured basilar–superior cerebellar artery aneurysm—case report. *Neurol Med Chir (Tokyo)* 1991; 31(8):526–528.
64. Harrison MJ, Hampton JR. Neurosurgical presentation of bacterial endocarditis. *British Medical Journal* 1967; 2(545):148.
65. Hart RG, Byer JA, Slaughter JR, Hewett JE, Easton JD. Occurrence and implications of seizures in subarachnoid hemorrhage due to ruptured intracranial aneurysms. *Neurosurgery* 1981; 8(4):417–421.
66. Hart RG, Kagan-Hallet K, Joerns SE. Mechanisms of intracranial hemorrhage in infective endocarditis. *Stroke* 1987; 18(6):1048–1056.
67. Hayashi M, Marukawa S, Fujii H, Kitano T, Kobayashi H, Munemoto S, Yamamoto S. Intracranial pressure in patients with diffuse cerebral arterial spasm following ruptured intracranial aneurysms. *Acta Neurochir (Wien)* 1978; 44(1–2):81–95.
68. Heros RC, Zervas NT, Varsos V. Cerebral vasospasm after subarachnoid hemorrhage: an update. *Ann Neurol* 1983; 14(6):599–608.
69. Heros RC, Zervas NT. Subarachnoid hemorrhage. *Annu Rev Med* 1983; 34:367–375.
70. Heros RC. Intracranial aneurysms. A review. *Minn Med* 1990; 73(10):27–32.
71. Hijdra A, van Gijn J, Stefanko S, Van Dongen KJ, Vermeulen M, Van Crevel H. Delayed cerebral ischemia after aneurysmal subarachnoid hemorrhage: clinicoanatomic correlations. *Neurology* 1986; 36(3):329–333.

72. Hijdra A, Vermeulen M, van Gijn J, van Crevel H. Rerupture of intracranial aneurysms: a clinicoanatomic study. *J Neurosurg* 1987; 67(1):29–33.
73. Hijdra A, Vermeulen M, van Gijn J, van Crevel H. Respiratory arrest in subarachnoid hemorrhage. *Neurology* 1984; 34(11):1501–1503.
74. Hillbom M, Kaste M. Alcohol intoxication: a risk factor for primary subarachnoid hemorrhage. *Neurology* 1982; 32(7):706–711.
75. Hongo K, Mizuno M, Oikawa S, Oya F, Kobayashi S. Subarachnoid hemorrhage presenting an "abnormal movement"—case report. *Neurol Med Chir (Tokyo)* 1993; 33(8):579–581.
76. Hunt WE, Hess RM. Surgical risk as related to time of intervention in the repair of intracranial aneurysms. *J Neurosurg* 1968; 28:14–19.
77. Inagawa T, Hirano A. Autopsy study of unruptured incidental intracranial aneurysms [see comments] *Surg Neurol* 1990; 34(6):361–365.
78. Iwama T, Andoh T, Sakai N, Iwata T, Hirata T, Yamada H. Dissecting and fusiform aneurysms of vertebro–basilar systems. MR imaging. *Neuroradiology* 1990; 32(4):272–279.
79. Jenkins A, Hadley DM, Teasdale GM, Condon B, Macpherson P, Patterson J. Magnetic resonance imaging of acute subarachnoid hemorrhage [see comments]. *Journal of Neurosurgery* 1988; 68(5)731–736.
80. Johnston SR, Hammond A, Griffiths L, Greenwood R, Clarke CR. Subarachnoid haemorrhage—can we do better? [see comments] *J R Soc Med* 1989; 82(12):721–724.
81. Jones Hr Jr, Siekert RG, Geraci JE. Neurologic manifestations of bacterial endocarditis. *Annals of Internal Medicine* 1969; 71(1):21–28.
82. Juvela S, Porras M, Heiskanen O. Natural history of unruptured intracranial aneurysms: a long–term follow–up study. In: *J Neurosurg* 1993; 79(2):174–182.
83. Juvela S. Minor leak before rupture of an intracranial aneurysm and subarachnoid hemorrhage of unknown etiology. *Neurosurgery* 1992; 30(1):7–11.
84. Kahn E, Markowitz J, Duffy L, Kenigsberg K, Davis JG, Daum F. Berry aneurysms, cirrhosis, pulmonary emphysema, and bilateral symmetrical cerebral calcifications: a new syndrome. *Am J Med Genet Suppl* 1987; 3:343–356.
85. Kamii H, Ogawa A, Sakurai Y, Kayama T. [Anterior inferior cerebellar artery aneurysm with a sudden onset of caudal cranial nerve symptoms] *No Shinkei Geka* 1989; 17(4):387–391 (Published in Japanese).
86. Kamrin RP. Temporal lobe epilepsy caused by unruptured middle cerebral artery aneurysms. *Arch Neurol* 1966; 14(4):421–427.
87. Karch SB. Upper gastrointestinal bleeding as a complication of intracranial disease. *J Neurosurg* 1972; 37:27–29.
88. Kashiwagi S, Tsuchida E, Shiroyama Y, Ito H, Yamashita T. Paraplegia due to a ruptured aneurysm of the distal posterior inferior cerebellar artery. *J Neurol Neurosurg Psychiatry* 1992; 55(9):836–837.
89. Kassell NF, Torner JC. Aneurysmal rebleeding: a preliminary report from the Cooperative Aneurysm Study. *Neurosurgery* 1983; 13(5):479–481.
90. Kettunen P. Subarachnoid haemorrhage and acute heart injury. *Clin Chim Acta* 1983; 134(1–2):123–127.

91. Kissel JT, Burde RM, Klingele TG, Zeiger HE. Pupil–sparing oculomotor palsies with internal carotid–posterior communicating artery aneurysms. *Ann Neurol* 1983; 13(2):149–154.
92. Kitahara T, Masuda T, Soma K. [The etiology of sudden cardiopulmonary arrest in subarachnoid hemorrhage] *No Shinkei Geka* 1993; 21(9):781–786 (Published in Japanese).
93. Kocan MJ. Electrocardiographic changes following subarachnoid hemorrhage. *J Neurosci Nurs* 1988; 20(6):362–365.
94. Kollegger H, Zeiler K, Oder W, Dal-Bianco P, Schmidbauer M, Deecke L. Subarachnoid haemorrhage: prognostic factors as related to working capacity. *Int Disabil Stud* 1989; 11(2):57–60.
95. Kreus K-E, Kemila SJ, Takala JR. Electrocardiographic changes in cerebrovascular accidents. *Acta Med Scand* 1969; 185:327–334.
96. Kudo T, Uno T. Ipsilateral hemiparesis caused by subarachnoid hemorrhage in a patient with a ruptured middle cerebral artery aneurysm: a case report. *Neurosurgery* 1984; 15(5):727–729.
97. Kudo T. Postoperative oculomotor palsy due to vasospasm in a patient with a ruptured internal carotid artery aneurysm: a case report. *Neurosurgery* 1986; 19(2):274–277.
98. Kutsuna M, Someda K, Morita K, Yamanouchi Y, Kurimoto T, Kawamura Y, Matsumura H. [Ischemic cerebral symptoms after subarachnoid hemorrhage due to aneurysmal rupture *No Shinkei Geka* 1978; 6(6):543–548 (Published in Japanese).
99. Kyoi K, Gega A, Tada T, Iida N, Tsunoda S, Utsumi S, Sakaki T, Morimoto T, Iwa H, Yokoyama K. [Carotid-ophthalmic aneurysms and visual abnormalities] *No Shinkei Geka* 1986; 14(10):1197–1204 (Published in Japanese).
100. Lanzino G, Andreoli A, Tognetti F, Limoni P, Calbucci F, Bortolami R, Lucchi ML, Callegari E, Testa C. Orbital pain and unruptured carotid–posterior communicating artery aneurysms: the role of sensory fibers of the third cranial nerve. *Acta Neurochir (Wien)* 1993; 120(1–2):7–11.
101. Laun A, Tonn JC. Cranial nerve lesions following subarachnoid hemorrhage and aneurysm of the circle of Willis. *Neurosurg Rev* 1988; 11(2):137–141.
102. Leblanc R, Winfield JA. The warning leak in subarachnoid hemorrhage and the importance of its early diagnosis. *Canadian Medical Journal* 1984; 131(10):1235–1236.
103. Lerner PI. Neurologic complications of infective endocarditis. *Med Clin North Am* 1985; 69(2):385–398.
104. Ljunggren B, Sonesson B, Saveland H, Brandt L. Cognitive impairment and adjustment in patients without neurological deficits after aneurysmal SAH and early operation. *J Neurosurg* 1985; 62(5):673–679.
105. Locksley HB. Natural history of subarachnoid hemorrhage, intracranial aneurysms and arteriovenous malformations. *Journal of Neurosurgery* 1966; 25(3):321–368.
106. Lundberg PO, Osterman PO. The benign and malignant forms of orgasmic cephalgia. *Headache* 1974; 14(3):164–165.
107. Lyrer P, Gratzl O. [Is early diagnosis possible in cerebral aneurysm? Symptoms of saccular cerebral aneurysms before the occurrence of massive subarachnoid

hemorrhage. Literature review and discussion] Gibt es eine Fruhdiagnose bei zerebralen Aneurysmen? Symptome sakkularer zerebraler Aneurysmen vor Auftreten einer massiven Subarachnoidalblutung. Literaturubersicht und Diskussion. *Schweiz Rundsch Med Prax* 1993; 82(1):3–8 (Published in German).

108. Mackenzie JM. The anatomy of aneurysm–bearing circles of Willis. *Clin Neuropathol* 1991; 10(4):187–189.
109. Matsumura H, Iwai F, Ichikizaki K. [Ischemic myocardial disorder in acute phase subarachnoid hemorrhage: clinical study of 52 patients] *No Shinkei Geka* 1991; 19(4):349–357 (Published in Japanese).
110. McFadzean RM, Gowan ME. Optochiasmal arachnoiditis after rupture of an anterior communicating artery aneurysm. *Trans Ophthalmol Soc U K* 1978; 98(4):490–493.
111. Meyer FB, Sundt TM Jr, Fode NC, Morgan MK, Forbes GS, Mellinger JF. Cerebral aneurysms in childhood and adolescence. *J Neurosurg* 1989; 70(3):420–425.
112. Mihara T, Asakura T, Kawamura H, Ogawa N, Kitamura K. [Postoperative psychiatric symptoms and electrocardiographic changes in aneurysm of the anterior communicating artery] *No To Shinkei* 1971; 23(11):1271–1280 (Published in Japanese).
113. Milhorat TH. Acute hydrocephalus after aneurysmal subarachnoid hemorrhage. *Neurosurgery* 1987; 20(1):15–20.
114. Misra BK, Whittle IR, Steers AJ, Sellar RJ. De novo saccular aneurysms. *Neurosurgery* 1988; 23(1):10–15.
115. Modesti LM, Binet EF. Value of computed tomography in the diagnosis and management of subarachnoid hemorrhage. *Neurosurgery* 1978; 3:151–156.
116. Molinari GF, Smith L, Goldstein MN, Satran R. Pathogenesis of cerbral mycotic aneurysms. *Neurology* 1973; 23(4):325–332.
117. Monsuez JJ, Vittecoq D, Rosenbaum A, Goujon C, Wolff M, Witchitz S, Modai J. Prognosis of ruptured intracranial mycotic aneurysms: a review of 12 cases. *Eur Heart J* 1989; 10(9):821–825.
118. Morawetz RB, Karp RB. Evolution and resolution of intracranial bacterial (mycotic) aneurysms. *Neurosurgery* 1984; 15(1):43–49.
119. Morinaga K, Hayashi S, Matsumoto Y, Omiya N, Mikami J, Ueda M, Sato H, Inoue Y, Okawara S. [Hyponatremia and cerebral vasospasm in patients with aneurysmal subarachnoid hemorrhage] *No To Shinkei* 1992; 44(7):629–632 (Published in Japanese).
120. Moskovichiute LI, Smirnov NA, Zograbian AS. [Memory disorders in patients with saccular aneurysms of the internal carotid arteries] Narushenie pamiati u bol'nykh s meshotchatymi anevrizmami vnutrennikh sonnykh arterii. *Vopr Neirokhir* 1978; (1):19–23 (Published in Russian).
121. Moskowitz MA, Rosenbaum AE, Tyler HR. Angiographically monitored resolution of cerebral mycotic aneurysms. *Neurology* 1974; 24(12):1103–1108.
122. Nathal E, Yasui N, Suzuki A, Hadeishi H. Ruptured anterior communicating artery aneurysm causing bilateral abducens nerve paralyses—case report. *Neurol Med Chir (Tokyo)* 1992; 32(1):17–20.
123. Nau R, Scheidt P, Gonska BD, Prange HW. [Subarachnoid hemorrhage with pul-

monary edema and electrocardiographic changes. The differential diagnosis of myocardial infarct] Subarachnoidalblutung mit Lungenodem und elektrokardiographischen Veranderungen. Differentialdiagnose des Myokardinfarkts. *Dtsch Med Wochenschr* 1992; 117(17):658–662 (Published in German).

124. Nehls DG, Flom RA, Carter AP, Spetzler RF. Multiple intracranial aneurysms: determining the site of rupture. *J Neursurg* 1985; 63:342–348.
125. Nishioka H. Report on the cooperative study of intracranial aneurysms and subarachnoid hemorrhage. VII. Pt. 1. Evaluation of the conservative management of ruptured intracranial aneurysms. *J Neurosurg* 1966; 25:574–592.
126. Noseworthy JH, Girvin JP. Sentinel tinnitus as symptom of acephalgic subarachnoid haemorrhage [letter] *Lancet* 1987; 1(8545):1315.
127. Oder W, Dal Bianco P, Kollegger H, Zeiler K, Binder H, Deecke L. Spontaneous subarachnoid hemorrhage. Prognostic factors for social readjustment. *Scand J Rehabil Med* 1990; 22(2):85–91.
128. Ogden JA, Mee EW, Henning M. A prospective study of impairment of cognition and memory and recovery after subarachnoid hemorrhage. *Neurosurgery* 1993; 33(4):572–587.
129. Ohaegbulam SC, Dujovny M, Ausman JI, Diaz FG, Malik GM. Ethnic distribution of intracranial aneurysms. *Acta Neurochir (Wien)* 1990; 106(3–4):132–135.
130. Okabe S, Ogane K, Suzuki S, Iwabuchi T, Ottomo M. [Disproportionately large communicating fourth ventricle with bilateral exotropia: report of two cases] *No Shinkei Geka* 1990; 18(10):969–973 (Published in Japanese).
131. Okazaki H. Fundamentals of Neuropathology: Morphologic Basis of Neurologic Disorders. 2nd ed. Tokyo: Igaku-Shoin Ltd, 1989.
132. Osler W. Gulstonian lectures on malignant endocarditis. *Lancet* 1885; 1:415–418, 459–464, 505–508.
133. Ostergaard JR, Bruun-Petersen G, Kristensen BO. The C3–F gene in patients with intracranial saccular aneurysms. *Acta Neurol Scand* 1986; 74(5):356–359.
134. Ostergaard JR. Risk factors in intracranial saccular aneurysms. Aspects on the formation and rupture of aneurysms, and development of cerebral vasospasm. *Acta Neurol Scand* 1989; 80(2):81–98.
135. Ostergaard JR. Headache as a warning symptom of impending aneurysmal subarachnoid haemorrhage. *Cephalalgia* 1991; 11(1):53–55.
136. Oyebode F, Kennedy S, Davison K. Psychiatric sequel of subarachnoid hemorrhage. *British Journal of Medicine* 1986; 36(2):104, 106–108.
137. Pakarinen S. Incidence, aetiology, and prognosis of primary subarachnoid haemorrhage. A study based on 589 cases diagnosed in a defined urban population during a defined period. *Acta Neurol Scand* 1967; 43(Suppl 29):1–28.
138. Pasqualin A, Mazza C, Cavazzani P, Scienza R, DaPian R. Intracranial aneurysms and subarachnoid hemorrhage in children and adolescents. *Childs Nerv Syst* 1986; 2(4):185–190.
139. Passeri S, Dalla Rosa V, Zampollo A. [Considerations on subarachnoid hemorrhage caused by pituitary adenoma. Presentation of an anatomo–clinical case] Considerazioni sull'emorragia sottoaracnoidea da adenoma ipofisario. Presentazione di una osservazionr anatomo–clinica. *Riv Patol Nerv Ment* 1968; 89(1):61–72 (Published in Italian).

140. Patel MK; Clarke MA. Lumbar puncture and subarachnoid haemorrhage. *Postgrad Med J* 1986; 62(733):1021–1024.
141. Perneczky A, Czech T. Prognosis of oculomotor palsy following subarachnoid hemorrhage due to aneurysms of the posterior communicating artery. *Zentralbl Neurochir* 1984; 45(3):189–195.
142. Pessin MS, Chimowitz MI, Levine SR, Kwan ES, Adelman LS, Earnest MP, Clark DM, Chason J, Ausman JI, Caplan LR. Stroke in patients with fusiform vertebrobasilar aneurysms. *Neurology* 1989; 39(1):16–21.
143. Petitti DB, Wingerd J. Ose of oral contraceptives, cigarette smoking, and risk of subarachnoid hemorrhage. *Lancet* 1978; 2(8083):234–5.
144. Phillips LH, Whisnant JP, Reagan TJ. Sudden death from stroke. *Stroke* 1977; 8(3):392–395.
145. Phillips LH 2d, Whisnant JP, O'Fallon WM, Sundt TM Jr. The unchanging pattern of subarachnoid hemorrhage in a community. *Neurology* 1980; 30(10):1034–1040.
146. Pia HW, Fontana H. Aneurysms of the posterior cerebral artery. Locations and clinical pictures. *Acta Neurochir (Wien)* 1977; 38(1–2):13–35.
147. Piazza P, Lisotto C, Querin F, Morassut S, Pomes A. [Usefulness of computerized tomography in the prognosis of subarachnoid hemorrhage] Utilita della tomografia computerizzata nella prognosi delle morragie subaracnoidee. *Radiol Med (Torino)* 1990; 79(6):585–589 (Published in Italian).
148. Pope FM, Nicholls AC, Narcisi P, Bartlett J, Neil-Dwyer G, Doshi B. Some patients with cerebral aneurysms are deficient in type III collagen. *Lancet* 1981; 1(8227):973–975.
149. Prim Capdevila J, Campillo Valero D, Coello Gomez F. [Hydrocephalus after subarachnoid hemorrhage] Hidrocefalia posthemorragia subaracnoidea. *Neurologia* 1990; 5(2):41–44 (Published in Spanish).
150. Pruitt AA, Rubin RH, Karchmer AW, Duncan GW. Neurologic complications of bacterial endocarditis. *Medicine* 1978; 57(4):329–343.
151. Raimondi AJ, Torres H. Acute hydrocephalus as a complication of subarachnoid hemorrhage. *Surg Neurol* 1973; 1(1):23–26.
152. Raja IA. Aneurysm–induced third nerve palsy. *J Neurosurg* 1972; 36(5):548–551.
153. Ramina R, Arruda WO, Prestes AC, Parolim MK. Severe optochiasmatic arachnoiditis after rupture of an internal carotid artery aneurysm. *Arq Neuropsiquiatr* 1989; 47(2):192–196.
154. Rappaport K. Subarachnoid hemorrhage: an unusual presentation of infective endocarditis. *Journal of the Iowa Medical Society* 1981; 71(5):197–199.
155. Reichenthal E, Savitz MH, Rothman AS, Katz SS, Malis LI. Ruptured intracranial aneurysms as a cause of subdural haematoma. Potential diagnostic pitfalls and the surgical management of the acute patient. *Neurochirurgia (Stuttg)* 1986; 29(6):219–224.
156. Roach MR, Drake CG. Ruptured cerebral aneurysms caused by microorganisms. *N Eng J Med* 1965; 273:240–244.
157. Rockswold GL, Seijeskog EL. Spontaneous subarachnoid hemorrhage. Initial presentation of brain tumors. *Minn Med* 1972; 55(9):805–806.

158. Rosenorn J, Eskesen V, Schmidt K, Ronde F. The risk of bleeding from ruptured intracranial aneurysms. *Journal of Neurosurgery* 1987; 67(3):329–332.
159. Rousseaux P, Scherpereel B, Bernard MH, Graftieaux JP, Guyot JF. Fever and cerebral vasospasms in ruptured intracranial aneurysms. *Surg Neurol* 1980; 14(6):459–465.
160. Ruben S, Afshar F. Visual failure following subarachnoid haemorrhage from rupture of an anterior communicating artery aneurysm [letter] *J Neurol Neurosurg Psychiatry* 1991; 54(11):1017–1018.
161. Salgado AV, Furlan AJ, Keys TF. Mycotic aneurysm, subarachnoid hemorrhage, and indications for cerebral angiography in infective endocarditis. *Stroke* 1987; 18(6):1057–1060.
162. Sanchez Echaniz J, Santiago Burruchaga M, Benito Fernandez J, Pocheville Guruceta I, Mendia Gutierrez M, Aramburu Bardesi N, Garaizar Axpe C, Prats Vinas JM. [Migraine in a pediatric emergency service] Migra~na en un servicio de urgencias pediatrico. *An Esp Pediatr* 1991; 34(4):267–271 (Published in Spanish).
163. Sandyk R. Facial myokymia—a false localizing sign in obstructive communicating hydrocephalus. A case report. *Eur Neurol* 1985; 24(2):112–114.
164. Sandyk R. Transient global amnesia: a presentation of subarachnoid haemorrhage [letter] *J Neurol* 1984; 231(5):283–284.
165. Sato J, Masuzawa H, Shiraishi K, Kanazawa I, Kamitani H. [New clinical grading in ruptured cerebral aneurysm] *No Shinkei Geka* 1986; 14(10):1183–1187 (Published in Japanese).
166. Schievink WI, Torres VE, Piepgras DG, Wiebers DO. Saccular intracranial aneurysms in autosomal dominant polycystickidney disease. *J Am Soc Nephrol* 1992; 3(1):88–95.
167. Sengupta RP, Saunders M, Clarke PRR. Unruptured Intracranial Aneurysms: An unusual source of epilepsy. *Acta Neurochir* 1978; 40:45–53.
168. Serizawa T, Satoh A, Miyata A, Kobayashi S, Odaki M, Nakamura H, Watanabe Y. Ruptured cerebral aneurysm associated with coarctation of the aorta—report of two cases. *Neurol Med Chir (Tokyo)* 1992; 32(6):342–345.
169. Shapiro SA. Sentinel symptoms and signs of intracranial aneurysms. *Indiana Med* 1990; 83(1):20–22.
170. Shiino A, Suzuki F, Nakazawa T, Matsuda M, Handa J. [Hydrocephalus after aneurysmal subarachnoid hemorrhage] *No Shinkei Geka* 1988; 16(5 Suppl):493–497 (Published in Japanese).
171. Shimoda M, Yamada S, Yamamoto I, Tsugane R, Sato O. Time course of CSF lactate in subarachnoid hemorrhage. Correlation with clinical grading and prognosis. *Acta Neurochir (Wien)* 1989; 99:127–134.
172. Solomon RA, Onesti ST, Klebanoff L. Relationship between the timing of aneurysm surgery and the development of delayed cerebral ischemia. *Journal of Neurosurgery* 1991; 75(1):56–61.
173. Soni SR. Aneurysms of the posterior communicating artery and oculomotor paresis. *J Neurol Neurosurg Psychiatry* 1974; 37(4):475–484.
174. Stehbens WE, Delahunt B, Hilless AD. Early berry aneurysm formation in Marfan's syndrome. *Surg Neurol* 1989; 31(3):200–202.

175. Stehbens WE. Pathology and pathogenesis of intracranial berry aneurysms. *Neurol Res* 1990; 12(1):29–34.
176. Stroinska-Kusiowa B, Filipczak D. [Symptoms preceding rupture of subarachnoid aneurysms: an analysis] Analiza objawow poprzedzajacych peknieecie tetniakow srodczaszkowych. *Neurol Neurochir Pol* 1978; 12(3):213–218 (Published in Polish).
177. Sundt TM. Surgical Techniques for Saccular and Giant Intracranial Aneurysms. Baltimore: Williams and Wilkins, 1990, p. 3.
178. Sundt TM Jr. Intracranial aneurysms and subarachnoid hemorrhage: a subject review for the clinician. *Mayo Clin Proc* 1970; 45(6):455–466.
179. Teasdale G, Jennett B. Assessment of coma and impaired consciousness. A practical scale. *Lancet* 1974; 2(872):81–84.
180. Theander S, Granholm L. Sequelae after spontaneous subarachnoid haemorrhage, with special reference to hydrocephalus and Korsakoff's syndrome. *Acta Neurol Scand* 1967; 43(4):479–488.
181. Thomas AM. Simultaneous presentation of two cerebral arterial aneurysms. *Postgrad Med J* 1984; 60(700):135–136.
182. Thygesen J, Rosenorn J. Transient bilateral blindness in relation to subarachnoid haemorrhage caused by spastic ischaemic changes in retina and optic nerve. *Acta Ophthalmol (Copenh)* 1982; 60(2):325–331.
183. Tomasello F, Albanese V, Picozzi P, Spadaro A, Conforti P. Relation of cerebral vasospasm to operative findings of subarachnoid blood around ruptured aneurysms. *Acta Neurochir (Wien)* 1982; 60(1–2):55–62.
184. Torvik A, Bhatia R, Murthy VS. Transitory block of arachnoid granulations following subarachnoid hemorrhage. A postmortem study. *Acta Neurochir* 1978; 41:137–146.
185. Toyama Y, Tanaka H, Nuruki K, Shirao T. Prinzmetal's variant angina associated with subarachnoid hemorrhage: A case report. *Angiology* 1979; 30(3):211–218.
186. Trentham DE. Letter: Berry aneurysms and lupus. *N Engl J Med* 1976; 295(2):114.
187. Anonymous. Unruptured aneurysms and ischemic attacks. *Arch Intern Med* 1979; 139(10):1081.
188. Venger BH, Aldama AE. Mycotic vasculitis with repeated intracranial aneurysmal hemorrhage. Case report. *J Neurosurg* 1988; 69(5):775–779.
189. Vermeulen M, van Gijn J. The diagnosis of subarachnoid haemorrhage. *J Neurol Neurosurg Psychiatry* 1990; 53(5):365–372.
190. Vidal BE, Dergal EB, Cesarman E, San Martin OM, Loyo M, Lugo BV, Ortega RP. Cardiac arrhythmias associated with subarachnoid hemorrhage: prospective study. Neurosurgery 1979; 5:657–680.
191. von Holst H, Mathiesen T. Electrolyte concentrations in serum and CSF following subarachnoid haemorrhage. *Br J Neurosurg* 1990; 4(2):123–126.
192. Waga S, Otsubo K, Handa H. Warning signs in intracranial aneurysms. *Surg Neurol* 1975; 3(1):15–20.
193. Wakai S, Fukushima T, Teramoto A, Sano K. Pituitary apoplexy: its incidence and clinical significance. *J Neurosurg* 1981; 55(2):187–193.
194. Walton JN. Subarahchnoid Hemorrhage. Edinbrugh: Livingstone, 1956.

195. Weir B, Grace M, Hansen J, Rothberg C. Time course of vasospasm in man. *J Neurosurg* 1978; 48(2):173–178.
196. Welty TE, Horner TG. Pathophysiology and treatment of subarachnoid hemorrhage. *Clin Pharm* 1990; 9(1):35–39.
197. Wenig C, Huber G, Emde H. Hydrocephalus after subarachnoid bleeding. A correlation of clinical findings, the results of radioisotope Cisternography and computer-assisted tomography. *Eur Neurol* 1979; 18(1):1–7.
198. Whisnant JP, Phillips LH 2nd, Sundt Jr. Aneurysmal subarachnoid hemorrhage: timing of surgery and mortality. *Mayo Clinic Proceedings* 1982; 57(8):471–475.
199. Whittle IR, Allsop JL, Halmagyi GM. Focal seizures: an unusual presentation of giant intracranial aneurysms. A report of four cases with comments on the natural history and treatment. *Surg Neurol* 1985; 24(5):533–540.
200. Wiebers DO, Torner JC, Meissner I. Impact of unruptured intracranial aneurysms on public health in the United States. *Stroke* 1992; 23(10):1416–1419.
201. Wiebers DO, Torres VE. Screening for unruptured intracranial aneurysms in autosomal dominant polycystic kidney disease [editorial; comment]. *New England Journal of Medicine* 1992; 327(13):953–955.
202. Wiebers DO, Whisnant JP, O'Fallon WM. The Natural history of unruptured intracranial aneurysms. *New England Journal of Medicine* 1981; 304:696–698.
203. Wiebers DO, Whisnant JP, Sundt TM, O'Fallon WM. The significance of unruptured intracranial aneurysms. *J Neurosurg* 1987; 66:23–29.
204. Wijdicks EF, Ropper AH, Hunnicutt EJ, Richardson GS, Nathanson JA. Atrial natriuretic factor and salt wasting after aneurysmal subarachnoid hemorrhage. *Stroke* 1991; 22(12):1519–1524.
205. Winn HR, Richardson AE, O'Brein W, Jane JA. The long–term prognosis in untreated cerebral aneurysms: II. Late morbidity and mortality. *Annals of Neurology* 1926; 4(5):418–426.
206. Wise BL. Syndrome of inappropriate antidiuretic hormone secretion after spontaneous subarachnoid hemorrhage: a reversible cause of clinical deterioration. *Neurosurgery* 1978; 3(3):412–414.
207. Yamanaka O, Fujiwara Y, Nakamura T, Miyakawa K, Kamishima G, Endoh M, Ichikawa F. [A case of subarachnoid hemorrhage with sick sinus and advanced AV block] *Kokyu To Junkan* 1992; 40(7):715–719 (Published in Japanese).
208. Yamaura A, Isobe K, Karasudani H, Tanaka M, Komiya H. Dissecting aneurysms of the posterior inferior cerebellar artery. *Neurosurgery* 1991; 28(6):894–898.
209. Zuccarello M, Iavicoli R, Pardatscher K, Fiore DL, Mingrino S. [The diagnostic value of the CT scan in subarachnoid hemorrhage from intracranial anurysms] Die diagnostische Bedeutung der CT bei subarachnoidaler Blutung aus Hirnarterienaneurysmen. *Neurochirurgia (Stuttg)* 1981; 24(2):47–50 (Published in German).

6
Intracranial Vascular Malformations

Robert D. Brown, Jr., David O. Wiebers, and David G. Piepgras
Mayo Clinic, Rochester, Minnesota

I. INTRODUCTION

Intracranial vascular malformations are the second most common identifiable cause of nontraumatic subarachnoid hemorrhage (SAH), accounting for approximately 10% of subarachnoid hemorrhages. Congenital arteriovenous malformations (AVMs) are the most common type of intracranial vascular malformation causing neurologic symptoms and are the most commonly recognized nonaneurysmal cause of subarachnoid hemorrhage [1,2]. Other types of vascular malformations may lead to neurologic disease including cavernous malformations, venous angiomas, and dural-based arteriovenous fistulae. From previous autopsy series, it has been reported that 60% of supratentorial and 40% of infratentorial vascular malformations are arteriovenous in type [3]. Clinical symptoms depend on the intracranial vascular malformation subtype involved, its arterial supply and venous drainage, and hemodynamic characteristics. In addition to intracranial hemorrhage, common manifestations of vascular malformations include seizures, headaches, and progressive neurologic deficit [4,5].

Definitive data on the incidence and prevalence of arteriovenous malformations are unavailable. The overall occurrence of intracranial AVMs has been reported to be about one-seventh as common as aneurysms [6]. In previous autopsy studies, Olivecrona found 46 AVMs among 3200 brain tumor patients for a frequency of 1.4% [7]. McCormick discovered 196 AVMs among 4530 consecutive autopsies reflecting a slightly higher frequency of 4.3% [8]; only 12.2% of the cases were symptomatic. Other stroke registry cohorts have indicated a 0.5–1.8% occurrence of arteriovenous malformation-related SAH among all patients with stroke [9,10,11]. In the Cooperative study of intracranial aneurysms and subarachnoid hemorrhage, arteriovenous malformations led to 8.6% of subarachnoid hemorrhages [12]. The concept that arteriovenous malformations cause subarachnoid hemorrhage is not without controversy [13–15]. In a review of head computerized tomography (CT) scans performed in the acute stage of arteriovenous malformation-related intracranial hemorrhage, 4% of patients had primarily subarachnoid hemorrhage, 8% had intraventricular hemorrhage, 26% had intracerebral hemorrhage with intraventricular hemorrhage, and 60% had intracerebral hemorrhage [15].

II. VASCULAR MALFORMATION SUBTYPES

Although the term arteriovenous malformation is typically used to describe all types of histologically abnormal arterial and venous malformations within the brain, it is more appropriate to consider arteriovenous malformations to be one of the main subcategories of intracranial vascular malformations. Arteriovenous malformations are the most common symptomatic vascular malformation within the brain. The other main types of vascular malformations include cavernous malformations, venous angiomas, telangiectases, varices, and dural arteriovenous fistulae.

A. Arteriovenous Malformations

Arteriovenous malformations are congenital abnormalities leading to a fistulous connection of arteries and veins without a normal intervening capillary bed, which usually occur as wedge-shaped lesions within the cerebral hemispheres. Although over 90% of lesions are supratentorial in location [12], lesions may also be noted within the cerebellar hemispheres, brainstem, and as primarily intraventricular malformations. Frequency of occurrence within each cortical lobe is related to size, with a range from 39% in the parietal lobe to 10% in the occipital lobe [12]. The lesions may vary in size from exceedingly small lesions visible only upon microscopic examination to those involving nearly an entire hemisphere.

The histological appearance is characteristic and consists of normal or dilated arteries with a variably developed histological appearance of structurally normal arteries. Wall thickness varies, and evidence of previous thrombosis and recanalization are frequently noted. Calcification in the surrounding parenchyma and evidence of prior hemorrhage are typical, and venous channels are commonly abnormal. The fistulous connection is irregularly sized and contains little elastic or muscular layering. The venous drainage system may also be dramatically enlarged and be termed a varix. Pathological delineation of the bleeding site is usually quite difficult [16,17].

Radiologic imaging studies frequently allow the documentation of an arteriovenous malformation prior to intracranial hemorrhage [4]. A CT scan without contrast may demonstrate a calcification and hypointensity of the surrounding brain parenchyma. Marked enhancement of the feeding arteries and draining veins usually follows the injection of contrast [18]. Magnetic resonance imaging reveals a signal void on T-1 and T-2 weighted sequences and may show the presence of prior subclinical intracranial hemorrhage surrounding the lesion, as indicated by the presence of hemosiderin or T-2 weighted changes in close proximity to the vascular malformation [19,20]. Cerebral angiography continues to be the gold standard for delineation of the size and nature of the arterial feeders and complete characterization of the venous drainage system. Since intracranial saccular aneurysms are also frequently associated with arteriovenous malformations [21–23], angiography may also allow the most sensitive method of delineating the potential presence of an associated aneurysm. Angiography demonstrates the characteristic appearance of enlarged feeding arteries and typically dilated draining veins with invariably rapid shunting of contrast from the arterial to venous system (Figures 1–3).

B. Dural Arteriovenous Fistulae

Most, if not all, dural arteriovenous fistula (AVF) are thought to be acquired lesions. They occur within the wall of a venous sinus or other smaller venous structure and are likely related to sinus thrombosis and venous hypertension [24]. The use of CT scanning both with and without contrast is often negative, although dilated venous drainage may be seen. Magnetic resonance imaging (MRI) and MR angiographic techniques are relatively insensitive to the diagnosis of a dural AVF, although MR imaging including 3-D time-of-flight may demonstrate the fistula site [25]. A cerebral angiographic image of the internal and external carotid arteries reveals arteriovenous fistulae and also characterizes the arterial feeder and draining venous systems. External carotid arteries are the most common arterial feeders, while venous drainage may be into a major venous sinus or into pial veins. Occlusion or other abnormalities of the major sinuses are often noted [1,24] (Figure 4).

C. Cavernous Malformations

Most of the intracranial vascular malformations that are angiographically occult are either cavernous malformations or thrombosed arteriovenous malformations [26–28]. A cavernous malformation is a distinct pathological entity consisting of thin-walled vascular channels without intervening neural parenchyma, surrounding astrogliosis, and possible vessel wall calcification, accounting for 16% of intracranial vascular malformations [16]. The vascular channels may be

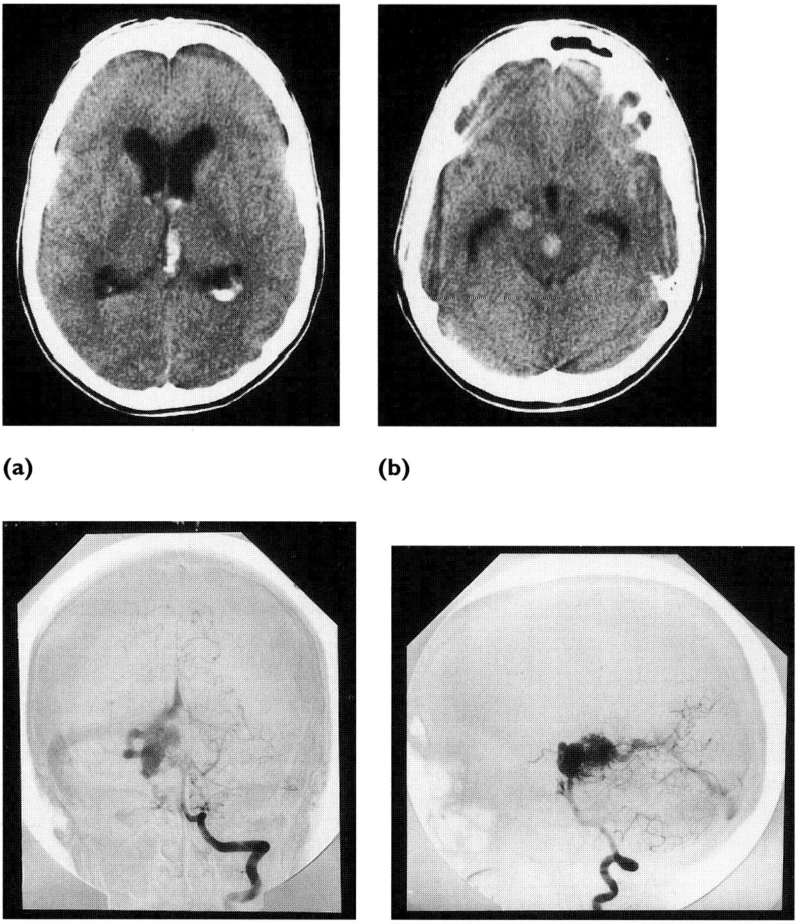

(a) (b) (c) (d)

Figure 1 A 32-year-old patient presented with the acute onset of headache and loss of consciousness. A CT scan without contrast revealed a hemorrhage lesion in the brainstem with blood in the third, fourth, and lateral ventricles. Cerebral angiography demonstrated a large arteriovenous malformation in the right perimesencephalic and diencephalic region. Numerous tortuous feeding vessels came from the right thalamogeniculate and thalamoperforating arteries. A large varix was also seen, and the major venous drainage was into the right basal vein of Rosenthal.

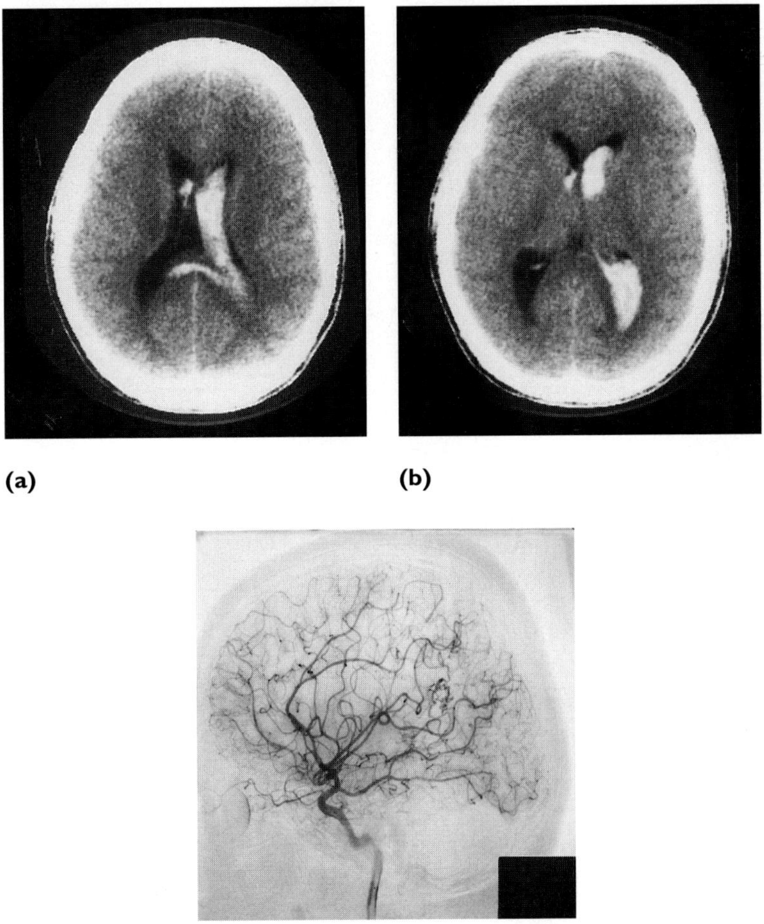

(a) (b) (c)

Figure 2 A 17-year-old male presented with lethargy, disorientation, and headache. A CT scan revealed an intraventricular hemorrhage. There was also a component of intraparenchymal blood with extension into the splenium of the corpus callosum. An angiogram showed a small tangle of abnormal vessels in the medial aspect of the left parietal lobe consistent with an arteriovenous malformation.

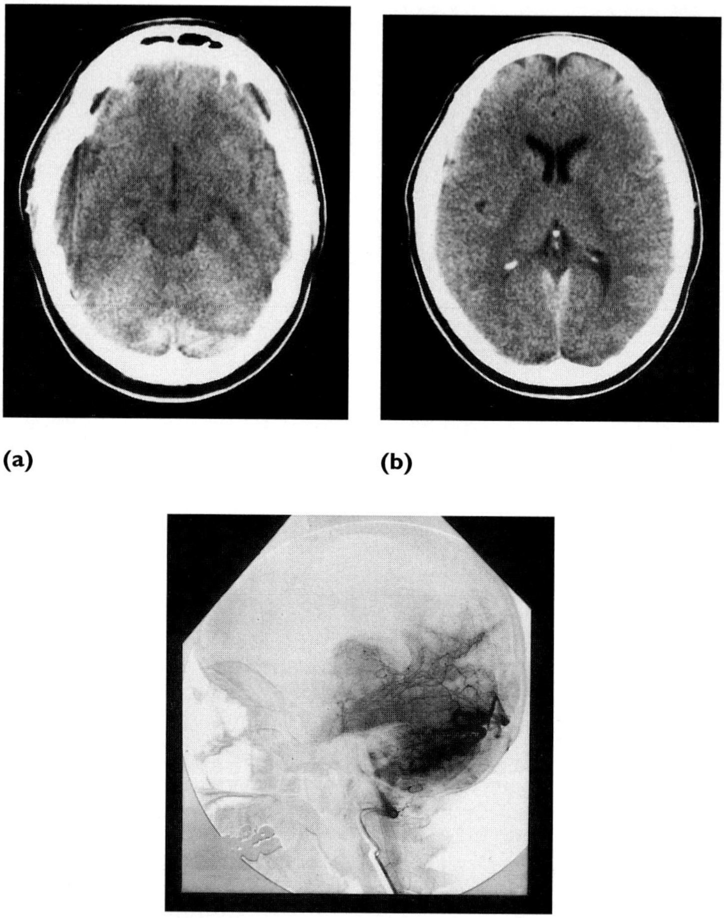

(a) (b)

(c)

Figure 3 A 28-year-old female presented with the acute onset of frontoparietal headache. A CT scan demonstrated a diffuse increased density under the tentorium in the posterior fossa with the question of subarachnoid hemorrhage. Spinal fluid examination was consistent with a subarachnoid hemorrhage. Angiography demonstrated a left cerebellar AVM fed by the inferior cerebellar arteries.

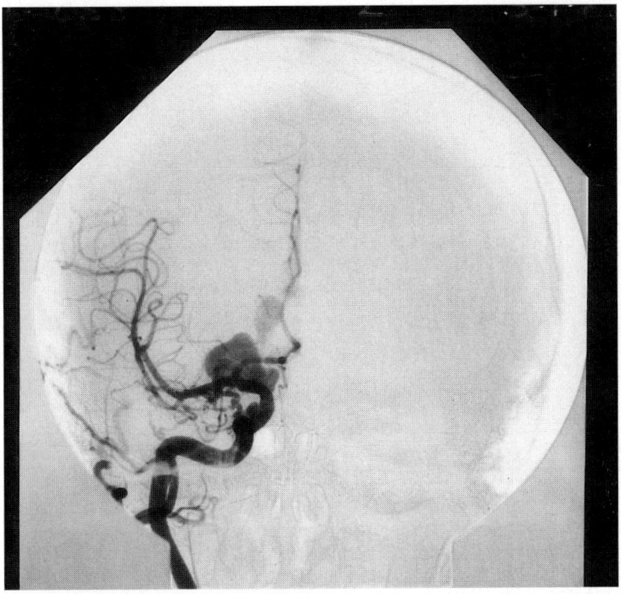

Figure 4 A 52-year-old man presented with mild headaches and a cranial bruit. Cerebral angiography revealed a large dural-based arteriovenous fistula located in the area of the right superior petrosal sinus with drainage into the vein of Galen and straight sinuses. The right superior petrosal sinus was occluded, and a large venous varix was present on the venous drainage system. Sixteen months following the initial presentation, the patient had a massive intracranial hemorrhage and died from the event.

thrombosed, and surrounding hemosiderin is usually present. While these lesions are angiographically occult, magnetic resonance imaging is leading to increased detection of these lesions before autopsy, although the scan cannot differentiate between occult arteriovenous malformations and cavernous malformations [29]. The characteristic MRI appearance includes a mixed high and low T-1 and T-2 weighted lesion with surrounding hypointensity [30,31]. Although these lesions have typically been considered an infrequent cause of clinically significant symptoms, more sophisticated radiologic studies have made it apparent that cavernous malformations may lead to serious neurologic symptoms and death (Figure 5).

Natural history information on the risk of hemorrhage in patients with an MRI appearance compatible with occult AVM or cavernous malformation is limited. Lesions most commonly present with seizures (40–52%), focal neurologic deficit (22–45%), and headaches (30%), although the lesions are asymptomatic

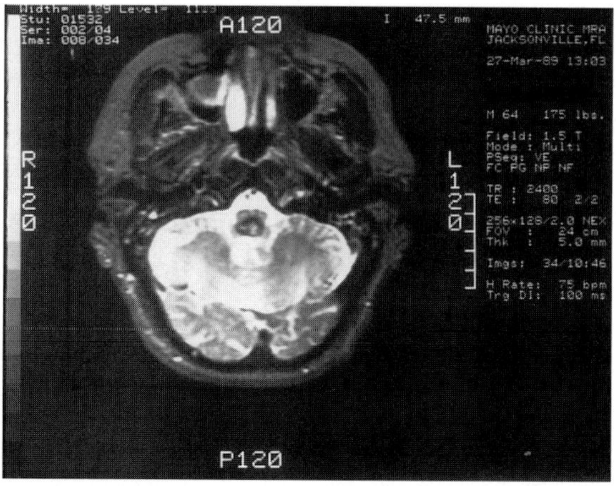

(a)

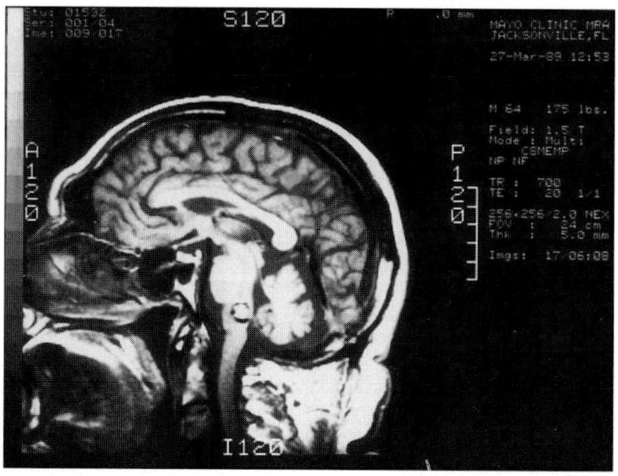

(b)

Figure 5 A 64-year-old male presented with sudden onset of right arm weakness and pain. An MRI scan showed a well-circumscribed lesion in the posterior medulla along the floor of the fourth ventricle with peripherally decreased and centrally increased signal intensity consistent with a cavernous malformation.

in 14–19% [32,33]. Among one group of 66 cases, only 7 of 57 symptomatic patients had symptoms caused by overt hemorrhage [32]. In another series, 9% of patients (3 of 32) had symptoms related to hemorrhage at diagnosis [33]. The overall bleeding rate during follow-up has ranged from 0.25–0.7% per year. Factors predicting future hemorrhage are not clearly defined, although lesions in the brainstem may lead to progressive symptoms or fatal hemorrhage [34–36].

D. Venous Angiomas

Venous angiomas consist of thin-walled venous channels with normal intervening neural parenchyma and rare evidence of prior hemorrhage. A CT scan may allow the delineation of a draining venous trunk, and an MRI scan may show a signal void consistent with a large draining vein or radial pattern of medullary veins [37]. Cerebral angiography reveals a distinct radial pattern with a subcortical venous trunk and enlarged veins over the cortical surface. The arterial phase should be normal [38]. Venous angiomas have been reported to be the most common vascular malformation noted at autopsy [39]. The clinical importance of the lesions is unclear with previous reports relating these lesions to intracranial hemorrhage and seizures [40–42], while others believe that the lesions are of little relevance [43] (Figure 6).

III. ARTERIOVENOUS MALFORMATIONS: CLINICAL PRESENTATION AND NATURAL HISTORY

Although many retrospective studies have helped clarify the natural history of intracranial arteriovenous malformations, the lack of prospective-based information has led to ongoing controversy [44–70]. Patient populations with conservatively managed unruptured arteriovenous malformations have been small, and other studies lack consistent long-term follow-up. The criteria used in the selection of patients for aggressive therapeutic intervention differ, making comparison of studies invalid. Radiologic features that may lead to increased risk of intracranial hemorrhage have been ascertained from relatively small groups of patients or have included those patients that have already experienced intracranial hemorrhage. Rapidly changing operative techniques, interventional neuroradiologic procedures, and radiation treatments have led to more frequent consideration of an aggressive approach for intracranial vascular lesions. The lack of clear understanding of the natural history of the lesions has made assessment of the therapeutic options difficult.

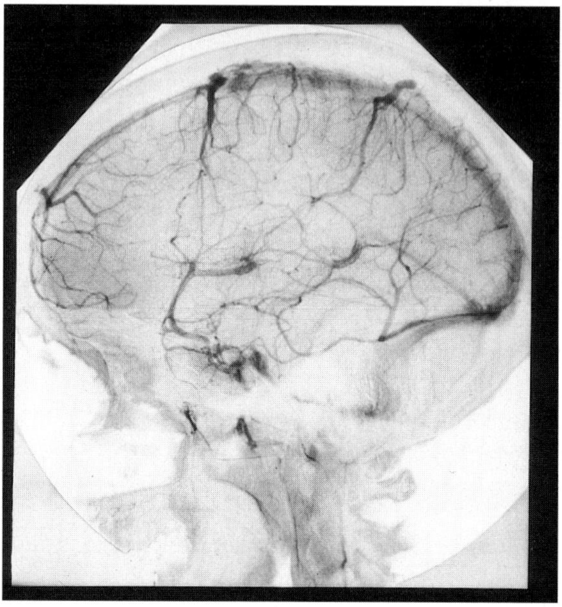

Figure 6 A 52-year-old patient presented with the abrupt onset of headache, and an intracranial hemorrhage was diagnosed on CT scan. Cerebral angiography demonstrated a venous angioma arising in the parasylvian right frontal lobe. The drainage was lateral via the right superficial middle cerebral vein.

A. Clinical Presentation

The overall frequency of AVM diagnosis may be slightly higher in males [4,5,44–48]. Although the lesions are uncommon in children, most AVMs present with symptoms before the age of 40 [4,44–48,55–56]. Approximately 50% of arteriovenous malformations that become symptomatic present as intracranial hemorrhage without any preceding warning [12,54,67,68]. Focal neurologic symptoms, severe headache, and loss of consciousness typically occur as a result of an intraparenchymal hemorrhage; subarachnoid hemorrhage and intraventricular hemorrhage are less common [4,5,44–48].

The clinical history of intracranial hemorrhage of any subtype does not aid the clinician in clearly differentiating an arteriovenous malformation from an aneurysmal or other etiology for the intracerebral hemorrhage. Because of the location of a typical arteriovenous malformation as a wedge-shaped lesion extending from the cortex down to the level of the ventricles, intraventricular or subarachnoid extension is commonly associated with a significant intraparenchymal component. Hemorrhage from cortical, surface vessels may cause subarachnoid hemorrhage, although it is often less severe than that noted with an aneurysmal rupture. A significant amount of hemorrhage at the base of the brain may lead to profound vasospasm mimicking that seen in aneurysmal subarachnoid hemorrhage [56,57], but significant vasospasm is uncommon.

In addition to intracerebral hemorrhage, other common presentations include seizures in 15–35% of the cases [4,5,12,45,48,53]. Seizures typically present in the young adult with either focal or generalized onset. A patient may present with seizures at the same time as hemorrhage, although seizure disorder may commence after subarachnoid hemorrhage. In the Cooperative study, seizures were noted in 28% of cases with supratentorial malformations. Among those patients for whom seizure type was specified, 44% had nonfocal seizures. The overall incidence of seizures was higher in patients with either a temporal or frontal lobe AVM, with generalized seizures most frequently seen with frontal lesions and focal seizures most commonly seen with parietal lesions [12]. Seizures may occur with lesions of the lateral ventricle, but in one series only 14% of the patients with lateral ventricle AVMs had nonhemorrhagic presentations.

The influence of presenting symptoms on risk of AVM rupture is unclear. Some have reported that patients presenting with convulsions may be at higher risk, although this has not been found consistently [4,48]. Approximately 25% of patients presenting with seizures eventually suffer an intracranial hemorrhage [47]. If patients with previous intracranial hemorrhage are excluded, approximately 57% of patients will present with some type of seizure disorder, with the risk of hemorrhage being similar to those presenting with headaches, progressive neurologic deficit, or in an asymptomatic state [4]. Graf had noted that without a previous history of seizures, the average yearly risk of hemorrhage was 2–3% [48]. A 25% risk of hemorrhage was noted over a 15-year period in another group of patients presenting with seizures [46].

Other common presentations for arteriovenous malformations in patients without prior intracranial hemorrhage include headaches related to the arteriovenous malformation, as seen in 15% of patients. Headaches are often ipsilateral to the lesion and may mimic migraine headaches, some with a preceding aura. Progressive neurologic deficit is uncommon, occurring in only 3% of patients without past hemorrhage. Focal neurologic spells related to vascular malformation steal phenomena are also uncommon [4].

Examination of patients with an AVM reveals a cranial or orbital bruit in 10–29% of those patients [4]. Presence of a bruit is not predictive of a differential hemorrhage risk. Larger size and high-flow characteristics of the lesion often are associated with an audible bruit.

B. Intracranial Hemorrhage: Risk, Morbidity, and Mortality

Recent evidence indicates that intracranial hemorrhage may occur in 18% of lesions presenting without prior intracranial hemorrhage. Over a mean follow-up period of 8.2 years, the mean risk of hemorrhage was 2.2% per year. The actuarial risk of bleed was 1.3% per year at one year, 1.7% per year at five years, 1.5% per year at ten years, and 2.2% per year at 15 years. Although nearly 60% of the hemorrhages occurred within the first ten years following diagnosis, a high risk of hemorrhage did persist over time. The mortality rate was noted to be 29%, and 23% of survivors had significant long-term morbidity [4].

Graf and others reported 15 of 134 patients suffering intracranial hemorrhage (11.2%) died as a result of the hemorrhage from the AVM. However, only 71 patients initially had an unruptured AVM, and among the 66 that could be followed, the risk of first hemorrhage was 2% at one year, 14% at five years, and 31% at ten years [48].

In the Cooperative study, 25 of 281 patients with a supratentorial malformation (8.9%) and five out of 26 with an infratentorial lesion (19%) died as a result of that hemorrhage. Fourteen percent of survivors were severely disabled, and an additional 26% were unable to work. The risk of hemorrhage among those presenting with seizures was 1% per year, with a 10% mortality rate [12]. Ondra and others have reported 166 prospective studied unoperated patients with symptomatic AVMs. Of 262 AVMs, 168 had no therapeutic intervention; 160 of those patients were then followed over a mean follow-up time of 23.7 years. Most of the patients (71%) had presented with hemorrhage; the overall yearly bleed rate among all patients was 4.0% with a nearly constant rate of hemorrhage during the initial 20 years of follow up. However, this bleed rate counted all hemorrhages, including recurrences; the risk of first hemorrhage was similar to that reported in other studies [4]. The first hemorrhage after follow up began was associated with a 23% risk of major morbidity or death. Overall, 23% of patients died as a result of AVM hemorrhage [59].

Other information comes from Svien [55], who reported an occurrence of ICH among 95 patients with intracranial AVM of 53%, and 6% of the patients died from the rupture. Forty (85%) of the survivors had a good outcome [55]. In another series, hemorrhage occurred in 27% of 26 patients presenting with seizures, and the mortality from AVM-related hemorrhage was 8%. A higher mortality was reported in those presenting with hemorrhage (14%), and the rebleeding rate was 67% [47].

C. Radiographic Features Predicting Hemorrhage

The small number of conservative-treatment patients followed has made the detection of radiologic predictors of hemorrhage difficult. A variety of angiographic features have been studied as useful indicators of AVM rupture. The size of the AVM was not found to be predictive of hemorrhage in a study of 168 patients with an unruptured AVM [4]. Others have noted that AVMs that are small in size may have a higher risk of rupture [48–51], with size measurements in maximum diameter [53] and AVM volume [61]. Graf noted that lesions less than 3 cm in maximal diameter have a higher risk of rupture. A similar influence was not seen for hemorrhage recurrence [48]. The AVM appearance may change acutely following rupture, including a decrease in size, although it is unclear if these changes persist [60]. Furthermore, AVM size may change over time irrespective of clinically apparent hemorrhage [61]; the frequency of AVM size increase is unknown.

The location of the AVM also has been reported to influence hemorrhage risk [48,57]. Right-sided lesions and temporal-lobe location have been associated with an increased risk of rupture. Others have noted that a periventricular or intraventricular site may be associated with hemorrhage [62,63], although this has not been confirmed in some series [64].

Hemodynamic characteristics that may be ascertained from angiography include degree of shunt and flow [4,54]. Parkinson has reported that lesions with high hemodynamic resistance may be at increased risk of hemorrhage, although others have not reported this finding [4,54].

The venous system may also be important in predicting rupture. Central venous drainage, intranidal aneurysm, or periventricular or intraventricular location were seen as important predictors of hemorrhage in one series [62]. Others have also found deep venous drainage to be a predictor of hemorrhage [71,72]. In the same studies, intranidal aneurysms, multiple aneurysms, feeding by perforators and location in the basal ganglia were predictors of presentation with hemorrhage. There may also be a correlation of increased occurrence of intracranial hemorrhage in deep brain AVMs with impaired venous outlets [72,73]. A single draining vein may also predict a higher risk of AVM rupture [72,74]. Others have not found site of venous drainage or the presence of a venous varix to be useful [4].

D. Recurrent Hemorrhage

It is likely that the risk of hemorrhage increases, at least transiently, following an initial intracranial hemorrhage. Graf and others reported that 24% of 134 patients with hemorrhage experienced a rebleed. The overall risk of rebleeding after the initial rupture was 6% during the first year and about 2% per year thereafter [48]. Among patients presenting with either epilepsy or surgery, a four-year recurrence risk of hemorrhage was 25%. Following a second hemorrhage, the one-year risk of another hemorrhage was 25%.

Among 47 survivors of initial hemorrhage from an AVM in the brain, 16 (34%) had a recurrent bleed with a 13% mortality rate from this recurrent hemorrhage; one in three patients with two bleeds suffered another recurrent bleed [44–45]. In the Cooperative study, 23% of 381 cases had recurrent hemorrhage with a mortality rate of 12% [12]. Forster noted a 25% chance of bleeding within four years in those patients suffering intracranial hemorrhage, while those patients that had bled twice had a one-year recurrent bleeding risk of 25% [46]. A rebleed rate of 4% per year among the subgroup of patients presenting with intracranial hemorrhage was reported in a series from Finland. The risk was unchanged over 20 years; the mean interval between hemorrhages was 7.7 years [49].

IV. ARTERIOVENOUS MALFORMATIONS IN CHILDREN

Symptomatic arteriovenous malformations are not commonly documented prior to the age of 20, yet they are the most common cause of hemorrhage stroke in children [75]. The percentage of patients with these congenital lesions that are diagnosed before adulthood is unknown. Clinical presentations in patients over the age of two years mimic those seen in adults, with hemorrhage apparently accounting for a higher percentage of initial symptoms, in 51–79% of cases [76–78]. In one series of 37 patients, 16 presented with either SAH or SAH with intraparenchymal hematoma. Chronic seizure disorder may be noted in 12–20% of cases and is the most common presentation in those patients without intracranial hemorrhage [79]. The clinical presentation in children under the age of two years is dependent on the high degree of shunt and size of the lesion. Congestive heart failure, an enlarging head due to hydrocephalus, and seizures are most commonly seen [76,79,80].

Mortality from the initial hemorrhage may be higher than that reported in adults [81,82] with 25% mortality in one series, although the mortality fell to 16% after the introduction of computed tomography. Cerebellar lesions that rupture may carry an increased mortality (57%) compared with hemispheric lesions (4.5%). Hemorrhage recurrence rate is similar to that reported in adults, with rebleed occurring in 5 of 23 (22%) of the patients treated conservatively [77]. In another series, the rate of hemorrhage recurrence was 70% among those that were not excised following the initial episode [79]. A fatal, ruptured arteriovenous malformation is an uncommon cause of sudden death in children, causing only one of ten sudden deaths in children in one series [83].

V. ANEURYSMS AND ARTERIOVENOUS MALFORMATIONS

Aneurysms are associated with intracranial arteriovenous malformations in 3.7–9% of patients [21–23,84,85]. Among 91 patients with unruptured intracranial arteriovenous malformations, 16 patients with 26 unruptured intracranial aneurysms were noted in one series [4]. Twenty-five of the aneurysms were on arteries feeding the malformation system with an equal number distributed proximally and distally. Eleven of the aneurysms were atypical in location, and all of those arose from primary or secondary branch feeders to a malformation. The risk of intracranial hemorrhage among patients with co-existing aneurysm and AVM was 7% per year at five years following diagnosis, compared to 1.7% for patients with AVM alone [21]. Previous reports had noted the frequent occurrence of the lesions in association with high-flow arteriovenous malformations. In the Mayo Clinic series, eleven (16%) of the 67 patients with high-flow AVMs had associated aneurysms compared with 5 (21%) of the 24 patients with low-flow AVMs [21]. It is apparent that intracranial AVMs are predisposed to aneurysm formation within AVM feeding systems, although the mechanism is not based simply on high blood flow or high arteriovenous shunt [21,22,85] (Figure 7).

VI. ARTERIOVENOUS MALFORMATIONS AND PREGNANCY

Subarachnoid hemorrhage is an uncommon complication of pregnancy but carries a high rate of maternal and fetal morbidity and mortality [87–94]. Approximately 2% of all SAHs occur during pregnancy [87], with saccular aneurysms causing between 56–75% and arteriovenous malformations between 25–50%. The rate during pregnancy among 451 women with intracranial AVM was reported to be 3.5% in one study. Pregnancy was not found to be a risk factor for hemorrhage in the same study [93], however the conclusions were obscured by difficulties in study design [94].

Almost half of patients with aneurysmal rupture during pregnancy had a previous pregnancy unassociated with hemorrhage, while AVMs often rupture in primiparous patients. In addition to primiparous patients, other differing characteristics of pregnancy-related hemorrhage in patients with AVMs include younger age and occurrence of bleed earlier, during the second trimester. Recur-

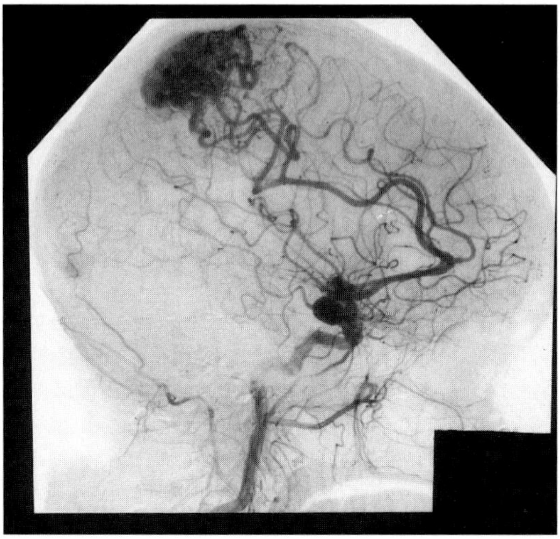

(a)

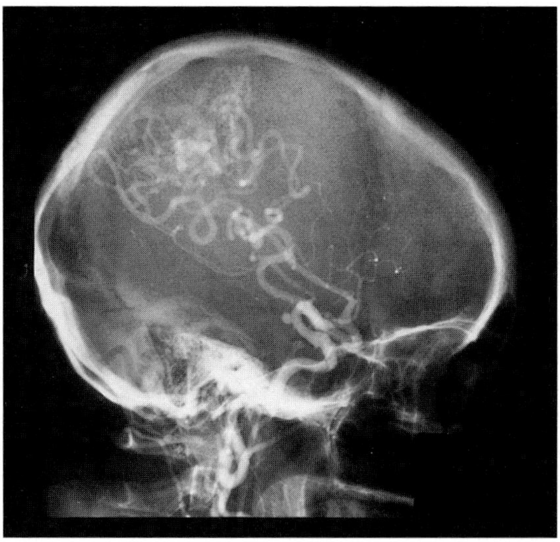

(b)

Figure 7 A 40-year-old female presented with a headache and cranial bruit. Cerebral angiography revealed a 5 × 5 cm high-flow, high-shunt, left parietal arteriovenous malformation with multiple enlarged feeders from the left anterior cerebral artery. Two saccular aneurysms were also noted. A 14 × 10 mm aneurysm was seen in the supraclinoid segment of the right internal carotid artery, and a 6 × 5 mm aneurysm was noted in the left internal carotid artery at the origin of the posterior communicating artery.

rent bleeds are typical during delivery or in subsequent pregnancies while aneurysmal rebleeds are noted after the initial hemorrhage or in the early postpartum period [83,90,92].

The mortality rates for mothers with AVM-related ICH is similar to those in nonpregnant patients [90]. Fetal mortality rates of 5–27% among mothers surviving the ICH [83,90] and a fetal complication occurrence of 49% have been reported [87]. Optimal treatment in the setting of intracranial hemorrhage during pregnancy may include surgical excision of AVM, if SAH occurs before the 35th week of gestation and the AVM is safely approachable. The pregnancy may then be allowed to go to full gestation. In cases of inoperable or partially excised AVM, elective cesarean section should be performed at 38 weeks gestation if the pelvis is proved inadequate. If the pelvis is adequate, vaginal delivery without Valsalva may be considered. Patients with hemorrhage occurring beyond 35 weeks gestation should be considered for cesarean section followed by AVM repair [92].

VII. DURAL ARTERIOVENOUS FISTULAE

Previous studies have examined the clinical presentation of dural arteriovenous fistulae, although the number of conservatively managed patients followed over time is small. Clinical data and limited natural history information are available from small series and literature reviews. In a long-term follow-up study of 54 patients diagnosed before intracranial hemorrhage, 5 of 52 patients experienced intracranial hemorrhage throughout the 6.6 year follow-up, for a crude risk of hemorrhage of 1.5% per year. Using actuarial methods, the risk of hemorrhage at the time of mean follow-up was 1.8% per year. There was an indication that lesions of the petrous sinus and straight sinus had a higher tendency to bleed, although the risk could not be documented independent of pial venous drainage. Dural AVMs with a venous varix on a draining vein also had an increased risk of hemorrhage, while no hemorrhages were seen in the 20 patients without a varix [95]. Previous reviews of the literature also reveal the potential for aggressive behavior including intracranial hemorrhage in the setting of dural arteriovenous malformation [95,96]. Awad and others noted the clinical course to be strongly affected by the dural AVM location, although the aggressive behavior could occur at any site [96]. Angiographic features associated with an aggressive prognosis included leptomeningeal drainage, retrograde venous drainage, variceal venous structures, and galenic venous drainage [97].

The site of intracranial hemorrhage associated with dural arteriovenous malformation depends on the site of the lesion and the structure from which the hemorrhage occurred. Subarachnoid hemorrhage and intraparenchymal are the most common types, although subdural hemorrhage and epidural hematomas may also be seen.

Other clinical manifestations occur in relation to a number of factors associated with the arteriovenous shunt. High venous flow, venous hypertension, arterial steal, cortical venous drainage, and hemorrhage all may lead to symptoms. Pulsatile tinnitus is the most common presenting symptom, while a cranial bruit is heard in 50% of cases. Severe traction headaches with diffuse elevation of intracranial pressure may be associated with papilledema and mental status change. Visual complaints may complicate lesions in the cavernous sinus, including loss of visual acuity, proptosis, diplopia, and conjunctival injection. Focal neurologic deficits of both central and peripheral etiology have also been reported [98].

VIII. SPINAL SUBARACHNOID HEMORRHAGE

Spontaneous spinal subarachnoid hemorrhage accounts for less than 1% of all cases of subarachnoid hemorrhage. Many cases may go undetected because of prominent intracranial symptoms and signs in spinal SAH [99]. Furthermore, signs and symptoms that localize a lesion to the spinal cord, cauda equina, or conus may be absent, discouraging aggressive evaluation of a potential spinal cord lesion.

Arteriovenous malformations are the most common cause of secondary spinal subarachnoid hemorrhage. Twelve to twenty-six percent of spinal AVMs may present with subarachnoid hemorrhage [100,101]. The spinal vascular malformations represent from 3–12% of spinal cord tumors [102]. In addition to spinal arteriovenous malformations, other vascular malformation subtypes may lead to spinal subarachnoid hemorrhage. Spinal tumors may also cause hemorrhage, including ependymoma, neurofibroma, meningiomas, and astrocytomas. Other rare causes include blood dyscrasias, anticoagulant drugs, infection, coarctation of the aorta, and polyarteritis nodosa [101–103].

Although saccular aneurysms are the most common cause of nontraumatic intracranial subarachnoid hemorrhage, arterial aneurysms in the spinal cord are exceedingly rare. The occurrence of aneurysm associated with a spinal AVM has been reported as high as 6% [104], but in a recent review of all cases of spinal AVM, cases were less commonly associated with arterial aneurysm.

IX. SPINAL ARTERIOVENOUS MALFORMATIONS AND SUBARACHNOID HEMORRHAGE

Overall occurrence of symptomatic spinal vascular malformations is higher in males, although the risk of hemorrhage may be higher in females. Nearly 50% of patients have clinical manifestations before the age of 30 years. Fifty-five percent of subarachnoid hemorrhages present in patients younger than 15 years old, and 85% have SAH as a presenting symptom [101]. The wide range of clinical symptoms depend on the localization of the lesion and the degree of intramedullary extension, the longitudinal dimensions of the lesion, the presence of venous stasis, the presence of either AVM distension or a high degree of shunting producing a steal phenomena, and the occurrence of thrombosis in the arterial or venous systems [2,101,103]. Well-localized symptoms are uncommon; weakness of the legs occurs in about one-third of cases and may be variable in severity from day to day. The weakness may be upper motor neuron in type, although a combination of upper and lower motor neuron distribution weakness may be seen [101,103]. Sensory phenomena in either a spinal or radicular distribution may be the initial presentation in 40% of patients. Sphincter disturbances are uncommon initial manifestations, although over 90% of patients have some sphincter disturbance by the time of diagnosis [103].

Spinal subarachnoid hemorrhage may be manifested by the sudden onset of back discomfort. The classical presentation of a stabbing severe back discomfort [105] is distinctly uncommon. If the SAH is associated with localizing spinal cord signs, the diagnosis may be made more easily.

The clinical presentation of spinal SAH may be broken down into three major groups [106]. One group of patients has primary spinal cord damage leading to myelopathic findings, while nerve root compression may lead to radiculopathy in the second group. Most of these subarachnoid hemorrhages are caused by vascular malformations that are at least in part intramedullary [101]. In another subgroup, intracranial symptoms including headache, mental status change, and loss of consciousness occur with intracranial extension of the hemorrhage [95,106,107]. The sudden, often recurrent episodes of severe back pain are produced by hemorrhage in the spinal subarachnoid space and lead to later signs of meningeal irritation [95,106].

Foix and Alajouanine described a syndrome of spinal vascular malformation producing subacutely to chronically progressive paraparesis, associated with venous stasis in the absence of arterial thrombosis [108]. Elevated venous pressure, transmitted through the high shunt from the arterial system, may lead to decreased arterial perfusion and progressive spinal cord infarction. Most of the cases have been associated with an AVM on the dura in the lower thoracic region, and a predominance of the lesions occur in males. The diagnosis is rarely made within six months after the onset of symptoms, and in over two-thirds of cases, the diagnosis is not made until symptoms have been present for over one year [109].

The delineation of a spinal or paraspinal bruit is a helpful clinical finding in the diagnosis of a spinal vascular malformation. Unfortunately, a bruit is uncommonly present. Aminoff reported that two of 12 patients that had adequate spinal auscultation in the setting of a spinal AVM had a bruit [100].

Spinal arteriovenous malformations may be subdivided based on the major arterial supplier, degree of flow, and type of shunt. While most malformations supplied by the anterior spinal artery have an intramedullary component, those supplied by posterior feeders are often extramedullary. Aminoff and others proposed the division of cases into those with posterior or anterior supply, with the anterior divisions further subdivided into intramedullary and the uncommon extramedullary lesions. They further noted that there is significant impact on the natural history based on the type of supply. All of the cases with subarachnoid hemorrhage had anterior supply with the exception of a single cervical lesion. Posterior malformations tended to follow a progressive course in 60% of cases. Other natural history characteristics that differentiate between the posterior- and anterior-supplied lesions include the age at onset, with 86% of patients noting symptoms before age 40 years having anterior-supplied lesions and 85% presenting after age 40 years with posterior-supplied lesions. A much higher percentage of the posterior-supplied lesions are male (87%) compared with intramedullary or mixed anterior-supplied lesions (57%) [100].

REFERENCES

1. McCormick WF. Pathology of vascular malformations of the brain. In: Wilson CB, Stein BM (Eds). Intracranial Arteriovenous Malformations. Baltimore, Maryland: Williams and Wilkins, 1984:44–63.
2. Jellinger K. Vascular malformations of the central nervous system: a morphological overview. *Neurosurg Rev* 1986; 9:177–216.
3. Stehbens WE. Telangiectases, hemangiomas, arteriovenous aneurysms, and allied disorders. In: Pathology of the Cerebral Blood Vessels. St. Louis: CV Mosby, 1972:471–558.
4. Brown RD Jr, Wiebers DO, Forbes G, O'Fallon WM, Piepgras DG, Marsh WR, et al. The natural history of unruptured intracranial arteriovenous malformations. *J Neurosurg* 1988; 68:352–357.
5. Wilkins RH. The natural history of intracranial vascular malformations: a review. *Neurosurgery* 1985; 16:421–430.
6. Michelson WJ. Natural history and pathophysiology of arteriovenous malformations. *Clin Neurosurg* 1978; 26:307–313.
7. Olivecrona H, Riives J. Arteriovenous aneurysms of the brain: their diagnosis and treatment. *Arch Neurol Psychiatry* 1948; 59:567–603.
8. McCormick WF, Schochet SS, Jr. Atlas of Cerebrovascular Disease. Philadelphia: WB Saunders Company, 1976:422.
9. Gross CR, Kase CS, Mohr JP, Cunningham SC, Baker WE. Stroke in south Alabama: incidence and diagnostic features—a population study. *Stroke* 1984; 15:249–255.
10. Furlan AJ, Whisnant JP, Elveback LR. The decreasing incidence of primary intracerebral hemorrhage: a population study. *Ann Neurol* 1979; 5:367–373.

11. Ingall TJ, Whisnant JP, Wiebers DO, O'Fallon WM. Has there been a decline in subarachnoid hemorrhage mortality? *Stroke* 1989; 20:718–724.
12. Perret G, Nishioka H. Report on the cooperative study of intracranial aneurysms and subarachnoid hemorrhage. Section VI. Arteriovenous Malformations. *J Neurosurg* 1966; 25:467–490.
13. Leblanc R, Ethier R, Little JR. Computed tomography findings in arteriovenous malformations of the brain. *J Neurosurg* 1979; 51:765–772.
14. Takahashi M, Sonobe M, Shirane R, Kubota Y, Kawakami H. Computed tomography of ruptured intracranial arteriovenous malformations in the acute stage. *Acta Neurochir* 1962; 66:87–94.
15. Aoki N. Do intracranial arteriovenous malformations cause subarachnoid hemorrhage? Review of computed tomography features of ruptured arteriovenous malformations in the acute stage. *Acta Neurochir* 1991; 112:92–95.
16. McCormick WF, Hardman JM, Boulter TR. Vascular malformations ("angiomas") of the brain, with special reference to those occurring in the posterior fossa. *J Neurosurg* 1968; 28:241–251.
17. McCormick WF. The pathology of vascular ("arteriovenous") malformations. *J Neurosurg* 1966; 24:807–816.
18. Kumar AJ, Fox MW, Vinuela F, Rosenbaum AE. Revisited old and new findings in unruptured larger arteriovenous malformations of the brain. *J Comput Assist Tomogr* 1984; 8:648–655.
19. Kucharczyk W, Lemme-Pleghos L, Uske A, Brant-Zawadzki M, Dooms G, Norman D. Intracranial vascular malformations: MR and CT imaging. *Radiology* 1985; 56:383–389.
20. Huston J, Rufenacht DA, Ehman RL, Wiebers DO. Intracranial aneurysms and vascular malformations: comparison of time-of-flight and phase-contrast MR angiography. *Radiology* 1991; 181:721–730.
21. Brown RD Jr, Wiebers DO, Forbes GS. Unruptured intracranial aneurysms and arteriovenous malformations: frequency of intracranial hemorrhage and relationship of lesions. *J Neurosurg* 1990; 73:859–863.
22. Miyasaka K, Wolpert SM, Prager RJ. The association of cerebral aneurysms, infundibula, and intracranial arteriovenous malformations. *Stroke* 1982; 13:196–203.
23. Batjer H, Suss RA, Sampson D. Intracranial arteriovenous malformations associated with aneurysms. *Neurosurgery* 1986; 18:29–35.
24. Houser OW, Campbell JK, Campbell RJ, Sundt TM Jr. Arteriovenous malformation affecting the transverse dural venous sinus—an acquired lesion. *Mayo Clin Proc* 1979; 54:651–661.
25. Chen J, Tsuruda JS, Halbach VV. Suspected dural arteriovenous fistula: results with screening MR angiography in seven patients. *Radiology* 1992; 183:265–271.
26. Becker DH, Townsend JJ, Kramer RA, Newton TH. Occult cerebrovascular malformations: a series of 18 histologically verified cases with negative angiography. *Brain* 1979; 102:249–287.
27. Warren RE Jr, Scheithauer BW, Laws ER Jr. Thrombosed arteriovenous malformations of the brain. *J Neurosurg* 1982; 57:520–526.
28. Wakai S, Ueda Y, Inoh S, Nagai M. Angiographic occult angiomas: a report of 13

cases with analysis of the cases documented in the literature. *Neurosurgery* 1985; 17:549–556.

29. Rapacki TFX, Brantley MJ, Furlow TW Jr, Geyer CA, Toro VE, George ED. Heterogeneity of cerebral cavernous hemangiomas diagnosed by MR imaging. *J Comp Assist Tomog* 1990; 14:18–25.
30. New PF, Ojemann RG, Davis KR, Rosen BR, Heros R, Kjellberg RN, et al. MR and CT of occult vascular malformations of the brain. *AJR* 1986; 147:985–993.
31. Rigamonti D, Drayer BP, Johnson PC, Hadley MN, Zabramski J, Spetzler RF. The MRI appearance of cavernous hemangiomas (angiomas). *J Neurosurg* 1987; 67:518–524.
32. Robinson JR, Awad IA, Little JR. Natural history of the cavernous angioma. *J Neurosurg* 1991; 75:709–714.
33. Curling OD Jr, Kelly DL Jr, Elster AD, Craven TE. An analysis of the natural history of cavernous angiomas. *J Neurosurg* 1991; 75:702–708.
34. Zimmerman RS, Spetzler RF, Lee KS, Zabramski JM, Hargraves RW. Cavernous malformations of the brainstem. *J Neurosurg* 1991; 75:32–39.
35. Abe M, Kjellberg RN, Adams RD. Clinical presentations of vascular malformations of the brainstem: comparison of angiographically positive and negative types. *J Neurol Neurosurg Psychiatry* 1989; 52:167–175.
36. Tung H, Giannotta SL, Chandrasoma PT, Zee Chi-Shing. Recurrent intraparenchymal hemorrhages from angiographically occult vascular malformations. *J Neurosurg* 1990; 73:174–180.
37. Rigamonti D, Spetzler RF, Drayer BP, Bojanowski WM, Hoda KJ, Rigamonti KH, et al. Appearance of venous malformations on magnetic resonance imaging. *J Neurosurg* 1988; 69:535–539.
38. Valavanis A, Wellauer J, Yasargil MG. The radiologic diagnosis of cerebral venous angiomas: cerebral angiography and computed tomography. *Neuroradiology* 1983; 24:193–199.
39. Sarwar M, McCormick WF. Intracerebral venous angioma: case report and review. *Arch Neurol* 1978; 35:323–328.
40. Moritake K, Handa H, Mori K, Ishikawa M, Morimoto M, Takebe Y. Venous angiomas of the brain. *Surg Neurol* 1980; 14:95–105.
41. Handa H, Moritake K. Venous angiomas of the brain. In: Fein JM, Flamm ES (Eds). Cerebrovascular Surgery. Volume 4. New York: Springer-Verlag; 1985:1139–1149.
42. Namaguchi Y, Kitamura K, Fukui M, Ikeda J, Hasuo K, Kishikawa T, et al. Intracranial venous angiomas. *Surg Neurol* 1982; 18:197–202.
43. Biller J, Toffol GJ, Shay JF, Fine M, Azar-Kia BN. Cerebellar venous angiomas: a continuing controversy. *Arch Neurol* 1985; 42:367–370.
44. Albert P. Personal experience in the treatment of 178 cases of arteriovenous malformations of the brain. *Acta Neurochir* 1982; 61:207–226.
45. Crawford PM, West CR, Chadwick DW, Shaw MD. Arteriovenous malformations of the brain: the natural history in unoperated patients. *J Neurol Neurosurg Psychiatry* 1986; 49:1–10.
46. Forster DMC, Steiner L, Hakanson S. Arteriovenous malformations of the brain. A long-term clinical study. *J Neurosurg* 1972; 37:562–570.

47. Fults D, Kelly DL. Natural history of arteriovenous malformations of the brain: a clinical study. *Neurosurgery* 1984; 15:658–662.
48. Graf CJ, Perret GE, Torner JC. Bleeding from cerebral arteriovenous malformations as part of their natural history. *J Neurosurg* 1983; 58:331–337.
49. Henderson WR, Gomez RLD. Natural history of cerebral angiomas. *Br Med J* 1967; 4:571–574.
50. Guidetti B, Delitala A. Intracranial arteriovenous malformations: conservative and surgical treatment. *J Neurosurg* 1980; 53:149–152.
51. Houser OW, Baker HL Jr, Svien HJ, Okazaki H. Arteriovenous malformations of the parenchyma of the brain: angiographic aspects. *Radiology* 1973; 109:83–90.
52. Jomin M, Lesoin F, Lozes G. Prognosis for arteriovenous malformations of the brain in adults based on 150 cases. *Surg Neurol* 1985; 23:362–366.
53. Morello G, Borghi GP. Cerebral angiomas. A report of 154 personal cases and a comparison between the results of surgical excision and conservative management. *Acta Neurochir* 1973; 28:135–155.
54. Parkinson D, Bachers G. Arteriovenous malformations. Summary of 100 consecutive supratentorial cases. *J Neurosurg* 1980; 53:285–299.
55. Svien JH, McRae JA. Arteriovenous anomalies of the brain: fate of patients not having definitive surgery. *J Neurosurg* 1965; 23:23–28.
56. Svien HJ, Olive I, Angulo-Rivero P. The fate of patients who have cerebral arteriovenous anomalies without definite surgical treatments. *J Neurosurg* 1956; 13:381–387.
57. Troupp H, Marttila I, Halonen V. Arteriovenous malformations of the brain. Prognosis without operation. *Acta Neurochir* 1970; 22:125–128.
58. Trumpy JH, Eldevik P. Intracranial arteriovenous malformations: conservative or surgical treatment? *Surg Neurol* 1977; 8:171–175.
59. Ondra SL, Troupp H, George UED, Schwab K. The natural history of symptomatic arteriovenous malformations of the brain: a 24–year follow-up assessment. *J Neurosurg* 1990; 73:387–391.
60. London D, Enzmann D. The changing angiographic appearance of an arteriovenous malformation after subarachnoid hemorrhage. *Neuroradiology* 1981; 21:281–284.
61. Waltimo O. The relationship of size, density, and localization of intracranial arteriovenous malformations to the type of initial symptoms. *J Neurol Sci* 1973; 19:21–27.
62. Marks MP, Lane B, Steinberg GK, Chang PJ. Hemorrhage in intracerebral arteriovenous malformations: angiographic determinants. *Radiology* 1990; 176:807–813.
63. Nagata S, Matsushima T, Fujii K, Takeshita I, Fukui M, Yasumori K. Lateral ventricular arteriovenous malformations: natural history and surgical indications. *Acta Neurochir* 1991; 112:37–46.
64. Pia HW. The acute treatment of cerebral arteriovenous angiomas associated with hematomas. In: Pia HW, Gleare JRW, Grote E, Zierski J, (eds). Cerebral Angiomas. New York: Springer, 1975:155–177.
65. Aminoff MJ. Treatment of unruptured cerebral arteriovenous malformations. *Neurology* 1987; 37:815–819.
66. Andersen EB, Petersen J, Mortensen EL, Udesen H. Conservatively treated patients with cerebral arteriovenous malformations: mental and physical outcome. *J Neurol Neurosurg Psychiatry* 1988; 51:1208–1212.

67. Mackenzie I. The clinical presentation of cerebral angioma: a review of 50 cases. *Brain* 1953; 76:184–214.
68. Olivecrona H, Riives J. Arteriovenous aneurysms of the brain. The diagnosis and treatment. *Arch Neurol Psychiatry* 1948; 59:567–602.
69. Nishimura K, Hawkins T. Cerebral vasospasm with subarachnoid hemorrhage from arteriovenous malformations of the brain. *Neuroradiology* 1975; 201–207.
70. Sasaki T, Mayanagi Y, Yano H, Kim S. Cerebral vasospasm with subarachnoid hemorrhage from cerebral arteriovenous malformations. *Surg Neurol* 1981; 16:183–187.
71. Turjman F, Massoud TJ, Vinuela F, Sayre JW, Guglielmi G, Duckwiler G. Correlation of the angioarchitectural features of cerebral arteriovenous malformations with clinical presentation of hemorrhage. *Neurosurgery* 1995; 37:856–862.
72. Miyasaka Y, Yada K, Ohwada T, Kitahara T, Kurata A, Irikura K. An analysis of the venous drainage system as a factor in hemorrhage from arteriovenous malformations. *J Neurosurg* 1992; 76:239–243.
73. Vinuela F, Nombela L, Roach MR, Fox AJ, Pelz DM. Stenotic and occlusive disease of the venous drainage system of deep brain AVM's. *J Neurosurg* 1985; 63:180–184.
74. Albert P, Salgado H, Polaina M, Trujillo F, Ponce de Leon A, Durand F. A study on the venous drainage of 150 cerebral arteriovenous malformations as related to haemorrhagic risks and size of the lesion. *Acta Neurochir* 1990; 103:30–34.
75. Sano K, Ueda Y, Saito I. Subarachnoid hemorrhage in children. *Childs Brain* 1978; 4:38–46.
76. Kelly JJ Jr, Mellinger JF, Sundt TM Jr. Intracranial arteriovenous malformations in childhood. *Ann Neurol* 1978; 3:338–343.
77. Kondziolka D, Humphreys RP, Hoffman JJ, Hendrick EB, Drake JM. Arteriovenous malformations of the brain in children: a forty–year experience. *Can J Neurol Sci* 1992; 19:40–45.
78. Suarez JC, Viano JC. Intracranial arteriovenous malformations in infancy and adolescence. *Childs Nerv Syst* 1989; 5:15–18.
79. Malik GM, Sadasivan B, Knighton RS, Ausman JI. The management of arteriovenous malformations in children *Childs Nerv Syst* 1991; 7:43–47.
80. Melville C, Walsh K, Sreeram N. Cerebral arteriovenous malformations in the neonate: clinical presentation, diagnosis, and outcome. *Int J Cardiol* 1991; 31:175–180.
81. Mori K, Murata T, Hashimoto N, Handa H. Clinical analysis of arteriovenous malformations in children. *Childs Brain* 1980; 6:13–25.
82. Celli P, Ferante L, Palma L, Cavedon G. Cerebral arteriovenous malformations in children: clinical features and outcome of treatment in children and adults. *Clin Neurol* 1984; 22:43–49.
83. Byard RW, Bourne AJ, Hanieh A. Sudden and unexpected death due to hemorrhage from occult central nervous system lesions: a pediatric autopsy study. *Pediatr Neurosurg* 1991–92; 17:88–94.
84. Paterson JH, McKissock W. A clinical survey of intracranial angiomas with special reference to their mode of progression and surgical treatment: a report of 110 cases. *Brain* 1956; 79:233–266.

85. Cronqvist S, Troupp H. The intracranial arteriovenous malformation and arterial aneurysm in the same patient. *Acta Neurol Scand* 1966; 42:307–316.
86. Suzuki J, Onuma T. Intracranial aneurysms associated with arteriovenous malformations. *J Neurosurg* 1979; 50:742–746.
87. Robinson JL, Hall CS, Sedzimir CB. Arteriovenous malformations, aneurysms, and pregnancy. *J Neurosurg* 1974; 41:63–70.
88. Sadasivan B, Malik GM, Lee C, Ausman JI. Vascular malformations and pregnancy. *Surg Neurol* 1990; 33:305–313.
89. Fox MW, Harms RW, Davis DH. Selected neurologic complications in pregnancy. *Mayo Clin Proc* 1990; 65:1595–1618.
90. Dias MS, Sekhar LN. Intracranial hemorrhage from aneurysms and arteriovenous malformations during pregnancy and the puerperium. *Neurosurgery* 1990; 27:855–866.
91. Robinson JL, Chir B, Hall CJ, Sedzimir CB. Subarachnoid hemorrhage in pregnancy. *J Neurosurg* 1972; 36:27–33.
92. Wiebers DO. Subarachnoid hemorrhage in pregnancy. *Semin Neurol* 1988; 8:226–229.
93. Horton JC, Chambers WA, Lyons SL, Adams RD, Kjellberg RN. Pregnancy and the risk of hemorrhage from cerebral arteriovenous malformations. *Neurosurgery* 1990; 27:867–872.
94. Wiebers DO. Pregnancy and the risk of hemorrhage from cerebral arteriovenous malformations. Review. *Neurosurgery* 1990; 27:872–873.
95. Brown RD Jr, Wiebers DO, Nichols DA. Intracranial dural arteriovenous malformations: a clinical radiologic, and long-term follow-up study. *Stroke* 1992; 23:157.
96. Awad IA, Little JR, Akrawi WP, Ahl J. Intracranial dural arteriovenous malformations: factors predisposing to an aggressive neurological course. *J Neurosurg* 1990; 72:839–850.
97. Malik GM, Pearce JE, Ausman JI, Mehta B. Dural arteriovenous malformations and intracranial hemorrhage. *Neurosurgery* 1984; 15:332–338.
98. Castaigne P, Bories J, Brunet P, Merland J, Meininger V. Les fistules arterioveineuses meningees pures a drainate veineux cortical. *Rev Neurol* 1976; 132:169–181.
99. Caroscio JT, Brannan T, Budabin M, Huang IP, Yahr MD. Subarachnoid hemorrhage secondary to spinal arteriovenous malformation and aneurysm. Report of a case and review of the literature. *Arch Neurol* 1980; 37:101–103.
100. Aminoff MJ, Logue V. The prognosis of patients with spinal vascular malformation. *Brain* 1974; 97:211–218.
101. Djindjian M. Clinical symptomatology and natural history of AVMs of the spinal cord. A study of the clinical aspects and prognosis based on 150 cases. In: Pia HW, Djindjian R (eds). Spinal Angiomas. Advances in Diagnosis and Therapy. Berlin, New York, Eidelberg: Springer, 1978; 75–83.
102. Odom GL. Vascular lesions of the spinal cord: malformations, spinal subarachnoid and extradural hemorrhage. *Clin Neurosurg* 1960; 8:196–234.
103. Aminoff MJ. Spinal angiomas. Oxford London Endenberg Melburn: Blackwell, 1976:43.

104. Miyamoto S, Kikuchi H, Karasawa J, Ikota T, Nagata I. Spinal cord arteriovenous malformations associated with spinal aneurysms. *Neurology* 1983; 13:577–580.
105. Michon PL. Le coup de poignard rachidien symptome initial de certaines hemorragies sousarachnoidiennes: essai sur les hemorragies meningees spinales. *Press Med* 1928; 36:964–966.
106. Henson RA, Croft PB. Spontaneous spinal subarachnoid hemorrhage. *QJ Med* 1956; 25:53–66.
107. Walton DN. Subarachnoid hemorrhage of unusual aetiology. *Neurology* 1953; 3:517–543.
108. Foix C, Alajouanine T. La myelite necrotique subaigue. *Rev Neurol* 1926; 2:1–42.
109. Mourier KL, Gelberg F, Rey A, Assouline E, George B, Reizine D, et al. Spinal dural arteriovenous malformations with perimedullary drainage: indications and results of surgery in 30 cases. *Acta Neurochir* 1989; 100:136–141.

7
Subarachnoid Hemorrhage Without Detectable Aneurysm

Gabriel J. E. Rinkel
University of Utrecht, The Netherlands

Eelco F. M. Wijdicks
Mayo Clinic, Rochester, Minnesota

I. INTRODUCTION

A nondiagnostic four-vessel angiogram occurs in 15 to 20 percent of patients with spontaneous subarachnoid hemorrhage [1]. The patients with a so-called angiogram-negative subarachnoid hemorrhage are often lumped together as a homogenous group and remain a diagnostic challenge. Numerous reports have emphasized that the prognosis in patients with angiogram-negative subarachnoid hemorrhage seems better than that in patients with a detected aneurysm. However, outcome is not invariably favorable; 10 to 30 percent of surviving patients do not recover to their previous state, and rebleeding, cerebral ischemia, and acute hydrocephalus have been reported in up to 20 percent of these patients [2–16].

In clinical practice, causes other than a hidden aneurysm should be considered, but most clinicians will remain extremely suspicious until follow-up angiograms have confirmed that no aneurysm can be detected. In recent years it has become clear that the outcome depends on the pattern of hemorrhage viewed with computerized tomography (CT). According to this pattern, patients with truly a benign prognosis can be set apart from patients who are at risk of complications and a poor outcome.

This chapter will review the possible diagnoses in subarachnoid hemorrhage with an initial normal angiogram and will give guidelines for the management of these patients.

II. THE PATTERNS OF HEMORRHAGE ON CT

The majority of patients without an aneurysm on the angiogram have a typical pattern of hemorrhage on CT, wherein the center of the bleeding is immediately anterior to the midbrain and the extravasated blood predominates in the perimesencephalic cisterns. There is no extension of blood to the lateral sylvian fissures or to the anterior interhemispheric fissure (Figure 1). Some sedimentation in the posterior horns may be seen, but frank intraventricular hemorrhage or extension into the parenchyma rule out that the patient belongs to this cate-

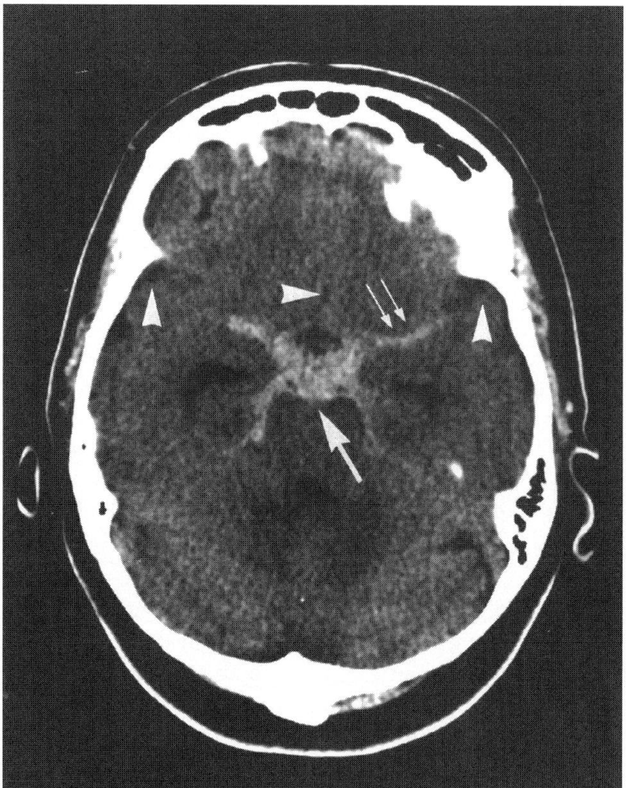

Figure 1 CT scan showing a perimesencephalic pattern of hemorrhage. The center of the bleeding is in the interpeduncular cistern (large arrow). There is some extension to the central parts of the sylvian fissures (small arrow), but not to the lateral part of the sylvian fissures or the anterior part of the interhemispheric fissure (arrowheads). There is no intraventricular blood.

gory [17]. Patients with this so-called perimesencephalic hemorrhage run an uncomplicated clinical course and invariably have an excellent prognosis.

The invariably good prognosis of patients with a perimesencephalic hemorrhage contrasts with the outcome of patients with diffuse or anteriorly located blood in the basal cisterns. In a recent report of 36 patients with diffuse or anteriorly located blood, three had a rebleed, five had symptomatic acute hydrocephalus, and one patient deteriorated from cerebral ischemia [18]. On long term follow-up another patient died from rebleeding. Ultimately, three of these 36 patients died and six were left disabled as the result of the hemorrhage [18]. In three other studies in which patients with angiogram-negative subarachnoid hemorrhage were subdivided according to the pattern of hemorrhage on CT [19,20,21], all patients with complications and poor outcome had hemorrhagic patterns different from the perimesencephalic pattern. In most poor-outcome patients in these studies, the center of the bleeding was located in the anterior interhemispheric fissure. The leading cause of hemorrhage in patients with a normal angiogram and a diffuse or anteriorly located hemorrhage in the basal cisterns is an occult aneurysm, but other causes should be considered as well.

Other patterns of hemorrhage are rare. Blood confined to the superficial cortical sulci is very common in patients with head injury. In a small minority of patients with trauma, the blood is confined to the posterior part of the ambient cistern at the level of the tentorial margin [22].

Although CT scans show blood in the vast majority of patients, a normal CT does not rule out subarachnoid hemorrhage [23]. We found only three patients with a normal CT in a personal series of 116 patients with subarachnoid hemorrhage and a normal angiogram. With these patients CT scans were made on the first or second day after the hemorrhage. All three had a good outcome after a median period of follow up of 55 months [24].

III. THE CLINICAL FEATURES AND DIAGNOSIS OF THE POSSIBLE CAUSES

A. Idiopathic Perimesencephalic Hemorrhage

Perimesencephalic hemorrhage constitutes approximately 10 percent of all patients with subarachnoid hemorrhage and two-thirds of those with a normal angiogram [17,19,25]. Most patients are in their sixth decade, but this type of hemorrhage can occur in younger patients and even in young children [26]. Conspicuously absent is a history of a warning headache and only few patients have a history of hypertension [27].

In one-third of the patients, strenuous activities precede the onset of symptoms [27]. The features at onset are often not as dramatic as in patients with aneurysmal rupture: the onset of the headache is gradual (minutes rather than seconds) in one-fourth of the patients, loss of consciousness is exceptional, and focal abnormalities have not been observed [25,27]. On admission, all patients are in perfect clinical condition, apart from their headache. Although 20 percent of patients have acute hydrocephalus on their admission CT scan, only few have symptoms from it, and even then an excellent outcome can be anticipated [28]. The clinical course is otherwise uneventful: delayed cerebral ischemia does not occur and rebleeds have not been documented thus far, even after a long interval in a large series of patients [18,27]. The period of convalescence is short and most patients are able to resume their previous lifestyle and work [29].

The diagnosis of perimesencephalic hemorrhage rests on the typical pattern of hemorrhage on CT and one normal angiogram. Within the category of perimesencephalic hemorrhage we include patients in whom the subarachnoid blood is confined to the prepontine cistern as well. Although the blood distribution in these patients is not perimesencephalic in the strict sense, the clinical features and outcome of these patients resemble those of patients with a genuine perimesencephalic hemorrhage [17]. A single angiogram is still obligatory since approximately 5 percent of patients with a perimesencephalic pattern of hemorrhage on CT have a ruptured basilar artery aneurysm [17,30,31]. The invariably good outcome and the absence of rebleeding on the long-term minimize the need for repeated angiograms. Moreover, the yield of repeated angiograms in these patients is negligible: in 40 patients with a perimesencephalic hemorrhage no single aneurysm was found on repeated studies [20, 21,32]. On the other hand, repeating the angiography of the posterior circulation is not without risks: in a recent study 3 of 16 patients had complications from a repeated angiography of the vertebral arteries [33]. Repeated angiography is therefore not indicated in patients with a perimesencephalic hemorrhage.

Perimesencephalic hemorrhage is no longer a mere esoteric peculiarity. In recent years one Japanese and several western-European studies have found patients with this particular pattern of hemorrhage and have confirmed the invariably good outcome in this subset of hemorrhage [19,20,30,31]. Similar observations have been made in North America [34]. These additional studies confirm that the perimesencephalic nonaneurysmal subarachnoid hemorrhage is a distinct clinical entity.

The definition of this variant of subarachnoid hemorrhage provisionally remains a descriptive one, since postmortem studies have not yet been obtained. The often mild clinical features, the limited extension of the blood on CT, and the normal angiograms in a large series of patients with this pattern of hemorrhage all argue against a ruptured aneurysm as source of the hemorrhage. Rupture of a dilated vein or a venous malformation in the prepontine or interpeduncular cistern seems a more reasonable hypothesis.

1. Occult Aneurysm

A quarter of patients with an aneurysmal pattern of hemorrhage on CT but a normal angiogram are in a poor clinical condition on admission and a quarter die or remain disabled as the result of the hemorrhage. These clinical features more closely resemble those of patients with a ruptured aneurysm than those of patients with a perimesencephalic hemorrhage. The high incidence of rebleeding in patients with an aneurysmal pattern of hemorrhage indicates that in at least some patients an aneurysm escaped radiological detection. Although it has been argued that repeating the angiogram is useless [2,35], combined data of seven studies on patients with angiogram-negative subarachnoid hemorrhage reveal that 135 repeated angiograms demonstrated no less than 22 aneurysms [7–10,12,13,32]. If one takes into account that patients with a perimesencephalic hemorrhage—who constitute two-third of patients without an aneurysm on the initial angiogram—were not excluded from these series, the yield of follow-up angiograms in patients with diffuse or anteriorly located hemorrhage on CT must be even higher. In a recent report of patients with an initially normal angiogram, a repeated study revealed an aneurysm in 7 of 10 patients with blood predominantly in the anterior interhemispheric fissure; one of three patients had blood predominantly in the sylvian fissure [32]. Few data exist on the yield of a third angiogram; in one series of 14 patients subjected to a third angiogram one aneurysm was found [10]. Anecdotal cases support the need for a third angiogram in selected patients [18,36,37]. The reasons for missing an aneurysm on angiography are not fully understood. Apart from more obvious reasons such as poor technique or insufficient projections, which probably account for a significant proportion of nonrevealing angiograms, several other explanations for false-negative angiograms have been proposed: 1. narrowing of vessels by vasospasm [38,39], 2. thrombosis of the aneurysm stalk or the entire sac [39,40,41], 3. microaneurysms too small to be detected on angiography [9,42,43], and (4) obliteration of the aneurysm by pressure of an adjacent hematoma. This latter possibility is supported by a recent report of two patients with a hematoma in the anterior interhemispheric fissure and with repeatedly normal angiograms, in whom exploratory craniotomy disclosed a patent anterior communicating artery aneurysm [44].

The substantial risk of a fatal rebleed, the several causes of nondetection of an aneurysm, and the relatively high yield of aneurysms on follow up angiograms favor a second angiography, despite its inherent risks.

2. Vertebral Artery Dissection

The proportion of vertebral artery dissections in patients with subarachnoid hemorrhage is unknown, but in a recent autopsy series a dissection was found in 5 of 110 patients with subarachnoid hemorrhage [36]. Most patients with a dissection are middle-aged, and approximately one-third is on treatment for hypertension [45]. The onset may be presaged by uncommon neck movements or by minor neck trauma. Some patients have biphasic headaches: a severe headache extending from the back of the neck, hours to days later followed by a sudden exacerbation of the headache. In patients with such biphasic headaches, the first episode may represent the beginning of the dissection and not meningeal irritation, as the initial headache can be indistinguishable from that of patients who develop brainstem infarcts and who have no subarachnoid blood on CT at that time [45]. In other patients, however, subarachnoid hemorrhage occurs immediately with the first symptoms [46]. On examination most patients only have meningeal irritation, but additional features may include lower cranial nerve palsies, Horner's syndrome, or more extensive lateral medullary syndromes [45,47]. Rebleeds are found in 30 percent of the patients, sometimes within hours of the initial hemorrhage but also after several weeks. These rebleeds are fatal in half the patients [45,46,47]. The clinical course can otherwise be complicated by hydrocephalus, hyponatremia, or pulmonary edema [47,48]. Approximately half the reported patients have a good outcome [45,47]. In some patients the dissection extends into the basilar artery; outcome is usually poor in those patients [47,48,49], although there are exceptions [50].

Blood throughout the cisterns is shown on CT scans and often intraventricular blood as well, with a predominance in the fourth and third ventricle [36,47]. In patients with a dissection, CT or magnetic resonance (MR) imaging may detect a thrombus within the false lumen of the dissection [51,52]. Angiographically the diagnosis rests on the demonstration of narrowing of the artery with signs of intimal flap, a pseudo-aneurysm, or a double lumen, but these features may be absent on an initial angiogram. In a series of 14 patients with a vertebral artery dissection, the first angiogram was normal in two and showed only nonspecific arterial narrowing in two others [48]. In these four patients only the second angiogram revealed the characteristic abnormalities. A second angiogram is not always diagnostic, since dissecting aneurysms may resolve spontaneously [48].

3. Carotid Artery Dissection

Only a few patients with subarachnoid hemorrhage from dissection of the intracranial portion of the carotid artery or its branches have been reported [53–57]. The presenting features are the same as in aneurysmal rupture: a severe headache of sudden onset, which may be accompanied by focal deficits; a depressed level of consciousness; or both. Rebleeds documented by CT have been reported [55]. The patterns of hemorrhage on CT of patients with dissection of the anterior or middle cerebral artery are indistinguishable from those of patients with a ruptured saccular aneurysm at these sites [55,57]. The diagnosis is made on the typical angiographic features, such as the double-lumen sign or a pseudoaneurysm. These features may not yet have developed on an early angiogram (within two weeks of the hemorrhage), which then only shows small filling defects that are easily overlooked or irregular narrowing that resembles vasospasm. Repeated angiograms after two or three months may disclose the true cause of the hemorrhage in these patients [55].

4. Dural Arteriovenous Malformation

Dural arteriovenous malformations (AVM) of the tentorium can give rise to a basal hemorrhage that is indistinguishable on CT from aneurysmal hemorrhage [58]. The anomaly is rare and can be found from adolescence up to old age. Rebleeding may occur in patients with dural AVMs; in a series of 5 patients presenting with subarachnoid hemorrhage, three had one or more rebleeds [59].

If CT scanning suggests a tentorial origin of the hemorrhage, repeated angiography should include visualization of the external carotid artery because branches of this artery can be the main or the sole feeders [60].

5. Arteriovenous Malformation of the Cervical Spine

Approximately 10 percent of patients with a spinal AVM present with a subarachnoid hemorrhage; in more than half of these patients the first hemorrhage occurs before the age of 20 [61,62]. Symptoms may start with a sudden and excruciating pain (*coup de poignard* or dagger thrust) in the lower part of the neck [62]. In other patients, pain radiating to the shoulders or arms points to a cervical origin of the hemorrhage [63]. If such clues are absent, the true origin of the hemorrhage emerges only when spinal cord dysfunction develops—after a delay that may be as short as a few hours or as long as a few years [62,64]. Rebleeds occur in half of the patients who survive the initial bleed [65], and eventually less than 10 percent of patients who have bled once remain asymptomatic thereafter [66]. Computerized tomography may show blood throughout the basal cisterns and ventricles [63]. Vertebral or spinal angiography can demonstrate the lesion. However, this procedure is not always diagnostic [62,64], is impractical without localizing signs or symptoms, and carries a risk of over 5 percent that persisting neurological deficit will ensue [67]. At present, MR imaging in the sagittal plane seems to be the first line of investigation.

6. Trauma

In most patients with trauma, the subarachnoid hemorrhage is located in the superficial cortical sulci, adjacent to a fracture or an intracerebral contusion, which obviates the lingering concern for a ruptured aneurysm. In patients with basal frontal contusions, however, the pattern of hemorrhage can resemble that of a ruptured anterior communicating artery aneurysm, and in patients with blood confined to the sylvian fissure, trauma can not be distinguished from aneurysmal rupture by the pattern of hemorrhage alone (Figure 2). In these patients adequate visualization of one or both carotid arteries is warranted.

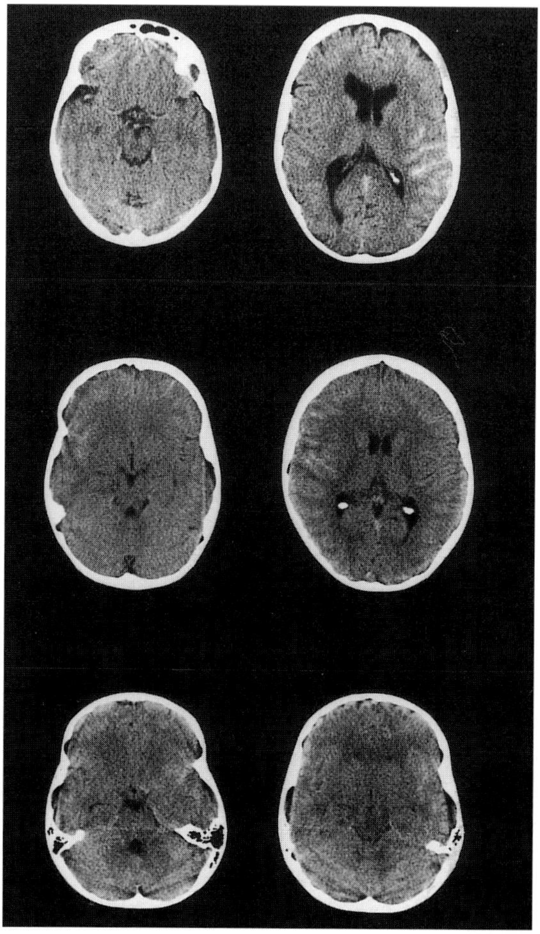

Figure 2 Traumatic versus aneurysmal subarachnoid hemorrhage. *Upper row:* A patient with a head injury and blood in the superficial sulci on the right but no blood in the sylvian fissure. Angiography is not indicated in patients with trauma and such a pattern of hemorrhage. *Middle row:* A patient with blood in the superficial sulci and sylvian fissure on the left. If the cause of the trauma is ambiguous in patients with such a pattern of hemorrhage, angiography is indicated to rule out that the trauma was provoked by aneurysmal rupture. *Lower row:* A patient with a small amount of blood in the sylvian fissure from a ruptured aneurysm.

In patients with direct trauma to the neck, or with head injury provoking vigorous neck movement, the trauma can immediately be followed by massive basal hemorrhage that results from a tear or even a complete rupture of one of the arteries of the vertebrobasilar circulation, which often is rapidly fatal [68,69].

In some patients with shearing injury, pronounced accumulation of blood can be found in the posterior part of the ambient cistern at the level of the tentorial margin [22]. The blood in the ambient cistern may be part of more extensive intracranial hemorrhage, but it can be the only site of hemorrhage [37]. Blood confined to the ambient cistern has also been reported in a patient with anticoagulant treatment and a relatively mild trauma (fall in the shower) [70]. The site of the hemorrhage makes a ruptured saccular aneurysm as source of the hemorrhage very unlikely.

7. Mycotic Aneurysms

The most frequent causes of mycotic aneurysms are infective endocarditis and aspergillosis. In patients with infective endocarditis most aneurysms are located on distal branches of the middle cerebral artery, but approximately 10 percent of the aneurysms are more proximally located [71]. Rupture of a mycotic aneurysm causes an intracerebral hematoma in most patients, but some have a pattern of hemorrhage indistinguishable on CT from that of a ruptured saccular aneurysm [72]. Rebleeds documented by CT have been reported [72]. Most patients present with valvular endocarditis before subarachnoid hemorrhage occurs, but rupture of a mycotic aneurysm can be the initial manifestation of infective endocarditis [73,74]. In older series, 10 percent of mycotic aneurysm were missed by angiography [75], but even nowadays the initial angiogram may be normal. The aneurysm in these patients can be found on repeated angiograms [72], but if angiography is repeated after too long an interval, it may be truly normal since mycotic aneurysms can resolve after antibiotic therapy [71].

Mycotic aneurysms in patients with aspergillosis are usually located on the proximal part of the basilar or carotid artery [76]. Rupture of such an aneurysm causes a massive subarachnoid hemorrhage in the basal cisterns, indistinguishable from that of a saccular aneurysm [77]. In some cases the initial angiogram is normal and only repeating the study reveals the aneurysm [77]. Aspergillosis is difficult to diagnose but should particularly be suspected in patients undergoing long-term treatment with antibiotics or immunosuppressive agents. Most patients with hematogenous dissemination have pulmonary lesions, but x-ray films of the chest may be normal early in the course [77,78]. Rupture of a mycotic aneurysm in patients with aspergillosis is often fatal [76].

8. Cocaine Abuse

In patients with subarachnoid hemorrhage related to the use of the alkaloid form of cocaine, half have no aneurysm on the angiogram [79]. The pattern of hemorrhage on CT may be indistinguishable from that of a ruptured saccular aneurysm [80], and the diagnosis rests on a confirmatory history or on the results of toxicologic tests. Rebleeds do occur, even in patients with a normal angiogram [81]. Outcome seems poor for these patients: four of five recently reported patients died after the cocaine-related subarachnoid hemorrhage [81]. The source of the hemorrhage in patients without an aneurysm is unknown. Although biopsy-proven vasculitis has been found in patients with cocaine abuse [82], angiograms of patients with subarachnoid hemorrhage related to cocaine abuse do not show changes suggestive of vasculitis [81,83].

9. Sickle Cell Disease

Subarachnoid hemorrhage is a rare complication of sickle cell disease [84]. Thirty percent of patients with sickle cell disease and subarachnoid hemorrhage are children [85]. In these children CT scans show blood in the superficial cortical sulci; angiograms reveal no aneurysm but often show multiple distal branch occlusions and leptomeningeal collateral circulation [85]. The subarachnoid hemorrhage is attributed to rupture of these collaterals. The outcome is poor: only three of the 11 recently reviewed children had a good outcome [85].

Most adult patients with sickle cell disease related subarachnoid hemorrhage have an aneurysm. The hemorrhage is located diffusely in the basal cisterns [86], and the outcome is comparable to that of patients with ruptured saccular aneurysms who have no sickle cell disease [85].

10. Coagulation Disorders

Anticoagulation-related subarachnoid hemorrhage seems rare. In a series of 116 patients with anticoagulant treatment and intracranial extracerebral hemorrhage, 7 had only subarachnoid hemorrhage. In two of these 7 patients the hemorrhage was associated with trauma, and in two other patients an aneurysm was found by angiography [87]. Thus, in only three of these patients no cause for the hemorrhage other than anticoagulation was found.

Severe coagulopathy other than by anticoagulant drugs is also a rare cause of hemorrhage confined to the subarachnoid space. In a recent series of 13 patients with intracranial hemorrhage after liver transplantation, only three had a subarachnoid hemorrhage on CT [88]. In all patients but one in this series the intracranial hemorrhage was associated with systemic bleeding [88].

11. Pituitary Apoplexy

Pituitary apoplexy has been proposed as one of the causes of subarachnoid hemorrhage of heretofore unknown cause [89]. The initial features are a sudden and severe headache, followed by nausea, vomiting, neck stiffness, and sometimes a depressed level of consciousness [90]. The hallmark of pituitary apoplexy is that most patients suffer a decrease in visual acuity: in one series of 15 patients, only two had normal visual acuity. Oculomotion is disturbed in most patients as well [91]. The pituitary fossa is the source of the hemorrhage as indicated by CT and MR scanning; in most instances the adenoma itself is also visible [91,92].

Table 1 Possible Causes and Diagnostic Strategy in Patients With Subarachnoid Hemorrhage and a Normal Angiogram

Cause of hemorrhage	Suggestive feature	Diagnosis by
Blood confined to cisterns around the midbrain		
Idiopathic perimesencephalic hemorrhage	Typical pattern of hemorrhage on CT	First normal angiogram
Trauma	Blood confined to ambient cistern	History
Diffuse or anteriorly located hemorrhage in the basal cisterns		
Occult aneurysm	Particularly with clots of blood in the anterior interhemispheric or sylvian fissure	Repeated angiography
Carotid or vertebral artery dissection	Recent trauma or uncommon neck movements; neck or facial pain; cranial nerve palsies; Horner's syndrome	Review angiogram; intraluminal thrombus on CT or MR; repeated angiography
Dural AVM	Old skull fracture	Review angiogram; repeated angiography
Cervical AVM	Pain radiating to shoulders or arms; spinal cord dysfunction; young age	MR imaging vertebral or spinal angiography
Trauma	Blood in superficial cortical sulci	History
Mycotic aneurysm	History; immunosuppression	Repeated angiography
Cocaine abuse	History	Toxicologic tests
Sickle cell disease	History; young age	Multiple distal branch occlusions
Coagulation disorders	History; systemic bleeding	Appropriate laboratory tests
Pituitary apoplexy	Poor or double vision	CT or MR images

12. Miscellaneous Causes

Other, exceedingly rare lesions that can give rise to subarachnoid hemorrhage in the basal cisterns are cervical tumors, such as a meningioma or a cavernous angioma [63,93], and rupture of a small circumferential artery in the pontine cistern [94]. These patients should be considered as clinical vignettes.

IV. GENERAL APPROACH IN PATIENTS WITH SUBARACHNOID HEMORRHAGE AND A NORMAL ANGIOGRAM

Patients with an aneurysm that goes undetected after the first angiogram are at risk of fatal rebleeds. It is therefore essential to minimize the number of patients with undetected aneurysms. This can be achieved by careful delineation of the angiography before the procedure is begun. The pattern of hemorrhage should direct the neuroradiologist to the offending vessel. In patients with intraparenchymal extension of the hemorrhage or with a localizing clot of subarachnoid blood, the prediction for the site of the ruptured aneurysm is correct in approximately 90% of the patients [95]. If no aneurysm is found at the predicted site after the routine frontal, lateral, and oblique projections, additional projections should be performed from the predicted site, before turning to other vessels or terminating the procedure. If no aneurysm is found on the initial angiogram after all, the further workup is directed by the history, the symptoms and signs, and the pattern of hemorrhage on CT.

The patient's history may already reveal a clue to the cause of the hemorrhage. Preceding uncommon neck movements (with painting the ceiling, for instance), or minor trauma such as chiropractic neck manipulation, should raise the suspicion of an intracranial artery dissection. Cocaine abuse should specifically be queried; long-term use of immunosuppressive agents or antibiotics may point to aspergillosis and pain radiating to the shoulders suggests a cervical origin of the hemorrhage.

On general examination, signs of trauma, drug abuse, systemic bleeding, or endocarditis may guide the clinician to the proper diagnosis. A decrease of visual acuity coming up with the hemorrhage points to a pituitary apoplexy. Lower cranial nerve palsies, Horner's syndrome, or more extensive lateral medullary syndromes point to a vertebral artery dissection [45,47]. Spinal cord dysfunction suggests a cervical AVM or a ruptured aneurysm of the distal posterior inferior cerebellar artery [96].

The pattern of hemorrhage is a powerful determinant for the diagnosis and prognosis. If the diagnosis of perimesencephalic hemorrhage has been confirmed by a normal angiogram, patients are no longer at risk of rebleeding or delayed cerebral ischemia. Treatment with calcium antagonists can then be discontinued and fluid replacement curtailed. Daily measurements of electrolytes and continuous EKG monitoring are no longer indicated. There is no need to keep these patients in an ICU, and we start to mobilize them as soon as possible. The invariably good outcome and absence of rebleeding obviate the need for a second angiography with its inherent risks. These patients can be discharged from the hospital after the period in which an acute hydrocephalus can develop and after the headache has subsided, the latter usually occurring in the second or third week. It is very important to reassure these patients that their bleeding was "innocent" and that they are not at risk for a second episode.

Patients with a single normal angiogram but an aneurysmal pattern of hemorrhage on CT are still at risk of rebleeding or delayed cerebral ischemia. Treatment of these patients should therefore be the same as the preoperative treatment of patients with a proven aneurysm. Particularly in patients with extensive extravasation of blood in the anterior interhemispheric fissure or in the sylvian fissure, a hidden aneurysm should be suspected. The first option in patients with accumulation of blood in the anterior interhemispheric fissure is MR imaging, since MR imaging has been reported to detect an anterior communicating artery aneurysm undetected by arteriography [97]. If this procedure is not diagnostic, we strongly advocate repeated angiography in these patients. In such patients even a second normal angiogram does not definitively exclude an aneurysm [18,44]. We therefore keep patients with two normal angiograms admitted and under close observation for 4 to 6 weeks. If rebleeding occurs within this period, we consider explorative craniotomy for patients with accumulation of blood in the anterior interhemispheric or the sylvian fissure. In one such patient we have found at operation an aneurysm of the middle cerebral artery, and recently three patients have been reported in whom an aneurysm of the anterior communicating artery was found at operation after two episodes of bleeding and two normal angiograms [41]. These four patients all had a good outcome despite their rebleeding. If no rebleeding occurs we perform a third angiogram three months after the hemorrhage. This strategy has never been consistently persued, but we have occasionally found aneurysms not seen on the two previous angiograms. If the third angiogram is negative again, and if other causes of subarachnoid hemorrhage have been excluded, we consider explorative craniotomy if the pattern of hemorrhage suggests an aneurysm of the anterior communicating or middle cerebral artery.

In patients with a pattern of hemorrhage suggestive of a lesion in the posterior circulation (marked intraventricular bleeding in the fourth and third ventricles with subarachnoid blood, if evident on the CT scan, centered around the midbrain and extending into the anteriorly located basal cisterns) [98,99], the angiogram should be reviewed for proper visualization of the branches of both vertebral arteries and for localized narrowing that may point to a vertebral artery dissection. The abnormalities suggesting an intracranial artery dissection may be very subtle in the first few days after the hemorrhage [36,57]. Before a second angiography, CT or MR imaging for detection of an intraluminal thrombus seems indicated. If a vertebral artery dissection has been demonstrated, we advise to keep these patients under close observation. Rebleeding occurs in 30% of these patients. These rebleedings are often accompanied by loss of consciousness and sometimes even by cardiopulmonary arrest, but as in patients with a ruptured aneurysm [100], complete recovery can occur with adequate resuscitation [48,46].

In patients in whom CT scanning suggests a tentorial origin of the hemorrhage and in whom the angiogram seems normal, the angiogram should be reviewed again, with the possibility of a tentorial AVM in mind. If again no lesion is found, repeated angiography is indicated, including visualization of the external carotid artery, because branches of this artery can be the main or the sole feeders [60]. If blood is confined to the ambient cistern, trauma is the most likely cause.

In patients with trauma, the presence of subarachnoid blood on the convexity without blood in the basal cisterns distinguishes head injury related hemorrhage from aneurysmal rupture. If patients with evidence of trauma have blood accumulated in the sylvian fissure as well, a limited angiographic study of the carotid circulation is indicated to rule out the possibility that the trauma was provoked by a rupture of an aneurysm on the middle cerebral artery (Figure 2). Blood confined to the superficial cortical sulci in children can occur with sickle cell disease. Appropriate laboratory investigations should be performed to rule out sickle cell disease and coagulation disorders in these children.

If CT is thought to be normal, it should be reviewed with particular attention to the prepontine cistern, because in some patients with a perimesencephalic hemorrhage this cistern is the only site where subarachnoid blood is found [17]. If no blood is found at all, the diagnosis of subarachnoid hemorrhage can be maintained only if the cerebrospinal fluid was xanthochromic after centrifugation [101]. The scarcity of data urges caution in advising about the management of these patients. If there are no features suggestive of a spinal AVM, repeat angiography is warranted, especially in patients with clinical features not compatible with a perimesencephalic hemorrhage.

REFERENCES

1. Kassell NF, Torner JC, Jane JA, Haley EC, Adams HP. The international cooperative study on the timing of aneurysm surgery. Part two: Surgical results. *J Neurosurg* 1990; 73:37–47.

2. Béguelin C, Seiler R. Subarachnoid hemorrhage with normal panangiography. *Neurosurgery* 1983; 13:409–411.
3. Velghe LE, de Wit P. Cryptogenic spontaneous subarachnoid haemorrhage. *Clin Neurol Neurosurg* 1983; 85:139–144.
4. Eskesen V, Sorensen EB, Rosenorn J, Schmidt K. The prognosis in subarachnoid hemorrhage of unknown origin. *J Neurosurg* 1984; 61:1029–1031.
5. Brismar J, Sundbärg G. Subarachnoid hemorrhage of unknown origin: prognosis and prognostic factors. *J Neurosurg* 1985; 63:349–354.
6. Barlow P. Incidence of delayed cerebral ischemia following subarachnoid haemorrhage of unknown cause. *J Neurol Neurosurg Psychiatry* 1985; 48:132–136.
7. Ruelle A, Lasio G, Boccardo M, Gottlieb A, Severi P. Long term prognosis of subarachnoid hemorrhage of unknown etiology. *J Neurol* 1985; 232:277–279.
8. Juul R, Frederiksen TA, Ringkjob R. Prognosis in subarachnoid hemorrhage of unknown etiology. *J Neurosurg* 1986; 64:359–362.
9. Spallone A, Ferrante L, Palatinsky E, Santoro A, Acqui M. Subarachnoid haemorrhage of unknown origin. *Acta Neurochir* 1986; 80:12–17.
10. Suzuki S, Kayama T, Sakurai Y, Ogawa A, Suzuki J. Subarachnoid hemorrhage of unknown cause. *Neurosurg* 1987; 21:310–313.
11. Jain VK, Hedge T, Easwaran RK, Das BS, Reddy GNN. Benign subarachnoid hemorrhage (Subarachnoid hemorrhage of unknown etiology). *Acta Neurochir* 1987; 86:89–92.
12. Giombini S, Bruzzone MG, Pluchino F. Subarachnoid hemorrhage of unexplained cause. *Neurosurgery* 1988; 22:313–316.
13. Cioffi F, Pasqualin A, Cavazzani P, Da Pian R. Subarachnoid haemorrhage of unknown origin: clinical and tomographical aspects. *Acta Neurochir* 1989; 97: 31–39.
14. Kawamura S, Yasui N. Clinical and long–term follow–up study in patients with spontaneous subarachnoid haemorrhage of unknown etiology. *Acta Neurochir* 1990; 106:110–114.
15. Oder W, Kollegger H, Zeiler K, Dal-Bianco P, Wessely P, Deecke L. Subarachnoid hemorrhage of unknown etiology: early prognostic factors for long term functional capacity. *J Neurosurg* 1991; 74:601–605.
16. Mehdorn HM, Dietrich U, Kalff R, Hoffmann B, Rauhut F, Grote W. Subarachnoid hemorrhage of unknown origin. Longterm prognosis. *Neurosurg Rev* 1992; 15:27–31.
17. Rinkel GJE, Wijdicks EFM, Vermeulen M, Ramos LMP, Tanghe HLJ, Hasan D, Meiners LC, van Gijn J. Nonaneurysmal perimesencephalic subarachnoid hemorrhage: CT and MR patterns that differ from aneurysmal rupture. *AJNR* 1991; 12:829–834, *AJR* 1991; 157:1325–1330.
18. Rinkel GJE, Wijdicks EFM, Hasan D, Kienstra G, Hageman L, Franke C, Vermeulen M, van Gijn J. Outcome in patients with subarachnoid haemorrhage and a negative angiography according to pattern of haemorrhage on computed tomography. *Lancet* 1991; 338:964–968.
19. Ferbert A, Hubo I, Biniek R. Non-traumatic subarachnoid hemorrhage with normal angiogram. Long term follow–up and CT predictors of complications. *J Neurol Sci* 1992; 107:14–18.

20. Farrés MT, Ferraz-Leite H, Schindler E, Muehlbauer M. Spontaneous subarachnoid hemorrhage with negative angiography: CT findings. *J Comput Assist Tomogr* 1992; 16:534–537.
21. van Calenbergh F, Plets C, Goffin L, Velghe L. Nonaneurysmal subarachnoid hemorrhage: prevalence of perimesencephalic hemorrhage in a consecutive series. *Surg Neurol* 1993; 39:320–323.
22. Takenaka N, Mine T, Suga S, Tamura K, Sagou M, Hirose Y, Ogino M, Okuno T, Enomoto K. Interpeduncular high–density spot in severe shearing injury. *Surg Neurol* 1990; 34:30–38.
23. van der Wee N, Rinkel GJE, Hasan D, van Gijn J. Detection of subarachnoid haemorrhage on early CT: is lumbar puncture still needed after a negative scan? *J Neurol Neurosurg Psychiatry* 1995; 58(3):357–359.
24. Rinkel GJE. Perimesencephalic nonaneurysmal hemorrhage. Amsterdam: Thesis publishers, 1991.
25. Van Gijn J, van Dongen KJ, Vermeulen M, Hijdra A. Perimesencephalic hemorrhage: a nonaneurysmal and benign form of subarachnoid hemorrhage. *Neurology* 1985; 35:493–497.
26. Schievink W, Wijdicks EFM, Piepgras DG, Nichols DA, Ebersold MJ. Perimesencephalic subarachnoid hemorrhage. Additional perspectives from four cases. *Stroke* 1994; 25(7):1507–1511.
27. Rinkel GJE, Wijdicks EFM, Vermeulen M, Hasan D, Brouwers PJAM, van Gijn J. The clinical course of perimesencephalic nonaneurysmal subarachnoid hemorrhage. *Ann Neurol* 1991; 29:463–468.
28. Rinkel GJE, Wijdicks EFM, Ramos LMP, van Gijn J. Progression of acute hydrocephalus in subarachnoid hemorrhage: a case report documented by serial CT scanning. *J Neurol Neurosurg Psychiatry* 1990; 53:354–355.
29. Rinkel GJE, Wijdicks EFM, Vermeulen M, Hageman LM, Tans JThJ, van Gijn J. Outcome in perimesencephalic (nonaneurysmal) subarachnoid hemorrhage: A follow up study in 37 patients. *Neurology* 1990; 40:1130–1132.
30. Pinto AN, Ferro JM, Canhao P, Campos J. How often is a perimesencephalic subarachnoid haemorrhage CT pattern caused by ruptured aneurysms. *Acta Neurochir* 1993; 124:79–81.
31. Kitahara T, Ohwada T, Tokiwa K, Kurata A, Miyasaka Y, Yada K, Kan S. Clinical study in patients with perimesencephalic hemorrhage of unknown etiology. *Neurol Surg* 1993; 21:903–908.
32. Iwanaga H, Wakai S, Ochai C, Narita J, Inoh S, Nagai M. Ruptured cerebral aneurysms missed by initial angiographic study. *Neurosurgery* 1990; 27:45–51.
33. Ronkainen A, Hernesniemi J. Subarachnoid haemorrhage of unknown aetiology. *Acta Neurochir* 1992; 119:29–34.
34. Kopitnik TA, Samson DS. Management of subarachnoid haemorrhage. *J Neurol Neurosurg Psychiat* 1993; 56:947–959.
35. Gilbert JW, Lee C, Young B. Repeat cerebral pan-angiography in subarachnoid hemorrhage of unknown etiology. *Surg Neurol* 1990; 33:19–21.
36. Sasaki O, Ogawa H, Koike T, Koizumi T, Tanaka R. A clinicopathological study of dissecting aneurysms of the intracranial vertebral artery. *J Neurosurg* 1991; 75:874–882.

37. Rinkel GJE, van Gijn J, Wijdicks EFM. Subarachnoid hemorrhage without detectable aneurysm: a review of the causes. Stroke 1993; 24:1403–1409.
38. Bohmfalk GL, Story JL. Intermittent appearance of a ruptured cerebral aneurysm on sequential angiograms. *J Neurosurg* 1980; 52:263–265.
39. Moritake K, Handa H, Ohtsuka, Hashimoto N. Vanishing cerebral aneurysm in serial angiography. *Surg Neurol* 1980; 16:36–40.
40. Edner G, Forster DMC, Steiner L, Bergvall U. Spontaneous healing of intracranial aneurysms after subarachnoid hemorrhage. *J Neurosurg* 1978; 48:450–454.
41. Jafar JJ, Weiner HL. Surgery for angiographically occult cerebral aneurysms. *J Neurosurg* 1993; 79:674–679.
42. Hayward RD. Subarachnoid haemorrhage of unknown etiology. A clinical and radiological study of 51 cases. *J Neurol Neurosurg Psychiatry* 1977; 40:926–931.
43. Sakai N, Yamada H, Ando T, Nishimura Y. Prevention of rebleeding after operation for subarachnoid hemorrhage of unknown cause. *Neurosurgery* 1985; 17:942–946.
44. Di Lorenzo N, Guidetti G. Anterior communicating aneurysm missed at angiography; report of two cases treated surgically. *Neurosurgery* 1988; 23:494–499.
45. Yamaura A, Watanabe Y, Saeki N. Dissecting aneurysms of the intracranial vertebral artery. *J Neurosurg* 1990; 72:183–188.
46. Aoki N, Sakai T. Rebleeding from intracranial dissecting aneurysm of the vertebral artery. *Stroke* 1990; 21:1628–1631.
47. Caplan LR, Baquis GD, Pessin MS, D'Alton G, Adelman LS, DeWitt LD, Ho K, Izukawa D, Kwan ES. Dissection of the intracranial vertebral artery. *Neurology* 1988; 38:868–877.
48. Friedman AH, Drake CG. Subarachnoid hemorrhage from intracranial dissecting aneurysm. *J Neurosurg* 1984; 60:325–334.
49. Alexander CB, Burger PC, Goree JA. Dissecting aneurysms of the basilar artery in 2 patients. *Stroke* 1979; 10:294–299.
50. Hosoda K, Fujita S, Kawaguchi T, Shose Y, Yonezawa K, Shirakuni T, Hamasaki M. Spontaneous dissecting aneurysms of the basilar artery presenting with subarachnoid hemorrhage. *J Neurosurg* 1991; 75:628–633.
51. Quint DJ, Spickler EM. Magnetic resonance demonstration of vertebral artery dissection. *J Neurosurg* 1990; 72:964–967.
52. Schwaighofer BW, Klein MV, Lyden PD, Hesselink JR. MR Imaging of vertebrobasilar vascular disease. *J Comput Assist Tomogr* 1990; 14:895–904.
53. Kunze S, Schiefer W. Angiographic demonstration of a dissecting aneurysm of the middle cerebral artery. *Neuroradiology* 1971; 2:201–206.
54. Adams HP Jr, Aschenbrener CA, Kassell NF, Ansbacher L, Cornell SH. Intracranial hemorrhage produced by spontaneous dissecting intracranial aneurysm. *Arch Neurol* 1982; 39:773–775.
55. Sasaki O, Koike T, Tanaka R, Ogawa H. Subarachnoid hemorrhage from a dissecting aneurysm of the middle cerebral artery. *J Neurosurg* 1991; 74:504–507.
56. Guridi J, Gállego J, Monzón F, Aguilera F. Intracerebral hemorrhage caused by transmural dissection of the anterior cerebral artery. *Stroke* 1993; 24:1400–1402.
57. Massoud TF, Anslow P, Molyneux AJ. Subarachnoid hemorrhage following spontaneous intracranial carotid artery dissection. *Neuroradiology* 1992; 34:33–35.

58. Lasjaunias P, Chiu M, ter Brugge K, Tolia A, Hurth M, Bernstein M. Neurological manifestations of intracranial dural arteriovenous malformations. *J Neurosurg* 1986; 64:724–730.
59. Halbach VV, Higashida RT, Hieshima GB, Goto K, Norman D, Newton TH. Dural fistulas involving the transverse and sigmoid sinuses: results of treatment in 28 patients. *Radiology* 1987; 163:443–447.
60. Aminoff MJ. Vascular anomalies in the intracranial dura mater. *Brain* 1973; 96:601–612.
61. Caroscio JT, Brannan T, Budabin M, Huang YP, Yahr MD. Subarachnoid hemorrhage secondary to spinal arteriovenous malformation and aneurysm. Report of a case and review of the literature. *Arch Neurol* 1980; 37:101–103.
62. Kandel EI. Complete excision of arteriovenous malformations of the cervical spinal cord. *Surg Neurol* 1980; 13:135–139.
63. Acciarri N, Padovani R, Pozzati E, Gaist G, Manetto V. Spinal cavernous angioma: a rare cause of subarachnoid hemorrhage. *Surg Neurol* 1992; 37:453–456.
64. Swann KW, Ropper AH, New PFJ, Poletti CE. Spontaneous spinal subarachnoid hemorrhage and subdural hematoma. *J Neurosurg* 1984; 61:975–980.
65. Aminoff MJ. Spinal Angiomas. Oxford: Blackwell Scientific Publications, 1976.
66. Aminoff MJ, Logue V. Clinical features of spinal vascular malformations. *Brain* 1974; 97:197–210.
67. Logue V. Angiomas of the spinal cord: review of the pathogenesis, clinical features and results of surgery. *J Neurol Neurosurg Psychiat* 1979; 42:1–11.
68. Harland WA, Pitts JF, Watson AA. Subarachnoid haemorrhage due to upper cervical trauma. *J Clin Pathol* 1983; 36:1335–1341.
69. Dowling G, Curry B. Traumatic basal subarachnoid hemorrhage: report of six cases and review of the literature. *Am J Forensic Med Pathol* 1988; 9:23–31.
70. Lavin PJM, Troost BT. Traumatic fourth nerve palsy: clinicoanatomic correlations with computed tomography scans. *Arch Neurol* 1984; 41:679–680.
71. Brust JCM, Dickinson PCT, Hughes JEO, Holtzman RNN. The diagnosis and treatment of cerebral mycotic aneurysms. *Ann Neurol* 1990; 27:238–246.
72. Steinberg GK, Guppy KH, Adler JR, Silverberg GD. Stereotactic, angiography–guided clipping of a distal, mycotic intracranial aneurysm using the Cosman–Roberts–Wells system: technical note. *Stroke* 1992; 30:408–411.
73. Salgado AV, Furlan AJ, Keys TF. Mycotic aneurysm, subarachnoid hemorrhage and indications for cerebral angiography in infective endocarditis. *Stroke* 1987; 18:1057–1060.
74. Vincent FM, Zimmerman JE, Auer TC, Martin DB. Subarachnoid hemorrhage: the initial manifestation of bacterial endocarditis. Report of a case with negative arteriography and computed tomography. *Neurosurgery* 1980; 7:488–490.
75. Ziment I. Nervous system complications in bacterial endocarditis. *Am J Med* 1969; 47:593–607.
76. Lau AHC, Takeshita M, Ishii N. Mycotic (Aspergillus) arteriitis resulting in fatal subarachnoid hemorrhage: a case report. *Angiology* 1991; 42:251–255.
77. Case Records of the Massachusetts General Hospital. Case 7–88. *N Engl J Med* 1988; 318:427–440.

78. Young RC, Bennet JE, Vogel CL, Carbone PP, de Vita VT. Aspergillosis: the spectrum of the disease in 98 patients. *Medicine* 1970; 49:147–173.
79. Levine SR, Brust JCM, Futrell N, Brass LM, Blake D, Fayad P, Schultz LR, Millikan CH, Ho KL, Welch KMA. A comparative study of the cerebrovascular complications of cocaine: alkaloidal versus hydrochloride: a review. *Stroke* 1991; 41:1173–1177.
80. Wojak JC, Flamm ES. Intracranial hemorrhage and cocaine use. *Stroke* 1987; 18:712–715.
81. Mangiardi JR, Daras M, Geller ME, Wetzner I, Tuchman AJ. Cocaine related intracranial hemorrhage. Report of nine cases and review. *Acta Neurol Scand* 1988; 77:177–180.
82. Krendel DA, Ditter SM, Frankel MR, Ross WK. Biopsy proven cerebral vasculitis associated with cocaine abuse. *Neurology* 1990; 40:1092–1094.
83. Levine SR, Brust JCM, Futrell N, Ho KL, Blake D, Millikan CH, Brass LM, Fayad P, Schultz LR, Selwa JF, Welch KMA. Cerebrovascular complications of the use of the "crack" form alkaloid cocaine. *N Engl J Med* 1990; 323:699–704.
84. Overby MC, Rothman AS. Multiple intracranial aneurysms in sickle cell anemia. *J Neurosurg* 1985; 62:430–434.
85. Carey J, Numaguchi Y, Nadell J. Subarachnoid hemorrhage in sickle cell disease. *Child's Nerv Syst* 1990; 6:47–50.
86. Love LC, Mickle JP, Sypert GW. Ruptured intracranail aneurysms in cases of sickle cell anemia. *Neurosurgery* 1985; 16:808–812.
87. Mattle H, Kohler S, Huber P, Rohner M, Steinsiepe KF. Anticoagulation–related intracranial extracerebral haemorrhage. *J Neurol Neurosurg Psychiatry* 1989; 52:829–837.
88. Estol CJ, Pessin MS, Martinez AJ. Cerebrovascular complications after orthotopic liver transplantation: a clinicopathologic study. *Neurology* 1991; 41:815–819.
89. Bjerre P, Videbaek H, Lindholm J. Subarachnoid hemorrhage with normal cerebral angiography: a prospective study on sellar abnormalities and pituitary function. *Neurosurgery* 1986; 19:1012–1015.
90. Reid RL, Quigly ME, Yen SSC. Pituitary apoplexy: a review. *Arch Neurol* 1985; 42:712–719.
91. McFadzean RM, Doyle D, Ramplin R, Teasdale E, Teasdale G. Pituitary apoplexy and its effect on vision. *Neurosurgery* 1991; 29:669–675.
92. Post JD, David NJ, Glaser JS, Safran A. Pituitary apoplexy: diagnosis by computed tomography. *Radiology* 1980; 134:665–670.
93. Scotti G, Filizzolo F, Scialfa G, Tampieri D, Versari P. Repeated subarachnoid hemorrhages from a cervical meningeoma. *J Neurosurg* 1987; 66:779–781.
94. Hochberg FH, Fisher CM, Roberson GH. Subarachnoid hemorrhage caused by rupture of a small superficial artery. *Neurology* 1974; 24:319–321.
95. Hillman J. Selective angiography for early aneurysm detection in acute subarachnoid haemorrhage. *Acta Neurochir* 1993; 121:20–25.
96. Kashiwagi S, Tsuchida E, Shiroyama Y, Ito H, Yamashita T. Paraplegia due to a ruptured aneurysm of the distal posterior inferior cerebellar artery. *J Neurol Neurosurg Psychiat* 1992; 55:836–837.

97. Pertuiset B, Haisa T, Bordi L, Abou Ouf S, Eissa M. Detection of a ruptured aneurysmal sac by MRI in a case of negative angiogram. Successful clipping of an anterior communicating artery aneurysm. *Acta Neurochir* 1989; 100:84–86.
98. Sadato N, Numaguchi Y, Rigamonti D, Salcman M, Gellad FE, Kishikawa T. Bleeding patterns in ruptured posterior fossa aneurysms: a CT study. *J Comput Assist Tomogr* 1991; 15:612–617.
99. Yeh HS, Tomsick TA, Tew JM. Intraventricular hemorrhage due to aneurysms of the distal posterior inferior cerebellar artery. *J Neurosurg* 1985; 62:772–775.
100. Hijdra A, Vermeulen M, van Gijn J, van Crevel H. Respiratory arrest in subarachnoid hemorrhage. *Neurology* 1984; 34:1501–1503.
101. Vermeulen M, Hasan D, Blijenberg BG, Hijdra A, van Gijn J. Xanthochromia after subarachnoid haemorrhage needs no revisitation. *J Neurol Neurosurg Psychiatry* 1989; 52:826–828.

8

Neurobehavioral Disorders After Subarachnoid Hemorrhage

Bradley F. Boeve
Mayo Clinic and Mayo Foundation, Rochester, Minnesota

Ronald C. Petersen
Mayo Clinic and Mayo Medical School, Rochester, Minnesota

I. INTRODUCTION

Mortality associated with subarachnoid hemorrhage has decreased significantly during the last few decades. With this decrease in mortality, attention has shifted to the cognitive impairment, emotional disturbances, and functional recovery that occur after the rupture and repair of intracranial aneurysms. Many patients who have undergone surgical repair of an aneurysm exhibit disorientation and impaired recent memory. Some of the patients may be combative, and others may fabricate bizarre stories. Anterograde and retrograde memory impairments may become evident postoperatively. Emotional changes can also occur, ranging from apathy to aggression or euphoria. These symptoms often abate, and in many cases, they resolve completely. However, in some patients, the emotional change may evolve into an anxiety or affective disorder that requires treatment. In still other patients, there remains a constellation of neurobehavioral problems of varying degrees that are permanent and disabling.

In this chapter, we first describe patients with a ruptured aneurysm of the anterior communicating artery and posterior communicating artery. These patients exemplify some of the possible neurobehavioral sequelae of aneurysmal subarachnoid hemorrhage. Next, we discuss the clinical features, frequency, and anatomy and pathophysiology of each of these disorders. Finally, we review the data about the cognitive outcome and functional recovery that occur after subarachnoid hemorrhage.

II. CASE REPORTS

A. Anterior Communicating Artery Aneurysm

Case 1 A 49-year-old left-handed homemaker with a high school education had a sudden, severe headache after arising from sleep and then experienced two generalized tonic-clonic convulsions. She was taken by ambulance to a local hospital, where she was noted to be drowsy but otherwise without focal neurologic findings. Computerized tomography (CT) showed extensive subarachnoid hemorrhage into the interhemispheric fissure, sylvian fissures, and basal cisterns and frontal intraparenchymal, and intraventricular hemorrhage with mild hydrocephalus (Hunt and Hess grade III [1], Fisher group 4 [2]). On arrival at the Mayo Clinic, she was still drowsy but oriented to person, place, and date. Other than for marked nuchal rigidity, the findings of the neurologic examination were normal. After she was given phenytoin, dexamethasone, and nimodipine, she underwent angiography. Four-vessel cerebral angiography showed an irregularly shaped anterior communicating artery aneurysm that was 18 × 14 × 12 mm, arose from the left side, and projected to the right, with no filling of the right A1 segment (Figure 1). Another aneurysm, 3 × 4 mm, was noted at the bifurcation of the right middle cerebral artery. No vasospasm was present.

The next day she underwent surgical repair of the aneurysm. After left pterional craniotomy and partial resection of the gyrus rectus, the aneurysm was isolated and partially dissected. A temporary clip was placed on the A1 segment and further dissection of the aneurysm was carried out so as not to disrupt any perforating vessels arising from the anterior cerebral artery/anterior communicating artery complex. A single Sugita bayonet clip was placed around the base of the aneurysm, and the temporary clip was removed. The aneurysm was opened and found to be completely occluded at its base.

Postoperatively, the patient was awake but disoriented and without focal signs. Volume expansion with intravenous saline was instituted, and treatment with nimodipine and phenytoin was continued, while dexamethasone was slowly tapered. Postoperative CT showed decreased attenuation in the mesial frontal areas bilaterally and a small amount of residual hemorrhage, but there was no hydrocephalus. Two days later she became unresponsive and later showed decerebrate posturing. Computerized tomography showed no change from the immediate postoperative study. Cerebral angiography showed complete obliteration of the aneurysm of the anterior communicating artery, no change in the aneurysm of the right middle cerebral artery, and no significant vasospasm. An intraventricular Camino intracranial pressure monitor revealed normal intracranial pressure. The exact cause of her deterioration was not clear, and her previous medical management was continued.

During the next two weeks, the patient's condition slowly and steadily improved. There was no evidence of any cranial nerve, motor, or sensory deficits,

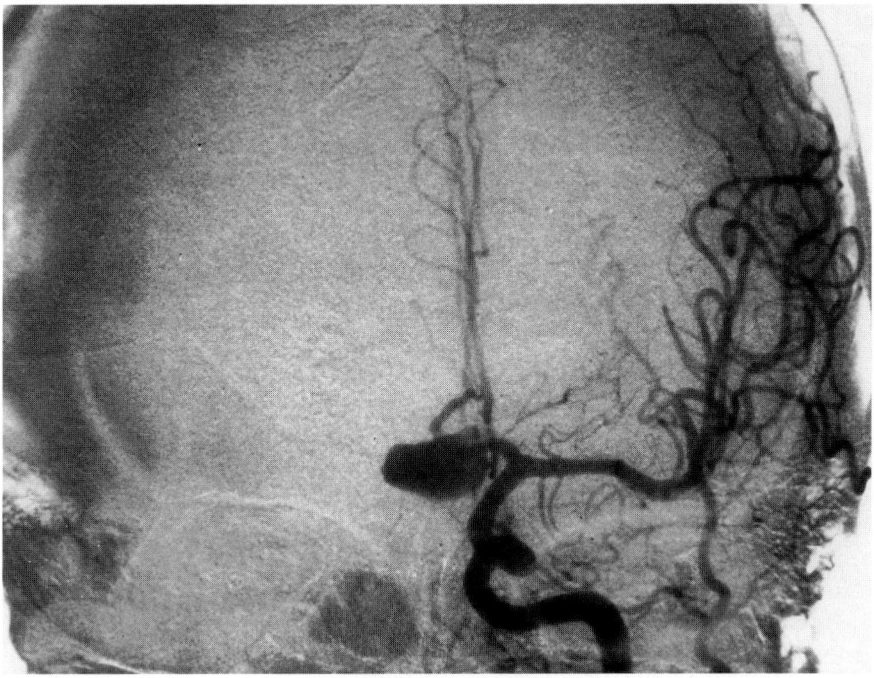

Figure 1 Cerebral angiogram (left common carotid artery injection) demonstrating an 18 × 14 × 12 mm aneurysm of the anterior communicating artery.

and she was able to ambulate with assistance. However, she did exhibit striking confabulation, easy distractibility, lack of concern, and memory impairment during casual conversations and bedside mental status testing. She was transferred to the rehabilitation unit about three weeks after the subarachnoid hemorrhage.

Despite intensive physical, occupational, speech, and cognitive therapy over the next seven weeks, her improvement was only mild. She had no evidence of aphasia or apraxia. She was able to ambulate and to transfer independently, and she performed most of the activities of daily living without cues. Her son had been hospitalized in the rehabilitation unit two years earlier after traumatic injury to the brain, and she was convinced that she was visiting him every day. She had no recollection of her recent operation or of events that occurred minutes or hours earlier. Her remote memory remained relatively intact. Her behavior was exceedingly impulsive and disruptive; for example, she bothered other patients in their rooms if she was unsupervised.

Formal neuropsychometric testing performed about eight weeks after the subarachnoid hemorrhage demonstrated the observations shown in Table 1. Her ability to learn and to retain verbal and visual/spatial information was markedly impaired. Testing showed markedly impaired recall of information after five minutes and complete loss of recall after a 30-minute delay. Verbal and nonverbal intellectual abilities were also impaired. Impairment of executive cognitive functions was apparent: she was impulsive, perseverative, and restricted in reasoning abilities, both behaviorally and in test performances.

Treatment with methylphenidate was not successful in decreasing her impulsiveness. She was subsequently dismissed home to the care of her family, who were very supportive and supervised her 24 hours a day.

A magnetic resonance imaging (MRI) scan performed four months after her hemorrhage showed signal changes consistent with bifrontal ischemic damage (Figure 2).

Her condition was reassessed 10 months after her hemorrhage. She was now independent in self-care, housecleaning, and cooking, but she was not able to manage her finances without assistance. Her memory for daily activities and current news events was minimally impaired. Her insight into her persistent cognitive difficulties was limited; for example, she saw no reason why her family and physicians restricted her from driving. Whereas she had been quite physically active before the hemorrhage, she now led a sedentary lifestyle and tended to indulge in sweets. She continued to experience difficulties in organizational abilities, such that learning complex, unstructured information was impaired. Neuropsychologic testing confirmed her functional deficits in attention/concentration, cognitive flexibility, and executive functions (Table 1). Anterograde memory function had improved considerably. These residual functional and cognitive deficits were consistent with bifrontal cerebral dysfunction. She participated in an outpatient brain-injury program and is currently independent with most activities of daily living but still too impaired to be gainfully employed.

B. Posterior Communicating Artery Aneurysm

Case 2 A 53-year-old right-handed female insurance agent with a ninth-grade education had a sudden severe frontal headache accompanied by nausea and vomiting. She did not seek medical attention until a similar episode occurred 11 days after the first one. Her local physician noted a dilated left pupil, and she was transferred to the Mayo Clinic for further evaluation. Neurologic examination at that time showed a dilated left pupil, full extraocular movements, and mild nuchal rigidity. No mental status, motor, sensory, or reflex abnormalities were noted. Computerized tomography of the head showed decreased sulcal markings but no intracerebral, intraventricular, or subarachnoid hemorrhage. Examination of the cerebrospinal fluid showed 166,400 erythrocytes and xanthochromia. Four-vessel cerebral angiography revealed a 10 × 3 mm lobulated aneurysm arising from the left posterior communicating artery (Figure 3). No vasospasm was evident.

Approximately 20 hours after angiography, her neurologic status was unchanged (Hunt and Hess grade II), and she underwent an uncomplicated left frontotemporal craniotomy. The aneurysm was clipped with a bayonet Sugita clip and then opened and found to be completely occluded at its base. The left anterior choroidal artery was not disturbed, but the left middle cerebral artery was surrounded by blood clot and appeared somewhat narrowed, suggestive of focal vasospasm.

Postoperatively, the patient was oriented to person and place but not to date or time, and she had diminished spontaneous and elicitable speech. Spontaneous movements in the right extremities were decreased. Volume expansion with saline given intravenously and treatment with nimodipine were instituted; however, nimodipine treatment was discontinued two days later because of hypotension. Disorientation, word-finding difficulties, and poor short-term memory persisted. Computerized tomography showed the aneurysm clip and a small amount of dependent blood in the lateral ventricles but no evidence of infarct. Transcranial Doppler ultrasonographic evaluation showed increased flow velocity in the proximal left middle cerebral artery consistent with vasospasm. Volume expansion was continued.

The weakness on the patient's right side gradually resolved. Eight days postoperatively, she underwent formal speech evaluation that showed defects in all language modalities, with relative sparing of repetition, and also marked response latencies, confabulatory speech, and flat affect. These findings are most consistent with transcortical aphasia with coexisting cognitive deficits. Except for cognitive and speech impairments, the results of neurologic examination were normal. She was transferred to the rehabilitation unit 11 days postoperatively.

The results of formal neuropsychometric testing performed four weeks postoperatively are shown in Table 1. These results demonstrated severe impairment in learning and in remembering new verbal information, but on testing visual-spatial information, her performance was much better. Also, her performance on tests of confrontational naming, verbal associative abilities, and reading comprehension was poor. Impairment in visual-spatial reasoning, problem-solving, attention, and arithmetic was only marginal. These findings are most consistent with left frontal and temporal cerebral dysfunction.

Her recovery was slow but steady during the rest of her hospitalization. She became completely independent in the activities of daily living. She used a memory journal as a compensatory aid when prompted. Initially, her affect was flat, but

Table 1 Neuropsychometric Data for Cases 1 and 2

	Case 1		Case 2	
Duration since SAH	8 wk	10 mo	4 wk	6 mo
Intellectual functioning				
WAIS-R results [3][a]				
Verbal IQ	82 (12)[b]	89 (23)		
Performance IQ	74 (4)	91 (27)		99
Full scale IQ	78 (7)	88 (21)		
Attention/concentration				
TMT [4]				
Part A		30		
Part B		152		
Stroop [5]				
Word		82	91	
Color		71	53	
Color-word		40	14	
Language functioning				
Naming (MLAE) [6]		50 (27)	36 (0)	
Token (MLAE) [6]		44 (82)	32 (<1)	
COWAT I [6]	11 (<1)	29 (12–22)	3 (<1)	
Visuospatial functioning				
JLO [7]			0 (1.5)	
Learning and memory				
WMS-R results [8]				
Logical memory				
Immediate	4	17	0	3
Delay	0	16	0	2
Retention	0%	94%	0%	67%
Visual reproduction				
Immediate	22	24	28	29
Delay	0	15	6	27
Retention	0%	63%	21%	93%
Verbal memory index	<50	79		<50
Visual memory index		78		78
General memory		74		<50
Attention/concentration index		109	101	97
AVLT/CVLT[c] [9,10]				
Learning curve	2 2 1 2 3	4 8 6 6 8	0 0 3 0 1	2 3 4 4 5
Short-term recall	0	6	0	0
Delayed recall	0	4	0	1
Retention	0%	40%	0%	20%
Planning, reasoning, problem solving				
WCST [11]				
Correct	42	58		
Errors	86	70		

Table 1 Continued

	Case 1		Case 2	
Duration since SAH	8 wk	10 mo	4 wk	6 mo
Perseverative responses	98	89		
Nonperseverative errors	13	3		
Perseverative errors	73	67		
Categories	0	3		
Failure to maintain set	1	0		

[a] AVLT, Auditory Verbal Learning Test; COWAT, Controlled Oral Word Association Test; CVLT, California Verbal Learning Test; IQ, Intelligence Quotient; JLO, Judgement of Line Orientation; MLAE, Multilingual Aphasia Examination; TMT, Trailmaking Test; WAIS-R, Weschler Adult Intelligence Scale-Revised; WCST, Wisconsin Card Sorting Test; WMS-R, Weschler Memory Scale-Revised.
[b] Numbers in parentheses are percentiles.
[c] Case 1 was administered the AVLT; case 2 was administered the CVLT.

she later exhibited appropriate humor. She showed no signs or symptoms of clinical depression. She performed familiar home management skills relatively well but did poorly when presented with unfamiliar or emergency situations. Her confabulation, anomia, memory impairment, and tangentiality slowly improved but were still present at six weeks postoperatively when she was dismissed and returned home, under 24-hour supervision by her family. Computerized tomography performed before dismissal showed a focus of decreased attenuation in the genu of the left internal capsule consistent with an infarct (Figure 4).

Follow-up evaluation six months postoperatively revealed marked improvement in her speech and cognitive function. She had already returned to part-time employment as a bookkeeper. On formal speech testing, her speech and language abilities were within normal limits, with no evidence of aphasia. On neuropsychometric testing (Table 1), her scores on tests of intellectual function and academic achievement were in the average range, which were improved significantly over her previous scores. Her scores on memory tests continued to demonstrate impaired memory for verbally presented information, with relative sparing of visual-spatial memory function.

III. NEUROBEHAVIORAL DISORDERS

A. Amnesia

1. Clinical Features

Although memory impairment has been described in association with posterior communicating artery aneurysms [12], amnesia occurring after subarachnoid

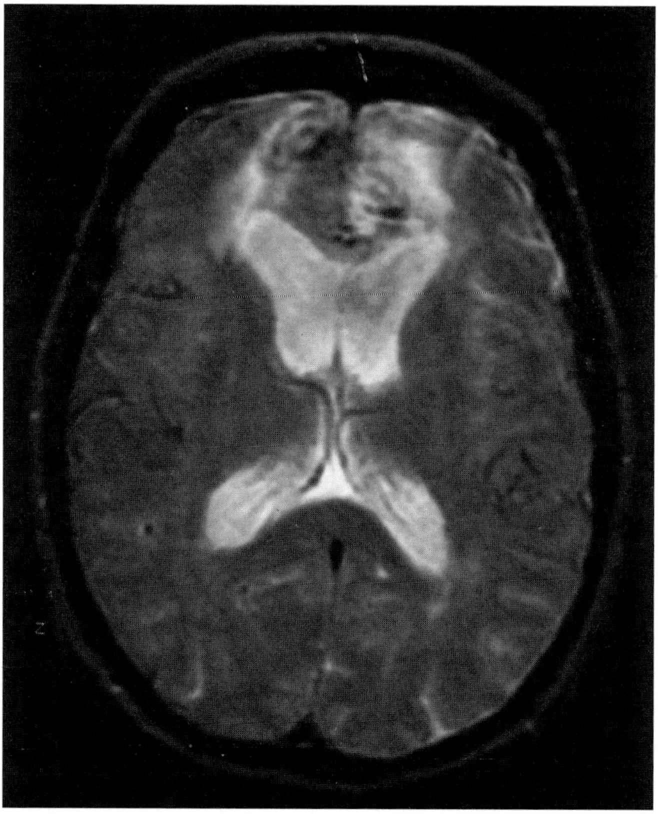

Figure 2 Magnetic resonance imaging scan of the brain (T_2-weighted axial view) showing residual bifrontal ischemic damage.

hemorrhage has been reported almost exclusively in association with rupture or repair (or both) of aneurysms of the anterior communicating artery [13–37]. Amnesia is typically part of the symptom complex of amnesia, confabulation, and personality changes, which Alexander and Freedman [25] have called "anterior communicating artery syndrome." Retrograde and anterograde components often coexist, and both tend to improve over time. The anterograde memory disturbances are global in nature, so that learning and recalling verbal material, visual material, movements, and actions are equally involved [16]. The patients with persistent amnesia typically have CT evidence of basal forebrain lesions (see below), which spare the diencephalon and medial temporal structures that are damaged in classic cases of amnesia [38,39]. Several investigators have attempted to characterize this apparently unique form of amnesia.

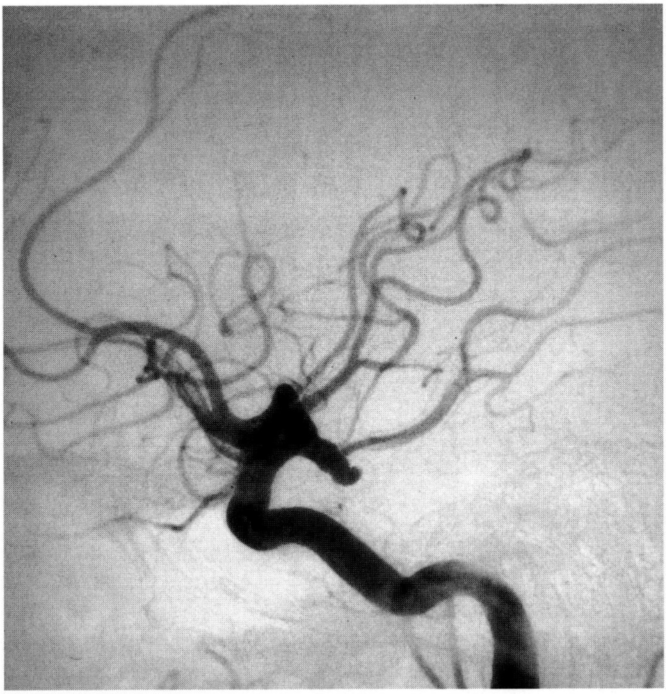

Figure 3 Cerebral angiogram (left common carotid artery injection) demonstrating a 10 × 3 mm lobulated aneurysm arising from the left posterior communicating artery.

Gade and Mortensen [40] studied remote memory of premorbid public events in patients with amnesia after repair of aneurysms of the anterior communicating artery. This form of amnesia is associated with dementia and is seen in other neurologic disorders (e.g., tumors, meningitis, and Korsakoff's syndrome). Patients with this form of amnesia, whether due to aneurysm of the anterior communicating artery or to another neurologic disorder, display a time-graded memory loss, in which recall and recognition for remote events are better than for recent premorbid events. This temporal gradient pattern is similar to that in Korsakoff's syndrome [41,42], which has been explained by the "continuity hypothesis," namely that slow and progressive anterograde amnesia in alcoholic patients would gradually hinder their ability to process and encode information, resulting in the temporal gradient for previous events [41]. However, as Gade and Mortensen [40] noted, a sudden process occurs in patients with aneurysm of the anterior communicating artery, which contradicts the continuity hypothesis as an explanation for a temporal gradient. Instead, their data supported the "episodic-semantic shift hypothesis," whereby remote episodic

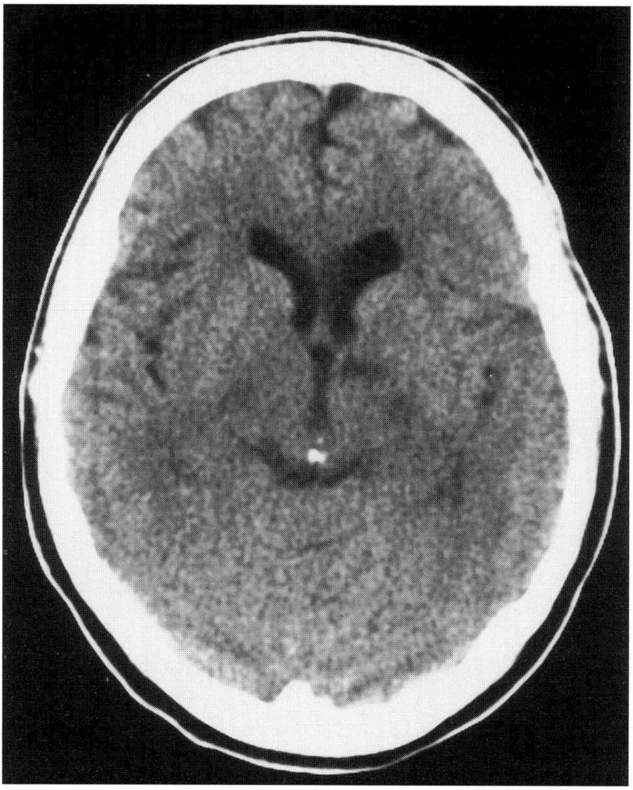

Figure 4 Computerized tomographic scan of the brain showing an infarct in the genu of the left internal capsule.

memories could be rehearsed and retold over time, gradually becoming more semantic in nature but losing the temporal and spatial relationships with which they were originally encoded [40]. Because memory loss for episodic memories is more severe than for semantic memories in amnesic patients [43], the remote memories would be recalled and recognized easier than recent, episodic memories if they are semantic in nature [40]. Gade and Mortensen [40] suggested that this episodic-semantic shift may represent a shift in the neural mechanisms underlying memory processing.

Several recent reports have described features of the anterograde amnesia in selected patients with aneurysm of the anterior communicating artery. Volpe and Hirst [24] studied two patients with amnesia that occurred after rupture and repair of anterior communicating artery aneurysms and found that several characteristics of the amnesia were similar to those described in cases of Korsakoff's syndrome, hypoxic brain injury, and herpes encephalitis, i.e., immediate memory is intact, free recall is poor, retrieval clues enhance recall, and susceptibility to interference is increased. The performance of these two patients on recognition tests was comparable to that of control subjects.

Patients with Korsakoff's syndrome and those with anterior communicating artery aneurysms have similar behavioral manifestations but possibly different neuropathologic lesions. Parkin et al. [30] studied a 42-year-old man with persistent memory impairment after rupture and repair of an anterior communicating artery aneurysm. His performance on a battery of psychometric tests (administered over two years after aneurysm repair) was compared with that of amnesic patients with Korsakoff's syndrome, patients with temporal lobe lesions, and normal control subjects. The most notable findings were marked sensitivity to proactive interference, impaired temporal discrimination, impaired free recall and source recall, and relatively preserved recognition and remote memory for faces. The sensitivity to proactive interference and impaired temporal discrimination and source recall were similar to that observed in patients with Korsakoff's syndrome [44,45], which the authors believe supports the role of frontal lobe dysfunction in these processes [30]. The preserved remote memory for faces and recognition is in contrast with the impaired remote memory in their patients with Korsakoff's syndrome and with other data showing that patients with Korsakoff's syndrome have impaired recognition [46]. The authors proposed that these qualitative differences of memory impairment in their patient are consistent with Schacter's hypothesis [47] that impaired "contextual chunking" occurs in frontal lobe dysfunction [30]. Clearly, the patient of Parkin et al. had features of cognitive impairment that are not only similar to but also in contrast with the typical findings in Korsakoff's syndrome. This is additional evidence that the dysfunctional neural mechanisms of memory processing in some patients with anterior communicating artery aneurysm are different from those in other amnesic disorders.

In sharp contrast to the cases mentioned above, Delbecq-Derouesne et al. [48] found impaired recognition but preserved recall in a patient after rupture and repair of an anterior communicating artery aneurysm. They proposed that the impaired recognition resulted from the patient's inability to subjectively "remember" the experience of remembering.

Damasio et al. [26] evaluated four patients after rupture of an aneurysm of the anterior cerebral artery-anterior communicating artery and one patient after resection of an arteriovenous malformation. On CT, all five patients had evidence of basal forebrain damage. All these patients were able to learn the generic aspects of separate stimuli, such as the name and face of a person, but they were unable to learn the contextual aspects of related stimuli, such as associating a person's name with that person's face. These five patients also had difficulty learning the temporal relationships of separate stimuli. As in the study of Volpe and Hirst [24], the performance of the patients on recall and recognition tasks was strongly enhanced by retrieval cues for retrograde and anterograde memories. Because retrograde and anterograde amnesia both improved with cuing, the authors stated that the defect in memory processing must primarily involve the retrieval process rather than the encoding and consolidation process [26]. In these patients with damage to the basal forebrain, the features of preserved generic memory processing, impaired contextual memory processing, relatively preserved consolidation, and impaired retrieval are in contrast with the features of the memory impairment associated with damage to the medial temporal lobe and dorsomedial thalamus, in which all of these memory processes are affected [26,38,39].

Damasio et al. [26] cited related reports to explain the unique features of amnesia due to lesions of the basal forebrain. The basal forebrain is connected directly with the amygdala (via the ventral amygdalofugal pathway) and hippocampus (via the fornix)—two structures in the medial temporal lobe that are arguably critical in memory function [49–53]. Positron emission tomography (PET) studies in patients with basal forebrain damage have shown diminished oxygen utilization in the medial temporal regions [54]. Thus, with basal forebrain damage, some degree of primary memory processing could continue in the medial temporal lobe structures, but the processing of stimulus relationships and temporal tagging would be impaired [26].

2. Frequency

In earlier studies, the frequency of amnesia after aneurysmal subarachnoid hemorrhage was based on qualitative descriptions of patients with various degrees of memory impairment, often as part of Korsakoff's syndrome and therefore included under the headings "psychiatric" or "psychologic" sequelae after subarachnoid hemorrhage [13,17,18,20–22,55,56]. Lindqvist and Norlen [13] noted Korsakoff's syndrome in 52% of patients with anterior communicating artery aneurysms treated surgically. Storey [55] observed "psychiatric" morbidity of some degree in 55% of patients with aneurysm treated or not treated surgically, and Short et al. [56] noted "psychiatric" morbidity in at least 67% of the patients in their series. Logue et al. [15] evaluated 79 patients who had rupture of an anterior cerebral artery-anterior communicating artery aneurysm. In 66 of the patients, the feeding anterior cerebral artery proximal to the aneurysm was clipped; the 13 other patients received conservative treatment. Retrograde amnesia was noted in 33% of the patients; in 9%, the amnesic gap was more than one week. Anterograde amnesia occurred in 87% of patients and persisted for longer than one year in 7% of patients.

Matsukado et al. [17] found "psychiatric" disorders primarily manifested as Korsakoff's syndrome in 20% of patients after aneurysmal subarachnoid hemorrhage. Nystrom [22] noted "mental disorders" in 29.9% of 1080 patients after subarachnoid hemorrhage. Follow-up evaluation of 501 of these patients 1 to 16 years later revealed that 3.3% had Korsakoff's syndrome. Maeda et al. [18] observed "psychiatric" symptoms in 47% of patients preoperatively and in 53% postoperatively. Hori and Suzuki [19] noted residual Korsakoff's syndrome and amnesia, with or without disorientation, in six of 303 patients (2%) with anterior communicating artery aneurysms treated surgically. Takaku et al. [20] reviewed 1000 cases of intracranial aneurysms treated surgically over a 15-year period and found that 4% of the patients had amnesia, 2% had Korsakoff's syndrome, and 1% had dementia at the time of hospital dismissal. Over a 9-year period, Okawa et al. [21] studied 95 patients after ruptured anterior communicating artery aneurysms and observed amnesia (alone or as part of Korsakoff's syndrome) in 45% of the patients who were conscious before surgical repair. Of these patients, 85 were examined two to three days postoperatively and 57 (62%) had amnesia. Of the 73 patients evaluated at least six months later, 19 (26%) still had memory difficulties. Sundt et al. [57] observed Korsakoff's syndrome in seven (4%) of 166 patients with anterior communicating artery aneurysm treated surgically. The syndrome was apparent preoperatively in three of the seven patients.

In several recent series, psychometric testing has been used to characterize the memory impairment in patients after aneurysmal subarachnoid hemorrhage [12,25,27,28,31,34–37,58–76]. Although descriptions of patients with severe amnesia are infrequent, psychometric evidence and subjective complaints of memory impairment were evident in most studies (the details of these studies are reviewed below) [12,25,27,28,31,34–37,58–63,65–67,69–76]. The decrease in the incidence of severe amnesia and in anterior communicating artery syndrome in recent studies has been attributed primarily to improved surgical techniques with the operating microscope and to better preservation of perforating branches from the anterior cerebral artery-anterior communicating artery complex (see below) [57,75–77].

3. Anatomy and Pathophysiology

The anatomical basis of the memory impairment that occurs after subarachnoid hemorrhage is a matter of debate. As DeLuca [36] has noted, the conflict about memory impairment associated with anterior communicating artery aneurysms involves those whose data best support the "diffuse cerebral injury hypothesis" versus the "focal lesion hypothesis." Proponents of the former view cite neuropsychometric evidence of memory impairment after subarachnoid hemorrhage, but no differences have been found in memory performance on neuropsychometric testing of patients with ruptured aneurysms of different vessels [12,37, 59–61,63,65,66,68,70,71]. Furthermore, no differences are apparent when test results between patients with aneurysmal subarachnoid hemorrhage and those with subarachnoid hemorrhage from an unknown source are compared [68]. Several methodologic inconsistencies in these and other studies (e.g., time of testing, method of investigation, and lack of control groups) make comparisons between studies difficult [36]. Methodologic limitations could favor the diffuse injury hypothesis [36]. Despite their limitations, these studies provide convincing evidence that a diffuse process may be responsible for the memory deficits that occur after subarachnoid hemorrhage. Some authors have proposed that the neurotoxic effects of blood in the subarachnoid space and meninges may produce a diffuse encephalopathy after subarachnoid hemorrhage (see below) [68,78].

Evidence for the focal lesion hypothesis is based primarily on radiologic, surgical, and autopsy data. Most of the cases involve ruptured aneurysms of the anterior communicating artery in which the basal forebrain—the nucleus basalis of Meynert, nucleus of the diagonal band of Broca, medial septal nuclei, nucleus accumbens—as well as the anterior cingulum and anterior hypothalamus is damaged [25,26,29]. Most of the patients studied by Alexander and Freedman [25] had CT evidence of unilateral or bilateral infarcts in the territory of the anterior cerebral artery. Damage to the basal forebrain showed on CT in all five patients evaluated by Damasio et al. [26]. Phillips et al. [29] found basal forebrain damage on postmortem examination of a man with anterograde amnesia that had persisted for five years after rupture and repair of an aneurysm of the anterior communicating artery.

A recent study by DeLuca [36] provided further support for the focal injury hypothesis. He compared the performance on various neuropsychometric tests of a group of patients with repaired aneurysms of the anterior communicating artery with that of a control group of patients who had intracranial hemorrhages in locations outside the distribution of the anterior communicating artery. The anterior communicating artery group performed worse than the control group on delayed verbal memory tests and on the Wisconsin Card Sorting Test but scored better than the control group on the Full Scale IQ of the WAIS-R. Almost all the patients in the anterior communicating artery group had CT evidence of frontal lobe involvement, whereas only one patient in the control group did. Unlike studies supporting the diffuse injury hypothesis, the study by DeLuca [36] included a control group and provided convincing evidence for the role of basal forebrain dysfunction in amnesia associated with aneurysms of the anterior communicating artery.

There is additional evidence in support of the role of the basal forebrain in memory. Several cholinergic groups of neurons in the basal forebrain (in the nucleus basalis of Meynert, the medial and lateral septal nuclei, and the vertical and horizontal nuclei of the diagonal band of Broca) project to the hippocampus, amygdala, and neocortex [79,80]. Memory dysfunction is a prominent feature of Alzheimer's disease, in which cholinergic neurons in the basal forebrain are selectively lost, especially in the nucleus basalis of Meynert [81]. Experimental studies suggest that damage to the medial septal nuclei rather than to the nucleus basalis is responsible for memory impairment [82]. Damage to the septal nuclei was presumably responsible for the amnesia that occurred after transcallosal excision of a subependymoma in the septum pellucidum [83]. Other cases have been reported recently of amnesia after isolated injury to the basal forebrain [84,85]. In the case described by Morris et al. [85], persistent anterograde and retrograde amnesia developed after resection of a low-grade glioma in the right basal forebrain. The lesion primarily involved the diagonal band of Broca, preoptic area, anterior hypothalamus, lamina terminalis, and paraterminal gyrus but spared the septal nuclei and nucleus basalis of Meynert. As noted above, damage to the basal forebrain could interrupt the ventral amygdalofugal pathway and fornix, thus disrupting memory processing in medial temporal lobe structures [49–53]. Morris et al. [85] proposed that disruption of the cholinergic pathways from the diagonal band of Broca to the hippocampus was responsible for the amnesia in their patients.

Despite the overwhelming evidence implicating basal forebrain damage in amnesia associated with aneurysms of the anterior communicating artery, isolated case reports of patients without radiologic evidence of parenchymal brain damage and a recent study by Irle et al. [35] warrant discussion. Lesions were not visualized on CT in four patients with anterior communicating artery syndrome in Alexander and Freedman's review [25] or in the two patients described by Volpe and Hirst [24]. Perhaps the resulting infarcts were not visualized because they were too small or obscured by the aneurysm clips. Persistent hypoperfusion through damaged but patent arteries could also alter the normal function of structures involved in memory. Additional postmortem examinations and PET and single-photon emission CT studies may clarify this issue.

Irle et al. [35] found that isolated lesions of the basal forebrain or striatum (as demonstrated on CT) did not produce amnesia in patients with ruptured aneurysms of the anterior communicating artery, whereas lesions of the basal forebrain in combination with those of the striatum did result in amnesia. These authors postulated that dysfunction of either the corticolimbic or corticostriate pathways permits compensatory recovery of memory function by the unaffected system, but dysfunction of both pathways is too overwhelming and amnesia ensues. The recent data of Irle [86,87] support this contention.

Several patients with CT evidence of basal forebrain damage had, on closer inspection, coexisting striatal or pallidal damage [26,29,36]. Two diseases that primarily involve the basal ganglia or dopaminergic dysfunction (or both) are Huntington's disease and Parkinson's disease. Memory impairment is a feature of Huntington's disease but is less frequent in Parkinson's disease [88–90]. Two recent reviews of patients with isolated lesions of the caudate nucleus noted memory impairment in several cases [91,92].

There are anatomical data that may explain the above findings. Several basal ganglia-thalamic-cortical circuits have been described, each of which has a presumed role in motor, oculomotor, or cognitive function [92–94]. The frontostriatal "cognitive loop" involves two circuits: 1. prefrontal cortex to ventral striatum to ventral pallidum to thalamic dorsomedial nucleus and back to prefrontal cortex and 2. amygdala to ventral striatum to ventral pallidum and back to amygdala [93–96]. Two other circuits, namely, the dorsolateral prefrontal cortical and the lateral orbitofrontal cortical circuits, involve dorsal striatal (i.e., caudate nucleus) and dorsal pallidal (i.e., globus pallidus) structures, which project to the thalamic dorsomedial nucleus [92,93]. Therefore, several circuits that interconnect cortical, basal ganglia, and limbic structures exist that, if disrupted, may result in memory impairment. A patient with amnesia that developed after injury to the mediobasal forebrain showed improvement on memory testing after treatment with bromocriptine [84]. This case supports the idea that the dopaminergic system has a role in memory function.

The neurotoxic effects of blood itself (as noted above) may result in diffuse encephalopathy, thereby causing cognitive impairment in many domains, including memory [68,78]. Progressive dementia is one of the features of superficial siderosis, an uncommon syndrome that presumably is the result of repeated and prolonged exposure to blood in the subarachnoid space [97]. Iron deposition and parenchymal cation dysfunction have been implicated in causing neuronal damage [68,78,97] and may be partly responsible for the spectrum of cognitive deficits associated with subarachnoid hemorrhage.

Focal brain damage can also impair memory function. Altered perfusion to structures supplied by the perforating branches of the anterior communicating artery is presumed to cause damage to the basal forebrain or basal ganglia (or both). Several anatomical studies have documented that in most persons perforating vessels from the anterior communicating artery perfuse the basal forebrain and surrounding structures [98–101]. The caudate nucleus is usually supplied by the recurrent artery of Heubner that often arises from the A2 segment near the junction of the anterior cerebral and anterior communicating arteries [99,102]. Disruption of these vessels by various means has been proposed as a cause of cognitive dysfunction.

The onset of amnesia with or without confabulation and personality changes is usually noted after surgical obliteration of an anterior communicating artery aneurysm, although some cases of this have been observed after rupture but before surgical repair [16,57]. Rupture of the aneurysm alone could cause hemorrhagic infarction or disruption of the perforating vessels. Gade [23] described 15 patients with amnesia after surgical repair of an anterior communicating artery aneurysm. Nine of the patients underwent "trapping" (both anterior cerebral arteries were ligated proximal to the aneurysm), and in the other six the neck of the aneurysm was clipped. He proposed that trapping obliterates the perforating vessels from the anterior communicating artery and that this leads to amnesia. Currently, standard neurosurgical management of aneurysms involves clipping the neck of the aneurysm and minimizing dissection around the aneurysm to lessen the risk of disrupting the perforating vessels [57,77]. In otherwise uncomplicated surgical procedures, prolonged intraoperative hypotension and especially vasospasm of the perforating vessels of the anterior communicating artery are probable causes of basal forebrain or basal ganglia damage. In cases in which infarcts are not seen radiographically, persistent hypoperfusion through damaged but patent arteries or simply fewer undamaged arteries could alter the normal function of the basal forebrain and basal ganglia. Therefore, theoretically, damage to structures critical for memory can occur at any time between rupture of the aneurysm and resolution of vasospasm, a period that often spans weeks.

B. Confabulation

1. Clinical Features

Confabulation occurring after subarachnoid hemorrhage is associated almost exclusively with aneurysms of the anterior communicating artery [13,14,16,21, 25–27,30,32,36,57,103–105]. As noted above, confabulation often coexists with amnesia and personality changes in anterior communicating artery syndrome [25]. Unlike amnesia and personality changes, confabulation usually resolves completely [13,21,25,30,103], although it may persist to some degree [14,21,26,103,104]. Many patients exhibit spontaneous, bizarre fabrications shortly after rupture or repair of the aneurysm [14,26,30,103–105]. Two patients described by Stuss et al. [103] had fabrications with morbid overtones. Damasio et al. [26] noted that a characteristic feature of the fabrications of their patients was that they appeared to be composed of current events intertwined in a seemingly logical manner with older, unrelated memories, similar to what seems to occur in dreaming. In subsequent conversations, some of the fabrications were used as if they had become incorporated into memory. As recovery progressed, the patients realized the bizarre and false nature of their fabrications. Paranoid features are notably absent in the reports on confabulation.

DeLuca and Cicerone [105] compared the frequency and severity of confabulations that occurred in a group of patients after repair of a ruptured anterior communicating artery aneurysm with those in a group of patients with intracranial hemorrhage elsewhere in the brain. The subjects were interviewed while oriented (oriented to person, place, and time on two consecutive occasions) and nonoriented (not fulfilling the definition of oriented). Confabulations were described as "severe" (spontaneous), "moderate" (provoked), or "absent." Confabulation was present in 100% of the patients with aneurysms of the anterior communicating artery, regardless of orientation status. This was in contrast with confabulation in only 41% of the control patients when nonoriented and 6% when oriented. These results suggest that transient confabulation in the control group was due to an acute confusional state, whereas persistent confabulation in the anterior communicating artery group was due to damage of the frontal lobe. In regard to severity, 67% of patients in the anterior communicating artery group exhibited severe (spontaneous) confabulations at some point during the interviews but none of the patients in the control group did. The distinction between spontaneous, or "fantastic," confabulation and provoked, or "momentary," confabulation has been the subject of several reports, and fantastic confabulation is believed to be a separate entity that signifies frontal lobe damage [103,104,106,107]. DeLuca and Cicerone [105] defined fantastic confabulation as "spontaneous fabrication of false memories with grandiose elaboration"; momentary confabulation was defined as "actual memories from the past displaced in temporal context." Because many patients have features of both forms of confabulation and because most patients who initially exhibit spontaneous and provoked confabulation later exhibit only the latter, DeLuca and Cicerone argued that these features of confabulation form a continuum rather than dichotomous poles.

Because confabulation and amnesia typically coexist, it may be reasonable to assume that confabulation is a manifestation of a primary memory deficit. Several other theories have been proposed about the underlying nature of confabulation. Mercer et al. [107] studied patients who had provoked confabulation in association with chronic alcoholism, anoxic encephalopathy, probable Alzheimer's disease, and normal-pressure hydrocephalus. The results of these investigators did not support the hypothesis that provoked confabulation was a direct manifestation of disorientation, suggestibility, or memory impairment; impaired memory processing was clearly a necessary co-contributor. They postulated that patients confabulate to questioning if 1. an answer is required but memory for the correct answer is impaired and 2. an alternative answer with highly overlearned or affectively significant features is available and self-corrective mechanisms are defective.

Stuss et al. [103] described the features of spontaneous confabulation in five patients, two of whom had frontal lobe lesions associated with surgical repair of an anterior communicating artery aneurysm. All the patients had impaired ability to inhibit responses, to monitor their behavior, and to use environmental cues. Memory dysfunction, impulsivity, and lack of concern were also obvious in each of the patients.

2. Frequency

Although cases of memory impairment without confabulation [27] and confabulation without amnesia [104] have been reported, most patients who confabulate after rupture or repair of an anterior communicating artery aneurysm are also amnesic [36]. Therefore, the frequency of confabulation parallels that of amnesia.

3. Anatomy and Pathophysiology

Radiologic evidence of frontal lobe damage is invariably present in patients with ruptured anterior communicating artery aneurysms who confabulate [25,26,30, 103–105]. Because these patients often have a combination of infarcts in the basal forebrain and the orbitofrontal cortex (i.e., in the distribution of the anterior cerebral artery), it has been debated whether isolated or combined lesions are necessary for confabulation. Confabulation has been observed in cases of an isolated lesion in the basal forebrain [29,83,85] but it was not observed in a patient with an anterior communicating artery aneurysm who had bifrontal infarcts [33]. Thus, damage to the basal forebrain with or without involvement of the orbitofrontal cortex seems to be the most plausible cause of confabulation [105].

Patients with a lesion in the frontal lobes have impairment in selective attention, in inhibiting distracting stimuli, and in planning and sequencing behavior. All these features are similar to those observed in patients with anterior communicating artery aneurysms who confabulate [103]. As Stuss et al. [103] noted, the frontal lobes have extensive connections with other cortical regions and the reticular activating system. Therefore, infarction of the orbitofrontal cortex or basal forebrain or both can disrupt these pathways and cause confabulation.

C. Emotional Changes

1. Clinical Features

Various emotional changes have been observed in patients after subarachnoid hemorrhage.* In some patients, emotional change is the most debilitating sequela and occasionally requires treatment. Despite relatively normal motor and cognitive functions, emotional recovery is far from optimal. The emotional

* The terms "personality," "psychologic," "psychiatric," and "emotional" have been used to describe the behavioral changes occurring after subarachnoid hemorrhage. For simplification, we have grouped all these changes under the term "emotional changes."

changes most commonly described after subarachnoid hemorrhage are listed in Table 2.

The most frequent emotional changes are apathy and fatigue. The functional significance of this "amotivational" condition is obvious: decreased work performance, lackluster attention to activities of daily living, and limited participation in recreational activities. At the other extreme, disinhibition and hypersociality may lead to such behavior as sexual indiscretions (e.g., masturbation in public) and incessant conversations with strangers in public places. Some patients become irritable and hostile, which often requires changes in the daily activities of their relatives so as to "not make him or her mad." Despite the low probability of another hemorrhage occurring after clipping of the aneurysm, some patients continue to ponder this possibility and other more mundane concerns. These feelings of anxiety and vulnerability may lead to social withdrawal. Some patients exhibit more severe sequelae, such as hallucinations, delusions, or suicidal ideation. Depression and mania can occur. Therefore, because of the emotional changes that occur after aneurysmal subarachnoid hemorrhage, a person may not only be a significant burden to the family but may also be a less productive member of society.

The negative connotations in most of these descriptions of patients imply that the condition of the patient is worse after subarachnoid hemorrhage. However, the spouses of 13 of the 261 (5%) patients reported by Storey [55] and of nine of the 79 (11%) patients reported by Logue et al. [15] noted "improved personalities" after aneurysm rupture or repair (or both). According to Logue et

Table 2 Emotional Changes That Frequently Occur After Subarachnoid Hemorrhage

Apathy	Vulnerability
Fatigue	Social withdrawal
Indifference	Decreased libido
Tolerance	Sleep disturbances
Euphoria	Hallucinations
Disinhibition	Delusions
Hypersociability	Dysphoria
Increased irritability	Depression
Selfishness	Mania
Hostility	Phobias
Emotional incontinence	Stereotypy
Anxiety	

Compiled from descriptions in references 12, 13, 15, 17, 18, 20, 21, 25, 27, 28, 31, 34, 35, 55, 56, 58–61, 64–66, 72, 73, 78, 108–112.

al. [15], "there had been a personality change for the better, of the type seen after a favourable leukotomy, although a price was usually paid for this in the form of a mild memory impairment."

2. Frequency

The reported frequency of emotional changes has ranged from 3.8% to 100% [12,13,15,17,18,20,21,25,27,28,31,34,35,55,56,58–61,64–66,72,73,78,108–112]. This wide range may be accounted for by various methodologic differences. Whereas in some studies patients and relatives were specifically asked to complete detailed questionnaires about emotional changes, other studies relied only on observations by examiners. It appears that emotional changes of some degree, whether noted by patients or their relatives or both, occur in a significant proportion of patients after aneurysmal subarachnoid hemorrhage.

3. Anatomy and Pathophysiology

The anatomy and pathophysiology underlying these emotional changes is less clear than for memory impairment and confabulation. Storey [55] noted severe anxiety and depressive symptoms in some patients who were without evidence of brain damage. Sonesson et al. [61] also noted anxiety, dysphoria, or social phobias in a large number of patients despite satisfactory neurologic outcomes. Anxiety and depressive states that develop during the recovery period after a life-threatening illness such as subarachnoid hemorrhage seem plausible. According to the current *Diagnostic and Statistical Manual of Mental Disorders* (4th edition) [113], many of these patients would be given the diagnosis of adjustment disorders.

Apathy and fatigue are especially frequent after rupture and repair of anterior communicating artery aneurysms [15,21,28,37,58,61,108,109]. Two recent studies of patients with lesions of the caudate nucleus described many of the same emotional changes as noted above: abulia, apathy, disinterest, disinhibition, euphoria, anxiety, depression, bipolar disorder, agoraphobia, paranoia, and auditory and visual hallucinations [91,92]. These behavioral changes could be due to disconnection of the dorsolateral frontal or orbitofrontal circuits (or both) by lesions of the caudate nucleus [91,93]. As in amnesia and Korsakoff's syndrome, the recurrent artery of Heubner may be involved in the pathogenesis of caudate lesions.

D. Alien-Hand Syndrome and Left-Limb Apraxia

1. Clinical Features

Rare cases of the alien-hand syndrome and left-limb apraxia associated with subarachnoid hemorrhage have been reported [114–118]. Both of these conditions are categorized as a disconnection or callosal syndrome, in which disruption of interhemispheric pathways produces impairment of limb function. The most notable feature of the alien-hand syndrome is competitive behavior between the left and right extremities, wherein the extremities on one side appear to resist the actions of those on the opposite side. Although one recently reported case of alien-hand syndrome involved the right hand [118], it is usually the left hand that is affected. Examples of this behavior are as follows: 1. the right hand turns on the faucet while the left hand turns it off [115]; 2. the left hand moves a checker, the right hand moves the checker back, and then the left hand moves it to its previous position on the checkerboard [117]; 3. the right hand turns the pages of a book while the left hand tries to close the book [117]; and 4. the right leg steps down the stairs as the left leg attempts to ascend the stairs [117]. Della Sala et al. [118] have suggested that this autonomous and disruptive behavior is more appropriately termed the "anarchic" rather than "alien" hand.

In left-limb apraxia, patients show impaired writing, object use, miming to command, and imitation with the left arm [114–117]. Other features of disconnection include poor naming of objects palpated by the left hand (tactile anomia), poor identification of speech on the left during dichotic listening, poor localization of tactile stimulation on the left, and impaired functioning of the left arm in the Block Design Test and Token Test [114–118]. Memory impairment, apathy, and akinesia, with or without mutism, have also been noted in these patients postoperatively.

2. Anatomy and Pathophysiology

Most of the patients described above had a ruptured aneurysm of either the anterior communicating artery [114,117,118] or the pericallosal artery [115,116]. However, one patient had a gunshot wound to the subfrontal structures [117] and another had rupture of a subfrontal arteriovenous malformation [115]. The anterior corpus callosum was damaged in all these patients. Because many functions of the left limbs require transfer of the information processed in the left hemisphere to the right hemisphere, disconnection of the interhemispheric pathways through damage of the anterior corpus callosum could result in left alien-hand syndrome and left-limb apraxia. The case described by Della Sala et al. [118] is noteworthy because the patient had apraxia, aphasic agraphia, and tactile anomia of the *left* hand as well as alien-hand syndrome of the *right* hand after rupture and repair of an anterior communicating artery aneurysm. These clinical signs persisted for three years postoperatively. Bilateral frontobasal paramedian infarcts demonstrated by CT were more extensive on the left and presumably involved the anterior corpus callosum and the supplementary motor area on the left. Because most cases of alien-hand syndrome improve with time and have radiologic evidence of damage to only the corpus callosum, Dellà Sala et al. [118] proposed that a combination of lesions of the corpus callosum and frontomesial cortex (possibly including the supplementary motor area) is responsible for the chronic signs of alien-hand syndrome. Thus, persistent signs of alien-hand syndrome are seen in the arm contralateral to the frontomesial cortical lesion.

E. Akinetic Mutism

Akinetic mutism is rarely observed in patients after subarachnoid hemorrhage. In the series of Logue et al. [15], eight patients were mute for 2 to 30 days postoperatively. Takaku et al. [20] noted akinetic mutism in 6 of 939 patients (0.6%) at the time of hospital dismissal. Okawa et al. [21] described a patient with akinetic mutism perioperatively whose condition subsequently improved. Four patients in the large series of Shephard had akinetic mutism [119]. Other sporadic cases of akinetic mutism associated with aneurysms of the anterior communicating and pericallosal arteries have been reported [25,75,116,118].

Akinetic mutism could be viewed as a condition at the extreme end of the spectrum of behavioral sequelae that includes apathy, loss of initiative, and fatigue. Damage to the ascending medial forebrain bundle [25] or caudate nucleus [91] could also cause akinetic mutism.

F. Aphasia

Aphasia is another rare neurobehavioral disorder that has been described in association with subarachnoid hemorrhage. Logue et al. [15] observed dysphasia in 38% of patients in their series. Takaku et al. [20] noted that 20 of 939 patients (2%) were aphasic at the time of dismissal. Follow-up review of 501 patients who received predominantly conservative treatment showed residual aphasia in 2.5% [22]. Other cases have been described briefly [21,118,119]. The specific characteristics of the language impairment were not described in any detail in these cases. As expected, aphasia was seen more frequently in association with aneurysms of the internal carotid artery and middle cerebral artery than of other cerebral arteries [20].

IV. COGNITIVE OUTCOME AND FUNCTIONAL RECOVERY

A. Cognitive Outcome

The neurobehavioral data that have been published to date involving subarachnoid hemorrhage and intracranial aneurysm repair are summarized in the Appendix at the end of this chapter. Several studies have used psychometric tests to characterize the cognitive impairment in patients after aneurysmal subarachnoid hemorrhage [12,15,25,27,28,31,34–37,58–76,109]. The wide range of results and conclusions in these studies is striking. For example, some authors have found minimal or no neuropsychometric deficits in patients with aneurysm in comparison with control subjects or normative data [58,64,70, 73,74,76,109]. In contrast, other authors have reported significant deficits [12,15,31,34–36,59,61,62,65–69,71,72]. Impairment has been found in all areas of cognitive function, including verbal and nonverbal memory, form perception, perceptual accuracy and speed, visuospatial construction, abstraction, concept formation, and cognitive flexibility. As noted above, the neurotoxic effects of the blood itself may be the cause of this diffuse spectrum of neuropsychometric deficits [68].

In many studies in which significant differences were found, control subjects or normative data were compared with patients with anterior communicating artery aneurysm (the group of patients most widely recognized to have cognitive deficits) [15,31,34,36,66,67,69]. The most consistent findings in patients with anterior communicating artery aneurysm were impaired performance on memory tests and relatively normal IQ scores. Some patients with anterior communicating artery aneurysm tended to perform worse on tests assessing memory and "frontal lobe functions" [36,62]. However, most studies did not find this tendency [59,61,64,67,69,70,73,74,76]. Despite the conflicting data, perhaps explained partly by methodologic inconsistencies among the studies, there clearly are some patients with marked neuropsychometric impairment after subarachnoid hemorrhage [25,26,28,32,34–36]. The negative findings in several studies are notable in that a significant proportion of patients have minimal cognitive sequelae after aneurysmal subarachnoid hemorrhage.

B. Prognostic Indicators of Cognitive Impairment and Functional Recovery

Investigators have also attempted to discover which clinical variables are correlated with cognitive outcome and functional recovery. Similar to the studies assessing the degree and pattern of neuropsychometric deficits after aneurysmal subarachnoid hemorrhage, data about prognostic indicators of cognitive impairment are also inconsistent. The following summarizes the clinical variables that have (or have not) been correlated with worse outcome on neuropsychometric testing and/or functional recovery.

1. Age

Some authors have found that worse outcome was associated with increased age [17,59,61,62], but others have found no such association [34,68,70,71, 73,74,109,122].

2. Aneurysm Location

As noted above, some authors found that the outcome was worse in association with aneurysms of the anterior cerebral and anterior communicating arteries [17,18,61,62,72,77]. However, other authors found no such association [20,37,59,64,65,67,69,70,73,74,76,109,122]. Furthermore, some authors reported that more psychologic, psychiatric, or personality changes were associated with middle cerebral artery aneurysms [55,108,121], carotid ophthalmic aneurysms [121], or vertebrobasilar and multiple aneurysms [20].

3. Preoperative Grade

Several authors have noted that a worse outcome is correlated with the severity of preoperative clinical grade, as determined with the classification of Botterell et al. [123], Hunt and Hess [1], or Fisher et al. [2,20,60,62,65,71,72,74,75, 109,111,112]. However, this association has not been observed by all authors [34,58,70,122].

4. Timing of Aneurysm Surgery

Although some authors found that a worse outcome is correlated with delayed surgical repair [65,109], others have noted the contrary [120]. According to one study, the highest incidence of "psychologic" symptoms occurred in patients operated on 3 to 7 days after subarachnoid hemorrhage rather than before 3 days or after 7 days [20]. Other investigators have found no association between the time of the operation and subsequent outcome [61,70,74].

5. Method of Aneurysm Obliteration

Gade [23] noted a higher incidence of amnesia in patients with anterior communicating artery aneurysm treated with aneurysm trapping rather than with neck ligation. No other studies have attempted to correlate the method of surgical repair with outcome.

6. Vasospasm

In several studies, worse outcome was associated with preoperative or postoperative vasospasm [17,19,34,37,70,109,111], although no such association was found in the study of Teissier du Cros and Lhermitte [58].

7. Nimodipine

No study to date has shown any beneficial effect of nimodipine with regard to cognitive outcome after subarachnoid hemorrhage [63,67].

8. Radiologic Data

Some authors have described patients with marked cognitive impairment despite normal findings on CT or MRI [24,25,69]. The converse has also been reported: patients with normal cognitive functioning yet abnormal CT or MRI findings [33,69]. One study noted worse outcome in patients with infarcts in the territory of the right anterior cerebral artery or bilaterally in the territory of that artery [25]. In another study, neuropsychometric deficits were related to infarction site and diffuse brain damage seen on CT [67]; yet another study found many inconsistencies between the location of aneurysms, lesions present on CT, and neuropsychometric deficits [12]. According to still another study, the combination of basal forebrain and striate nucleus lesions, rather than either one alone, causes memory impairment [35].

9. Other Factors

Worse outcome has also been associated with increased blood pressure [111,112], posterior projection of anterior communicating artery aneurysms [109], hematoma [109], multiple ruptures [18,21], prolonged loss of consciousness [18,19,21], bifrontal surgical approach [57], operations performed without use of an operating microscope [21], resection of the gyrus rectus [58], and perioperative complications [31,72,73,122].

Factors worthy of further study include diabetes insipidus and increased intracranial pressure. Because the diabetes insipidus that occurs after subarachnoid hemorrhage is presumed to be the result of hypothalamic dysfunction and because the hypothalamus and basal forebrain are in proximity, anterior communicating artery syndrome may be encountered frequently in patients with this abnormality. Communicating and noncommunicating hydrocephalus are well-known complications of aneurysmal subarachnoid hemorrhage and may be overlooked if the diagnosis of symptomatic hydrocephalus is based only on the findings of postoperative CT scans. Symptomatic hydrocephalus typically causes diffuse rather than focal cognitive abnormalities and may be responsible for the diffuse encephalopathy observed in some patients after subarachnoid hemorrhage.

C. Treatment of Neurobehavioral Disorders

Improvement in the neurobehavioral disorders that develop after subarachnoid hemorrhage often occurs with time. Patients who have residual emotional changes can benefit from counseling and pharmacologic treatment. Amnesia is a particularly disabling problem, for which few treatments appear to be effective. A recent study demonstrated improvement after treatment with bromocriptine, but not physostigmine, for amnesia that developed in a patient with an iatrogenically induced basal forebrain lesion [84]. Alternatively, cholinergic agents may be helpful if the nucleus basalis of Meynert, septal nuclei, nucleus of the diagonal band of Broca, or their projections are damaged.

REFERENCES

1. Hunt WE, Hess RM. Surgical risk as related to time of intervention in the repair of intracranial aneurysms. *J Neurosurg* 1968; 28:14–20.
2. Fisher CM, Kistler JP, Davis JM. Relation of cerebral vasospasm to subarachnoid hemorrhage visualized by computerized tomographic scanning. *Neurosurgery* 1980; 6:1–9.
3. Wechsler D. Wechsler Adult Intelligence Scale–Revised. San Antonio: The Psychological Corporation, 1981.
4. Reitan R. Validity of the Trail–Making Test as an indication of organic brain damage. *Percept Mot Skills* 1958; 8:271–276.
5. Comalli P Jr, Wapner S, Werner H. Interference effects of Stroop Color–Word Test in childhood, adulthood, and aging. *J Gen Psychol* 1962; 100:47–53.
6. Benton A, Hamsher KD. Multilingual Aphasia Examination. Iowa City, Iowa: University of Iowa, 1976.
7. Benton AL, Hamsher KD, Varney N, Spreen O. Contributions to Neuropsychological Assessment: A Clinical Manual. New York: Oxford University Press, 1983.
8. Wechsler D. Wechsler Memory Scale–Revised. San Antonio: The Psychological Corporation, 1987.
9. Rey A. L'examen Clinique en Psychologie. Paris: Presses Universitaires de France, 1958.
10. Delis D, Kramer J, Kaplan E, Ober B. The California Verbal Learning Test. New York: The Psychological Corporation, 1987.
11. Heaton R. Wisconsin Card Sorting Test Manual. Odessa, Florida: Psychological Assessment Resources, Inc., 1981.
12. Barbarotto R, De Santis A, Laiacona M, Basso A, Spagnoli D, Capitani E. Neuropsychological follow–up of patients operated for aneurysms of the middle cerebral artery and posterior communicating artery. *Cortex* 1989; 25:275–288.
13. Lindqvist G, Norlen G. Korsakoff's syndrome after operation on ruptured aneurysm of the anterior communicating artery. *Acta Psychiatr Scand* 1966; 42:24–34.
14. Talland GA, Sweet WH, Ballantine HT Jr. Amnesic syndrome with anterior communicating artery aneurysm. *J Nerve Ment Dis* 1967; 145:179–192.
15. Logue V, Durward M, Pratt RT, Piercy M, Nixon WL. The quality of survival after rupture of an anterior cerebral aneurysm. *Br J Psychiatry* 1968; 114:137–160.
16. Luria AR. The neuropsychology of memory. Washington, DC: VH Winston and Sons, 1976:255–297.
17. Matsukado Y, Kitamura K, Shida K, Takamatsu I. Psychiatric disorders after surgery of anterior communicating and internal carotid aneurysms. *No To Shinkei* 1968; 20:557–564.

18. Maeda S, Okawa M, Aiba T. Psychiatric symptoms of intracranial arterial aneurysms—pre- and post-surgical conditions and follow–up observations. *Rinsho Shinkeigaku* 1974; 14:1–9.
19. Hori S, Suzuki J. Early and late results of intracranial direct surgery of anterior communicating artery aneurysms. *J Neurosurg* 1979; 50:433–440.
20. Takaku A, Tanaka S, Mori T, Suzuki J. Postoperative complications in 1,000 cases of intracranial aneurysms. *Surg Neurol* 1979; 12:137–144.
21. Okawa M, Maeda S, Nukui H, Kawafuchi J. Psychiatric symptoms in ruptured anterior communicating aneurysms: social prognosis. *Acta Psychiatr Scand* 1980; 61:306–312.
22. Nystrom S. Psychodynamics in Subarachnoid Hemorrhage. A Study Based on 1,183 Patients. Helsinki, Finland: TA Sahalan Kirjapaino Oy, 1973:39–47.
23. Gade A. Amnesia after operations on aneurysms of the anterior communicating artery. *Surg Neurol* 1982; 18:46–49.
24. Volpe BT, Hirst W. Amnesia following the rupture and repair of an anterior communicating artery aneurysm. *J Neurol Neurosurg Psychiatry* 1983; 46:704–709.
25. Alexander MP, Freedman M. Amnesia after anterior communicating artery aneurysm rupture. *Neurology* 1984; 34:752–757.
26. Damasio AR, Graff-Radford NR, Eslinger PJ, Damasio H, Kassell N. Amnesia following basal forebrain lesions. *Arch Neurol* 1985; 42:263–271.
27. Vilkki J. Amnesic syndromes after surgery of anterior communicating artery aneurysms. *Cortex* 1985; 21:431–444.
28. Steinman DR, Bigler ED. Neuropsychological sequelae of ruptured anterior communicating artery aneurysm. *Int J Clin Neuropsych* 1986; 8:135–140.
29. Phillips S, Sangalang V, Sterns G. Basal forebrain infarction. A clinicopathologic correlation. *Arch Neurol* 1987; 44:1134–1138.
30. Parkin AJ, Leng NR, Stanhope N, Smith AP. Memory impairment following ruptured aneurysm of the anterior communicating artery. *Brain Cogn* 1988; 7:231–243.
31. Fasanaro AM, Valiani R, Russo G, Scarano E, De Falco R, Profeta G. Memory performances after anterior communicating artery aneurysm surgery. *Acta Neurol (Napoli)* 1989; 11:272–278.
32. Youngjohn JR, Altman IM, Van Doren J. Amnesia following anterior communicating artery aneurysm surgery (abstract). *J Clin Exp Neuropsychol* 1989; 11:61.
33. DeLuca J. Predicting behavioral patterns following anterior communicating artery aneurysm (abstract). *Arch Phys Med Rehabil* 1990; 71:777.
34. Stenhouse LM, Knight RG, Longmore BE, Bishara SN. Long–term cognitive deficits in patients after surgery on aneurysms of the anterior communicating artery. *J Neurol Neurosurg Psychiatry* 1991; 54:909–914.
35. Irle E, Wowra B, Kunert HJ, Hampl J, Kunze S. Memory disturbances following anterior communicating artery rupture. *Ann Neurol* 1992; 31:473–480.
36. DeLuca J. Cognitive dysfunction after aneurysm of the anterior communicating artery. *J Clin Exp Neuropsych* 1992; 14:924–934.
37. Drumm D, Greene K, Marciano F, Prigatano G, Spetzer R. Neurobehavioral deficits following rupture of anterior communicating (ACoA) aneurysms: The ACoA aneurysm syndrome. *BNI Quarterly* 1993; 9:2–12.

38. Scoville WB, Milner B. Loss of recent memory after bilateral hippocampal lesions. *J Neurol Neurosurg Psychiatry* 1957; 20:11–21.
39. Milner B, Corkin S, Teuber H-L. Further analysis of the hippocampal amnesic syndrome: 14–year follow–up study of H. M. *Neuropsychologia* 1968; 6:215–234.
40. Gade A, Mortensen EL. Temporal gradient in the remote memory impairment of amnesic patients with lesions in the basal forebrain. *Neuropsychologia* 1990; 28:985–1001.
41. Albert MS, Butters N, Levin J. Temporal gradients in the retrograde amnesia of patients with alcoholic Korsakoff's disease. *Arch Neurol* 1979; 36:211–216.
42. Squire LR, Cohen N. Memory and amnesia: resistance to disruption develops for years after learning. *Behav Neural Biol* 1979; 25:115–125.
43. Warrington EK, McCarthy RA. The fractionation of retrograde amnesia. *Brain Cogn* 1988; 7:184–200.
44. Butters N, Cermak LS. Alcoholic Korsakoff's Syndrome: An Information–Processing Approach to Amnesia. New York: Academic Press, 1980.
45. Parkin A. Memory and Amnesia: An Introduction. Oxford: Blackwell, 1987.
46. Squire LR. Comparisons between forms of amnesia: some deficits are unique to Korsakoff's syndrome. *J Exp Psychol Learn Mem Cogn* 1982; 8:560–571.
47. Schacter D. Memory, amnesia, and frontal lobe dysfunction. *Psychobiology* 1987; 15:21–36.
48. Delbecq-Derouesne J, Beauvois MF, Shallice T. Preserved recall versus impaired recognition. A case study. *Brain* 1990; 113:1045–1074.
49. Van Hoesen GW. The cortico–cortical projections of the posterior parahippocampal area in the rhesus monkey (abstract). *Anat Rec* 1980; 196:195A.
50. Rosene DL, Van Hoesen GW. Hippocampal efferents reach widespread areas of cerebral cortex and amygdala in the rhesus monkey. *Science* 1977; 198:315–317.
51. Aggleton JP, Burton MJ, Passingham RE. Cortical and subcortical afferents to the amygdala of the rhesus monkey (*Macaca mulatta*). *Brain Res* 1980; 190:347–368.
52. Amaral DG, Cowan WM. Subcortical afferents to the hippocampal formation in the monkey. *J Comp Neurol* 1980; 189:573–591.
53. Price JL, Amaral DG. An autoradiographic study of the projections of the central nucleus of the monkey amygdala. *J Neurosci* 1981; 1:1242–1259.
54. Volpe BT, Herscovitch P, Raichle ME. Positron emission tomography defines metabolic abnormality in mesial temporal lobes of two patients with amnesia after rupture and repair of anterior communicating artery aneurysm (abstract). *Neurology* 1984; 34:188.
55. Storey PB. Psychiatric sequelae of subarachnoid haemorrhage. *Br Med J* 1967; 3:261–266.
56. Short MJ, Wilson WP, Odom GL. Psychiatric sequelae of subarachnoid hemorrhage. *South Med J* 1968; 61:87–91.
57. Sundt TM Jr, Kobayashi S, Fode NC, Whisnant JP. Results and complications of surgical management of 809 intracranial aneurysms in 722 cases. Related and unrelated to grade of patient, type of aneurysm, and timing of surgery. *J Neurosurg* 1982; 56:753–765.
58. Teissier du Cros J, Lhermitte F. Neuropsychological analysis of ruptured saccular

aneurysms of the anterior communicating artery after radical therapy (32 cases). *Surg Neurol* 1984; 22:353–359.

59. Ljunggren B, Sonesson B, Saveland H, Brandt L. Cognitive impairment and adjustment in patients without neurological deficits after aneurysmal SAH and early operation. *J Neurosurg* 1985; 62:673–679.
60. Saveland H, Sonesson B, Ljunggren B, et al. Outcome evaluation following subarachnoid hemorrhage. *J Neurosurg* 1986; 64:191–196.
61. Sonesson B, Ljunggren B, Saveland H, Brandt L. Cognition and adjustment after late and early operation for ruptured aneurysm. *Neurosurgery* 1987; 21:279–287.
62. Bornstein RA, Weir BK, Petruk KC, Disney LB. Neuropsychological function in patients after subarachnoid hemorrhage. *Neurosurgery* 1987; 21:651–654.
63. Saveland H, Sonesson B, Ljunggren B, Ryman T, Brandt L. Does intravenous nimodipine treatment influence cognition in patients subjected to early aneurysm operation? *Acta Neurol Scand* 1988; 77:54–59.
64. McKenna P, Willison JR, Phil B, Lowe D, Neil-Dwyer G. Cognitive outcome and quality of life one year after subarachnoid haemorrhage. *Neurosurgery* 1989; 24:361–367.
65. De Santis A, Laiacona M, Barbarotto R, et al. Neuropsychological outcome of patients operated upon for an intracranial aneurysm: analysis of general prognostic factors and of the effects of the location of the aneurysm. *J Neurol Neurosurg Psychiatry* 1989; 52:1135–1140.
66. Laiacona M, De Santis A, Barbarotto R, Basso A, Spagnoli D, Capitani E. Neuropsychological follow–up of patients operated for aneurysms of anterior communicating artery. *Cortex* 1989; 25:261–273.
67. Vilkki J, Holst P, Ohman J, Servo A, Heiskanen O. Cognitive deficits related to computed tomographic findings after surgery for a ruptured intracranial aneurysm. *Neurosurgery* 1989; 25:166–172.
68. Sonesson B, Saveland H, Ljunggren B, Brandt L. Cognitive functioning after subarachnoid haemorrhage of unknown origin. *Acta Neurol Scand* 1989; 80:400–410.
69. Romner B, Sonesson B, Ljunggren B, Brandt L, Saveland H, Holtas S. Late magnetic resonance imaging related to neurobehavioral functioning after aneurysmal subarachnoid hemorrhage. *Neurosurgery* 1989; 25:390–396.
70. Richardson JT. Performance in free recall following rupture and repair of intracranial aneurysm. *Brain Cogn* 1989; 9:210–226.
71. Ogden J, Levin P, Mee E. Long–term neuropsychological and psychosocial effects of subarachnoid hemorrhage. *Neuropsych Neuropsychol Behav Neurol* 1990; 3:260–274.
72. Stegen G, Freckmann N. Outcome and rehabilitation after aneurysmal subarachnoid haemorrhage. *Zentralbl Neurochir* 1991; 52:37–39.
73. Maurice-Williams RS, Willison JR, Hatfield R. The cognitive and psychological sequelae of uncomplicated aneurysm surgery. *J Neurol Neurosurg Psychiatry* 1991; 54:335–340.
74. Richardson JT. Cognitive performance following rupture and repair of intracranial aneurysm. *Acta Neurol Scand* 1991; 83:110–122.
75. Awad IA, Little JR. Perioperative management and outcome after surgical treatment of anterior cerebral artery aneurysms. *Can J Neurol Sci* 1991; 18:120–125.

76. Hutter BO, Gilsbach JM. Cognitive deficits after rupture and early repair of anterior communicating artery aneurysms. *Acta Neurochir (Wien)* 1992; 116:6–13.
77. Krayenbuhl HA, Yasargil MG, Flamm ES, Tew JM Jr. Microsurgical treatment of intracranial saccular aneurysms. *J Neurosurg* 1972; 37:678–686.
78. Ropper AH, Zervas NT. Outcome 1 year after SAH from cerebral aneurysm. Management morbidity, mortality, and functional status in 112 consecutive good-risk patients. *J Neurosurg* 1984; 60:909–915.
79. Mesulam MM, Van Hoesen GW. Acetylcholinesterase–rich projections from the basal forebrain of the rhesus monkey to neocortex. *Brain Res* 1976; 109:152–157.
80. Mesulam MM, Mufson EJ, Levey AI, Wainer BH. Cholinergic innervation of cortex by the basal forebrain: Cytochemistry and cortical connections of the septal area, diagonal band nuclei, nucleus basalis (substantia innominata), and hypothalamus in the rhesus monkey. *J Comp Neurol* 1983; 214:170–197.
81. Whitehouse PJ, Price DL, Struble RG, Clark AW, Coyle JT, Delon MR. Alzheimer's disease and senile dementia: loss of neurons in the basal forebrain. *Science* 1982; 215:1237–1239.
82. Zola-Morgan S, Squire LR. Neuroanatomy of memory. *Annu Rev Neurosci* 1993; 16:547–563.
83. Berti A, Arienta C, Papagno C. A case of amnesia after excision of the septum pellucidum. *J Neurol Neurosurg Psychiatry* 1990; 53:922–924.
84. Dobkin BH, Hanlon R. Dopamine agonist treatment of antegrade amnesia from a mediobasal forebrain injury. *Ann Neurol* 1993; 33:313–316.
85. Morris MK, Bowers D, Chatterjee A, Heilman KM. Amnesia following a discrete basal forebrain lesion. *Brain* 1992; 115:1827–1847.
86. Irle E. Lesion size and recovery of function: some new perspectives. *Brain Res* 1987; 434:307–320.
87. Irle E. An analysis of the correlation of lesion size, localization and behavioral effects in 283 published studies of cortical and subcortical lesions in old–world monkeys. *Brain Res Brain Res Rev* 1990; 15:181–213.
88. Butters N, Albert MS, Sax D. Investigations of the memory disorders of patients with Huntington's disease. *Adv Neurol* 1979; 23:203–213.
89. Diamond R, White RF, Myers RH, et al. Evidence of presymptomatic cognitive decline in Huntington's disease. *J Clin Exp Neuropsychol* 1992; 14:961–975.
90. Massman PJ, Delis DC, Butters N, Levin BE, Salmon DP. Are all subcortical dementias alike? Verbal learning and memory in Parkinson's and Huntington's disease patients. *J Clin Exp Neuropsychol* 1990; 12:729–744.
91. Mendez MF, Adams NL, Lewandowski KS. Neurobehavioral changes associated with caudate lesions. *Neurology* 1989; 39:349–354.
92. Caplan LR, Schmahmann JD, Kase CS, et al. Caudate infarcts. *Arch Neurol* 1990; 47:133–143.
93. Alexander GE, DeLong MR, Strick PL. Parallel organization of functionally segregated circuits linking basal ganglia and cortex. *Annu Rev Neurosci* 1986; 9:357–381.
94. Nauta WJH. Circuitous connections linking cerebral cortex, limbic system, and corpus striatum. In: Doane BK, Livingston KE, (eds). The Limbic System: Functional Organization and Clinical Disorders. New York: Raven Press, 1986:43–54.

95. Haber SN, Groenewegen HJ, Grove EA, Nauta WJ. Efferent connections of the ventral pallidum: Evidence of a dual striato pallidofugal pathway. *J Comp Neurol* 1985; 235:322–335.
96. Caselli RJ, Yanagihara T. Memory disorders in degenerative neurological diseases. In: Yanagihara T, Petersen RC, (eds). Memory Disorders: Research and Clinical Practice. New York: Marcel Dekker, 1991:369–395.
97. Hughes JT, Oppenheimer DR. Superficial siderosis of the central nervous system. A report on nine cases with autopsy. *Acta Neuropathol (Berl)* 1969; 13:56–74.
98. Dunker RO, Harris AB. Surgical anatomy of the proximal anterior cerebral artery. *J Neurosurg* 1976; 44:359–367.
99. Perlmutter D, Rhoton AL Jr. Microsurgical anatomy of the anterior cerebral–anterior communicating–recurrent artery complex. *J Neurosurg* 1976; 45:259–272.
100. Crowell RM, Morawetz RB. The anterior communicating artery has significant branches. *Stroke* 1977; 8:272–273.
101. Vincentelli F, Lehman G, Caruso G, Grisoli F, Rabehanta P, Gouaze A. Extracerebral course of the perforating branches of the anterior communicating artery: microsurgical anatomical study. *Surg Neurol* 1991; 35:98–104.
102. Gorczyca W, Mohr G. Microvascular anatomy of Heubner's recurrent artery. *Neurol Res* 1987; 9:259–264.
103. Stuss DT, Alexander MP, Lieberman A, Levine H. An extraordinary form of confabulation. *Neurology* 1978; 28:1166–1172.
104. Kapur N, Coughlan AK. Confabulation and frontal lobe dysfunction. *J Neurol Neurosurg Psychiatry* 1980; 43:461–463.
105. DeLuca J, Cicerone KD. Confabulation following aneurysm of the anterior communicating artery. *Cortex* 1991; 27:417–423.
106. Berlyne N. Confabulation. *Br J Psychiatry* 1972; 120:31–39.
107. Mercer B, Wapner W, Gardner H, Benson DF. A study of confabulation. *Arch Neurol* 1977; 34:429–433.
108. Storey PB. Brain damage and personality change after subarachnoid haemorrhage. *Br J Psychiatry* 1970; 117:129–142.
109. Sengupta RP, Chiu JSP, Brierley H. Quality of survival following direct surgery for anterior communicating artery aneurysms. *J Neurosurg* 1975; 43:58–64.
110. Rasmussen P, Busch H, Haase J, et al. Intracranial saccular aneurysms. Results of treatment in 851 patients. *Acta Neurochir (Wien)* 1980; 53:1–17.
111. Artiola i Fortuny L, Prieto-Valiente L. Long-term prognosis in surgically treated intracranial aneurysms. Part 2: Morbidity. *J Neurosurg* 1981; 54:35–43.
112. Oder W, Kollegger H, Zeiler K, Dal-Bianco P, Wessely P, Deecke L. Subarachnoid hemorrhage of unknown etiology: early prognostic factors for long–term functional capacity. *J Neurosurg* 1991; 74:601–655.
113. American Psychiatric Association. Diagnostic and Statistical Manual of Mental Disorders: DMS–IV, 4th ed. Washington, DC: American Psychiatric Association, 1994.
114. Beukelman DR, Flowers CR, Swanson PD. Cerebral disconnection associated with anterior communicating artery aneurysm: Implications for evaluation of symptoms. *Arch Phys Med Rehabil* 1980; 61:18–23.

115. Levin HS, Goldstein FC, Ghostine SY, Weiner RL, Crofford MJ, Eisenberg HM. Hemispheric disconnection syndrome persisting after anterior cerebral artery aneurysm rupture. *Neurosurgery* 1987; 21:831–838.
116. Graff-Radford NR, Welsh K, Godersky J. Callosal apraxia. *Neurology* 1987; 37:100–105.
117. Banks G, Short P, Martinez J, Latchaw R, Ratcliff G, Boller F. The alien hand syndrome. Clinical and postmortem findings. *Arch Neurol* 1989; 46:456–459.
118. Della Sala S, Marchetti C, Spinnler H. Right–sided anarchic (alien) hand: a longitudinal study. *Neuropsychologia* 1991; 29:1113–1127.
119. Shephard RH. Ruptured cerebral aneurysms: Early and late prognosis with surgical treatment. A personal series, 1958–1980. *J Neurosurg* 1983; 59:6–15.
120. Adams CB, Loach AB, O'Laoire SA. Intracranial aneurysms: analysis of results of microneurosurgery. *Br Med J* 1976; 2:607–609.
121. Sengupta RP, McAllister VL, Sastry Kolluri VR. Results of surgical treatment of intracranial aneurysms. In: Sengupta RP, McAllister VL, (eds). Subarachnoid Haemorrhage. Berlin: Springer–Verlag, 1986:237–267.
122. Tidswell P, Dias PS, Sagar HJ, Moyes AR, Battersby RD. Cognitive outcome after aneurysm rupture: relationship to aneurysm site and perioperative complications. *Neurology* 1995; 45:875–882.
123. Botterell EH, Lougheed WM, Scott JW, Vandewater SL. Hypothermia, and interruption of carotid, or carotid and vertebral circulation, in the surgical management of intracranial aneurysms. *J Neurosurg* 1956; 13:1–42.

APPENDIX Review of Neurobehavioral Findings in Patients After Subarachnoid Hemorrhage or Repair of Intracranial Aneurysms or Both

Study	Number of patients	Aneurysm location[a]	Neuropsychometrical results	Functional/cognitive/emotional status	Comment
Lindqvist and Norlen, 1966 [13]	33	ACoA	Performed but no detail	17 (52%) pts with Korsakoff's syndrome; memory impairment persisted several months later in 5 pts; "flattening of ambitions" and "emotional shallowness" persisted in some after memory impairment resolved	Procedures: aneurysm neck ligation, trapping, wrapping, or electrocoagulation
Storey, 1967 [55]	261	All	Not performed	Followup of 209 pts 6 mo–6 yr after treatment: 1. 115 (55%) pts had "psychiatric" morbidity of some degree, 27 (13%) pts had severe/very severe "psychiatric" morbidity; 2. 13 (6%) pts were regarded to have "improved personality," of whom 8 had ACA or ACoA aneurysms	Procedures: common carotid ligation, proximal ACA ligation, or direct aneurysm surgery in 60%, or conservative therapy; no microscope used "Psychiatric" morbidity correlated with MCA aneurysms treated surgically,[b] and ACoA and PCA aneurysms treated conservatively
Logue et al., 1968 [15]	79	ACA/ACoA	Performed 6 to 101 mo postop in 65 pts: mean WAIS scores near normal, mean MQ less than VIQ[d]	Followup all pts 6–101 mo after treatment: 44 (56%) returned to previous work level; 26 (33%) had retrograde amnesia of some degree after treatment (lasting > 1 week; in 7 [9%]); 69	Procedure: ACA ligation (84%) or conservative therapy; no microscope used Authors noted 9 pts had improved personality but most also had mild memory impairment

				(87%) had anterograde amnesia of some degree after treatment (lasting (87%) had anterograde am- mt 1 yr in 6 [8%]); 18 (23%) confabulated after treatment (confabulation noted at followup in 6 [8%]); 8 (10%) were totally mute for 2 to 30 days after treatment; 30 (38%) had dysphasia after treatment (32 [41%] made dysphasic errors on NP tests); 15 (19%) reported elevation of mood and 10 (13%) were more depressed; 25 (32%) worried less after treatment and 9 (11%) worried more; 14 (18%) had affective flattening; 30 (38%) had emotional lability; 9 (11%) thought to have "improved personality"	
Short et al., 1968 [56]	29	All	Not performed	Followup of all pts 2 mo–7 yr after SAH: 8 (28%) had objective memory loss; 18 (62%) had affective disability and 6 had medical care and 1 other was hospitalized; 5 (17%) noted hallucinations; 15 (52%) returned to previous work level	Procedures: Crutchfield clamp application in 21, "open operation" in 8 Authors noted emotional and intellectual disabilities rather than physical disabilities were greatest impediment to recovery

APPENDIX Continued

Study	Number of patients	Aneurysm location[a]	Neuropsychometrical results	Functional/cognitive/emotional status	Comment
Matsukado et al., 1968 [17]	70	All	Performed but no details given	Of 57 pts (8 with ACA or ACoA aneurysms) treated surgically, 11 (19%) had "psychiatric disorders" postop, primarily Korsakoff's syndrome	Procedures: aneurysm clipping, wrapping, or trapping in 57 pts Authors noted "psychiatric disorders" occurred more frequently in pts with ACA or ACoA aneurysm and in pts with increased age and vasospasm
Storey, 1970 (Extension of 1967 study) [108]	261	All	Performed but no details given	Followup of all pts 6 mo–6 yr postop: 145 (56%) returned to previous work level; 108 (41%) had "personality impairment" of some degree (common reported symptoms were less vitality in 70 [27%], greater irritability in 58 [22%], more easily worried, 51 [20%]); 13 (5%) were regarded to have "improved personality" (8 of whom had ACA or ACoA aneurysms)	Surgical details not described; 30 (11%) pts had no aneurysm on angio Author concluded 1. "personality impairment" most common with MCA aneurysm, the commonest changes were increased anxiety and irritability and loss of vitality; 2. personality change without intellectual impairment more common with ACoA aneurysms
Krayenbuhl et al., 1972 [77]	250	All	Not performed	Followup (duration not noted): 191 (83%) of 231 surviving pts returned to	Procedure: aneurysm clipping with operative microscope Authors noted only influence

				previous work (part- or full-time); 58 (61%) with ACoA aneurysm had confusion and memory deficits pre- or postop (permanent in 6 [6%] of them)	of aneurysm location on surgical results was presence of confusion and memory deficits in many pts with ACoA aneurysm
Nystrom, 1973 [22]	1080	All	Not performed	After SAH, 323 (30%) pts had "mental disorders" and 175 (16%) had aphasia Followup (1–16 yr) of 501 pts after SAH: 16 (3%) had Korsakoff's syndrome, 12 (2%) had aphasia, 8 (2%) had depression, 3 (0.6%) had anxiety, and 1 (0.2%) had "general psychosis"	Associations noted between 1. Korsakoff's syndrome and ACoA and dominant hemisphere MCA aneurysms, 2. aphasia and dominant hemisphere MCA aneurysms, and 3. "general psychosis" and ACoA and pericallosal aneurysms
Maeda et al., 1974 [18]	102	All	Not performed	"Psychiatric" symptoms noted in 47% of pts preop and 53% postop; Korsakoff's syndrome common with ACoA aneurysm Followup of 29 pts: confabulation improved within 2–6 mo, memory deficits and "personality impairments" tended to persist	Surgical details not given Authors noted pts with ACoA aneurysm had highest "psychiatric morbidity," "psychiatric disturbances" tended to be more severe with repeated SAH and in pts with longer duration of disturbed consciousness, nature of "psychiatric disturbances" was identical preop and postop

APPENDIX Continued

Study	Number of patients	Aneurysm location[a]	Neuropsychometrical results	Functional/cognitive/emotional status	Comment
Sengupta et al., 1975 [109]	32	ACoA	Performed 4–33 mo postop in 26 pts: mean WAIS and WMS scores near normal	Work level not noted Many with residual loss of interest, initiative, and energy	Procedures: aneurysmal neck clipping, wrapping, or both; no microscope used Worse outcome[c] correlated with poor clinical grade at operation, delayed surgery, posterior projection of aneurysm, generalized vasospasm, hematoma Authors concluded no evidence of postop intellectual impairment, but personality changes were present in many patients
Adams et al., 1976 [120]	100	All	Not performed	Followup of 85 surviving pts 6 mo postop: 64 (75%) returned to previous work level (64% of original series)	Procedures: aneurysm clipping or wrapping, all with operative microscope
Hori and Suzuki, 1979 [19]	346	ACoA	Not performed	Followup of 303 pts: 256 (84%) capable of working; 6 had residual Korsakoff's syndrome, amnesia, or disorientation	338 pts had ruptured and 8 had unruptured ACoA aneurysms Procedures: ligation, clipping, trapping, resection and suture, wrapping, or combination of these; no microscope used

					Authors noted all 6 pts with "psychiatric symptoms" had been transiently unconscious and had either intracerebral hematoma or vasospasm; in 5 pts, symptoms were present preop
Takaku et al., 1979 [20]	1000	All	Not performed	Of 939 surviving pts at discharge, 107 (11%) had "psychologic" symptoms: disorientation in 88 (9%), amnesia in 41 (4%), "personality impairment" in 36 (4%), Korsakoff's syndrome in 22 (2%), dementia in 11 (1%), hallucinations in 9 (1%), akinetic mutism in 6 (0.6%), emotional instability in 2 (0.2%), stereotypy in 1 (0.1%); 20 (2%) also were aphasic at dismissal	Surgical details not described Authors noted "psychologic" symptoms more common with ACoA, VB, and multiple aneurysms, worse preop grade, and surgery 3–7 days after SAH; these symptoms improved in 63% of pts
Rasmussen et al., 1980 [110]	851	All	Not performed	Followup of 435 surviving pts 2–7 yr postop: 218 (50%) had "normal functional capacity," 167 (38%) noted impaired memory, 124 (29%) noted fatigue, 111 (26%) noted "changes in character"	Procedures: aneurysm clipping, ligature, trapping, coating, or carotid ligature in 67% or conservative therapy; use of microscope not noted Authors noted dementia, "character changes," head aches, and generalized fatigue were most incapacitating factors in surviving pts

APPENDIX Continued

Study	Number of patients	Aneurysm location[a]	Neuropsychometrical results	Functional/cognitive/emotional status	Comment
Okawa et al., 1980 [21]	95	ACoA	Not performed	"Psychiatric" symptoms noted in 54 (61%) pts preop, in 60 (71%) conscious pts postop, in 25 (34%) of 73 pts at followup 6 mo–9 yr postop; disorientation, confabulation, and amnesia were most common 60 (82%) pts returned to "normal lives," 2 had severe Korsakoff's syndrome 7 yr postop, 1 had aphasia	Procedures: 36% with operating microscope; psychiatric morbidity reduced in this group[e] Authors noted repair may exacerbate "psychiatric" symptoms in pts with multiple ruptures, prolonged loss of consciousness, transient neurologic symptoms; personality changes are greatest obstacle to social rehabilitation
Artiola i Fortuny and Prieto-Valiente, 1981 [111]	265	All	Not performed	Followup of 204 surviving pts 18–66 mo postop; 171 (84%) were physically independent, 132 (65%) returned to premorbid social activities, 132 (65%) had normal psychiatric profiles, 104 (51%) returned to same work level, 83 (41%) felt as well as before operation	Operative microscope used for all pts Authors noted worse outcome on different variables[c] correlated with postop vasospasm, increased age (especially 50–59 yr), increased blood pressure at admission, and poorer preop neurologic status
Sundt et al., 1982 [57]	722	All	Not performed	Followup of 644 surviving pts at least 6 mo postop: 553 (86%) had normal mentation and employment Korsakoff's syndrome devel-	Operative microscope used on all pts, including 466 with recent SAH and 178 with symptoms but no recent SAH (78 died preop)

				oped in 7 (4%) pts with ACoA aneurysms (3 preop, 4 postop), 3 of the 7 had normal mentation and employment at followup	Authors noted Korsakoff's syndrome was either a complication of the initial hemorrhage or from surgical trauma but not vasospasm
Gade, 1982 [23]	48	ACoA	Performed 3–24 mo postop in all pts but no details given	Followup of all pts 3 mo postop: 15 (31%) had amnesia, 9 of 11 (82%) who had trapping and 6 of 37 (16%) who had aneurysmal neck ligation had amnesia	Author concluded trapping invariably disrupts the blood supply through the ACoA perforating branches and should be avoided if possible
Shephard, 1983 [119]	815	All	Not performed	Followup of 501 surviving pts at various times postop: 376 (75%) had "normal working capacity," dementia, psychiatric disorders, impaired memory, dysphasia, or akinetic mutism noted in several pts	Procedures: aneurysm clipping, ligation, wrapping, trapping, carotid ligation or a combination in 75% or conservative therapy; use of microscope not noted
Ropper and Zervas, 1984 [78]	112	All	Not performed	Followup of all pts at least 1 yr postop: 52 (46%) were fully recovered, 28 (25%) reported bothersome emotional or psychologic disturbances, 50 (45%) returned to same work level	Procedures: aneurysm surgery with microscope (100 pts), conservative treatment (12 pts) All pts categorized as Hunt & Hess grade I or II Authors noted, in majority of pts, deteriorated work capacity caused by psychologic or emotional disturbances rather than physical deficits

APPENDIX Continued

Study	Number of patients	Aneurysm location[a]	Neuropsychometrical results	Functional/cognitive/emotional status	Comment
Teissier du Cros and Lhermitte, 1984 [58]	32	ACoA	Performed 12–50 mo postop in all pts: mean WMS and WAIS scores near normal; serious impairment noted in 6 (19%) on mental control, 9 (28%) on Rey-Osterrieth Complex Figure	Followup of all pts 12–50 mo postop: 27 (84%) returned to work; 4 (13%) unable to work because of cognitive impairment or personality changes, 10 (31%) noted weariness and memory loss, 11 (34%) noted lowered initiative	Procedure: all pts had aneurysm neck clipping with operative microscope Authors noted that the only correlation between NP, neurologic, and surgical factors was worse MQ score correlated with resection of gyrus rectus[c]
Alexander and Freedman, 1984 [25]	11	ACoA	Performed 6 weeks–11 yr postop in all pts: 6 (55%) had MQ scores < 85, all pts tested were impaired on immediate recall, delayed recall, and AVLT, 9 (82%) had very poor word-list generation	Followup of all pts 6 weeks–11 yr postop: none returned to previous work level; 4 (36%) institutionalized; 10 (91%) had confabulation (persistent and "extraordinary" in 4); all pts had flat, jocular, and/or irritable affect	Surgical details not known No CT evidence of infarction in 4 (36%) pts Authors concluded that amnesia and personality changes are due to ACoA territory infarction and gross frontal lobe infarction is not required for syndrome (authors coined term "ACoA syndrome")
Ljunggren et al., 1985 [59]	40	All	Performed 14 mo–7 yr postop in all pts: 15 (38%) had short-term memory deficits, 33 (83%) had some memory deficit	Followup of all pts 14 mo–7 yr postop: 12 (30%) noted fatigue and lack of initiative; 20 (50%) noted social maladjustment; 23 (58%) noted	Procedure: all pts had aneurysmal clipping with microscope Authors noted worse cognitive impairment correlated with

				short-term memory difficulty; 30 (75%) noted emotional adjustment difficulty	increased age but not aneurysm location Authors concluded that the wide spectrum of cognitive dysfunction demonstrated the presence of a diffuse SAH-induced encephalopathy in all pts
Damasio et al., 1985 [26]	5	ACA, ACoA, or AVM	Performed at different times postop in all pts: each pt scored poorly on various memory tests	All pts had memory impairment, confabulation, emotional changes	All pts had basal forebrain damage (4 after rupture and repair of ACoA aneurysms and 1 after AVM resection) Authors concluded basal forebrain damage caused atypical amnesic syndrome in their pts
Vilkki, 1985 [27]	5	ACoA	Performed 8 days–8 mo postop in all pts (10 normal controls also tested): mean scores on several WAIS subtests and tests of verbal memory similar to controls, but several pts scored poorly on isolated tests; mean scores on tests of visual, incidental, and imaginatory memory worse than controls[b]	One pt returned to previous work level Memory impairment noted postop in all 5 pts, confabulation in 2, apathy and stereotyped movements in 1	Procedures: aneurysm clipping or trapping, use of microscope not noted CT evidence of frontal lobe lesion in 3 pts, they had more severe deficits Author presumed 1. amnesia with ACoA aneurysm caused by ischemic periventricular diencephalic lesion and 2. persistent confusion, lack of initiative, and disinhibition of irrelevant associations caused by superimposed frontal lobe lesions

APPENDIX Continued

Study	Number of patients	Aneurysm location[a]	Neuropsychometrical results	Functional/cognitive/emotional status	Comment
Steinman and Bigler, 1986 [28]	7	ACoA	Performed 11 mo–9 yr postop in 6 pts (1 pt disphasic): mean scores on WAIS subtests near norms, mean WMS MQ score much lower than mean IQ scores in 5 pts	Followup 11 mo–9 yr postop: families of all pts reported decreased self-criticism, impatience and impulsivity, decreased initiative, impaired judgment, increased dependency, reduced learning capacity, apathy	Procedure: aneurysm clipping in all pts; microscope use not noted Authors concluded that although some cognitive functions were relatively spared, behavioral and personality disturbances are common in pts with ruptured ACoA aneurysms
Sengupta et al., 1986 [121]	500	All	Not performed	Of 446 survivors not lost to followup at least 6 mo postop: 73% returned to work; 12.5% were capable but unemployed; 14.5% were unfit for employment	Procedures: aneurysm clipping, ligature, trapping, wrapping, or proximal carotid ligation; microscope use not noted Authors noted worse functional recovery more frequent in pts with carotid ophthalmic and MCA aneurysms; ACoA aneurysm pts least disabled
Saveland et al., 1986 [60]	78	All	Performed at least 1 yr postop in 31 pts but no details	Followup of 31 pts at least 1 yr postop: 31 (100%) with "good or fair neurologic outcome" noted psychosocial	Procedure: all pts had aneurysm clipping with operative microscope, some also received nimodipine

				or cognitive incapacitation to some degree (in 10 [32%] incapacitation was severe), 26 (33%) of original series were regarded to have achieved "good physical and psychologic outcome"	Good outcome correlated with better preoperative grade Authors concluded few pts recover with minimal sequelae after aneurysmal SAH
Sonesson et al., 1987 [61]	93	All	Performed at least 1 yr postop in 55 ES and in 38 LS pts, all with "good" neurologic status; in LS group, 34 (89%) had memory impairment (68% with verbal and 60% with nonverbal deficits), 23 (61%) had attentional deficits, 15 (39%) had perceptual deficits, 13 (34%) had impaired concept formation and abstract thinking	55% ES and 55% LS, fatigue; 24% ES and 29% LS, sleep disturbances; 32% ES and 32% LS, anxiety; 30% ES and 30% LS, irritability; 31% ES and 21% LS, dysphoria; 31% ES and 42% LS, vulnerability; 29% ES and 24% LS, social withdrawal and insecurity; 22% ES and 21% LS, developed social phobias; 55% ES and 55% LS, memory disturbances; 31% ES and 31% LS, impaired concentration; 26% of all pts, impaired working capacity	Surgical details not described (presumably same as in references 59 and 60) Authors noted no differences in cognitive or psychosocial sequelae between ES and LS pts, but decreased tempo and perceptual vigilance more common in pts with ACoA aneurysm Authors concluded cognitive malfunction and psychosocial disturbances were similar in ES and LS pts, supporting concept that initial hemorrhage is responsible for residual cognitive disturbances after SAH
Bornstein et al., 1987 [62]	48	All	Performed 1–66 mo postop in 37 pts with "good" and in 9 with "poor" neurologic outcome	Followup of 46 pts at various times postop: 32 (70%) returned to previous work level, 26 (57%) pts with	Surgical details not described Authors noted worse NP outcome correlated with increased age,[d] ACoA aneu-

APPENDIX Continued

Study	Number of patients	Aneurysm location[a]	Neuropsychometrical results	Functional/cognitive/emotional status	Comment
			27 pts (56%) classified as normal or mildly impaired on NP tests, only 1 of whom had poor neurologic outcome	"good" neurologic outcome had normal or mild impairment on psychometric tests, 4 (9%) had severe impairment	rysm,[d] preoperative grade; significant NP deficits occurred less frequently than in earlier reports
Saveland et al., 1988 [63]	56	All	Performed at least 2 yr postop in all pts; results of nimodipine and placebo groups compared	No details given	Procedures: 21 nimodipine-treated and 35 placebo-treated pts had repair, but no details given No significant NP characteristics emerged between two groups Authors concluded nimodipine is without cognitive protective effects and cognitive deficits result from initial hemorrhage
Fasanaro et al., 1989 [31]	10	ACoA	Performed 10–14 mo postop in all pts: 6 (60%) had NP evidence of memory impairment	Followup of all pts 10–14 mo postop: 6 (60%) reported behavioral disorders	Procedures: all pts had "early" aneurysmal neck clipping; microscope use not noted Authors noted worse NP outcome correlated with intraoperative aneurysm rupture
McKenna et al., 1989 [64]	100	All	Performed 1 yr postop in 70 pts without neurologic deficits, in 13 with neurologic deficits, in 34 controls 1 yr after MI; mean scores on several WAIS subtests, memory tests, and the WCST	Followup of 83 aneurysm pts and 34 post-MI pts at 1 yr: 56 (80%) pts without neurologic deficits and 28 (82%) post-MI pts had some impairment in quality of life; after extracting factors not	Procedures: of original 100 pts, 86 had LS (81 with aneurysm and 5 with AVM), surgical details not described Authors concluded no significant reduction in intel-

			WCST similar to normals in group without neurologic deficits and MI group, but group with neurologic deficits scored lower	relating to SAH or MI, 13 (19% pts without neurologic deficits and 18 (53%) post-MI pts had some reduction in quality of life attributable to insult	lectual ability or quality of life in pts with uncomplicated course after SAH
De Santis et al. 1989 [65]	114	All	Performed 7–115 mo postop in all pts; NP impairment present if >1 "pathologic" score on 13 subtests; 32 (31%) pts with "good recovery" on GOS and 6 (13%) without deteriorated working capacity, social habits, or emotional life classified as NP impaired	Followup of all pts 7–115 mo postop: 103 (90%) had "good recovery"; 11 (10%) were "moderately disabled" on GOS; 45 (39%) were without deteriorated working capacity, social habits, or emotional life; 47 (41%) had mild, 18 (16%) had moderate, 4 (4%) had severe impairment in these factors	Procedure: all pts had aneurysmal neck clipping with operative microscope Authors noted worse NP outcome correlated with "late" surgery[d] and possibly preop neurologic grade, not correlated with aneurysm location Authors concluded "late" surgery has negative influence on NP outcome and several pts with good neurologic outcome had NP deficits
Laiacona et al., 1989 (Subset of pts in De Santis study [65]) [66]	43	ACoA	Performed 7–115 mo postop in all pts; NP impairment present if >1 "pathologic" score on 15 subtests; 25 (58%) pts with various degrees of NP impairment in memory, language, intelligence, and spatial ability	Followup of all pts 7–115 mo postop: 39 (91%) had "good recovery"; 4 (9%) were "moderately disabled" on GOS; 23 (53%) were without deteriorated working capacity, social habits, or emotional life; 16 (37%) had mild, 4 (9%) had moderate impairment in these factors	Procedure: all pts had aneurysmal neck clipping with operative microscope Authors concluded a wide range of NP deficits demonstrates lack of constant or typical pattern of NP impairment with ACoA aneurysm, suggesting diffuse rather than focal brain damage (possibly causing attentional deficit) is responsible for variation in NP deficits

APPENDIX Continued

Study	Number of patients	Aneurysm location[a]	Neuropsychometrical results	Functional/cognitive/emotional status	Comment
Barbarotto et al., 1989 (Subset of pts in DeSantis [65] study) [12]	54	27 MCA 27 PCoA	Performed 7–115 mo postop in all pts NP impairment present if >1 "pathologic" scores on 15 subtests; 3 pts (30%) with L MCA, 6 (35%) with R MCA, 2 (17%) with L PCoA, and 5 (33%) with R PCoA had NP impairment	Followup of all pts 7–115 mo postop In MCA group: 25 (93%) had "good recovery" and 2 (7%) were "moderately disabled" on the GOS; 7 (26%) had no deteriorated working capacity, social habits, or emotional life; 12 (44%) had mild, 4 (15%) had moderate, and 4 (15%) had severe impairment in these factors In PCoA group, 25 (93%) had "good recovery" and 2 (7%) were "moderately disabled" on the GOS; 15 (56%) had no deteriorated working capacity, social habits, or emotional life; 10 (37%) had mild, 2 (7%) had moderate impairment in these factors	Procedure: all pts had aneurysmal neck clipping with operative microscope LMCA and PCoA pts more impaired on naming, verbal fluency, and verbal short-term memory; R MCA and PCoA pts more impaired on short-term and long-term spatial memory and discrimination of line orientation; several pts had NP deficits inconsistent with aneurysm side Authors concluded about 1/3 of L and R MCA and PCoA pts had persistent cognitive sequelae; pattern of sequelae tends to agree with hemispheric specialization; because several pts had NP and CT deficits inconsistent with aneurysm side, a more diffuse process may be present

Vilkki et al., 1989 [67]	118	ACA, ACoA, ICA, MCA	Performed 1 yr postop in 96 pts; NP results then compared with presence or absence of diffuse brain damage and presence or absence of infarction in frontomedial, R lateral, or L lateral areas or no infarction on CT Frontomedial group performed poorly on Object Memory, but not Fluency, Stroop II/I Category Identification, and Sorting R lateral group, only those with associated diffuse brain damage, performed poorly on Rey-Osterrieth Complex Figure L lateral group performed poorly on all verbal tests	Poor score on GOS correlated with low memory scores in frontomedial group, deficient categorical reasoning in R lateral group, and slow performances on color naming and verbal fluency in L lateral group	Surgical details not described 56 pts randomized in double-blinded, placebo-controlled nimodipine trial; no difference in NP results between placebo and nimodipine groups Authors concluded NP deficits are related to infarction site and diffuse brain damage on CT 1 yr after aneurysmal SAH; infarction from delayed ischemia may be more important than that caused by hemorrhage and surgical repair Data do not confirm that pts with ACoA aneurysm have poorer NP outcome or those with frontomedial damage have inflexible behavior and disinhibition of habitual response tendencies on "frontal lobe" tests
Sonesson et al., 1989 [68]	20	Unknown	Performed 14 mo–8 yr postop in all pts; results compared with 93 pts after aneurysmal SAH and normative data; 11 pts (55%) had NP	Followup of all pts 14 mo–8 yr postop: 18 pts (90%) returned to previous work capacity	All pts had SAH from unknown source (cerebral angio negative in all cases) Worse outcome not correlated with increased age

APPENDIX Continued

Study	Number of patients	Aneurysm location[a]	Neuropsychometrical results	Functional/cognitive/emotional status	Comment
			evidence of memory impairment; other NP deficits noted in several pts only mean scores on NP tests of memory and concept formation/abstraction were lower than normative values;[b] essentially no difference in mean scores on NP tests between this group and aneurysmal SAH group		Authors noted pts with SAH of unknown cause may have less catastrophic sequelae, significant cognitive disturbances may still occur Authors concluded blood anywhere in subarachnoid space may affect cognitive functions
Romner et al., 1989 [69]	20	ACoA, ICA, MCA	Performed 13–77 mo postop in all pts; NP results then compared with tissue loss seen on MRI (performed 3.5–10 yr postop); 18 pts (90%) had verbal or nonverbal memory impairment (or both); most pts had deficits on several NP tests	Followup of all pts at least 2 yr postop: no neurologic or obvious psycho-organic defects	Procedure: all pts had "early" aneurysmal neck clipping; operative microscope use not noted (presumably used) No significant correlations found between NP deficits and MRI tissue loss, amount of extravasated blood on preoperative CT, and aneurysm location Authors concluded normal cognitive functioning does not exclude pathologic MRI findings (or vice versa)

Richardson, 1989 [70]	76	All	Performed 6 weeks and 6 mo postop (62 pts in 1st session, 39 in 2nd session, 32 in both); mean MQ and Full Scale IQ scores similar to norms for each aneurysm location; controls performed better in Free Recall than aneurysm pts,[f] more words recalled in initial than in final tests[g]	No details given	Procedure: all pts had aneurysm clipping, wrapping, or common carotid ligation with operative microscope Results on initial and final tests suggested aneurysm pts have reduced working-memory capacity and long-term memory dysfunction Of several clinical variables, only occurrence of postoperative vasospasm was associated with poorer NP outcome Author concluded that the similar degree of NP impairment among pts with different aneurysm sites suggests deficits due to diffuse cerebral damage
Ogden et al., 1990 [71]	16	All	Performed 55–62 mo after SAH in all pts; results compared among 10 pts with aneurysmal SAH, 6 with SAH from unknown source, and with normative values all pts were impaired on at least 1 of the 8 NP tests administered; impairment on	Followup of all pts 55–62 mo after SAH: 11 (69%) had increased irritability, 10 (63%) had sensitivity to noise, 8 (50%) had depression, 8 (50%) had social withdrawal, 8 (50%) had inability to resume premorbid occupation, 7 (44%) had	Procedures: 10 pts had aneurysmal neck clipping, in other 6, cerebral arteriography was negative Worse NP outcome correlated with preoperative neurologic grade Nonaneurysm pts had poorer outcome on categories of re-

APPENDIX Continued

Study	Number of patients	Aneurysm location[a]	Neuropsychometrical results	Functional/cognitive/emotional status	Comment
			Rey-Osterrieth Complex Figure most frequent Aneurysm group performed worse than nonaneurysm group only on the modified WCST	anxiety, 6 (38%) had fatigue, 6 (38%) had decreased leisure activities	turn to work, leisure activities, and fatigue, for which authors propose psychologic rather than NP factors were responsible Authors noted only 6 pts (38%) were considered to have good NP recovery despite all being rated as having good neurologic recovery
Stegen and Freckmann, 1991 [72]	108	All	Performed 12 mo postop in 87 pts: 43 (49%) had visual memory dysfunction in comparison with controls	Followup of 87 pts 12 mo postop: 81 (93%) had no neurologic deficits; 24 (28%) noted diminished intellectual abilities (noted by relatives in 39 [45%]); 44 (51%) noted increased depression, anxiety, or restlessness (noted by relatives in 24 [28%]); 85 (98%) had lack of social contact; 69 (79%) had recurrence of SAH; 71 (82%) were discontent with local postop care	All pts underwent "early" surgery, with continuous nimodipine infusion; other surgical details not described Worse outcome on some NP tests correlated with poorer operative grades and presence of postop complications; emotional changes more frequent in ACA aneurysm pts Authors concluded psychologic problems after aneurysmal SAH delayed rehabilitation; recommended involving a psychologist in first 12 mo postop

Maurice-Williams et al., 1991 [73]	31	All	Performed 1 day preop, before hospital dismissal, and 1 yr postop in 27 pts: 5 (19%) pts clearly worse on NP tests at dismissal; 4 recovered to preoperative status at 1 yr	Followup of 27 pts 12–16 mo postop: 24 (89%) returned to premorbid level of functioning, 24 (89%) neurologically intact; relatives reported no psychologic changes in 20 (74%); 16 (59%) reported as psychologically unchanged	Procedures: "late" aneurysm clipping or wrapping with operative microscope No correlation found between many clinical variables (including aneurysm location) and NP or psychologic outcome Authors concluded aneurysm repair itself does not threaten higher intellectual function unless specific complication occurs
Oder et al., 1991 [112]	41	Unknown	Not performed	Followup 25–143 mo after SAH: 24 of 28 survivors (86%) who did not retire because of age were working part- or full-time; 22 (54%) had various degrees of "organic mental syndrome" (i.e., memory deficits, reduced reasoning ability, mental slowing, and emotional changes)	All pts had SAH from unknown source (cerebral angio negative in all cases) Worse functional outcome correlated with history of hypertension, focal neurologic deficits on admission, Hunt & Hess grade III or greater on admission, and presence of "organic mental syndrome" on discharge Authors concluded pts without above factors have a benign course
Richardson, 1991 [74] (Extension of 1989 study)	76	All	Performed 6 weeks and 6 mo postop (62 pts in 1st session, 39 in 2nd session, 32 in both)	No details given	Procedures: all pts had aneurysm clipping, wrapping, or common carotid ligation with operative microscope

APPENDIX Continued

Study	Number of patients	Aneurysm location[a]	Neuropsychometrical results	Functional/cognitive/emotional status	Comment
			Mean MQ and Full Scale IQ scores similar to norms for each aneurysm location At 6-week assessment, pts impaired on information, vocabulary, fluency, face recognition, object naming, and delayed free recall; at 6-mo assessment, pts impaired on fluency, object naming, and delayed free recall only		Worse outcome on NP tests at 6-week assessment correlated with postop arterial spasm, and at 6-mo assessment, correlated with admission and operative neurologic grade; no correlations present for several other clinical variables (including aneurysm location) Author concluded minimal NP deficits at 6-mo assessment indicate little evidence of any residual generalized cognitive impairment postop of ruptured aneurysms
Stenhouse et al., 1991 [34]	27	ACoA	Performed 12–84 mo postop in 25 pts and 20 controls; mean scores compared between groups: mean WAIS IQ scores lower for the aneurysm group but not significant; mean WMS MQ,[d] LM,[d] and AL[d] scores lower for aneurysm group; mean WCST scores showed aneurysm group made fewer successful category shifts[d] and	Followup of 27 pts 12–84 mo postop: 11 (41%) had no demonstrable social, psychologic, or cognitive sequelae; 6 (22%) had NP results suggesting "pervasive global impairment"; 6 (22%) had NP results suggesting "focal frontal deficits"	Procedure: all pts had aneurysmal neck clipping; microscope use not noted Worse NP outcome correlated with preoperative vasospasm[f] but not age or preoperative neurologic grade Authors concluded that after memory deficits resolve, marked functional impairment attributable to frontal lobe damage may remain,

			more perseverative responses[d] Some pts had severe deficits on NP tests		especially after vasospasm of vessels supplying frontal structures
Awad and Little, 1991 [75]	38	ACA	Performed at least 6 mo postop in some pts; no details given	Followup of all pts 6 mo postop: 29 (76%) resumed former occupation or had subtle difficulties not requiring assistance; 5 (13%) required occasional assistance; and 4 (11%) required major assistance or were vegetative or dead	Procedures: 28 ruptured and 10 unruptured aneurysms were clipped with operative microscope; nifedipine and later nimodipine also given 5 pts (17%) with "good" outcome had mild neurocognitive sequelae Authors noted overall outcome correlated with preoperative grade
Hutter and Gilsbach, 1992 [76]	48	All	Performed 1–5 yr after SAH in 18 pts with ACoA aneurysm (ACoA group) and in 21 with ruptured aneurysm in other locations and 9 pts with SAH of unknown cause (non-ACoA group) NP results compared between the two groups: 6 (33%) in ACoA group and 2 (7%) in non-ACoA group had no NP deficits; 9 (50%) in ACoA group and 15 (50%) in non-ACoA group had ≥ 3 (of 19) NP deficits	Followup of all pts 6 mo after SAH showed: 14 (78%) of ACoA group and 25 (83%) of non-ACoA group had minimal or no deficits ("good" outcome on GOS); 4 (22%) in ACoA group and 5 (17%) in non-ACoA group had mild deficits but were still independent ("fair" outcome on GOS)	Procedures: 18 in ACoA group and 21 in non-ACoA group had "early" aneurysm surgery with operative microscope; nimodipine also given No significant difference in number of cognitive deficits observed between the 2 groups: ACoA group tended to have more deficits in verbal long-term and figural short-term memory, non-AcoA group tended to have more deficits in language and concentration Authors concluded memory problems are not more fre-

APPENDIX Continued

Study	Number of patients	Aneurysm location[a]	Neuropsychometrical results	Functional/cognitive/emotional status	Comment
					quent in ACoA pts than in those with SAH from other origin, suggesting modern microsurgical techniques and postop management minimize residual cognitive deficits in SAH pts
Irle et al., 1992 [35]	87	Primarily ACoA, normal controls	Performed 1–5 yr postop in 30 pts with CT lesions (27 with ACoA aneurysms), in 27 with no CT lesions (all with ACoA aneurysms), and 30 normal controls; NP results compared among subgroups with different CT lesions, aneurysm pts with no CT lesions, and normal controls NP memory tests showed pts with combined basal forebrain and striate lesions on CT had memory deficits; either lesion in isolation did not produce amnesia	Results on the MMPI and POMS showed pts with higher scores more likely than not to have striate lesions on CT; coexisting basal forebrain or ventral frontal lesions tended to ameliorate, not aggravate, emotional changes	Surgical details not given Authors concluded basal forebrain and striatum involved in mnemonic processing by different pathways; destruction of one pathway may not cause memory deficits because of compensatory mechanism by other pathway, but combined dysfunction may produce marked memory deficit
DeLuca, 1992 [36]	24	ACoA, controls	Performed 1–11 mo postop in 11 pts with ACoA aneurysm (ACoA group) and 1–4 mo	No details given	Procedures: all in ACoA group had aneurysm clipping, surgical details not given

			after SAH (from aneurysms in other locations) and/or intraparenchymal hemorrhage in 13 control pts (ICH group); NP results compared between groups: ACoA group scored better on Full Scale IQ,[b] but more perseverative errors on WCST,[f] reduced number of categories on WCST,[b] worse performance on Logical Memory Delay test[d] (all in ACoA group scored 0)		Author concluded marked delayed verbal memory deficits in ACoA group support "focal" rather than "diffuse" model of cerebral damage underlying cognitive impairment in pts with ACoA aneurysm
Drumm et al., 1993 [37]	90	ACoA, controls	Psychometric tests not performed Observed behaviors were graded in 40 pts after ACoA surgery (35 of whom had SAH and 5 who were discovered incidentally), and 50 pts after repair of aneurysms in other locations (32 of whom had SAH and 18 were discovered incidentally)	Not described in detail	Procedure: all pts had aneurysm clipping with operative microscope Pts with incidental aneurysms had fewer neurobehavioral deficits than those with SAH Pts with SAH had similar neurobehavioral scores regardless of aneurysm site Pts with SAH and vasospasm had impaired memory function regardless of aneurysm site ACoA pts who had vasospasm had decreased "initiation" during testing Authors concluded initial hemorrhage and complications

APPENDIX Continued

Study	Number of patients	Aneurysm location[a]	Neuropsychometrical results	Functional/cognitive/emotional status	Comment
					of SAH rather than surgical repair are more likely to account for neurobehavioral deficits after aneurysm rupture and repair
Tidswell et al., 1995 [122]	37	ACoA, PCoA, MCA, OA	NP tests performed 6–45 mo after surgery NP performance compared between ACoA aneurysm ($n=20$) and non-ACoA aneurysm ($n=17$) groups Relationship of cognitive performance to preoperative, surgical, and postoperative factors was analyzed	Six (16%) scored higher than 13 on BDI Functional status not described in detail	All pts underwent aneurysm clipping using operative microscope No differences in cognitive outcome between ACoA and non-ACoA groups were found Postoperative neurologic events (hemiparesis, dysphasia, hyponatremia, hydrocephalus) were strongest predictors of cognitive outcome

[a] Abbreviations: ACA, anterior cerebral artery; ACoA, anterior communicating artery; AL, Associate Learning; AVLT, Auditory Verbal Learning Test; AVM, arteriovenous malformation; BDI, Beck Depression Inventory; CT, computerized tomography; ES, early surgery; GOS, Glasgow Outcome Scale; ICA, internal carotid artery; IQ, intelligence quotient; L, left; LM, Logical Memory; LS, late surgery; MCA, middle cerebral artery; MMPI, Minnesota Multiphasic Personality Inventory; MQ, memory quotient; MRI, magnetic resonance imaging; NP, neuropsychologic(al); OA, ophthalmic artery; P, performance; pts, patients; PCA, posterior cerebral artery; PCoA, posterior communicating artery; POMS, Profile of Mood States; R, right; SAH, subarachnoid hemorrhage; V, verbal; VB, vertebrobasilar; WAIS, Wechsler Adult Intelligence Scale; WCST, Wisconsin Card Sorting Test; WMS, Wechsler Memory Scale.

[b] $P<0.05$.

[c] Several correlations with statistically significant results; degree of statistical significance dependent on each variable.

[d] $P<0.01$.

[e] $P<0.02$.

[f] $P<0.005$.

[g] $P<0.001$.

9

Computerized Tomography and Magnetic Resonance Imaging of Subarachnoid Hemorrhage and Intracranial Aneurysms

Bob Lefsrud and Gary M. Miller
Mayo Clinic, Rochester, Minnesota

I. INTRODUCTION

Computerized tomography (CT) and magnetic resonance (MR) imaging have revolutionalized the detection and the diagnosis of subarachnoid hemorrhage and aneurysms that often went unrecognized or incompletely evaluated by angiography alone. This chapter will emphasize a basic approach to subarachnoid hemorrhage and aneurysms from a cross sectional imaging point of view. The angiographic appearance of these conditions will be covered in the surgical and vascular interventional chapters of this monograph.

II. CT IMAGING OF SUBARACHNOID HEMORRHAGE

Computerized tomography is the imaging modality of choice for identifying acute subarachnoid hemorrhage with a detection rate reported from 60 to 100% [1,2]. The CT is readily available, fast, relatively inexpensive, compatible with all life support systems, lacks the contraindications of MRI, and rarely misses acute surgical abnormalities. The CT is more sensitive to small amounts of acute subarachnoid blood than conventional spin echo and gradient echo sequences [3,4]. Computerized tomography has the advantage of identifying small calcifications that may be associated with vascular lesions. These calcifications may be easily overlooked with MRI due to a paucity of mobile protons. Contrast enhancement is usually not used initially when looking for intracerebral hemorrhage to avoid confusion with bright calcification or contrast enhancement. Contrast should be administered to make vessels more apparent when looking for aneurysms or vascular malformations after a nonenhanced study has been performed. Contrast should be avoided in patients with prior contrast reactions, medical contraindications, or possibly if emergency angiography is being considered. Electron density is the only intrinsic factor that determines image contrast. Technical factors such as slice thickness, Mas, window width, slice angle, as well as location, volume, and relation to surrounding structures, will all affect the appearance of blood on CT.

Acute blood is bright on CT, although rarely it may be isodense with a low hematocrit (less than 23%) or in patients with severe coagulopathy or on anticoagulation medications in whom acute blood clots do not form. Subarachnoid hemorrhage (SAH) quickly diffuses throughout the cerebrospinal fluid (CSF) spaces and the attenuation of the blood decreases as the volume of the CSF mixing with the blood increases (Figure 1). Subarachnoid fluid will remain isodense to CSF or brain until blood replaces more than 70% of the CSF in a location [4]. In extensive SAH, the cranial nerves and blood vessels may appear as filling defects in the dense subarachnoid blood giving a "cisternogram" effect. Usually, SAH is confined to a few sulci or fissures and may give a "feathered" effect. The increased attenuation usually persists from one day to one week. By the end of the first week, up to 50% of SAH can still be detected [5–8]. However, if after the first week SAH is still prominent, rehemorrhage should be considered [9]. If blood accumulates too quickly, an unretracted semiliquid clot forms, resulting in a hypodense area within a generalized hyperdense acute hematoma or clot. This is called the "swirl sign" [10].

With faulty clot retraction or abnormal clotting function, fluid-fluid levels may occur. This has been reported in up to 50% of patients when hemorrhage results from a coagulopathy [11]. Fluid-fluid levels can also be seen with rehemorrhage when blood products of different ages layer out. If the volume of hemorrhage is large enough, reflux of blood will often be seen in the ventricular system. Blood often layers dependently in the occipital horns and fourth ventricle.

A negative CT exam does not exclude the possibility of SAH. There is no apparent correlation between the volume of blood in the intracranial versus the intraspinal subarachnoid space [12].

As the attenuation of blood decreases with time and breakdown of the clot, the SAH becomes isointense to brain parenchyma resulting in an apparent obliteration of the cortical sulci and basal cisterns. This finding may simulate diffuse cerebral edema or increased intracranial pressure. If small amounts of blood are present, it may just obliterate the dependent CSF spaces. The most

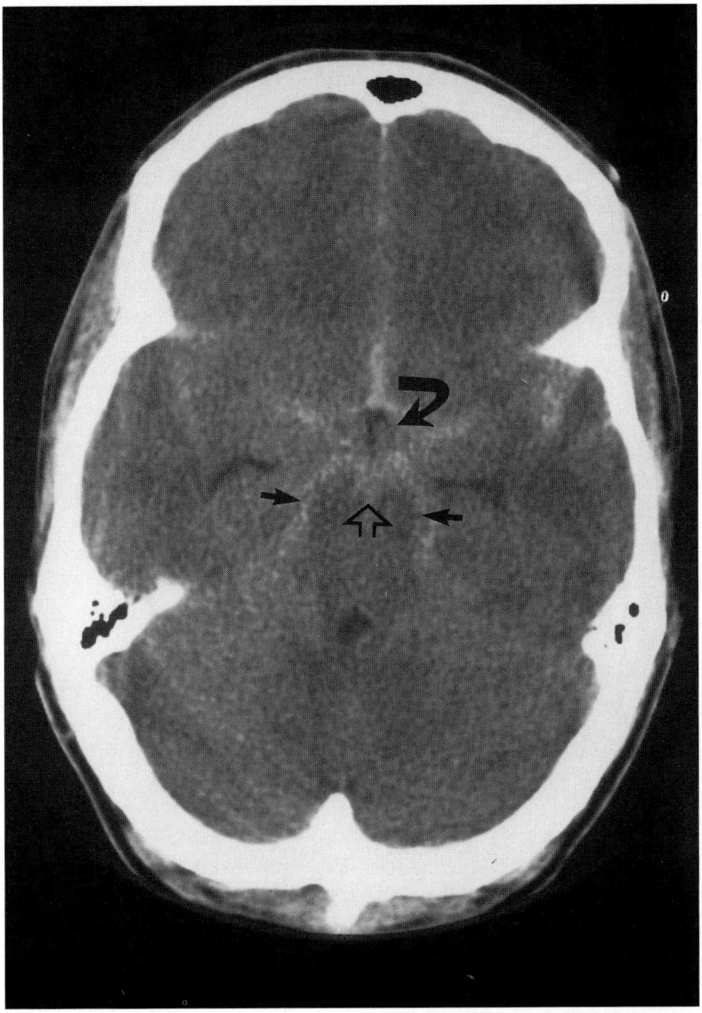

Figure 1 Perimesencephalic subarachnoid hemorrhage. Acute hyperdense blood is present in the intrapeduncular cistern (open arrowhead), perimesencephalic cisterns (small black arrows), and within the suprasellar cistern (black curved arrow) on the nonenhanced CT image.

sensitive indicator of a small volume of SAH may be filling of the interpeduncular cistern. After several more days, the fluid decreases in the attenuation to become isointense with the CSF and becomes undetectable by noncontrast CT imaging.

Contrast enhanced CT images obtained during the isodense or hypodense stage may reveal leptomeningeal enhancement in the areas affected by hemorrhage. Diffuse enhancement may be seen within the cortical sulci and fissures with apparent thickening of the tentorium or falx. Care must be taken not to confuse this appearance with diffuse leptomeningeal inflammation, infection, or neoplasm (Figure 2).

Diffuse cerebral edema may result in a "pseudo-subarachnoid hemorrhage" with decreased attenuation of the brain and dura with the circulating

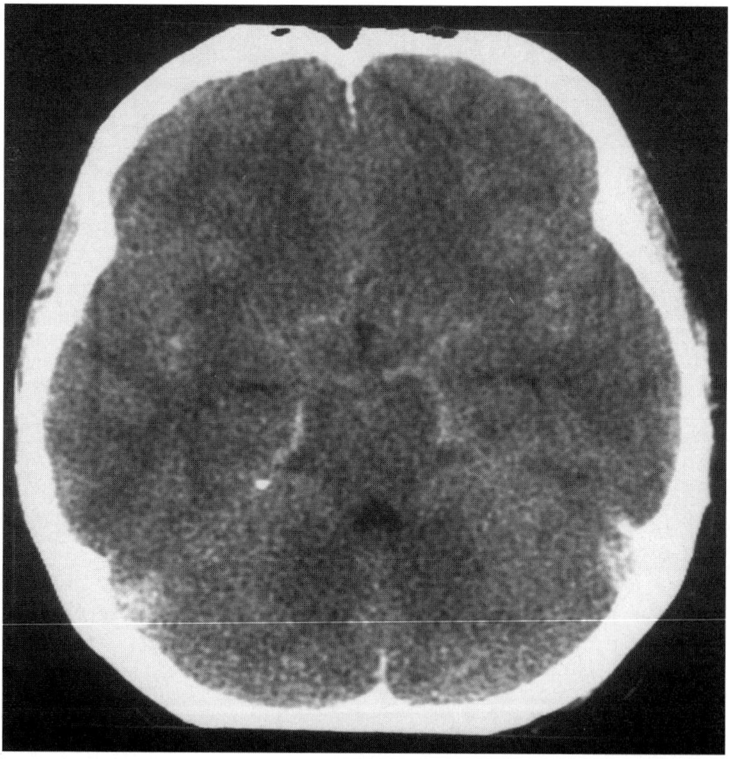

Figure 2 SAH mimic. Enhanced head CT shows increased density in the basilar cisterns with filling of the cerebral and cerebellar sulci not unlike subarachnoid blood. This, however, is a case of bacterial meningitis with enhancement and thickening of the leptomeninges.

blood appearing hyperdense in comparison to the adjacent brain parenchyma [13].

III. MR IMAGING OF SUBARACHNOID HEMORRHAGE

The appearance of blood on MRI is one of the most complicated and controversial areas in neuroradiology. The intensity is time dependent and the appearance usually follows a predictable pattern. Intrinsic factors such as the sequential breakdown of hemoglobin, lysis of the clot, protein concentration, red blood cell morphology, size, and location of the hematoma, as well associated edema may all vary the intensity of blood. Extrinsic factors such as the choice of pulse sequences and field strength have significant effects on the MRI signal. Several articles and reviews are available to discuss this complex and sometimes controversial subject [14–16].

The MR appearance of hemorrhage on spin echo sequences can usually be broken down by time into five discrete stages. A hemorrhagic focus may display two or more different stages at the same time, which may give a complex appearance. The appearance of hemorrhage on gradient recall echo (GRE) sequences is usually hypointense. Table 1 represents this simplified approach to the appearance of blood on MR imaging.

The appearance of flowing blood on MRI is also multifactorial depending on factors such as pulse sequence, application of saturation bands, flow direction, flow-related enhancement, echo rephasing, diastolic pseudogating, velocity, and turbulence. In general, flowing blood is dark due to time-of-flight phe-

Table 1 MRI Appearance of Hemorrhage

Stage	Time	Hemoglobin state	T_1	T_2
Hyperacute	0–6 hours	Oxyhemoglobin	↔	↑
Acute[a]	7 hours–3 days	Deoxyhemoglobin	↔	↓
Subacute[a]		Methoglobin		
Early[a]	4–7 days	intracellular	↑	↓
Late[a]	1–4 weeks	extracellular	↑	↑
Chronic	Months to years	Ferritin and Hemosiderin	↓	↓↓

[a] Surrounding edema is usually present appearing T_1 ↓ and T_2 ↑.
Abbreviations: ↔ isointense, ↑ hyperintense, ↓ hypointense, and ↓↓ hypointense with "blooming." All relative to cerebral white matter.
Note: Hemoglobin on GRE studies is usually hypointense.

nomena on conventional spin echo (SE) sequences and bright on GRE sequences due to flow-related enhancement. A common artifact is bright blood on the first and/or last images of the sequence with SE sequences due to inflow of fresh blood not affected by the pulse sequence. Analysis of different pulse sequences and MR angiography may be needed to exclude thrombosis from flowing blood [17,18].

The degree of sensitivity of MR for acute subarachnoid hemorrhage is disputed. Ogawa et al. reported that MR is extremely sensitive, specific, and highly accurate for depicting the presence of SAH (96–100%) [19]. This degree of accuracy has been called into question [2]. There is no doubt that MR studies of acute SAH require more careful inspection and analysis than CT studies. Comparing 30 cases of acute SAH, Satoh et al. found that three out of four SAH that appeared normal on CT showed high intensity on T2 weighted images indicative of blood. They concluded that MRI is very helpful in diagnosing SAH, particularly if the clinical suspicion is high and the CT is negative [20].

While CT is currently the modality of choice for evaluating acute SAH, MR imaging may eventually replace CT for the diagnosis as exam times are shortened, new pulse sequences are developed, and as further technical developments occur. A preliminary study with 20 patients demonstrated high signal from acute SAH using a new pulse sequence called fluid attenuated inversion recovery (FLAIR) that nulls the signal from CSF and causes heavy T2-weighting [21,22]. This sequence has proven useful in a wide variety of other central nervous system diseases. The FLAIR sequence appears particularly useful to detect SAH in the posterior fossa, which is difficult to detect with CT because of beam hardening artifact. As this sequence becomes more readily available commercially, its role will become better defined.

Pulsation effects on vessels may artificially make them appear larger than they are, whereby stenosis is usually overestimated with MRI [17]. Fast flowing CSF may create a flow void and give the false appearance of a vessel. Bone and air have few mobile protons and are low intensity on all MRI sequences so if these are contiguous with vessels demonstrating flow void, this could give the appearance of a vessel abnormality. Aeration of the anterior clinoid will create a signal void and can mimic an aneurysm of the supraclinoid internal carotid artery [23].

Larger recurrent subarachnoid hemorrhage may result in intra- and extracellular deposition of hemosiderin in the leptomeninges, subpial tissue, cranial nerves, the lining of the ventricles, and epithelium of the choroid plexus. This is called superficial siderosis (SS) or hemosiderosis. A wide variety of etiologies may produce this recurrent bleeding with the most common causes being bleeding secondary to tumors (especially ependymomas), vascular malformations, prior surgery, trauma (especially nerve root avulsion), and neonatal intraventricular hemorrhage [24,25]. In one quarter of the cases no evidence of bleeding is found, even at autopsy [24] (Figure 3). The classic triad of clinical findings includes hearing loss, cerebellar dysfunction, and pyramidal track signs. Progressive mental deterioration and myelopathy may be seen in more severe cases. The clinical findings reflect the area of greatest histopathologic destruction, which involves the superior cerebellar vermis, the cisternal segment of the eighth cranial nerve, and superficially the area around the brainstem and cord.

The imaging modality best suited to look for SS is MRI, due to the magnetic susceptibility of blood breakdown products. High field strength magnets are most sensitive as magnetic susceptibility is proportional to the square of the magnetic field strength. Gradient recall echo (GRE) sequences should be more sensitive than spin-echo series but this did not make a noticeable difference in the cases reviewed by Bracchi [25]. Marginal hypointensity around the basal cerebral surfaces, cranial nerves, cerebellum, brainstem, and cord are the findings expected on T2W or GRE sequences. A hypointense rim is rarely noted on T1W sequences or on CT, which typically shows cerebellar atrophy in more advanced cases. Fast spin-echo sequences, which are less sensitive to magnetic susceptibility effects, can cause an artifactually low signal margin between coronal tissue and adjacent subarachnoid space that can mimic SS. If in question, heavily weighted T2 or GRE sequences should also be reviewed to avoid overcalling this condition [26].

Ferromagnetic aneurysm clips are a contraindication to MRI as they may be torqued off the aneurysm or tear the neck, which can result in death [27]. As well, significant artifact may be produced by the clip. Most aneurysm clips currently being placed during surgery are MRI compatible. A patient with an aneurysm clip should not be placed in a MRI unit unless the type of clip and its ferromagnetic properties are known. This should be documented on the operative report if the patient or referring physician does not know for sure. If in doubt, the study should be deferred.

Other than ferromagnetic aneurysm clips, other ferromagnetic implants, materials or devices are contraindicated because of the risk of movement and/or dislodgment of the object. Induction of electric current, heating, or artifact produced by these objects can occur. Patients with electrically, magnetically, or mechanically activated implants or devices should not undergo MRI because the electromagnetic fields could adversely affect the operation of the implant or device and result in injury. Such devices would include cardiac pacemakers, implantable cardiac defibrillators, hearing aids, cochlear implants, magnetic dental implants, neurostimulators, bone growth stimulators, and implantable drug infusion pumps. Shellock and Kanal have written an excellent book discussing magnetic resonance bioeffects, safety, and screening [28].

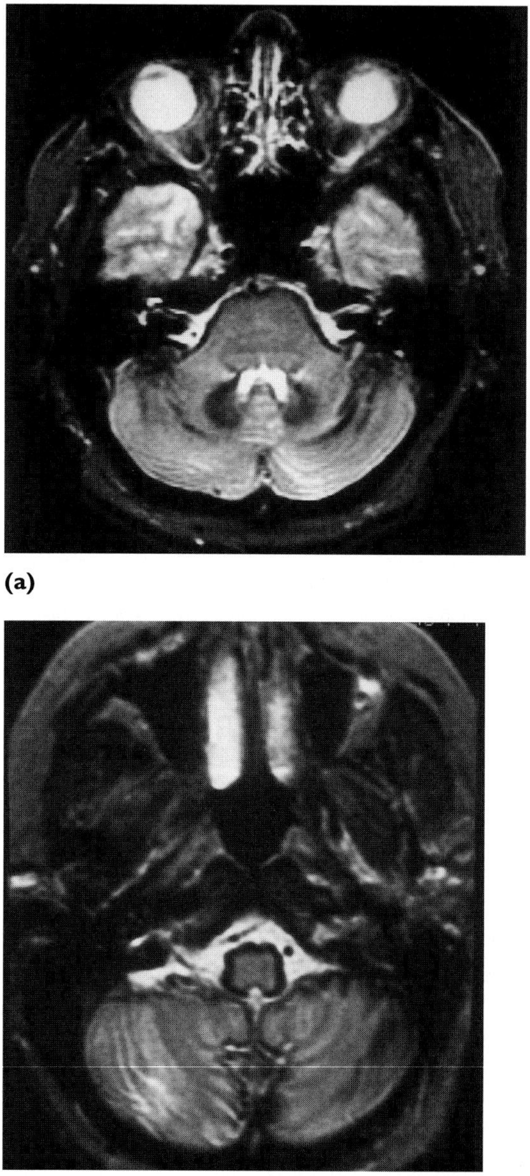

(a)

(b)

Figure 3 Superficial siderosis (SS) of unknown etiology. (a) Decreased signal along the surfaces of the pons, middle cerebral peduncles, and cerebellar folia are typical for SS on this T2-weighted spin echo sequence. (b) On a lower slice, a thick rim of low signal surrounds the medulla and to a lesser extent, the inferior vermis and cerebellar folia.

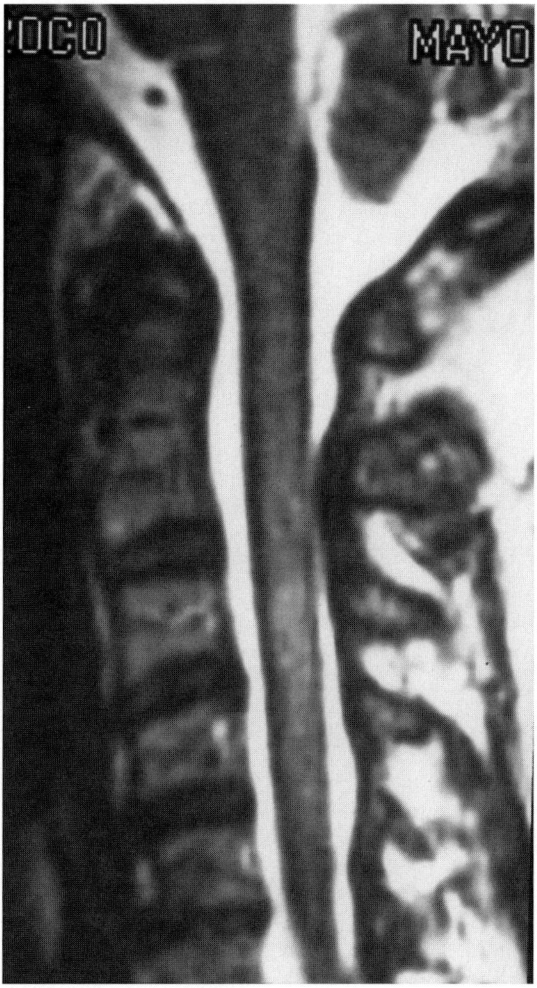

(c)

Figure 3 Continued.
(c) A rim of subpial decreased signal surrounds the upper cervical cord and medulla indicative of SS on this mid sagittal T2-weighted image.

A. CT and MR Imaging of Intracranial Aneurysms

Aneurysms account for approximately 80% of spontaneous subarachnoid hemorrhages; therefore, any SAH must be considered a consequence of a ruptured aneurysm until proven otherwise [29,30]. About 50% of patients with aneurysmal SAH will die or suffer severe disability as a result of the initial hemorrhage and another 25–35% will die as a direct result of subsequent hemorrhage if untreated [31]. Rehemorrhage will occur in up to 50% of ruptured aneurysms during the first six months if untreated [32]. Early diagnosis and treatment is necessary to reduce the risk of rehemorrhage. While angiography remains the gold standard for evaluating the location and morphology of aneurysms, CT and MRI have an important role in detecting subarachnoid hemorrhage, occasionally characterizing the aneurysm and identifying complicating factors. Nonruptured aneurysms are frequently identified while evaluating the patient for other intracranial pathology (Figure 4).

IV. CLASSIFICATION OF INTRACRANIAL ANEURYSMS

Three morphologic types of intracranial aneurysms can be recognized with cross-sectional imaging: saccular (berry aneurysms), fusiform (atherosclerotic, serpiginous), and dissecting aneurysms. The pathology and etiology of these types are distinct and have differing clinical courses.

Saccular aneurysms are focal and usually round or oval. These outpouchings usually arising at arterial bifurcations due to a deficiency in the internal elastic lamina and muscularis at the aneurysm neck [33] (Figure 5). Over 90% are felt to be degenerative in nature due to abnormal stress. This theory is supported by the appearance of flow-related aneurysms, which are the second most common cause of saccular aneurysms after degeneration [34]. Mycotic aneurysms account for up to 4.5% of all intracranial aneurysms [35]. Streptococcus viridans is the most common etiologic agent, usually seen in patients with subacute bacterial endocarditis or drug abuse. Mycotic aneurysms may be saccular or fusiform and likely start in the adventitia. Most cases are treated acutely with antibiotics. Serial angiograms or MRA should be performed to document effectiveness of medical therapy. Surgery can be difficult because mycotic aneurysms may be very friable. Surgery is usually reserved for SAH, or antibiotic treatment failure to reduce the aneurysm size after four to six weeks [36]. Traumatic aneurysms make up less than 1% of intracranial aneurysms and are often seen peripherally, contiguous to skull fractures, or along the anterocerebral artery due to impaction against the falx [37]. Oncotic aneurysms are rare. There is an increased risk for aneurysm occurrence in some families.

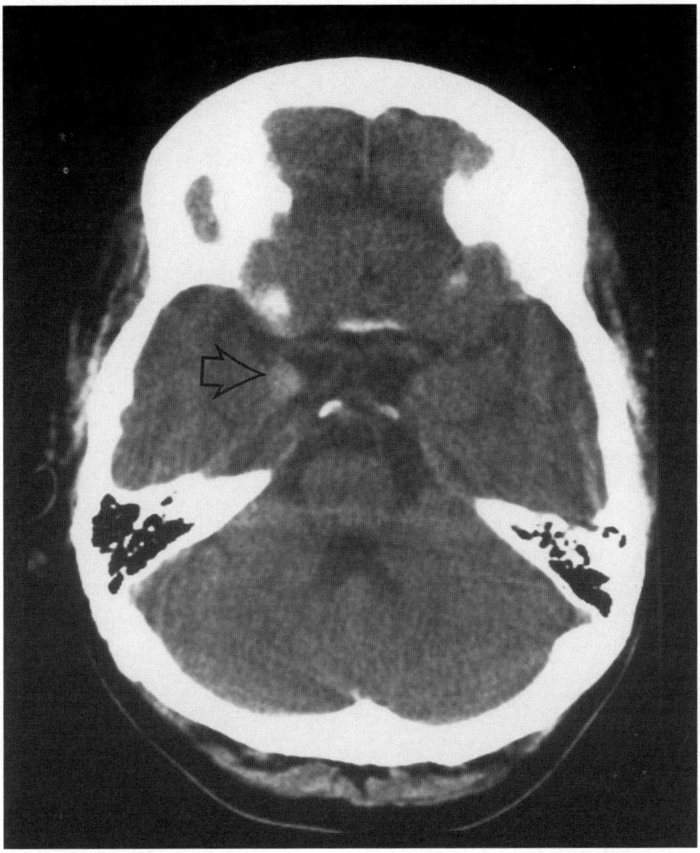

Figure 4 Incidental right posterior communicating cerebral artery aneurysm in a 24-year-old female. Nonenhanced CT demonstrates a hyperdense patent 1.0-cm aneurysm (open arrow) of the MCA at the right lateral aspect of the suprasellar cistern.

Multiple intracranial aneurysms may be seen with the figures ranging from 14 to 45% [38]. There is a strong female predominance for multiple aneurysms. When multiple, 75% of patients have two aneurysms, 15% have three, and 10% have more than three aneurysms [34].

Ninety percent of intracranial aneurysms are found in the anterior circulation with the remaining ten percent occurring in the vertebral basilar circulation. In angiographic series, roughly one-third of cases involve the anterior communicating artery, one-third involve the posterior communicating artery,

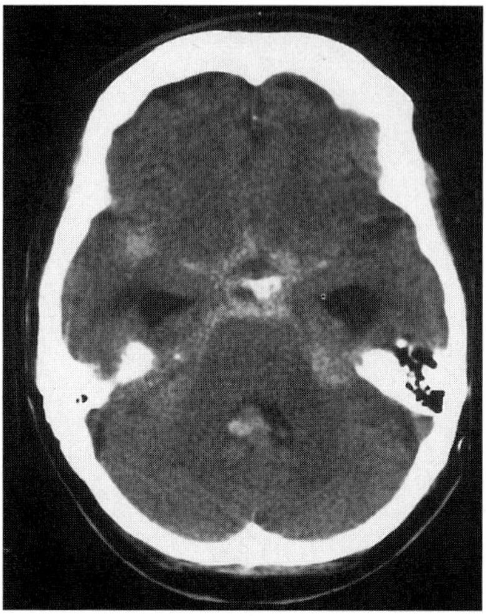

(a)

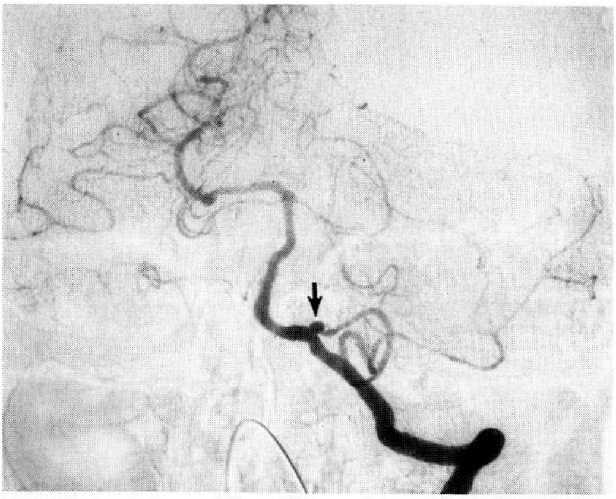

(b)

Figure 5 Subarachnoid hemorrhage from PICA origin aneurysm. (a) Nonenhanced CT demonstrates subarachnoid hemorrhage in the basilar cisterns, cerebellopontine angles, and inferior right Sylvian fissure. Dilated temporal horns, blood in the distended fourth ventricle, and effaced sulci indicates significant hydrocephalus. (b) PICA origin aneurysm (small black arrow) is demonstrated on this mid-arterial phase left vertebral angiogram in the Towne's position.

and 20% occur at the middle cerebral bifurcation. However, in autopsy series, MCA is the most common aneurysm with the next most common site being at the bifurcation of the supraclinoid internal carotid artery [39].

Subarachnoid hemorrhage is the most common clinical presenting symptom occurring in about 90% of patients. Cranial neuropathy, seizure, and TIA are less common. The risk of aneurysm rupture in part relates to the size of the aneurysm and increases with size, but is roughly 1% per year in asymptomatic patients [31].

Fusiform or serpiginous aneurysms are secondary to degenerative change weakening the arterial wall with resultant arterial dilation and elongation. These lesions represent severe vessel ectasia. This commonly occurs in older patients with other areas of vasculopathy. When symptomatic, the aneurysms may rupture, although most result in cranial neuropathies, brainstem infarction, or hydrocephalus. This type of aneurysm is most commonly found in the vertebrobasilar circulation [34].

A dissecting aneurysm is an extension of an arterial dissection with intramural hematoma extending into the subadventitial plane or the other layers of the media in the extracranial vessels. The intramural hematoma is located between the internal elastic lamina and the media in most intracranial arterial dissections. Pseudoaneurysms may also form if the adventitia is breached. This condition may be spontaneous, related to trauma or fibromuscular dysplasia. Horner's syndrome may be seen if the sympathetic nerves are compressed. Most dissecting aneurysms occur just below the skull base in both the internal carotid and vertebral arteries [40] (Figure 6). Intracranial dissections are uncommon with most occurring in the mid supraclinoid internal carotid artery segment [41]. Spontaneous dissections resulting in SAH are largely confined to the posterior fossa. A review of the literature by Tanaka in 1989 showed that only 14% of dissections resulting in SAH were in the anterior circulation [42]. No specific MRI or CT appearance has been described for dissecting aneurysms and the diagnosis is confirmed by angiography.

Aneurysms greater than 2.5 cm (one inch) are by definition called giant aneurysms [43]. They may be saccular or fusiform. Giant aneurysms constitute 5–13% of all intracranial aneurysms. Females are three times more likely to have this type of aneurysm [44]. Most of these patients present with signs and symptoms related to mass effect from the aneurysm rather than SAH. In a series of 174 giant aneurysms by Drake, 35% presented as hemorrhage while 10% showed evidence of remote bleeding [45]. Cross-sectional imaging is especially useful for pretreatment planning as an angiogram may underestimate the size of the lesion due to thrombosis and wall thickening and is not as sensitive to calcium within the wall [Figure 7]. Due to thrombosed intraluminal contents, a significant number of giant aneurysms may be missed or misdiagnosed on CT. Contrast enhancement may suggest an enhancing tumor. Adjacent edema or

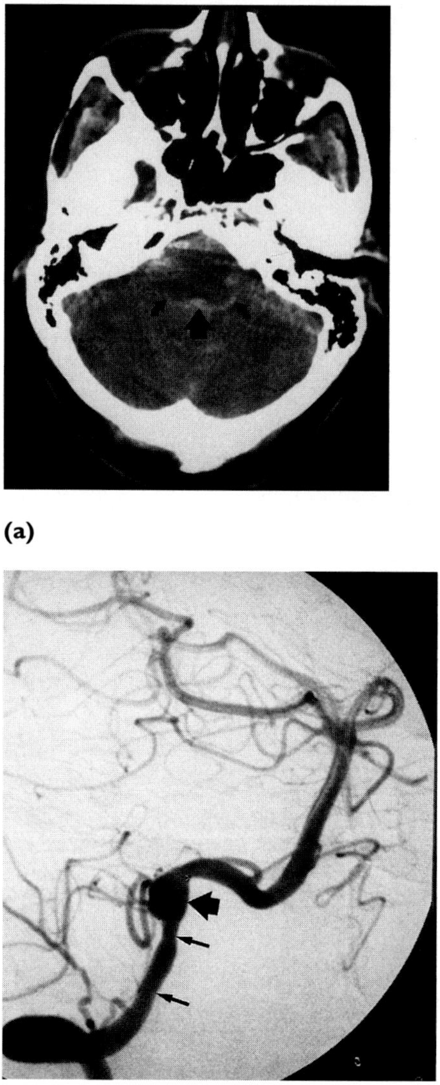

(a)

(b)

Figure 6 Subarachnoid hemorrhage from a vertebral artery dissection. (a) Subarachnoid hemorrhage is present in the perimedullary cisterns, between the cerebellar folia, within the foramen of Luschka bilaterally (small curved black arrows), and within the fourth ventricle (large black straight arrow) on this nonenhanced CT. (b) Irregular luminal narrowing is noted between C2 and the skull base (small thin black arrows). Saclike focal outpouching represents the dissecting aneurysm at the skull base (large thick black arrow) on this early arterial phase vertebral injection in a frontal oblique projection. This is the most common site for vertebral dissecting aneurysms.

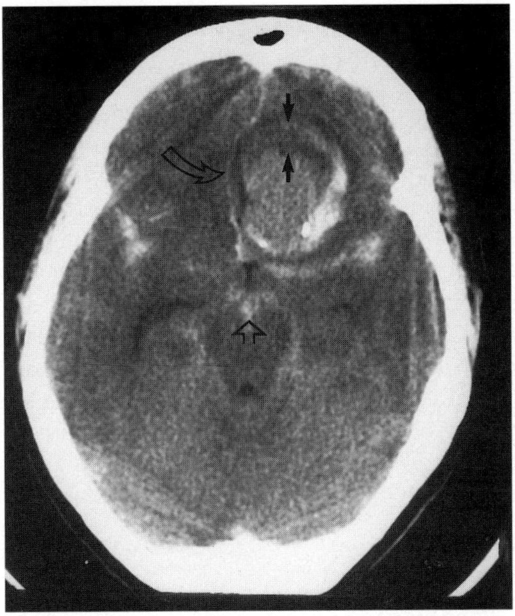

(a)

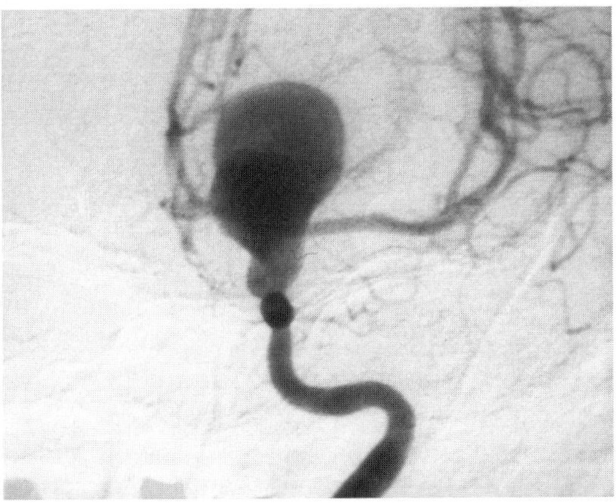

(b)

Figure 7 Giant ICA aneurysm. (a) Hyperdense subarachnoid blood is present in the basilar cisterns and intrapeduncular cistern (small open arrow). A large partially thrombosed aneurysm is noted with peripheral hypodense thrombus (between small black arrows). The patent lumen is slightly hyperdense. The lateral wall is thickened and calcified. Moderate mass effect from the aneurysm results in subfalcine herniation to the left (curved open arrow) on this nonenhanced CT. (b) Giant left ICA aneurysm is shown on this left carotid angiogram in a frontal projection. Note that the mural thrombosis, wall thickening, and calcifications are not apparent on the angiogram.

ischemia may reinforce this misinterpretation. A high index of suspicion must be maintained in order to include an aneurysm in the differential diagnosis of any circular or fusiform lesion on cross-sectional imaging.

Up to 95% of SAH caused by ruptured aneurysms may be identified within 48 hours by noncontrast CT study [46,47]. The distribution of blood may give a useful clue to the origin of the ruptured aneurysm as the area of thickest blood clot is usually located near the rupture site [47]. Interhemispheric fissure hemorrhage is common with anterior communicating artery aneurysms. Sylvian fissure blood is frequently seen with middle cerebral artery aneurysms. Fourth ventricular hemorrhage is frequent with posterior fossa aneurysms. Frontal horn blood is typically seen with anterior communicating artery lesions [48]. Focal clot location is of assistance when multiple aneurysms are present. In up to 10% of cases, blood clot may actually outline the aneurysm [49]. About 5% of ruptured aneurysms result in subdural hematomas [50].

V. CT IMAGING OF INTRACRANIAL ANEURYSMS

The appearance of an aneurysm will vary depending if it is patent, partially, or fully thrombosed. On noncontrast CT, patent aneurysms appear as circular or oval, iso to slightly hyperintense lesions contiguous to their parent vessels, and are usually located within the suprasellar cistern or sylvian fissure. These enhance avidly with the administration of intravenous contrast material. Schmidt, using enhanced high-resolution axial CT, demonstrates 97% accuracy in diagnosing cerebral aneurysms 3 mm and greater in size [51].

Partially thrombosed aneurysms may demonstrate a hypo- or hyperdense wall due to atherosclerotic debris or calcification, respectively. Enhancement may be seen in the residual lumen and outer wall with contrast administration. Completely thrombosed aneurysms are often slightly hyperdense and may show rim enhancement with contrast administration (Figure 8).

Serpentine or fusiform aneurysms often demonstrate calcification within the thickened wall. Frequently edema is seen in the surrounding parenchyma. Bleeding and scarring within the wall often leads to a lamellated appearance. With contrast enhancement, the surrounding parenchyma enhance secondary to inflammation. Occasionally, hyperdense acute thrombosis may be noted. In long-standing lesions near the skull base, bone erosion may be evident.

Fischer's grading system assessing the thickness of blood clot on CT following aneurysmal rupture is useful in predicting the development of vasospasm, which is the major cause of delayed morbidity and mortality [52]. Only the Grade 3 type hemorrhage with focal or diffuse clot greater than 1 mm in vertical dimension predisposes to significant vasospasm.

Hydrocephalus may be seen in up to 21% of patients following aneurysmal rupture due to obstructive or nonobstructive causes [53]. Ischemia may be seen acutely due to aneurysmal rupture or after three days due to vasospasm in 20–30% of patients [54]. Computerized tomography is useful in assessing other complications of SAH such as the intraparenchymal hemorrhage noted in 20–40% of cases, intraventricular hemorrhage in 15–30% of cases, and subdural hemorrhage in 2–5% of cases [55] (Figure 9).

VI. MR IMAGING OF INTRACRANIAL ANEURYSMS

Magnetic resonance (MR) imaging is playing an increasing role in defining the normal and pathologic cerebrovascular anatomy, as well as the detection and management of cerebral aneurysms. It is important to consider the capabilities, pitfalls, and artifacts associated with each MR pulse sequence. Traditional spin echo (SE), gradient recall echoe (GRE) and fluid attenuated inversion recovery (FLAIR) sequences, as well as MRA, can all give unique information that can help to sort out these often complex images. The appearance of aneurysms may be highly variable due to selection of pulse sequence, flow characteristics, fibrosis, calcification, as well as the presence and age of clot.

In general, patent aneurysms will be identified as outpouchings contiguous with a vessel and will contain the same signal characteristics as the vessel. On spin echo sequences, this usually will be a signal void. With GRE sequences, flowing blood is usually bright. Unruptured aneurysms smaller than 5 mm cannot always be visualized due to limitations in spatial resolution. If in doubt, thinner slices through the area of interest can be obtained, as can orthogonal series for further characterization. Enhancement is usually not seen in patent vessels with the administration of intravenous contrast material; however, phase-encoding artifacts from the rapidly flowing blood will increase after contrast, which may add confidence to the diagnosis of a patent aneurysm [Figure 10]. Pulsation artifact may also help distinguish a giant aneurysm from a solid or cystic lesion. Signal within the aneurysm may be variable due to slow or turbulent flow.

Partially thrombosed aneurysms often have a complex signal pattern due to multilaminated clot and slow or turbulent blood flow. A dark rim due to hemosiderin within a fibrous capsule is often present, aiding the diagnosis [56]. Gadolinium enhancement may be helpful in demonstrating slower turbulent flow, as well as in further defining the aneurysmal wall, which often enhances. Peripheral lamellated clot in the wall is usually more apparent with MRI, while calcification and enhancement of the patent lumen is usually demonstrated better by CT (Figure 11).

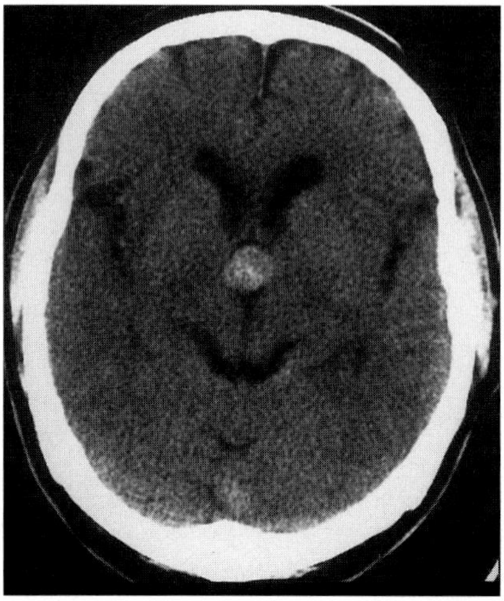

(a)

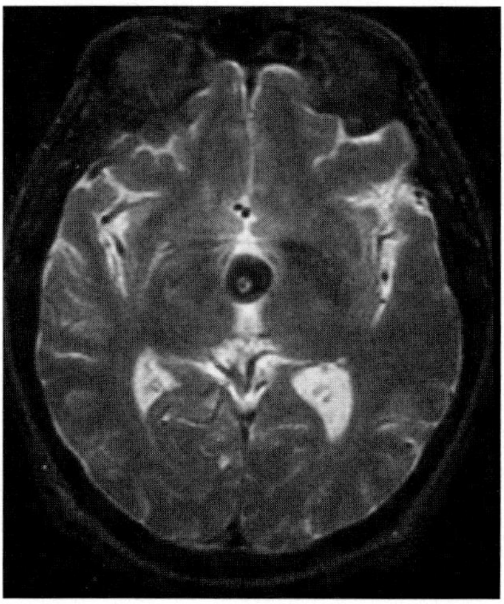

(b)

Figure 8 Basilar tip aneurysm. (a) A 1.5-cm hyperdense mass fills the anterior third ventricle on this nonenhanced CT. This appearance is consistent with an aneurysm, although a colloid cyst or exophytic suprasellar mass could have a similar appearance. (b) Bright slow flowing blood is present within the central third of the aneurysm on this T2-weighted MR image. The dark signal which composes the outer two-thirds of the aneurysm sac is due to peripheral intraluminal thrombus.

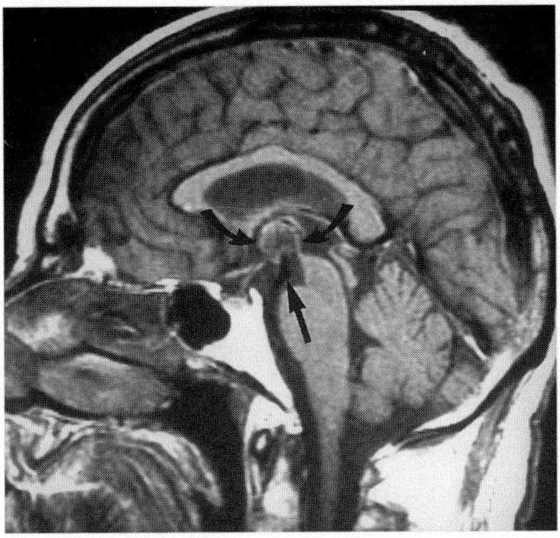

(c)

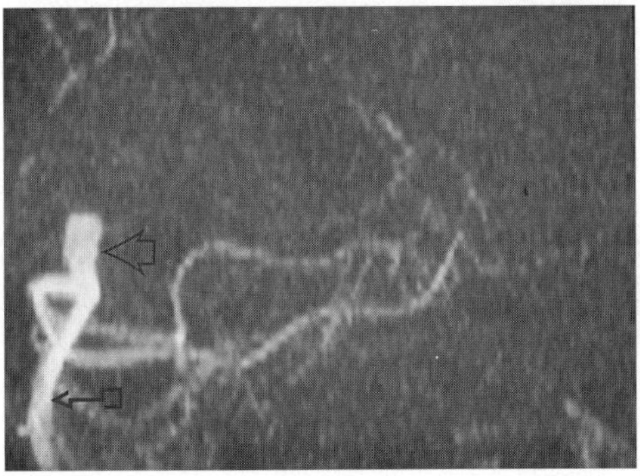

(d)

Figure 8 Continued.
(c) Sagittal T1-weighted image demonstrates flow voids (straight black arrow) in the basilar artery plus the inferior and central aspect of the partially thrombosed aneurysm (curved black arrows), which extend into the third ventricle. (d) A partition image of the basilar artery (arrow with square tail) and its branches in a lateral projection from a 3D time-of-flight (TOG) MR angiogram demonstrates central flow within the aneurysm (large open arrow). Note that the peripheral thrombus is not apparent on this flow-sensitive study.

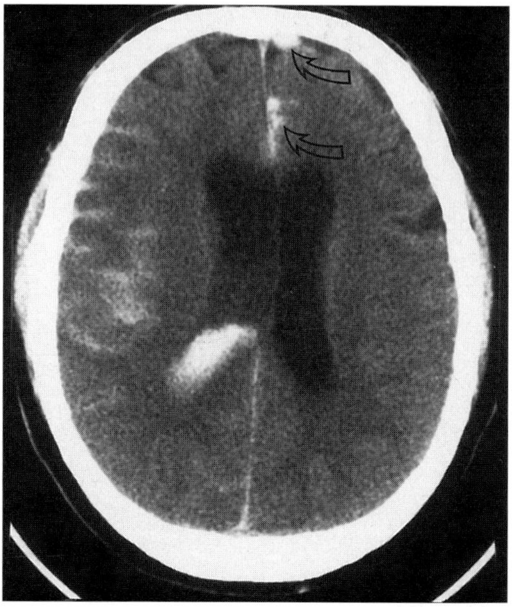

(a)

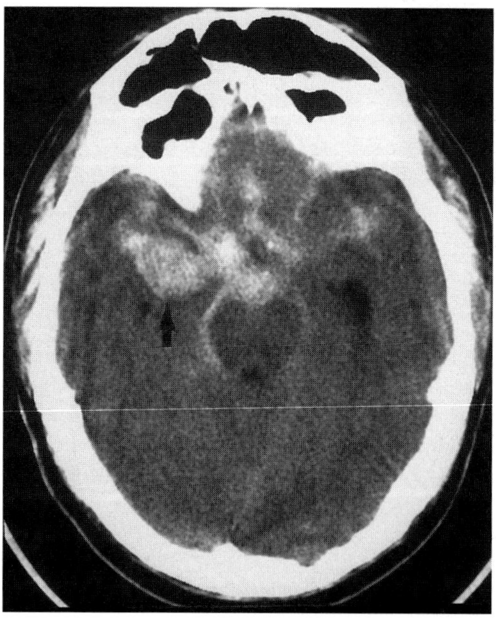

(b)

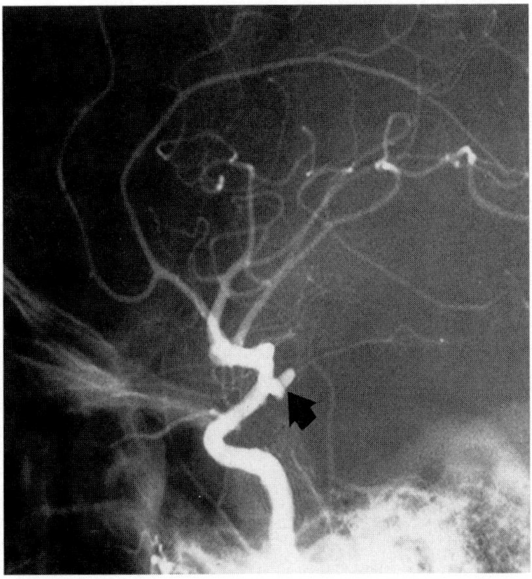

(c)

Figure 9 Extensive SAH and intraparenchymal hematoma from a right posterior communicating artery aneurysm. (a) Nonenhanced CT image through the level of the midbrain demonstrates extensive basilar subarachnoid hemorrhage with associated right temporal lobe parenchymal hematoma (small black arrow). Dilated left temporal horn indicates associated hydrocephalus. (b) A. higher CT image at the level of the lateral ventricles demonstrates SAH over the right mid frontal convexity with focal clots in the left anterior interhemispheric fissure (curved open arrows). Dependent intraventricular blood is present in the right atrium. (c) Lobulated posterior communicating artery origin aneurysm (thick black arrow) is noted on this lateral early arterial right-carotid angiogram.

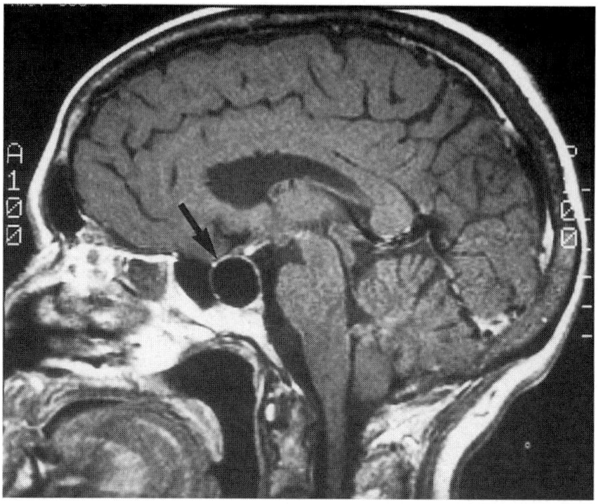

(a)

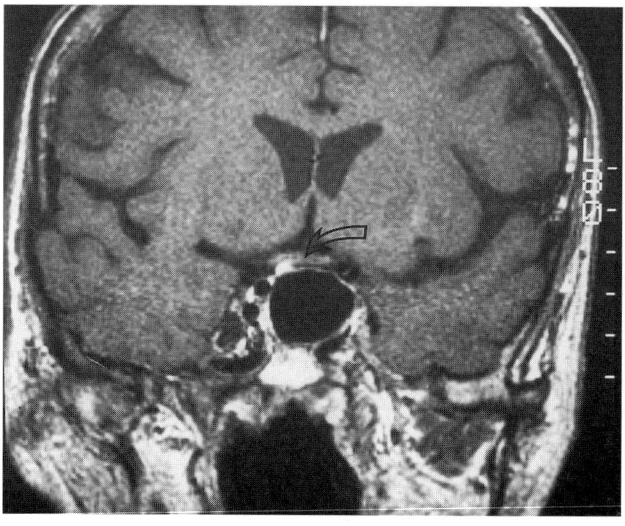

(b)

Figure 10 Patent intrasellar aneurysm. (a) Sagittal enhanced T1-weighted midline image demonstrates a patent aneurysm with a thin enhancing wall (black arrow). (b) Coronal enhanced T1-weighted sequence demonstrates elevation of the optic chiasm (curved open arrow). Horizontally-oriented phase or "ghosting" artifacts are subtly demonstrated, indicating flow within the aneurysm, which is dark due to time-of-flight phenomenon.

Complete thrombosis of an aneurysm may have several different appearances depending on the age of the thrombus, which may be multilayered. Thrombosis is common and is often variable due to the dynamic process of organization and lysis. Acute hemorrhage may be isointense with adjacent brain tissue and can be difficult to distinguish on both the T1 and T2 sequences. In the case of a negative angiogram in a patient with SAH, cervical or entire spine MRI may be useful to exclude a spinal cord hemorrhagic lesion.

The major complication of aneurysmal rupture is vasospasm. This is identified in 30–70% of angiograms, usually between the third and twelfth day, and becomes symptomatic in 20–30% of patients [54]. As vasospasm is rarely observed before three days, if clinical deterioration occurs in this time period. CT should be obtained to exclude the possibility of rehemorrhage, infarction due to embolism from the aneurysm, or progression of acute hydrocephalus. Ischemia may be indicated by decreased attenuation on CT or T2 hyperintensity on MRI. Pial enhancement on CT or MRI after three days may be observed, suggesting increased permeability of the blood/brain barrier.

Acute hydrocephalus may be seen on admission CT in 15% of SAH patients, with 40% of these being symptomatic [57]. This may be due to communicating or noncommunicating hydrocephalus. Posterior circulation aneurysm rupture has a higher incidence of hydrocephalus than does anterior circulation ruptures. Acute hydrocephalus does not always progress into chronic hydrocephalus.

A. Nonaneurysmal Subarachnoid Hemorrhage

Trauma is the most common cause of SAH. This may be associated with other intra- or extra-axial hemorrhage or may be seen in isolation. Other etiologies include perimesencephalic SAH, vascular malformations, spinal cord lesion hemorrhage, vasculitis, coagulation disorders, and arterial dissection.

The perimesencephalic type of nonaneurysmal subarachnoid hemorrhage (PMSAH) is a recently described clinical and radiologic entity with a good outcome [58,59]. A normal cerebral angiogram is present in 10–15% of patients with spontaneous SAH. One-half to two-thirds of these patients will demonstrate a perimesencephalic pattern of hemorrhage with blood predominately confined to the cisterns around the midbrain, usually located immediately anterior to the brainstem (Figure 12). The lateral sylvian and anterior intrahemispheric fissures are never completely filled with blood. Interventricular blood is uncommon and if seen is only in the fourth ventricle due to reflux. This pattern may be due to the lower pressure of bleeding seen with this condition. The likelihood of finding an aneurysm with a PMSAH distribution on early studies varies from 0–2.7% [60]. Angiography, however, remains essential to rule out a posterior circulation aneurysm.

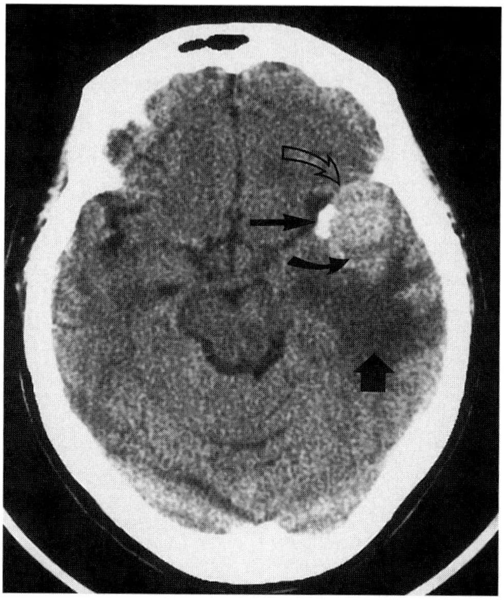

(a)

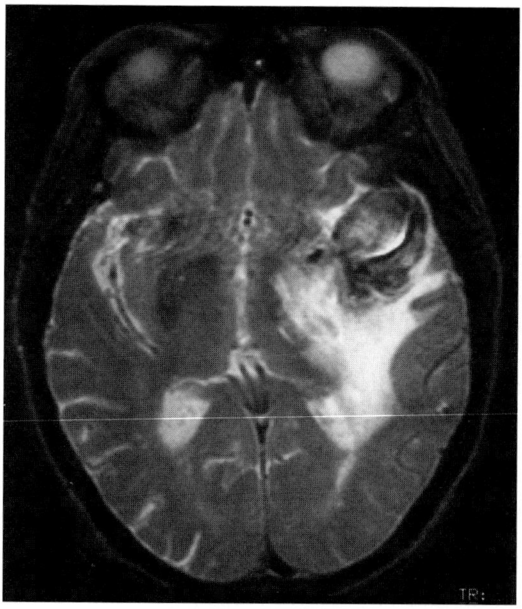

(b)

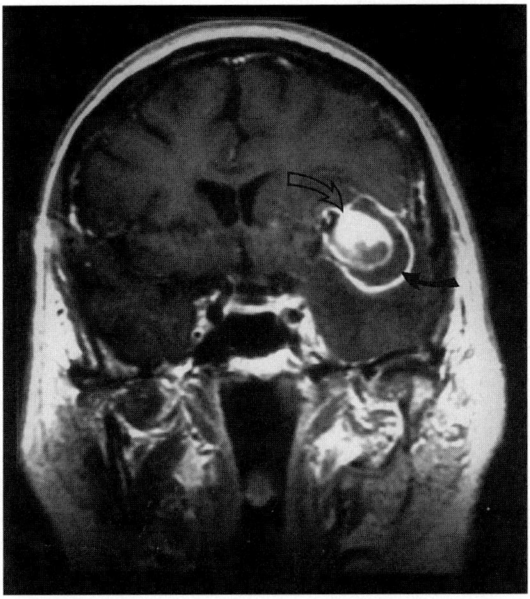

(c)

Figure 11 Giant left MCA aneurysm with distal ischemic change. (a) Nonenhanced CT demonstrates rim thrombus (black curved arrow) and mural calcification (small black arrow) partially surrounding the largely patent giant aneurysm (open curved arrow). Distal ischemic change is noted in the temporal lobe manifested by the decreased density and mass effect (large black arrow). (b) Axial T2-weighted MR image demonstrates similar findings on a slightly higher slice. Note pulsation artifacts horizontally in the phase-encoding direction at the same level indicating a patent lumen. (c) Enhanced coronal T1-weighted MRI through the giant aneurysm demonstrates enhancement within the patent lumen (curved open arrow) and within the thickened vessel wall (black curved arrow). Pulsation artifacts are present.

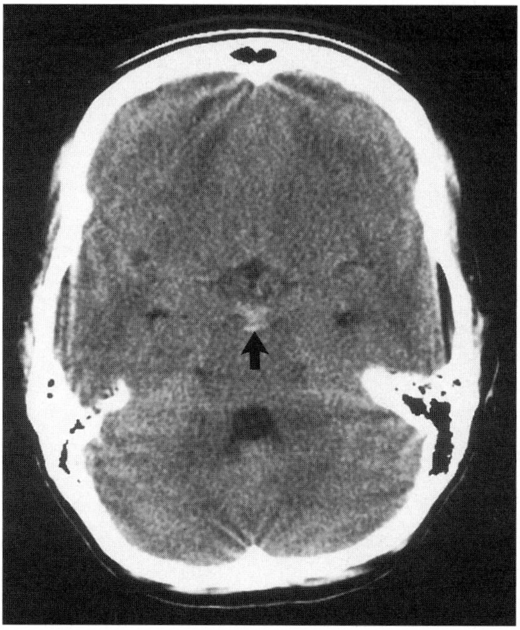

Figure 12 Perimesencephalic SAH in a 40-year-old female with negative angiogram and MRI. CT demonstrates hyperdense clot in the interpeduncular cistern (black arrow) with little, if any, blood in the other basilar cisterns. Early hydrocephalus with dilation of the temporal horns and fourth ventricle.

In Rinkel's study of 65 patients with PMSAH, none of the patients rebled or had delayed cerebral ischemia [61]. However, in 40 consecutive patients with PMSAH pattern, 11 patients developed hydrocephalus [62]. In all of these patients, the perimesencephalic cisterns were completely filled with blood. Only three patients (5%) developed clinical signs of acute hydrocephalus with two of these requiring ventricular shunting. All patients had a favorable outcome after three months. The cause of this benign disorder remains unknown but the likely source is venous or capillary bleeding.

It appears now that two distinct subsets of patients with angiogram negative subarachnoid hemorrhage are present. Those with the PMSAH pattern have an excellent prognosis, while those without this pattern demonstrated a 25% morbidity and mortality rate. Rankle et al. conclude that patients with a PMSAH pattern do not need a repeat angiography to search for an occult aneurysm after an initial negative angiogram [63].

ACKNOWLEDGMENTS

The authors wish to acknowledge the secretarial skills of Debbie Roach who made this chapter possible. We also thank John Atkinson, M.D., for his suggestions and support.

REFERENCES

1. Sadato N, Numaguchi T, Rigamonti D, et al. Bleeding patterns in ruptured posterior fossa aneurysms: a CT study. *J Comp Asst Tomogr* 1991; 15:612–617.
2. Atlas SW. MR imaging is highly sensitive for acute subarachnoid hemorrhage . . . not! *Radiology* 1993; 186:319–322.
3. Grossman RI. Magnetic resonance imaging of hemorrhage. In: Taveras JM, Ferrucci JT (eds). Radiology: Diagnosis–Imaging–Intervention. Philadelphia: Lippincott, 1990:ch 46.
4. Chakeres DW, Bryan RN. Acute subarachnoid hemorrhage: In vivo comparison of magnetic resonance and computed tomography. *AJNR* 1986; 7:223–228.
5. Inoui Y, Saiwai S, Miyamato T, et al. Post contrast computed tomography in subarachnoid hemorrhage from ruptured aneurysms. *J Comput Asst Tomogr* 1981; 5:341–344.
6. Ghoshhajra K, Scotti L, Marasco J, et al. CT detection of intracranial aneurysm in subarachnoid hemorrhage. *AJR* 1979; 132:613–616.
7. Liliequist B, Lindquist M, Valdimarsson E. Computed tomography and subarachnoid hemorrhage. *Neuroradiology* 1977; 14:21–26.
8. Lim ST, Sage DJ. Detection of subarachnoid blood clot and other thin flat structures by computed tomography. *Radiology* 1977; 123:79–84.
9. Tarr RW, Hecht ST, Horton JA. Nontraumatic intracranial hemorrhage. In: Latchaw RE (ed). MR and CT Imaging of the Head, Neck, and Spine. 2nd ed. St. Louis: Mosby Year Book, 1991:267.
10. Cohen WA, Wayman LA. Computed tomography of intracranial hemorrhage. *Neuroimaging Clinics N Amer* 1992; 2:75–87.
11. Pfleger MJ, Hardee EP, Hayman LA. Fluid/fluid levels in intracerebral hematoma: A sign of coagulopathy. Reported at the 30th Annual Scientific Meeting of the American Society of Neuroradiology. St. Louis, Missouri, May 31–June 5, 1992.
12. Davis JM, Ploetz J, Davis KR, et al. Cranial computed tomography in subarachnoid hemorrhages: relationship between blood detected by CT and lumbar puncture. *J Comput Asst Tomogr* 1980; 4:794–796.
13. Osborn AG. Diagnostic Neuroradiology. St. Louis: Mosby Year Book, 1994:212.
14. Bradley WG Jr. MR appearance of hemorrhage in the brain. *Radiology* 1993; 198:15–26.
15. Bradley WG Jr. Hemorrhage and hemorrhagic infections in the brain. *Neuroimaging Clinics N Amer* 1994; 4:707–731.
16. Osborn AG. Diagnostic Neuroradiology. St. Louis: Mosby Year Book, 1994:154–198.

17. Axel L. Blood flow effects in magnetic resonance imaging. *AJR* 1984; 143:1157–1166.
18. Bradley WG Jr. Flow phenomena in MR imaging. *AJR* 1988; 150:983–994.
19. Ogawa T, Inugami A, Shimosegawa E, et al. Subarachnoid hemorrhage: evaluation with MR imaging. *Radiology* 1993; 186:345–351.
20. Satoh S, Kadoya S. Magnetic resonance imaging of subarachnoid hemorrhage. *Neuroradiology* 1988; 30:361–366.
21. Noguchi K, Ogawa T, Inugami A, Toyoshima H, Okudera T, Uemura K. MR of acute subarachnoid hemorrhage: a preliminary report of fluid–attenuated inversion recovery pulse sequences. *AJNR* 1994; 15:1940–1943.
22. Noguchi K, Ogawa T, Inugami A. Acute subarachnoid hemorrhage: MR imaging with fluid–attenuated inversion recovery pulse sequences. *Radiology* 1995; 196:773–777.
23. Gean AD, Pile-Spellman J, Heros RC. A pneumatized anterior clinoid mimicking an aneurysm on MR imaging. *J Neurosurg* 1989; 71:128–132.
24. Bourgouin PM, Tampieri D, Melancon D, del Carpio R, Ethier R. Superficial siderosis of the brain following unexplained subarachnoid hemorrhage: MRI diagnosis and clinical significance. *Neuroradiology* 1992; 34:407–410.
25. Bracchi M, Savoiardo M, Triulzi F, et al. Superficial siderosis of the CNS: MR diagnosis and clinical findings. *AJNR* 1993; 14:227–236.
26. Osborn AG. Diagnostic Neuroradiology. St. Louis: Mosby Year Book, 1994:184.
27. Kanal E, Shellock FG. MR imaging of patients with intracranial aneurysm clips. *Radiology* 1993; 187:612–614.
28. Shellock FG, Kanal E. Magnetic resonance: Bioeffects, Safety, and Patient Management. New York: Raven Press Ltd, 1994.
29. Cioffi F, Pasgalin A, Cavazzsani P, Da Pian R. Subarachnoid hemorrhage of unknown origin: clinical and tomographical aspects. *ACTA Neurochir (Wein)* 1989; 97:31–39.
30. Rinkel G, van Gijn J, Wijdickj E. Subarachnoid hemorrhages without detectable aneurysms: a review of the causes. *Stroke* 1993; 24:1403–1409.
31. Camarata PJ, Latchaw RE Jr, Ruffenacht DA, Heros RC. Intracranial aneurysms. *Invest Radiol* 1993; 28:373–382.
32. Brott T, Mandybur TI. Case–control study of clinical outcome after aneurysmal subarachnoid hemorrhage. *Neurosur* 1986; 19:891–895.
33. Stehbens WE. Etiology of intracranial berry aneurysms. *J Neurosurg* 1989; 70:823–831.
34. Osborn AG. Intracranial aneurysms: clinicopathologic correlations. Core Curriculum Course in Neuroradiology. Part I: Vascular lesions and degenerative diseases. Reported at the Annual Scientific Meeting of the American Society of Neuroradiology. Chicago, Illinois, April 21–22, 1995.
35. Barami K, Ko K. Ruptured mycotic aneurysm presenting as an intraparenchymal hemorrhage and nonadjacent acute subdural hematoma: case report and review of the literature. *Surg Neurol* 1994; 41:290–293.
36. Bingham WF. Treatment of mycotic intracranial aneurysms. *J Neurosurg* 1977; 46:428–437.

37. Buckingham MJ, Crone KR, Ball WS, et al. Traumatic intracranial aneurysms in childhood: two cases and a review of the literature. *Neurosurgery* 1988; 22:398–408.
38. Wilson FMA, Jaspan T, Holland IM. Multiple cerebral aneurysms: a reappraisal. *Neuroradiology* 1989; 31:232–236.
39. Osborn AG. Intracranial aneurysms. In: Diagnostic Neuroradiology. St. Louis: Mosby, 1994:248–283.
40. Berger MS, Wilson CB. Intracranial dissecting aneurysms of the posterior circulation: report of six cases and review of the literature. *J Neurosurg* 1984; 61:882–894.
41. Massoud TF, Anslow P, Molyneux AJ. Subarachnoid hemorrhage following spontaneous intracranial carotid artery dissection. *Neuroradiology* 1992; 34:33–35.
42. Tanaka K, Waga S, Kojima T, Kubo Y, Shimizu T, Niwa S. Non-traumatic dissecting aneurysms of the intracranial vertebral artery: report of six cases. *Acta Neurochir* 1989; 100:62–66.
43. Bull J. Massive aneurysms at the base of the brain. *Brain* 1969; 92:535–570.
44. Atlas SW, Grossman RI, Goldberg HI, Hackney DB, Bilaniuk LT, Zimmerman RA. Partially thrombosed giant intracranial aneurysms: correlation of MR and pathologic findings. *Radiology* 1987; 162:111–114.
45. Drake CG. Giant intracranial aneurysms: experience with surgical treatment in 174 patients. *Clin Neurol* 1979; 26:12–95.
46. Kassell NF, Torner JC, Haley EC Jr, Jain JA, Adams HP, Kongable GL. An international cooperative study on the timing of aneurysm surgery. I: Overall management results. *J Neurosurg* 1990; 73:18–36.
47. Vermeulen M, van Gijn J. The diagnosis of subarachnoid hemorrhage. *J Neurol Neurosurg Psychiatry* 1990; 53:365–372.
48. Osborn AG. Diagnostic neuroradiology. St. Louis: Mosby Year Book, 1994:226.
49. Tomsick TA. Aneurysm: CT, angiography, MR/MRA. Core Curriculum Course in Neuroradiology. Part I: Vascular lesions and degenerative diseases. Reported at the Annual Scientific Meeting of the American Society of Neuroradiology. Chicago, Illinois, April 21–22, 1995.
50. Eggers R, Tomsick T, Lukin R, Chamber A. Recognition of subdural hematoma secondary to ruptured aneurysm by computerized tomography. *Comput Radiol* 1982; 6:309–313.
51. Schmidt UD, Steiger HJ, Huber P. Accuracy of high resolution computed tomography in direct diagnosis of cerebral aneurysms. *Neuroradiology* 1987; 29:152–159.
52. Fisher CM, Kistler JP, Davis JM. Relation of cerebral vasospasm to subarachnoid hemorrhage visualized by computerized tomographic scanning. *Neurosurgery* 1980; 6:1–9.
53. Milhorat TH. Acute hydrocephalus after aneurysmal subarachnoid hemorrhage. *Neurosurgery* 1987; 20:15–20.
54. Kassell NF, Sasaki T, Colohan ART, et al. Cerebral vasospasm following aneurysmal subarachnoid hemorrhage. *Stroke* 1985; 16:562–572.
55. Greenberg MS. Handbook of Neurosurgery. 3rd ed. Lakeland, Florida: Greenberg Graphics, Inc., 1994: 711.

56. Hahn FJ, Ong E, McComb R, Leibrock L. Peripheral signal void ring in giant vertebral aneurysm: MR and pathology findings. *J Comp Asst Tomogr* 1986; 10:1036–1038.
57. Graff-Radford N, Torner J, Adams HP, et al. Factors associated with hydrocephalus after subarachnoid hemorrhage. *Arch Neurol* 1989; 46:744–752.
58. van Gijn J, van Dongen KJ, Vermeulen M, Hijdra A. Perimesencephalic hemorrhage: a nonaneurysmal and benign form of subarachnoid hemorrhage. *Neurology* 1985; 35:493–497.
59. Rinkel GJ, Wijdicks EF, Vermeulen M, et al. Nonaneurysmal perimesencephalic subarachnoid hemorrhage: CT and MR patterns that differ from aneurysmal rupture. *AJNR* 1991; 12:829–834.
60. Pinto AN, Ferro JM, Canhao P, Campos J. How often is a perimesencephalic subarachnoid haemorrhage CT pattern caused by ruptured aneurysms? *Acta Neurochir (Austria)* 1993; 124:79–81.
61. Rinkel GJ, Wijdicks EF, Vermeulen M, Hasan D, Brouwers PJ, van Gijn J. The clinical course of perimesencephalic nonaneurysmal subarachnoid hemorrhage. *Ann Neurol* 1991; 29:463–468.
62. Rinkel GJ, Wijdicks EF, Vermeulen M, Tans JT, Hasan D, van Gijn J. Acute hydrocephalus in nonaneurysmal perimesencephalic hemorrhage: evidence of CSF block at the tentorial hiatus. *Neurology* 1992; 42:1805–1807.
63. Rinkel GJ, Wijdicks EF, Hasan D, et al. Outcome in patients with subarachnoid haemorrhage and negative angiography according to pattern of haemorrhage on computed tomography. *Lancet* 1991; 338:964–968.

10

Computerized Tomography and Magnetic Resonance Imaging of CNS Vascular Malformations

Bob Lefsrud and Gary M. Miller
Mayo Clinic, Rochester, Minnesota

I. INTRODUCTION

Several, often confusing, terminologies and classifications have been used to describe vascular malformations. Four basic types can usually be recognized pathologically and with cross-sectional diagnostic imaging: 1. arteriovenous malformations (AVMs), 2. capillary malformations, 3. cavernous angiomas, and 4. venous malformations.

Some investigators consider capillary malformations and cavernous hemangiomas as a spectrum, while others feel that cavernous angiomas should be lumped with venous malformations [1,2]. Another category of mixed (pathologically heterogenous) lesions has been proposed that demonstrates two or more morphologically distinct areas within the vascular malformation [3]. McCormick adds a fifth group splitting varices from the venous malformation group [4].

Intracranial vascular malformations not fitting neatly into the above basic types that will be reviewed in this chapter include angiographically occult vascular malformations (AOGM), vascular abnormalities of the vein of Galen, dural arteriovenous fistulae (DAVF), and carotid cavernous fistulae (CCF). We conclude with an approach to vascular malformations in the spinal cord.

II. ARTERIOVENOUS MALFORMATIONS

Pathologically, AVMs have no intervening capillary bed with blood shunting from engorged abnormal thick-walled vascular channels that are neither purely arterial or entirely venous in type. Usually the arteries and veins of the adjacent normal brain tissue remain uninfluenced and establish no collateral channels with the malformation. Eighty-five to ninety percent of parenchymal AVMs are found in the cerebral hemispheres [1]. Ninety-eight percent are solitary. Multiple AVMs may be found in the syndromes of Weber-Mason and Rendu-Osler-Weber. The prevalence of AVM in the general population is 0.02–0.05%, or roughly one-tenth of that of saccular aneurysms [5].

Dural vascular malformations make up 10% of intracranial AVMs [6]. Pathologically, they usually represent a complex of microfistulae within the wall of a venous sinus, usually without a discrete nidus, unlike brain parenchymal AVMs. In this case, they are called dural arteriovenous fistulae (DAVFs) [6]. These are felt to be acquired, possibly due to prior venous sinus thrombosis [7]. Most dural vascular malformations involve the skull base and make up one-third of posterior fossa AVMs [8]. The cavernous sinus is the second most common site for DAVFs, followed by the superior sagittal and straight sinuses [9]. These are discussed later in the chapter.

Intracranial hemorrhage is the most common presenting symptom in 50–70% of patients with AVMs, which is usually intraparenchymal, although subarachnoid hemorrhage may be seen in up to one-third of cases [10–13]. Brain AVMs are the second most common cause of spontaneous subarachnoid hemorrhage in adults and the most common symptomatic type of vascular malformation [14]. The risk of initial hemorrhage is about 2–3% per year. The incidence of rehemorrhage in the first year is 6% and then 3% a year thereafter [15].

Central venous drainage, periventricular or intraventricular location, and intranidal aneurysm have shown to be associated with increased risk of hemorrhage [16]. Angiomatous changes appear to decrease the chance of hemorrhage; the additional dilated arterial collateral supply within angiomatous lesions may lower the perfusion pressure of the AVM [16].

Conventional angiography is no longer needed for initial diagnosis and characterization of AVMs and may obviate the need of angiography for inoperable lesions. Angiography, however, is mandatory in the planning of surgical or endovascular therapy. The Spetzler–Martin AVM grading system may be used to compare AVM series [17]. This five-point system is based on lesion size, eloquence of adjacent brain tissue, and pattern of venous drainage. A separate Grade 6 is reserved for inoperable lesions that would be associated with disabling deficit or death [18]. A grading system may be helpful for interseries comparison. However, each AVM is unique in its own characteristics and intervention requires more than a cookbook approach. Therefore, each lesion must be assessed individually.

The association of cerebral AVMs and aneurysms has been noted to have prevalence varying from 3–23%, although a recent superselective angiographic assessment in 58 patients by Turjman demonstrates flow-related aneurysms in nearly 60% of cases [19]. These flow-related aneurysms are thin walled and may be more prone to rupture. Eighty percent of AVMs that bleed harbor flow-related aneurysms [20].

Parenchymal AVMs are typically a cortically-based, wedge-shaped tangle of vessels with little or no mass effect unless there has been recent bleeding. These vascular malformations may be focal or diffuse, the latter sometimes involving an entire lobe or hemisphere.

III. CT IMAGING OF ARTERIOVENOUS MALFORMATIONS

On nonenhanced CT studies, the most common pattern of AVMs is a mixed density lesion in 50–60% of cases with uniform isointense lesions being recognized in 15–30% of cases. Uniformly high-density lesions may be seen in 10–15% of cases [21] and AVMs may not be visualized in 10–23% of plain CT scans. Serpiginous vessels are often seen. Hyperintensity may be due to acute hemorrhage, thrombosed vessels, or the calcifications that are seen in 25–30% of cases [22]. Areas of low attenuation are usually due to adjacent brain atrophy due to steal phenomena or ischemia. In a study by Kumar et al. of 60 patients with clinically unruptured intracranial AVMs, 33 patients (55%) demonstrated local or distant mass effects with a degree of mass effect proportional to the size of the AVM [23]. The enlarged vessels contributed to the mass effect in one-quarter of cases while edema was the predominant component in only two cases.

With the administration of contrast material, serpiginous dense enhancement is noted in up to 80% of cases [24]. No enhancement will be observed in the uncommon thrombosed AVMs. Linear enhancement or thickening of adjacent leptomeninges may be present. In the study by Terbrugge, 23% of AVMs that were isodense were missed on plain film but picked up after the injection of intravenous contrast material [21].

IV. MR IMAGING OF ARTERIOVENOUS MALFORMATIONS

The MR appearance of patent parenchymal AVMs is variable depending on the pulse sequence, flow rates, and presence of hemorrhage. Adjacent atrophy and gliosis or mass effect may be present with increased T2 signal [22,23]. Dilated feeding and draining vessels are the hallmark of this lesion [24] (Figure 1). Thrombosed AVMs with hemorrhage usually contain a dark hemosiderin ring that may help to differentiate these from hemorrhagic neoplasms.

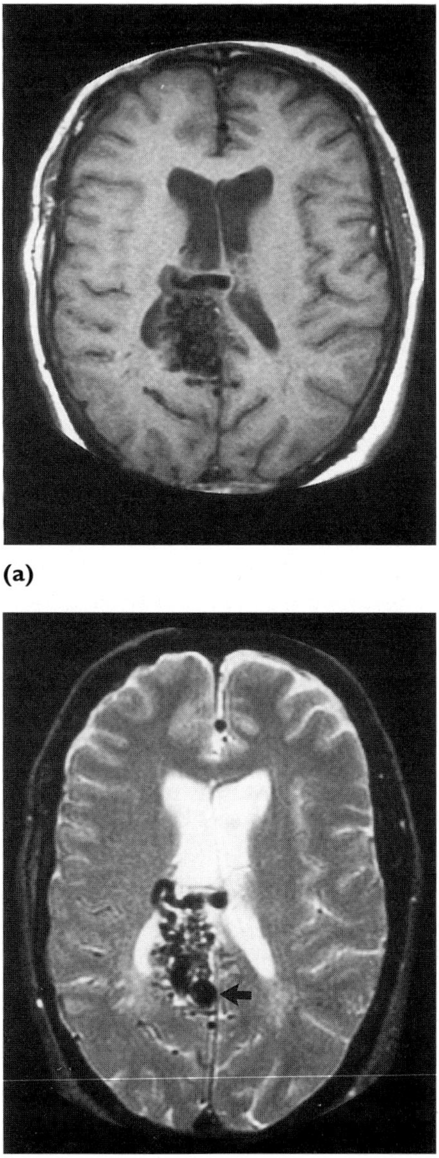

(a)

(b)

Figure 1 Right parietal AVM. (a) The complex tangle of dilated vessels is typical for a parenchymal AVM on this axial T1-weighted nonenhanced image. (b) T2-weighted spin echo sequence at the same level demonstrates the vessels slightly better. Note a posterior dilated venous varix (black arrow). This lesion demonstrates little or no mass effect.

The MR appearance of dural-based AVMs and AVFs is nonspecific but may be suggested by dilated cortical veins without the appearance of a parenchymal nidus [9]. Although angiography is necessary for confirmation of diagnosis, MRA may be helpful.

Although it is less sensitive in identifying small calcified AVMs, MRI is superior to conventional angiography and CT in demonstrating the anatomic relation of the nidus, feeding vessels, and draining veins [25,26]. The MRI technique is also more sensitive in demonstrating associated parenchymal abnormalities and MRI is also superior in demonstrating occlusion of vessels of the nidus following endovascular embolization or spontaneous thrombosis [27]. The CT technique may better demonstrate acute hemorrhage. Hemosiderin is manifest by decreased intensity, and blooming on T2 sequences is seen in 63% of patients with spin echo sequences and up to 95% of patients with gradient echo imaging [28]. This suggests asymptomatic bleeding or chronic RBC diapedesis. Intranidal aneurysms and angiomatous change may be seen but cannot be reliably identified with MR [28]. The administration of gadolinium is usually not necessary for diagnosis and characterization, although it may be helpful for the detection of slow flowing veins (Figure 2).

A. Capillary Malformations

Capillary telangiectasias are composed of a tangle of dilated and variable capillary blood vessels, usually but not invariably separated by normal brain parenchyma and often accompanied by enlarged draining veins that are morphologically normal otherwise [1]. Most of these are small and clinically silent. Rarely are they associated with hemorrhage. They infrequently reach the surface of the brain. No abnormal feeding vessels are present. The pons is the most common location followed in descending order by the cerebral cortex, cortical white matter, middle cerebral peduncle, dentate, and nucleus [29]. Multiple lesions are not infrequent. Capillary telangiectasias may coexist with cavernous hemangiomas [2].

Nonenhanced studies are usually normal unless there has been prior hemorrhage or adjacent gliosis [29]. Uniform contrast enhancement is seen more often on MRI than on CT, demonstrating a well-defined faint to moderate circumscribed lesion. If hemorrhage has occurred, the appearance may be identical to angiographically occult vascular malformations (AOVMs).

Radiation induced telangiectasia is a condition of endothelial hyperplasia and dilation of capillary channels is a recognized complication of radiation therapy. This hemorrhagic focus results in MR features similar to those described for AOVMs, with the majority of the lesions appearing hypointense on T2, indicative of hemosiderin deposition [30]. Twenty-five percent of patients demonstrate evidence of frank intracranial hemorrhage. These foci are usually small

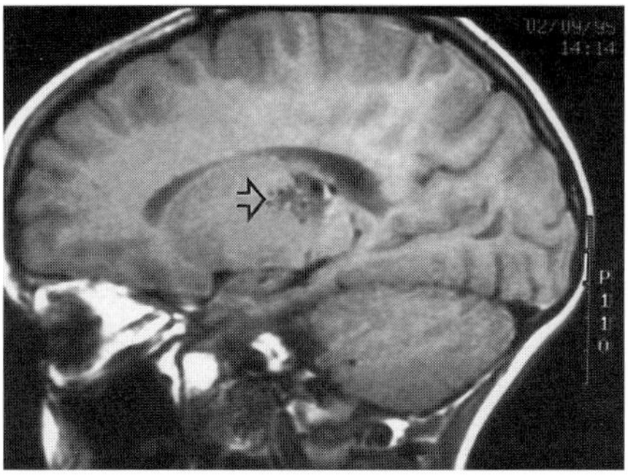

(a)

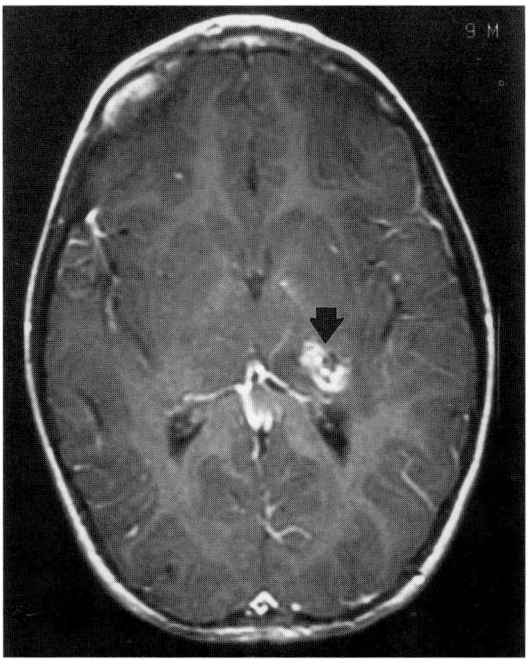

(b)

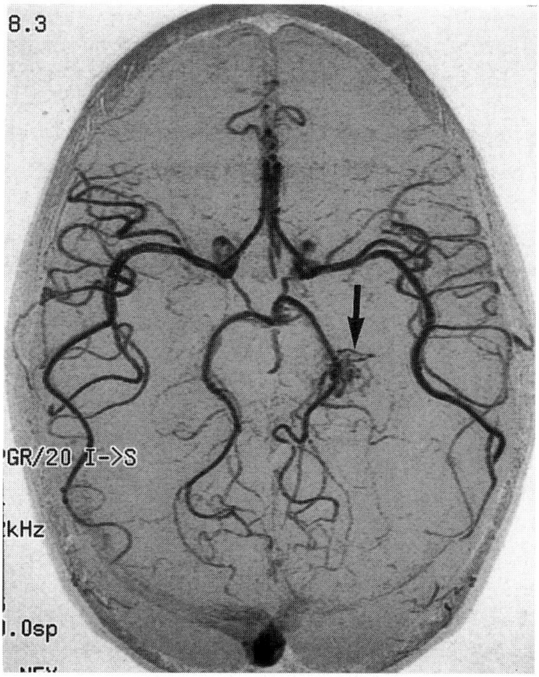

(c)

Figure 2 AVM of the left thalamus. (a) Flow voids and decreased signal in the thalamus represent an AVM on this sagittal nonenhanced T1-weighted sequence (open arrow). (b) The lesion demonstrates marked contrast enhancement within the slow flowing vessels (large black arrow) on this axial enhanced T1-weighted sequence. (c) Prominent arterial feeders are demonstrated from the left P2 segment on this collapsed view from a three-dimensional time-of-flight circle of Willis magnetic resonance study.

(<5 mm) and multiple in 45% of cases [30]. The changes are likely due to endothelial injury with subsequent vascular thrombosis, although mineralization, fibrosis, hyalinization, and endothelial swelling have been proposed [30]. Differential diagnosis would include other causes of multiple hemorrhagic foci, including cavernous malformations, amyloidosis, and multiple hemorrhagic metastases.

B. Cavernous Angiomas

Cavernous angiomas (cavernous malformations, cavernous hemangiomas, cavernomas, cavernous venous malformations) represent endothelial-lined sinusoidal spaces without intervening parenchymal tissue [2,31]. Clot within different spaces and with different stages of evolution is usually seen. A peripheral hemosiderin ring is common. These lesions grossly are multilobulated with surrounding and interdigitating fibers and granulation tissue. Vascular channels lack muscular or elastic fibers. Fiber septi may contain hemosiderin, calcifications, or both. Intravascular thrombosis is common, likely due to the slow flow. Lesions are well circumscribed due to a pseudocapsule [1] and size is usually less than 3 cm. Multiple lesions may be found in the familial form, up to 73% compared with 10–15% for the sporadic form. The familial occurrence is observed more frequently in persons of Hispanic origin [32,33]. Eighty percent are supratentorial, more commonly in the frontal and temporal lobes, in the deep white matter or at the cortical medullary junction. The pons and cerebellar hemispheres are the most common location within the posterior fossa [34]. Cavernous angiomas may occur in the cord where they may coexist with brain lesions [35] (Figure 3).

Extracerebellar cavernous hemangiomas have been described in the subarachnoid, subdural, extradural, dural sinus and intraventricular spaces and may have the typical popcorn appearance or demonstrate uniform homogeneous enhancement resembling a meningioma [36]. Cavernous angiomas are the most common brain vascular lesion identified on MRI, and they have an annual risk of hemorrhage less than 1% [34]. Seizures are the presenting symptom in about half of patients with one out of six coming to medical attention due to hemorrhage or progressive neurological symptoms [37].

Hoang and Hasso have characterized three components of the cavernoma to help understand their CT and MR imaging appearance [29]. The three parts include a vascular component with slowly flowing or thrombosed blood in sinusoidal spaces; a connective tissue component with irregular intersecting septae separating the sinusoidal spaces; and a peripheral gliotic component, often containing blood breakdown products. On unenhanced CT, the circular to multinodular lesion is usually mild to moderately hyperdense with calcifications seen in up to one-third of cases. Hypointense, nonenhancing areas may be present due to old blood or cystic change. Intravenous contrast enhancement is seen in 70–94% of cases. The adjacent brain parenchyma is usually normal and the lesion is well circumscribed unless recent hemorrhage has occurred, when mass effect and edema may be noted. The typical mulberry or popcorn-like appearance is characteristic, although not specific; other lesions such as thrombosed AVMs, hemorrhagic capillary telangiectasias, gliomas, or metastatic lesions (especially melanoma) may have an identical appearance [29,38] (Figure 4).

The MR appearance mimics the heterogeneous pathologic character with a complex mixed-signal core representing hemorrhage in different stages of evolution [39]. A low-signal hemosiderin ring usually completely surrounds the lesion, which becomes more prominent on T2W or GRE sequences [32]. To look for multiple lesions which may not be visualized with standard spin echo sequences gradient echo sequences should always be performed when a solitary intracranial hemorrhage lesion is identified. Even with conventional T2W spin-echo sequences, in some studies MRI demonstrated 60% more lesions than CT [32,40]. Fast spin echo sequences should be used with caution as they are even less sensitive than traditional spin echo sequences to detect hemosiderin. Hemosiderin is also less conspicuous on lower field strength units. Enhancement following contrast administration is variable from none to intense.

C. Venous Malformations

Venous malformations or developmental venous abnormalities (DVAs) are likely developmental anatomic variants due to arrested growth of the fetal venous system. Venous development occurs later than the brain arterial supply [41]. These retained primitive embryologic medullary veins radially drain into a single large vein with a "spoke-wheel" or "caput medusa" appearance (Figure 5). Normal intervening brain parenchyma is present and neither capillaries nor arteries are involved with this process. Up to one-third of venous malformations are associated with cavernous angiomas [42]. Associated focal neuronal migration abnormalities have also been reported, a finding consistent with the theory of arrested venous development [43]. This is the most common vascular malformation noted in some autopsy series, occurring in 3% of autopsies [4]. The frontal lobe is the most common location (40%), followed by the cerebellum (20%). Two-thirds are supratentorial. Most venous angiomas are solitary although multiple lesions may be seen in the blue rubber bleb nevus syndrome [44]. Venous angiomas are usually asymptomatic with the most common symptoms being seizures and headaches [45]. Hemorrhage is uncommon and when this occurs is often associated with a coexisting cavernous angioma [43]. In McCormick's autopsy series, three (15%) of 20 cerebellar venous angiomas showed evidence of prior hemorrhage [4]. There may be a positive correlation

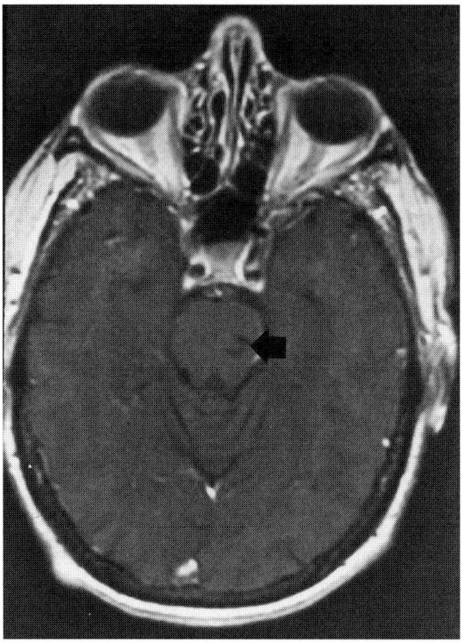

(a)

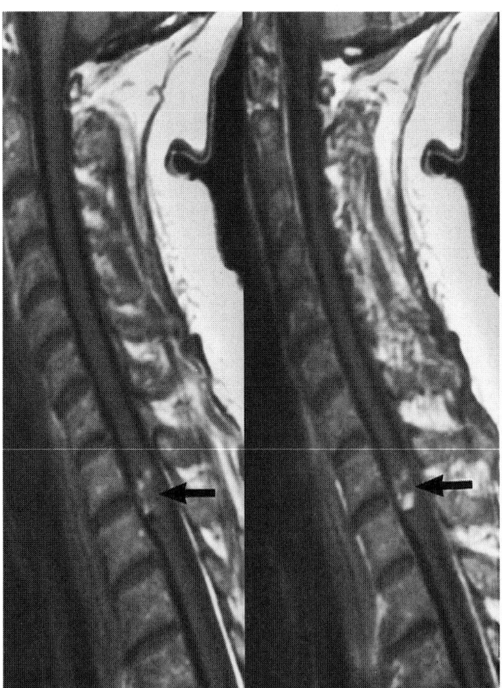

(b)

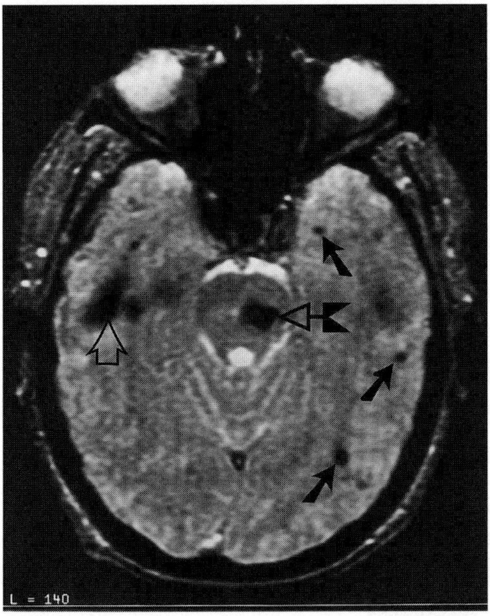

(c)

Figure 3 Multiple cavernous hemangiomas in the same patient. (a) Sagittal enhanced T1-weighted images demonstrate a multilobulated intramedullary lesion with central heterogeneous increased signal in a surrounding rim of low signal at the T1-2 level due to hemosiderin (thin black arrows). Note cord expansion at this level. (b) Enhanced T1-weighted axial image suggests a left mid pontine lesion with a low-intensity rim that does not enhance (thick back arrow). (c) T2-weighted gradient recalled echo image at the same level as "b." The pontine cavernous hemangioma is much more conspicuous (arrow with tail) and at least three more lesions are noted in the left temporal lobe at the same level (black angled arrows). Susceptibility artifact is present from the petrous ridge on the right (large open arrow). This pulse sequence is much more sensitive to the paramagnetic effects of hemosiderin and blood products.

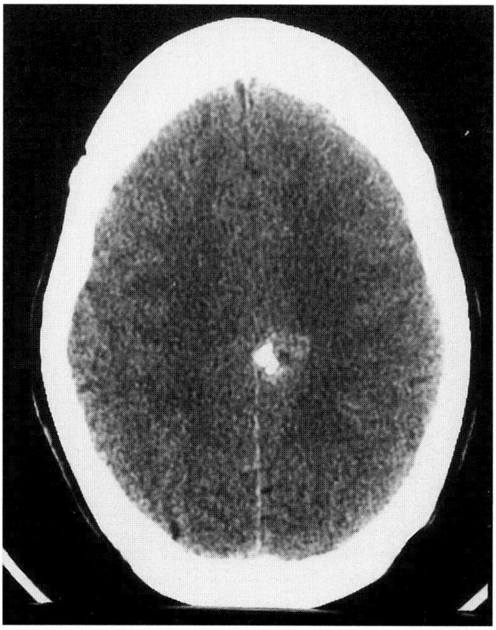

(a)

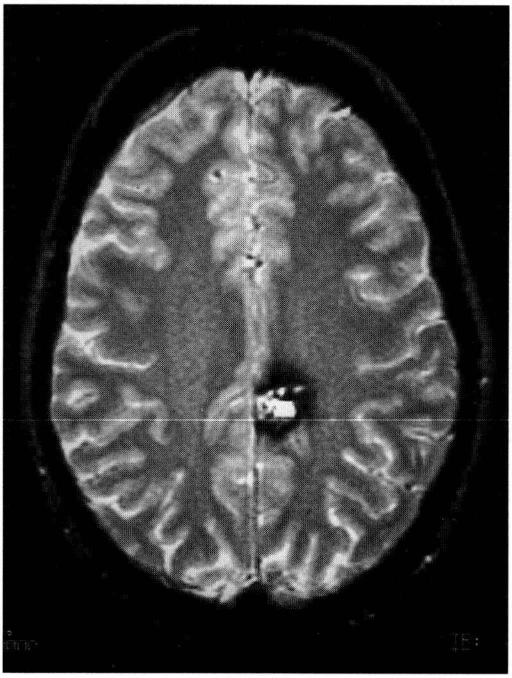

(b)

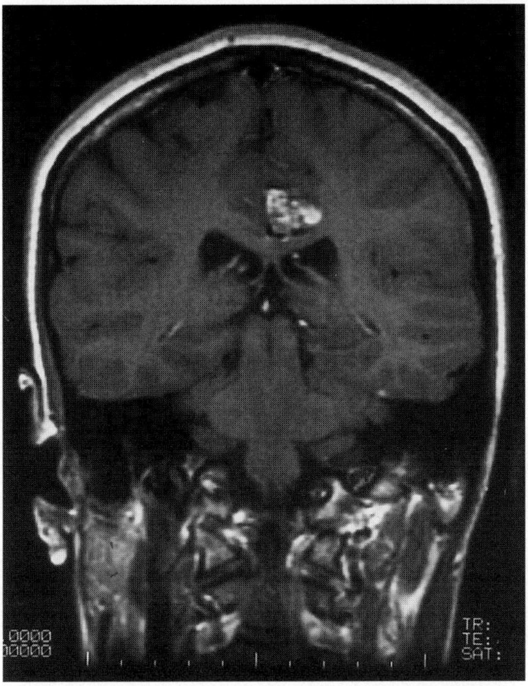

(c)

Figure 4 Cavernous hemangioma of the left posterior cingulate gyrus. (a) Chunk-like calcification and heterogeneous hyperdensity is noted on this nonenhanced CT of a lesion that abuts the falx. The CT appearance is nonspecific and the differential diagnosis would include neoplasms such as a meningioma or oligodendroglioma, infectious process such as tuberculosis or other healed granuloma, or a vascular malformation. (b) A dark hemosiderin ring surrounds a central bright signal focus on this T2-weighted axial MR image. This appearance is typical for a cavernous hemangioma. (c) Coronal enhanced T1-weighted sequence demonstrates a lobulated cavernoma with bright central signal occupying the cingulate gyrus. Note that the hemosiderin ring is less apparent than on the T2 sequence.

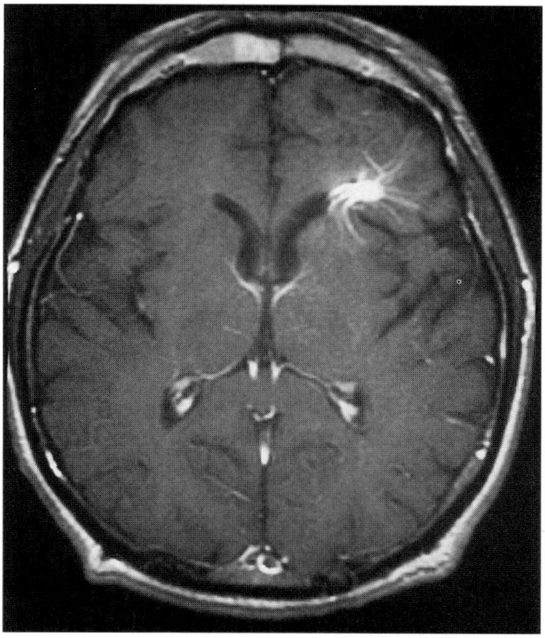

Figure 5 Venous angioma. Dilated curvilinear radially oriented enhancing veins drain into an enlarged central vein giving the typical appearance of a venous angioma on this enhanced axial T1-weighted MR image. THe frontal lobe is the most common site for this type of malformation.

between the size of the DVA and frequency of hemorrhage [46]. However, most series suggest that solitary venous angiomas rarely are symptomatic and if there is associated hemorrhage, strong suspicion of coexistent cavernous malformation must be explored.

In reviewing the literature, Valavanis found that about 70% of DVAs drained into the superficial venous system, while 22% drained deep to the subependymal venous system. The remaining venous malformations contributed to both systems [47].

Sinus pericranii is an anomalous communication or subperiosteal venous angioma connecting the intracranial and extracranial venous circulation. This is usually found in males less than the age of 30 [44]. Congenital post-traumatic or spontaneous etiologies have been proposed. Patients are usually asymptomatic, although clinically a soft mass is often present that increases in size with the head-down position or with Valsalva maneuver. Sinus pericranii should enhance to the same degree as other intracranial venous structures following the intravenous injection of contrast material. Overlying bone defect or erosion is noted with imaging [48].

Sturge-Weber syndrome (encephalo-trigeminal angiomatosis) is a leptomeningeal capillary venous angioma from persistence of a usually transitory stage of vessel development normally associated with underlying cortical hemiatrophy due to anoxia from preferential superficial blood flow [49]. This results in underlying cortical calcifications that usually have a typical tram-track appearance on opposing gyri. Ipsilateral thickening of the skull, orbits, and enlarged sinuses are present. Associated facial telangiectasia in the trigeminal region, mental retardation, and crossed hemiparesis are often seen, as well as contralateral hemiatrophy. Associated marked bleeding is rare. With contrast administration, enhancement is noted in the pial angioma, gyri, ipsilateral enlarged choroid plexus, and from very prominent medullary and subependymal veins [50,51].

V. IMAGING OF VENOUS MALFORMATIONS

Nonenhanced CT images of venous angiomas are usually normal or demonstrate prominent draining veins with a hairlike appearance of converging, enlarged, deep white-matter veins. Enhanced CT usually detects a linear or curvilinear attenuating vessel [43]. Calcification, edema, or mass effect are rare. Enhanced or plain CT studies of 51 MR-documented venous angiomas demonstrated only 16 and 6 lesions, respectively [52].

Magnetic resonance scans usually demonstrate a flow void or paradoxically flow-related enhancement in venous angiomas [53]. Truwit observed that hyperintensity on proton and T2W images noted in early reports was likely due to spatial misregistration artifact when the draining vein is neither parallel nor perpendicular to the phase encoding direction [43]. Enhancement of parenchyma adjacent to a venous malformation may be due to venous restrictive disease of the draining vein and it is thought that these lesions may be more prone to hemorrhage [43]. The T2 imaging approach is more successful in showing these lesions than a T1-weighted series [54,55]. Gliosis or hemorrhage may be seen in up to 15% of cases [56]. Approximately one-third of venous angiomas are discovered only after administration of gadolinium due to pooling of contrast in the slow-flowing veins [57].

A. Angiographically Occult Vascular Malformations (AOVMs)

Cryptic vascular malformations or AOVMs are composed of partially or completely thrombosed AVMs, cavernous malformations, venous angiomas, capillary telangiectasias, or mixed lesions. Possible factors for angiographic nonvisualization of such vascular malformations would include spontaneous or secondary thrombosis with hyaline degeneration, obliteration subsequent to rupture, compression by adjacent clot or gliotic scar, or the slow flow through it necessitating very late films to visualize a small lesion [58]. Cavernous angiomas may constitute up to 62% of AOVMs with mixed lesions making up the next most common group [58]. Other studies state that AVMs constitute over 50% of AOVMs [59,60]. The histopathology of cryptic malformations did not seem to have a prognostic significance in a study by Sigal of 20 AOVMs retrospectively studied over a mean period of 18 months. The study showed progressive bleeding in 20% of the cases and regression in 20% of the cases [61].

In a study of 188 consecutive patients, AOVMs presented with clinically significant bleeds more times than AVMs (61.7% versus 15.6%), leading to a higher nonoperative morbidity. However, mortality associated with hemorrhage was twice as high in AVM patients (7.5% vs. 3.6% of the cases) [62].

The CT and MRI findings are nonspecific and identical to that ascribed in cavernous hemangiomas [58,63]. Hyperdensity on CT may represent hemorrhage or calcium. Enhancement is variable. The appearance is characteristic but not pathognomonic and further assessment with MRI is usually warranted if picked up on CT to exclude a neoplasm [64].

The appearance on MRI is usually more specific than that of CT although calcifications may be less apparent [64]. Enhancement is usual although not always seen. The different stages of hematoma are better assessed with MRI than with CT. In a study by Kida, none of the 22 nonsymptomatic lesions demonstrated enhancement effects with Gd-DTPA [65]. This characteristic may be helpful in distinguishing which lesion is symptomatic if several vascular malformations are present.

B. Vascular Abnormalities of the Vein of Galen

Vein of Galen vascular abnormalities are a heterogeneous group of lesions with different clinical presentations and outcomes based on enlarged deep venous structures of the galenic system and an "aneurysm" of a midline venous structure [66]. Garcia-Monaco et al., after reviewing more than 100 cases, were able to describe two main types of vein of Galen abnormalities: 1. Vein of Galen aneurysmal malformation (VGAM) and 2. Vein of Galen aneurysmal dilation (VGAD) [67]. Vein of Galen aneurysmal malformations are vascular lesions with shunting in the wall of the embryologic venous precursor to the vein of Galen, called the median prosencephalic vein (MPV). The later developing normal vein of Galen does not exist with this abnormality. Two types may be distinguished depending on the location of the fistula. In the "choroidal type" of VGAM, the shunt is extracerebral in the subarachnoid space and corresponds to the normal arteries supplying the choroidal structures. The less common "mural type" of

VGAM is located in the wall of the median prosencephalic vein and usually is supplied by the collicular and/or posterior choroidal arteries.

In the vein of Galen aneurysmal dilation group, the dilated vein is the fully developed vein of Galen. Three types of VGAD can be identified: 1. a parenchymal AVM with VGAD is due to a subpial AVM that drains into a tributary of the dilated vein of Galen, which often demonstrates outflow obstruction; 2. a DAVF with VGAD is an acquired lesion with a shunt in the wall of the vein of Galen (blood supply arises from falcotentorial arteries with venous dilation related to stenosis or thrombosis of the straight sinus); and 3. a varicose VGAD, due to dilation of the vein of Galen secondary to outflow obstruction without a concomitant vascular abnormality [67].

Yasargil divides vein of Galen aneurysms into four categories [68,69]. Type I contains pure fistulas between arteries and the vein of Galen extrinsic to the brain parenchyma. Type II includes thalamus perforator arteries that supply and travel through normal brain parenchyma and give branches to the vein of Galen. Type III is a mixture of Type I and II lesions. Type IV lesions are vascular malformations proximal to the vein of Galen that drain into veins that secondarily empty into the veins of Galen (Figure 6). Quisling and Mickle have modified this classification based on the lesion's complexity, afferent supply, and efferent venous drainage. As well, they add a grading system for the venous component of the malformation that corresponds to venous pressure within the malformation [70]. These observations may be useful for providing a rationale for attempts to treat galenic malformations but may be more cumbersome than other classifications.

The clinical presentation is dependent on the patient's age and the type of vein of Galen abnormality. Congestive heart failure, cranial bruit, hydrocephalus, craniomegaly, failure to thrive, headaches, exercise syncope, seizures, hemiparesis, visual deterioration, and subarachnoid hemorrhage may all contribute to the clinical presentation [69]. Turner's syndrome and blue rubber bleb nevus syndrome have both been reported to occur in association with vein of Galen vascular abnormalities [71,72]. Other associated vascular abnormalities include transposition of the great vessels and aortic stenosis [73,74].

Color Doppler ultrasound is a useful method for screening and evaluating vein of Galen vascular malformations, both in utero and in the perinatal period [69]. Bidirectional flow in a dilated midline vein, along with enlarged feeding vessels and obstructive hydrocephalus, is often noted. The flow characteristics may be helpful in assessing therapy. Computerized tomography imaging often reveals a round oval mass lying posterior to the third ventricle, which avidly enhances with the administration of contrast material. Enhancement of the wall may be noted if the malformation is thrombosed, resulting in a "target sign" [75]. Calcification of the wall is noted in 14% of patients [76] (Figure 7). Compared to CT, MR provides improved depiction of both arterial and venous anatomy [69]. The ability of MR to image in the sagittal, coronal, and axial planes

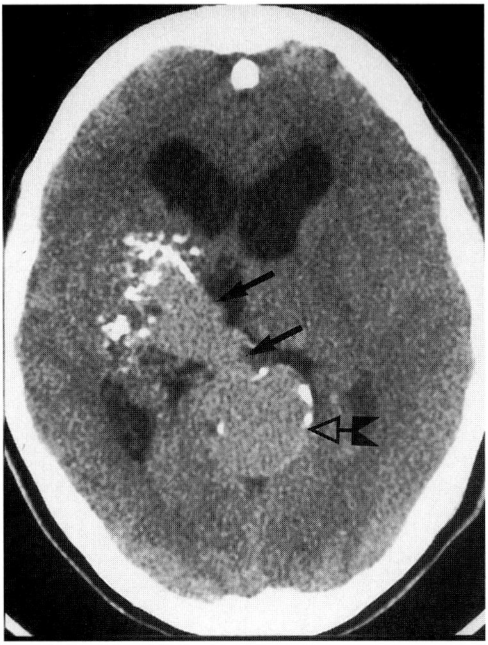

Figure 6 Vein of Galen aneurysmal dilation (VGAD)—Yasargil type IV malformation. An AVM of the right basal ganglia, demarcated by numerous calcifications, drains into massively dilated basal vein of Rosenthal (black arrow). This subsequently drains into the partially rim-calcified true vein of Galen (arrow with tail) as seen in this nonenhanced CT. Note the long-standing hydrocephalus due to partial obstruction of the posterior third ventricle.

makes characterization of the arterial and venous structures, as well as the malformation's position and size, more apparent. An MR angiography may be helpful for vascular delineation, although catheter angiography is necessary if endovascular intervention is considered for treatment.

C. Dural Arteriovenous Fistulae

1. Classification of Dural Arteriovenous Fistulae

Dural arteriovenous fistulae (DAVFs) are shunting vascular malformations that are located within the dura itself [77,78]. These are fed by dural arteries and drain either into cortical veins and/or into dural sinus [79]. These account for 10–15% of all intracranial arteriovenous malformations [80]. Within the posterior fossa, the AVFs account for 35% of arteriovenous malformations, usually

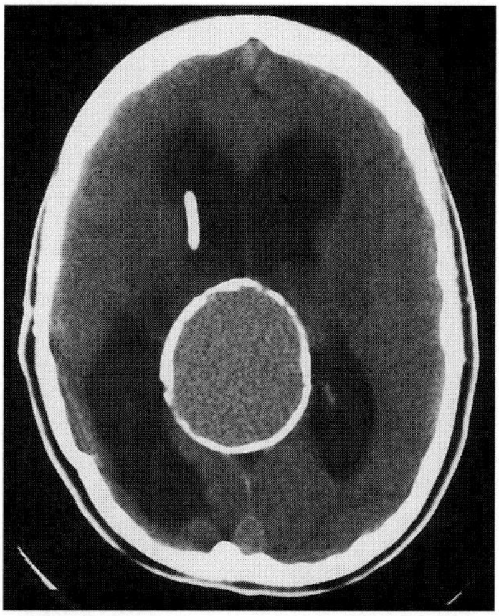

(a)

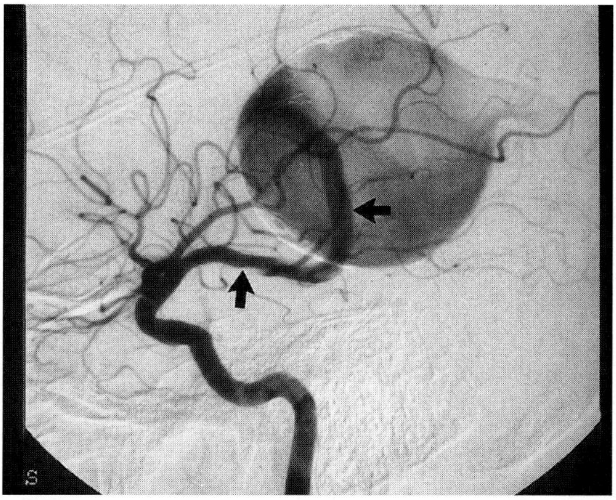

(b)

Figure 7 Vain of Galen aneurysmal malformation of the "choroidal type" (Yasargil type I). (a) A large rimmed, calcified, otherwise uniformly hyperdense mass is present on this nonenhanced CT, centered in the posterior third ventricle region resulting in marked ventricular dilation, which is typical for a vein of Galen vascular anomaly. A right frontal horn ventricular shunt tube is present. (b) A high-flow shunt is present into the "aneurysm" via an enlarged branch of a choroidal artery (arrows) on this early arterial phase of a carotid injection in the lateral projection. Note that most of the intracerebral flow feeds the malformation.

involving the transverse or sigmoid sinus [80]. Houser et al., at the Mayo Clinic, demonstrated that the type of venous drainage of the DAVF had a large influence on its clinical presentation [77]. Cognard et al. have recently expanded the classification of dural AVFs proposed in 1978 by Djindjian et al. [81,82]. Based on a series of 205 consecutive patients, the system is intended to help evaluate the risk of symptoms according to five types of venous drainage. Type I DAVF is located in the main sinus dural venous with antigrade of flow and has a benign course. Type II DAVF empties into the main sinus dural venous with retrograde flow (IIA), resulting in intracranial hypertension in 20% of cases, or into the cortical veins (IIB), resulting in hemorrhage in 10% of cases, or both (IIA and B). Type III DAVF demonstrate direct cortical venous drainage without venous ectasia of more than 5 mm and result in a hemorrhage in 40% of cases. Type IV DAVF have direct cortical venous drainage with venous ectasia and result in hemorrhage in 65% of cases. Type V DAVFs demonstrate spinal venous drainage and produce progressive myelopathy in 50% of cases. This classification system provides a framework for decision making about appropriate therapy.

The DAVFs, contrary to the other brain vascular malformations, are acquired lesions [78,79]. This is usually secondary to venous thrombosis, which may be idiopathic, or secondary to venous obstruction (trauma, infection, surgery, pregnancy, tumor, vascular disease, congenital abnormalities). Angiogenesis at the site of clot probably results in formation of the DAVF or alternatively, a tear in the basal membrane of the vessels may contribute to neovascularity. Tentorial and foramen magnum fistulas have a worse prognosis possibly because the majority of these lesions drain into subarachnoid veins [83] (Figure 8). Intracranial DAVF is also a rare cause of myelopathy leading to tetraparesis, which is thought to be due to venous congestion in the brain stem or spinal cord [84].

In DAVF Group I patients with pure sinus drainage, CT and MRI studies are usually negative. Group II through IV lesions drain into cortical veins, which may be dilated, and are usually detected with either CT or MRI, especially when contrast enhancement is used [Figure 9]. Secondary atrophy due to steal phenomena, gliosis, focal edema, or hydrocephalus (likely due to prior SAH) may also be visualized and are most conspicuous on T2W images [79]. Therapeutic options include vascular compression, transarterial or venous embolization, surgical vascular clipping of the draining vein, and embolization following surgery [83].

2. Carotid Cavernous Fistulae

Carotid cavernous fistulae (CCF) are a type of DAVF that represent abnormal drainage between the intracavernous portion of the internal carotid artery (ICA) or branches of the external carotid artery (ECA) and venous channels of the cavernous sinus (CS) [85]. Carotid cavernous fistulae have been classified etiologically as traumatic or spontaneous, hemodynamically as high flow or low flow fistula, and angiographically as direct or indirect fistulae [86]. Barrow et al. in 1985 proposed four types of CCF based on clinical and angiographic findings: Type A are direct high-flow shunts between the ICA and CS, which produce early signs and symptoms; Type B are shunts between meningeal branches of the ICA and CS; Type C are shunts between the meningeal branches of the ECA and CS; and Type D are shunts that occur between branches of both the ICA and ECA to the CS [87]. Types B, C, and D are dural-based fistulae with low flow and tend to present and occasionally resolve spontaneously [86]. Acquired CCF are traumatic in origin in up to 80% of cases [88,89]. Palestine et al., at the Mayo Clinic, found that 53% were related to MVA trauma with facial trauma accounting for 71% of these cases [90]. It is speculated that many spontaneous CCFs are secondary to rupture of a preexisting ICA aneurysm, which results in a high-flow direct fistula. Connective tissue disorders, hypertension, and arteriosclerotic vascular disease have also been implicated [86].

Computerized tomography of the brain with and without contrast enhancement often reveals a dilated cavernous sinus and/or engorged superior ophthalmic vein (Figure 10). Proptosis or effusions may be present if venous pressure is elevated (Figure 11). Use of the bone-window algorithm may demonstrate associated basal skull fractures. Intracranial hemorrhage may also be present, although not usually seen unless draining cortical veins are present [86].

Better anatomic resolution of the cavernous sinus, superior ophthalmic vein, and adjacent cortical veins is provided by MRI, but MRI will less readily pick up bone fractures. Magnetic resonance angiography may be useful for further evaluation, particularly with phase contrast (PC) MRA, which can demonstrate the direction of flow within the superior ophthalmic vein and cavernous sinus.

Cerebral angiography is the definitive diagnostic study and is necessary if treatment is contemplated. Type A, high-flow fistula spontaneously resolve in only 5% of cases [91]. Alternatively, Type B, C, and D CCF spontaneously resolve in up to 60% of cases without treatment [92]. DeBrun recommends emergent intervention in cases of acute clinical deterioration, such as hemiplegia due to steal phenomena; herniation of the CCS into the sphenoid sinus, which carries a risk of massive epistasis; recruitment of cortical venous drainage, which carries an increased risk of SAH; or with intraocular pressure greater than 40 mm of mercury, due to risk of monocular blindness or glaucoma [93]. Less emergent indications for treatment include progressive loss of vision, diplopia, patient intolerance of a bruit, malignant proptosis with corneal exposure or hemorrhage [86]. Most CCFs can be treated with endovascular techniques, ei-

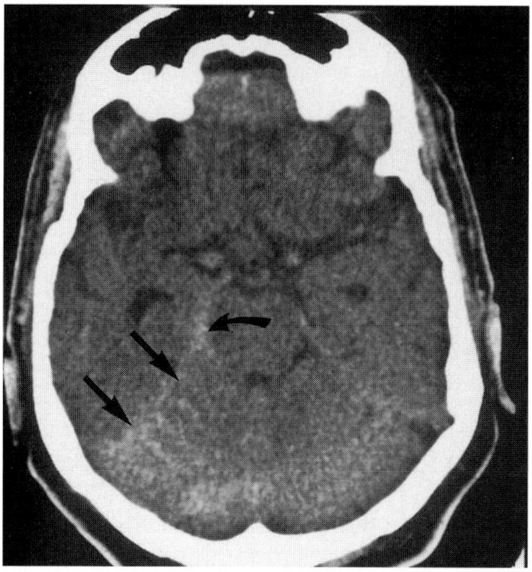

(a)

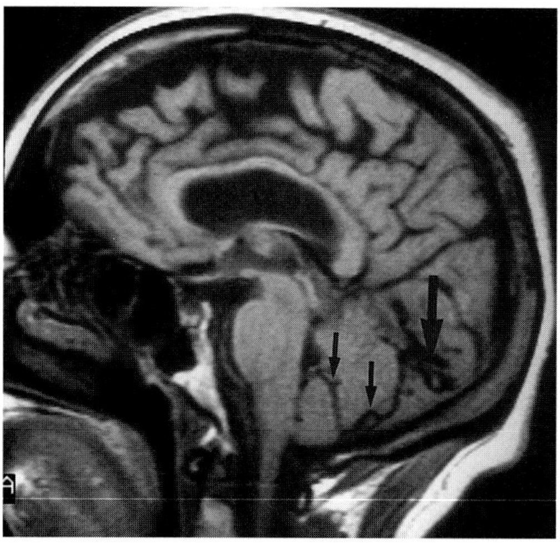

(b)

Figure 8 SAH from a posterior fossa Type III DAVF in an 80-year-old female. (a) Bright blood fills the right perimesencephalic cistern (curved black arrow) and is present under the tentorium (black straight arrows) as seen on this plain CT. (b) Nonenhanced sagittal T1-weighted image demonstrates a dilated PICA (thin black arrows), as well as prominent posterior subtentorial vessels (large black arrow).

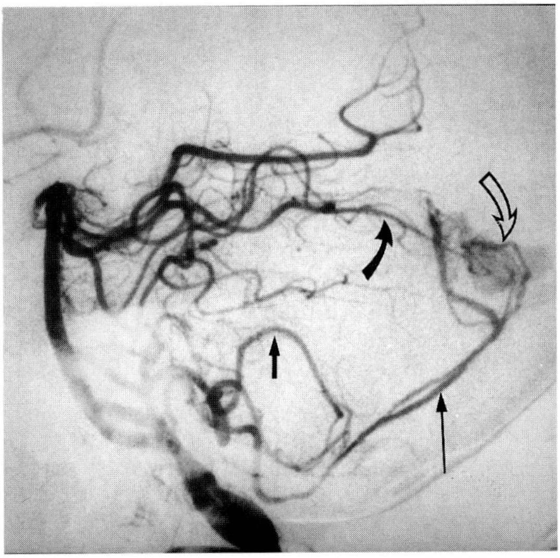

(c)

Figure 8 Continued.
(c) Lateral vertebral angiogram shows a tentorial DAVF with a blush indicating the area of shunt (curved open arrow). The vascular malformation is fed by an enlarged occipital meningeal artery, the PICA, and superior cerebellar artery branches (thin black arrow, short black arrow, and curved black arrow, respectively). Venous drainage is into mildly dilated subarachnoid and parenchymal veins which in turn drain into the straight sinus and torcula.

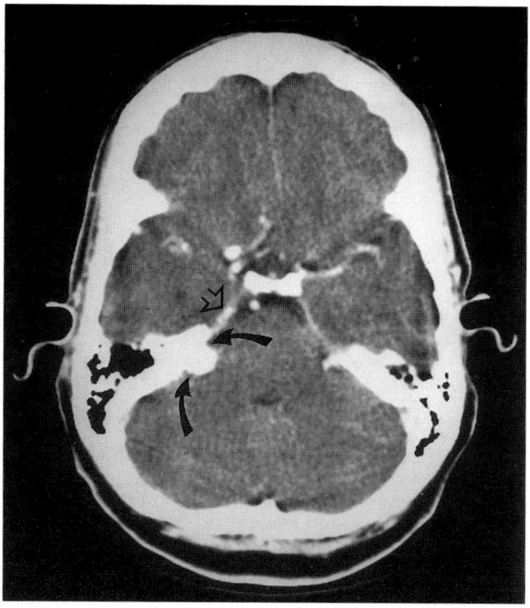

(a)

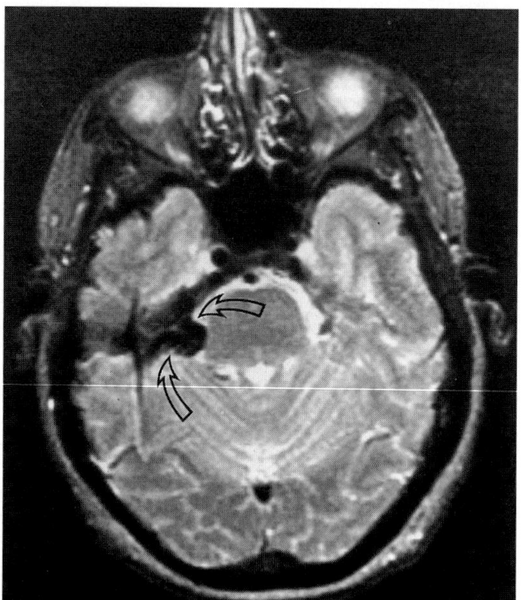

(b)

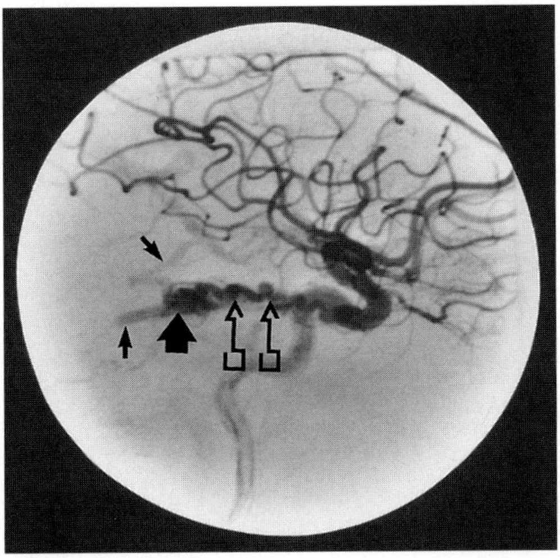

(c)

Figure 9 Type III dural AVF of the right tentorial incisura simulating a meningioma. (a) A uniformly-enhancing mass-like lesion is present with a broad base arising from the tentorial incisura or petrous apex (black arrows) as seen on this enhanced CT. (a) There is also thickening of the petroclinoid ligament (small open straight arrow). (b) On the axial T2-weighted spin echo sequence, the lesion (open curved arrow) demonstrates low signal along with thickening of the petroclinoid ligament. (c) A right carotid angiogram in the lateral projection demonstrates a dilated hypertrophied dural artery from the meningohypophysial trunk (open square-tailed arrows), feeding a tentorial-based fistula nidus (large black arrow). Shunting is demonstrated by early nondilated cortical draining veins (small straight black arrows).

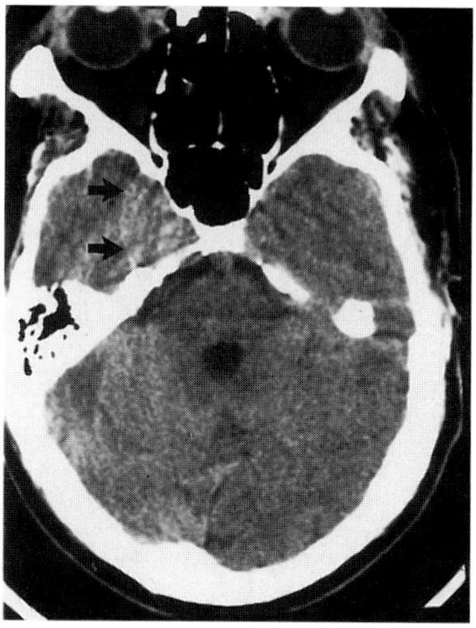

(a)

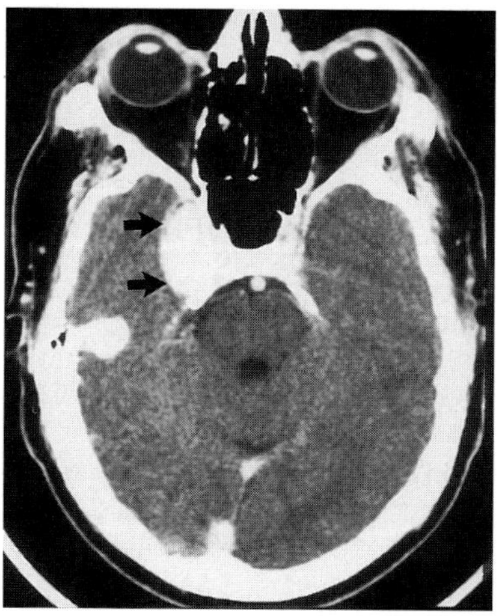

(b)

Figure 10 Direct, high flow, Type I, carotid cavernous fistula. (a) Note enlargement and lateral convex bowing of the right cavernous sinus (black arrows) as seen on this nonenhanced CT. (b) Marked uniform enhancement of the right cavernous sinuses is present (black arrows). This appearance is nonspecific and the differential diagnosis would also include a meningioma, schwannoma, or extraparenchymal dural cavernous hemangioma.

ther arterial or venous. Surgery is now usually reserved for failed endovascular therapy [93].

D. Arteriovenous Malformations and Aneurysms in the Spinal Cord

Spinal vascular malformations are uncommon and represent about 4% of primary intraspinal masses [94]. Spinal aneurysms are rare and if present are usually associated with intramedullary spinal cord AVMs [95]. These spinal aneurysms are usually located on the anterior spinal artery feeding the AVM with the usual presentation of hemorrhage in 85% of cases. Angiography is usually necessary for diagnosis of spinal aneurysms [95].

Most spinal cord malformations are arteriovenous fistulae (AVFs) or arteriovenous malformations (AVMs). Capillary telangiectasia and cavernous angiomas are even less common, with venous angiomas rarely reported [96]. Spinal cord malformations, including AVMs with a true nidus and AVFs with small direct shunts to venous outflow tracks, have been divided into four types based on their clinical presentation, location, and imaging characteristics [97].

1. Classification of Arteriovenous Malformations in the Spinal Cord

Type I vascular malformation of the cord is the dural arteriovenous fistulae (DAVF). This group represented 38% of 210 patients treated for AVMs in a series by Mourier [98], although 63% of 97 spine vascular malformations in a recent Mayo Clinic series were Type I DAVFs [99]. The lesion is more typical in males between the ages of 40 and 80. Patients usually present with slowly progressive myelopathy or radiculopathy of the lower extremities. Bowel and bladder dysfunction occurs late and if the lesion is untreated patients can develop into paraplegia or quadriparesis. These symptoms are often puzzling and many of these patients have had prior laminectomies without relief of symptoms [100,101]. These lesions are thought to be spontaneous in 60% of cases with 40% having had associated trauma [102]. The fistula nidus is usually located in the dural sleeve of an exiting thoracic or lumbar nerve root but up to 8% of fistulae may arise from an intracranial nidus and 9% arise from a sacral nidus [101]. This has important angiographic implications. The venous drainage is into a dilated radicular vein with retrograde flow into the coronal venous plexus surrounding the cord, resulting in chronic venous hypertension and ischemia [103] (Figure 12).

Type II vascular malformations of the cord are the so-called "glomus" malformations. These intramedullary AVMs have a compact vascular nidus and are supplied by multiple spinal artery feeders. These usually present with intramedullary hemorrhage in younger patients, usually in the dorsal cervical cord [97].

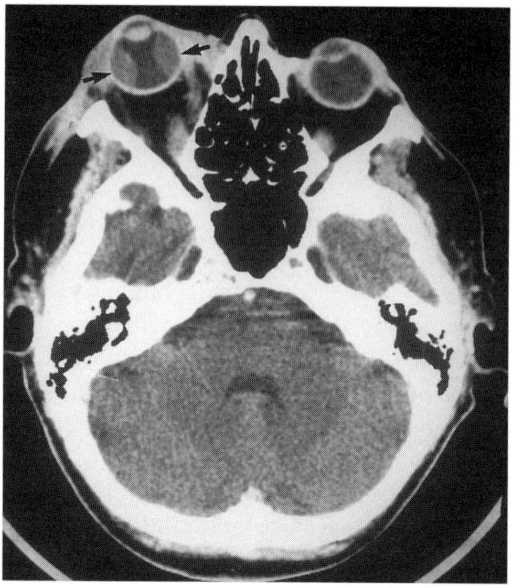

(a)

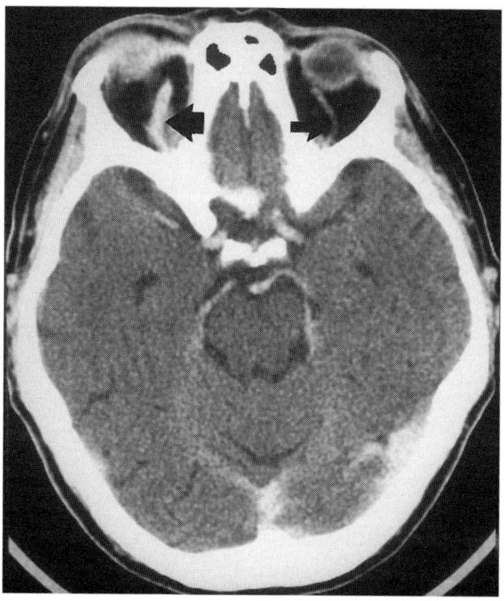

(b)

Figure 11 Type B carotid cavernous fistula. (a) Enhanced CT demonstrates orbital proptosis, peri-orbital soft-tissue swelling, and subchoroidal effusions (arrows) within the right globe due to elevated intravenous pressure. (b) A higher slice in the same series shows the dilated right superior ophthalmic vein (SOV) (large black arrow). Note the normal-sized SOV on the left (small black arrow).

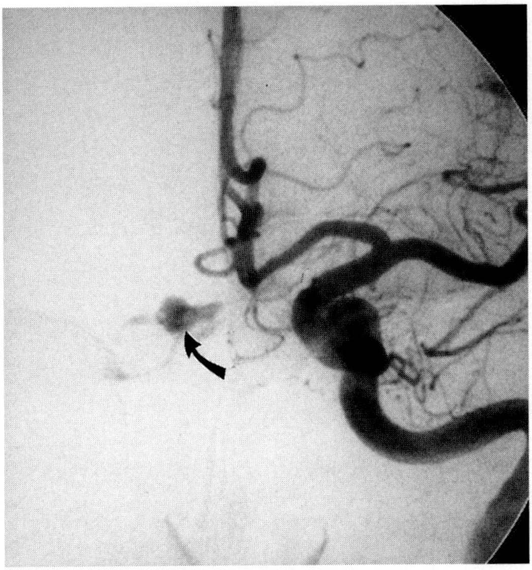

(c)

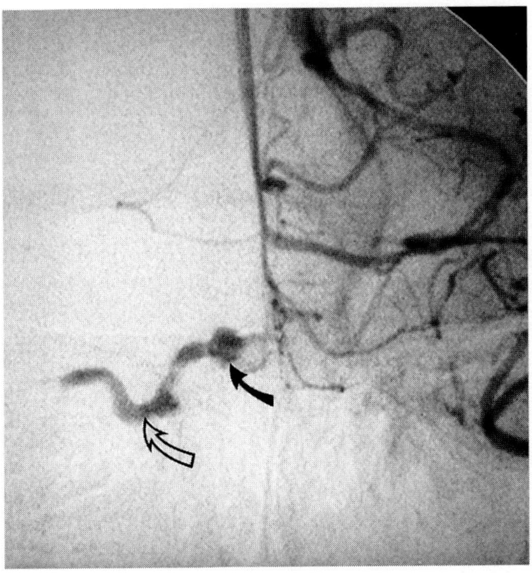

(d)

Figure 11 Continued.
(c) Left carotid angiogram in the frontal projection demonstrates filling of the right cavernous sinus (black curved arrow) from small internal carotid meningeal branches. (d) A venous phase image from the same injection as "C" demonstrates retrograde flow from the cavernous sinus (black curved arrow) into the superior ophthalmic vein (open curved arrows).

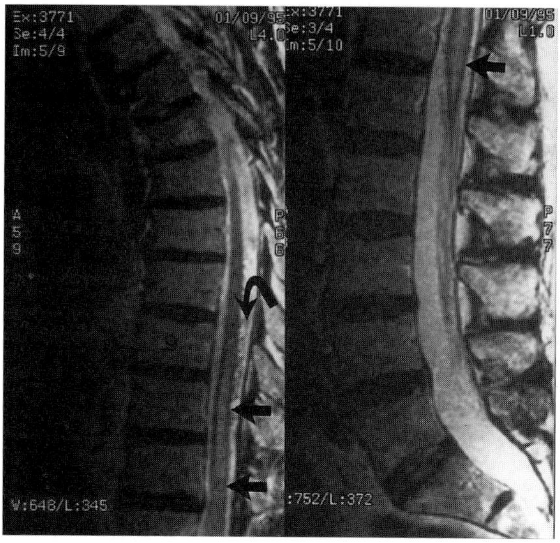

(a)

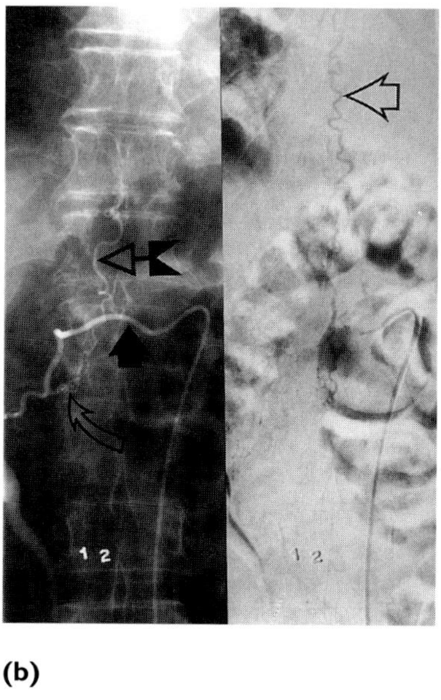

(b)

Figure 12 Spinal dural AVF Type I. (a) Sagittal thoracic and lumbar spine T2-weighted images demonstrate increased T2 signal within the lower thoracic cord and conus medullaris (black straight arrows). Note the dorsally located veins in the draining coronal plexus (black curved arrow). (b) Right T12 intercostal injection (large black arrowhead) demonstrates the fistula in the exiting nerve root sleeve (curved open arrow). Cephalad retrograde venous drainage is into the radiculomedullary vein (arrow with tail). The later subtraction image demonstrates contrast in the draining serpiginous coronal venous plexus (open arrowhead).

Type III vascular malformations have also been called "juvenile" type spinal vascular malformations and are the rarest of the spinal malformations. In this large complex vascular mass, the nidus involves not only the intramedullary compartment but often expands into the intradural, epidural, or even extraspinal spaces. This vascular mass is usually fed from several different levels by multiple arterial feeders [96] (Figure 13).

Type IV spinal vascular malformations represent intradural perimedullary arteriovenous fistulae. These lesions are characterized by the presence of a direct arteriovenous shunt located on the pial surface of the cord without a nidus. They are fed by spinal arteries and drain into dilated perimedullary veins. These lesions have been subdivided into three types by Merland et al. according to their anatomic, angiographic, and hemodynamic features [104,105,106]. This classification, while complex, reflects practical difficulties in diagnosis and treatment. Clinically, the patients with Type IV AVMs are younger than those with dural AVFs. Acute onset of symptoms or subarachnoid hemorrhage may be seen but in most cases patients present with progressive conus medullaris and cauda equina syndrome [97].

2. CT Imaging of Arteriovenous Malformations in the Spinal Cord

Diagnostic imaging procedures include myelography, CT myelography, MR, and angiography. Supine and prone entire spine myelography has been the screening method of choice for demonstrating dilated and tortuous medullary veins. The cord contour is nonspecific, may be normal, expanded due to edema, or decreased due to atrophy. Tomomyelography may be helpful for better identification of vascular filling defects in questionable cases. Computerized tomography myelography is also very sensitive to intradural extramedullary vessels although it is limited to selected axial slices and not as useful for screening of the entire spine as this would be cumbersome, time-consuming, and exposes the patient to excessive radiation. Computerized tomography is inferior to MR in both sensitivity and specificity in the demonstration of spinal vascular malformations [103]. Casazza et al. have reported a case of spinal myoclonus and clinical deterioration in a patient with a spinal cord AVM that may have been due to contrast leakage into the surrounding cord parenchyma through a defective spinal cord/blood barrier [107].

3. MR Imaging of Arteriovenous Malformations in the Spinal Cord

Magnetic resonance imaging is considered the screening modality of choice when a vascular malformation of the cord is suspected [99,100,103]. The appearance will vary with the type of malformation and pulse sequence utilized. The most common finding is likely an indirect line of T2 signal hyperintensity due to chronic venous ischemia, edema, and atrophy. In the recent series by

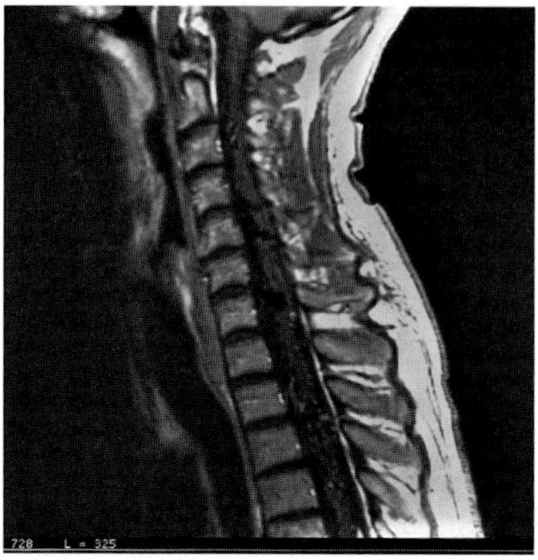

(a)

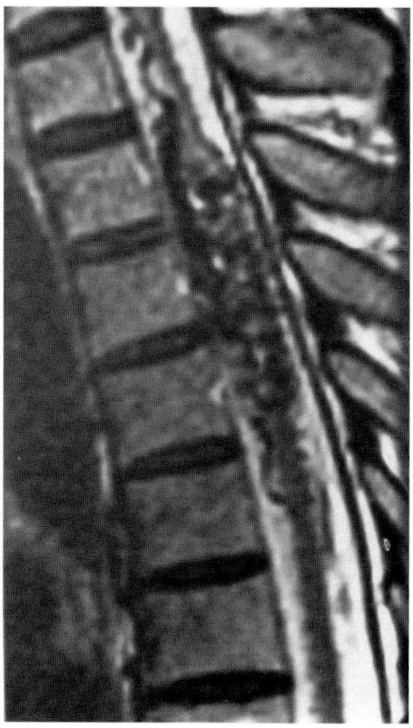

(b)

Figure 13 Type III or "juvenile" type spinal vascular malformation. (a) Sagittal enhanced T1-weighted image demonstrates numerous intramedullary and extramedullary vessels in the cervical and upper thoracic spinal canal manifest by flow voids and areas of enhancement due to flow-related enhancement and slow flow. (b) Magnified sagittal T2-weighted image of the upper thoracic spine shows a tangle of vessels from T2 through T5 within the expanded cord.

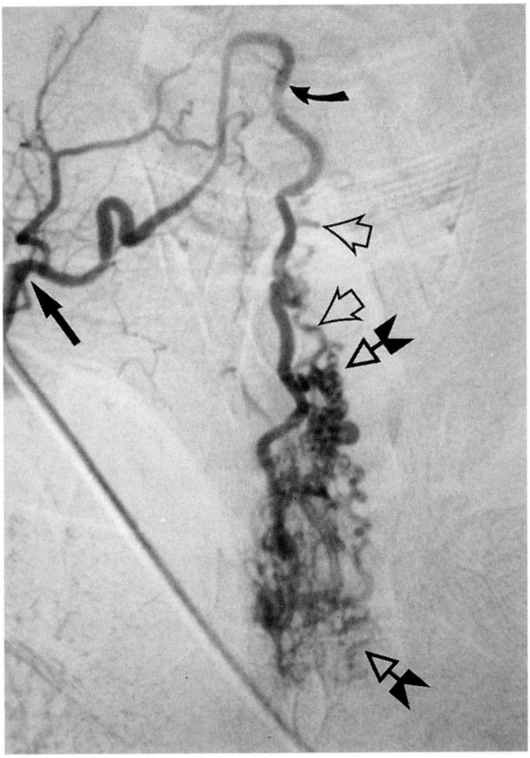

(c)

Figure 13 Continued.
(c) Selective subtraction angiogram with injection into the right costocervical trunk (large black arrow) demonstrates filling of the enlarged anterior spinal artery (black curved arrow), which in turn partially supplies the complex intramedullary and extramedullary vascular malformation (between arrows with tails). Arterial supply also came from the right third, fourth, sixth, and left sixth, and eighth intercostal arteries (not shown). The predominant venous drainage was via a large serpiginous vein (large open arrows) along the anterior aspect of the cord draining intracranially into the anterior pontomesencephalic vein.

Gilbertson et al. of 66 patients with Type I AVF, all 66 cases demonstrate T2 signal abnormalities within the cord extending over an average length of seven vertebral bodies [99]. Pial flow voids from the dilated coronal venous plexus were seen in less than half of the cases, usually better with T2 sequences. These were sometimes difficult to distinguish from CSF flow-void artifact. Mass effect was present in about half of the cases.

Hemorrhage has been seen in about half of the Type II, III, and IV vascular malformations of the spinal cord but has not been reported in the DAVF group (Type I) [99,108]. Magnetic resonance imaging is the best modality for assessing spinal intraparenchymal and spinal subarachnoid hemorrhage. The appearance will vary with the age of the hemorrhage, as mentioned earlier. Chronic hemorrhage resulting in superficial siderosis is characterized by pial and subpial decreased signal intensity due to hemosiderin-laden macrophages. It is best visualized with a heavy T2-weighted technique or GRE images.

Magnetic resonance imaging also has the advantage of detecting thrombosed vessels. Marked neurologic deterioration can occur with spontaneous thrombosis of vascular malformations and has been called the Foix-Alajouanine syndrome. Clinically, this may mimic acute myelitis, transverse myelitis, or spondylosis. MRA of the spinal cord appears to be a promising technique to assess for dilated vessels.

A definitive presurgical diagnosis of a spinal vascular malformation may sometimes be achieved only by complete selective angiography of the spinal cord, which necessitates catheterization of all feeding pedicles, including the brachiocephalic and iliac vessels. It is necessary to assess the hemodynamic effects and flow patterns of the feeding vessels and draining veins so that the appropriate treatment can be planned [97]. The treatment of choice is variable, depending on the type of vascular malformation, location, and expertise of the treating physicians. Endovascular treatment, surgery, or a combination of these may be used in selected cases [98–100,108].

ACKNOWLEDGMENTS

The authors wish to acknowledge the secretarial skills of Debbie Roach who made this chapter possible. We also thank John Atkinson, M.D., for his suggestions and support.

REFERENCES

1. Okazaki H. Cerebrovascular disease. In: Fundamentals of Neuropathology. New York: Igaku-Shoin, 1989:27–94.

2. Rigamonti D, Johnson PC, Spetzler RF, Hadley MN, Drayer BP. Cavernous malformations and capillary telangiectasia: a spectrum within a single pathological entity. *Neurosurgery* 1991; 28:60–64.
3. Awad IA, Robinson JR Jr, Mohanty S, Estes ML. Mixed vascular malformations of the brain: clinical and pathogenetic considerations. *Neurosurgery* 1993; 83:179–188.
4. McCormick WF. The pathology of vascular ("arteriovenous") malformations. *J Neurosurg* 1966; 24:807–816.
5. Osborn AG. Diagnostic neuroradiology. St. Louis: Mosby Year Book, 1994:284–329.
6. Newton TH, Cronqvist S. Involvement of the dural arteries in intracranial arteriovenous malformations. *Radiology* 1969; 93:1071–1078.
7. Houser OW, Campbell JK, Campbell RJ, Sundt TM. Arteriovenous malformations affecting the transverse dural venous sinus: an acquired lesion. *Mayo Clinic Proc* 1979; 54:651–661.
8. Newton TH, Weidner W, Greitz T. Dural arteriovenous malformations in the posterior fossa. *Radiology* 1968; 90:27–35.
9. De Marco JK, Dillon WP, Halbach VV, Tsuruda JS. Dural arteriovenous fistulas: evaluation with MR imaging. *Radiology* 1990; 175:193–199.
10. Fults D, Kelly DL. Natural history of arteriovenous malformations of the brain: a clinical study. *Neurosurgery* 1984; 15:658–662.
11. Jomin M, Lesoin F, Lozes G. Prognosis for arteriovenous malformations of the brain in adults based on 150 cases. *Sugr Neurol* 1985; 23:362–366.
12. Morgan MK, Johnston I. Intracranial arteriovenous malformations: an 11–year experience. *Med J Aust* 1989; 148:65–68.
13. Ondra SL, Troupp H, George ED, Schwab K. The natural history of symptomatic arteriovenous malformations of the brain: a 24–year follow–up assessment. *J Neurosurg* 1990; 73:387–391.
14. Vinuela F. Update on intravascular functional evaluation and therapy of intracranial arteriovenous malformations. *Interventional Neuroradiology* 1992; 2:279.
15. Graf CJ, Perret GE, Torner JC. Bleeding from cerebral arteriovenous malformations as part of their natural history. *J Neurosurg* 1983; 58:331–337.
16. Marks MP, Lane B, Steinberg GK, Chang PJ. Hemorrhage in intracerebral arterio venous malformations: angiographic determinants. *Radiology* 1990; 176:807–813.
17. Spetzler RF, Martin NA. A proposed grading system for arteriovenous malformations. *J Neurosurg* 1986; 65:476–483.
18. Greenberg MS. Handbook of Neurosurgery. Florida: Lakeland, 1994:755.
19. Turjman F, Massoud TF, Vinuela F, et al. Aneurysms related to cerebral arteriovenous malformations: superselective angiographic assessment in 58 patients. *AJNR* 1994; 15:1601–1605.
20. Osborn AG. Intracranial aneurysms: clinicopathologic correlations. Core Curriculum Course in Neuroradiology. Part I: Vascular lesions and degenerative diseases. Reported at the Annual Scientific Meeting of the American Society of Neuroradiology. Chicago, Illinois, April 21–22, 1995.

21. Terbrugge K, Scotti G, Ethier R, Melancon D, Tchang S, Milner C. Computed tomography in intracranial arteriovenous malformations. *Radiology* 1977; 122:703–705.
22. Osborn AG. Diagnostic neuroradiology. St. Louis: Mosby Year Book, 1994:294.
23. Kumar AJ, Vinuela F, Fox AJ, Rosenbaum A. Unruptured intracranial arteriovenous malformations do cause mass effect. *AJNR* 1985; 6:29–32.
24. Grayson T. Arteriovenous Malformation. Baltimore, Maryland: Williams and Wilkins, 1991:136.
25. Pott M, Huber M, Assheuer J, Bewermeyer H. MRI of angiographically occult vascular malformations. *AJR Am J Roentgenol* 1986; 146(6):1223–1228.
26. Leblanc R, Levesque M, Comair Y, Ethier R. Aneurysms and vascular malformations. *Top Magn Reson Imaging* 1989; 2(1):49–62.
27. Smith HJ, Strother CM, Kikuchi Y, et al. MR imaging in the management of supratentorial intracranial AVMs. *AJR* 1988; 150:1143–1153.
28. Chappell PM, Steinberg GK, Marks MP. Clinically documented hemorrhage in cerebral arteriovenous malformations: MR characteristics. *Radiology* 1992; 183:719–724.
29. Hoang T-A, Hasso AN. Intracranial vascular malformations. *Neuroimaging Clinics of North America* 1994; 4:823–847.
30. Gaensler EHL, Dillon WP, Edwards MSB, Larson DA, Rosenau W, Wilson CB. Radiation–induced telangiectasia in the brain simulates cryptic vascular malformations at MR imaging. *Radiology* 1994; 193:629–636.
31. Atlas SW. Intracranial vascular malformations and aneurysms. Current imaging applications. *Radiol Clin North Am* 1988; 26:821–837.
32. Rigamonti D, Hadley MH, Drayer BP, et al. Cerebral cavernous malformations. *New England Journal of Medicine* 1988; 319:343–347.
33. Malik S, Cohen BH, Robinson J, Fried A, Sila A. Progressive vision loss. *Arch Neurol* 1992; 49:170–173.
34. Robinson JR, Awad IA, Little JR. Natural history of the cavernous angioma. *J Neurosurg* 1991; 75:709–714.
35. Nonogaki Y, Ishii M, Oda N, HNagashima C. Coexistence of intracranial and spinal cavernous angiomas: case report. *No Shinkei Geka (Japan)* 1992; 20(12):1277–1281.
36. Shen WC, Lee SK. CT and MRI of parasellar cavernous hemangioma in two cases. *J Formos Med Assoc (Hong Kong)* 1992; 91(Suppl 2):S165–169.
37. Brophy BP, Sweeney C, Phipps S, Perrett LV, Sandhu A, Albertyn LE. Cavernous haemangiomas (angiomas) of the brain: clinically significant lesions. *Australas Radiol (Australia)* 1993; 37(2):147–155.
38. Yasargil MG. Microneurosurgery. New York: Thieme Medical Publishers, 1987.
39. Preul MC, Villemure JG, Leblanc R, Del Carpio-O'Donovan R. MRI diagnosis of brainstem cavernous angiomas presenting as tumours. *Can J Neurol Sci (Canada)* 1992; 19(3):376–382.
40. Farmer JP, Cosgrove GR, Villemure JG, Meagher-Villemure K, Tampieri D, Melanson D. Intracerebral cavernous angiomas. *Neurology* 1988; 38(11):1699–1704.

41. Goulao A, Alvarez H, Garcia Monaco R, Pruvost P, Lasjaunias P. Venous anomalies and abnormalities of the posterior fossa. *Neuroradiology (Germany, West)* 1990; 31(6):476–482.
42. Ostertun B, Solymosi L. Magnetic resonance angiography of cerebral developmental venous anomalies: its role in differential diagnosis. *Neuroradiology (Germany)* 1993; 35(2):97–104.
43. Truwit CL. Venous angioma of the brain: history, significance, and imaging findings. *AJR* 1992; 159:1299–1307.
44. Sherry RG, Walker ML, Olds MV. Sinus pericranii and venous angioma in the blue–rubber bleb nevus syndrome. *AJNR* 1984; 5:832–834.
45. Wilms G, Marchal G, Van Hecke P, Van Fraeyenhoven L, Decrop E, Baert AL. Cerebral venous angiomas. MR imaging at 1.5 tesla. *Neuroradiology* 1990; 32:81–85.
46. Rothfus WE, Albright AL, Casey KF, Latchaw RE, Roppolo HMN. Cerebellar venous angioma: "benign" entity? *AJNR* 1984; 5:61–66.
47. Valvanis A, Wellauer J, Yasargil MG. The radiological diagnosis of cerebral venous angioma: cerebral angiography and computed tomography. *Neuroradiology* 1983; 24:193–199.
48. Sadler LR, Tarr RW, Jungreis CA, Sekhar L. Sinus pericranii: CT and MR findings. *JCAT* 1990; 14(1):124–127.
49. Smirniotopoulos JG, Murphy FM. The phakomatoses. *AJNR* 1992; 13:725–746.
50. Elster D, Chen MYM. MR imaging of Sturge-Weber syndrome. *AJNR* 1990; 11:685–689.
51. Osborn AG. Diagnostic neuroradiology. St. Louis: Mosby Year Book, 1994:98–101.
52. Vielvoye GJ, Pijl ME. Magnetic resonance imaging of the so–called cerebral cryptic angiomas. *Clin Neurol Neurosurg (Netherlands)* 1992; 94:S171–175.
53. Toro VE, Geyer CA, Sherman JL, Parisi JE, Brantley MJ. Cerebral venous angiomas: MR findings. *JCAT* 1988; 12(6):935–940.
54. Augustyn GT, Scott JA, Olson E, Gilmor RL, Edwards MK. Cerebral venus angiomas: MR imaging. *Radiology* 1985; 156:391–395.
55. Uchino A, Imada H, Ohno M. Magnetic resonance imaging of intracranial venous angiomas. *Clin Imaging* 1990; 14:309–314.
56. Wilms G, Demaerel P, Marchal G, Baert AL, Plets C. Gadolinium–enhanced MR imaging of cerebral venous angiomas with emphasis on their drainage. *JCAT* 1991; 15(2):199–206.
57. Kyoshima K, Nakazawa T, Nakasu S, Handa J. Angiographically occult vascular malformations in the posterior fossa. *Nippon Geka Hokan (Japan)* 1989; 58(2):257–264.
58. Robinson JR Jr, Awad IA, Masaryk TJ, Estes ML. Pathological heterogeneity of angiographically occult vascular malformations of the brain. *Neurosurgery* 1993; 33(4):547–554.
59. Rapacki TF, Brantley MJ, Furlow TW Jr, Geyer CA, Toro VE, George ED. Heterogeneity of cerebral cavernous hemangiomas diagnosed by MR imaging. *JCAT* 1990; 14(1):18–25.

60. Ebeling JD, Tranmer BI, Davis KA, Kindt GW, De Masters BK. Thrombosed arteriovenous malformations: a type of occult vascular malformation. Magnetic resonance imaging and histopathological correlations. *Neurosurgery* 1988; 23(5):605–610.
61. Sigal R, Krief O, Houtteville JP, Halimi P, Doyon D, Pariente D. Occult cerebrovascular malformations: follow–up with MR imaging. *Radiology* 1990; 176(3):815–819.
62. Lobato RD, Rivas JJ, Gomez PA, Cabrera A, Sarabia R, Lamas E. Comparison of the clinical presentation of symptomatic arteriovenous malformations and occult vascular malformations. *Neurosurgery* 1993; 32(5):876–878.
63. New PF, Ojemann RG, Davis KR, et al. MR and CT of occult vascular malformations of the brain. *AJR Am J Roentgenol* 1986; 147(5):985–993.
64. Lemme-Plaghos L, Kucharczyk W, Brant-Zawadzki M, et al. MRI of angiographically occult vascular malformations. *AJR Am J Roentgenol* 1986; 146(6):1223–1228.
65. Kida Y, Kobayashi T, Tanaka T, Oyama H, Iwakoshi T. Clinical presentations and MRI findings of angiographically occult vascular malformations. *No Shinkei Geka* 1994; 22(2):141–145.
66. Seidenwurm D, Berenstein A, Hyman A, Kowalsi H. Vein of Galen malformation: correlation of clinical presentation, arteriography, and MR imaging. *AJNR* 1991; 12:347–354.
67. Garcia-Monaco R, Lasjaunias P, Berenstein A. Therapeutic management of vein of Galen aneurysmal malformations. In: F. Vinuela (ed). Interventional Neuroradiology: Endovascular Therapy of the Central Nervous System. New York: Raven Press 1992:113–127.
68. Yasargil MC. Microsurgery IIIB. New York: Theme Medical Publishers, 1988:323–357.
69. Horowitz MB, Jungreis CA, Quisling RG, Pollack I. Vein of Galen aneurysms: a review and current perspective. *Am J Neurorad* 1994; 15:1486–1496.
70. Quisling RG, Mickle JP. Venous pressure measurements in vein of Galen aneurysms. *Am J Neurorad* 1989; 10:411–417.
71. Jarrell HR, Schochet SS Jr, Krous H, Barnes P. Turner's syndrome and vein of Galen aneurysm: a previously unreported association. *Acta Neuropathol* 1981; 55:189–191.
72. Rosenblum WI, Nakoneczna I, Konderding HS, Nochlin D, Ghatak NR. Multiple vascular malformation in the "blue rubber bleb naevus" syndrome: a case with aneurysm of vein of Galen and vascular lesions suggesting a link to the Weber–Osler–Rendu syndrome. *Histopathology* 1978; 2:301–311.
73. Eide J, Folling M. Malformation of the great vein of Galen with neonatal heart failure: report of two cases. *Acta Paediatr Scand* 1978; 67:529–532.
74. Gomez JR, Whitten CF, Nolke A, Bernstein J, Meyer JS. Aneurysmal malformation of the great vein of Galen causing heart failure in early infancy. *Pediatrics* 1983; 31:400.
75. Skirkhoda A, Whaley RA, Boone SC, Scatliff JH, Schnapf D. Varied CT appearance of aneurysms of the vein of Galen in infancy. *Neuroradiology* 1981; 21:265–270.

76. Chapman S, Hockley AD. Calcification of an aneurysm of the vein of Galen. *Pediatr Radiol* 1989; 19:541–542.
77. Houser OW, Baker HL, Rhoton AL, Okazaki H. Intracranial dural arteriovenous malformations. *Radiology* 1972; 105:55–64.
78. Chaudhary MY, Sachdev VP, Cho SH, Weitzner I Jr, Puljic S, Huang YP. Dural AV malformation of the major venous sinus: an acquired lesion. *Am J Neurorad* 1982; 3:13–19.
79. Rodesch G, Lasjaunias P. Physiopathology and semeiology of dural arteriovenous shunts. *Neuroradiologia* 1992; 5:11–21.
80. Newton TH, Weidner W, Greitz T. Dural arteriovenous malformations in the posterior fossa. *Radiology* 1968; 90:27–35.
81. Djindjian R, Merland JJ. Super–Selective Arteriography of the External Carotid Artery. New York, NY: Springer-Verlag, 1977:606–628.
82. Cognard C, Gobin YP, Pierot L, et al. Cerebral dural arteriovenous fistulas: clinical and angiographic correlation with a revised classification of venous drainage. *Radiology* 1995; 194:671–680.
83. Pierot L, Chiras J, Meder J-F, Rose M, Rivierez M, Marsault C. Dural arteriovenous fistulas of the posterior fossa draining into subarachnoid veins. *AJNR* 1992; 13:315–323.
84. Gaensler EH, Jackson DE, Halbach VV. Arteriovenous fistulas of the cervicomedullary junction as a cause of meylopathy: radiographic finding in two cases. *AJNR* 1990; 11:518–521.
85. Dandy WE. Carotid–cavernous aneurysms (pulsating exophthalmos). *Zentralbl Neurochir* 1937; 2:77–113,165–204.
86. Jimenez DF, Gibbs SR. Carotid–cavernous sinus fistulae in craniofacial trauma: classification and treatment. *J Cranio-Maxillofacial Trauma* 1995; 1:7–15.
87. Barrow DL, Spector RH, Braun IF, et al. Classification and treatment of spontaneous carotid–cavernous sinus fistulas. *J Neurosurg* 1985; 62(2):248–256.
88. Love L, Marsan RE. Carotid cavernous fistula. *Angiology* 1974; 25(4):231–236.
89. Morley TP. Appraisal of various forms of management in 41 cases of carotid–cavernous fistula. In: Current Controversies in Neurosurgery. Philadelphia: WB Saunders Company 1976; 217–236.
90. Palestine AG, Younge BR, Peipgras DG. Visual prognosis in carotid–cavernous fistula. *Arch Ophthalmol* 1981; 99(9):1600–1603.
91. Newton TH, Hoyt WF. Dural arteriovenous shunts in the region of the cavernous sinus. *Neuroradiology* 1970; 1:71–81.
92. Nishijima M, Iwai R, Horie Y, et al. Spontaneous occlusion of traumatic carotid-cavernous fistula orbital venography. *Surg Neurol* 1985; 23(5):489–492.
93. Debrun G. Management of traumatic carotid–cavernous fistulas. In: F. Vinuela (ed). Interventional Neuroradiology: Endovascular Therapy of the Central Nervous System. New York: Raven Press 1992; 107–112.
94. Youmans JR. Neurological Surgery. 2nd ed. Philadelphia: W.B. Saunders, 1982.
95. Biondi A, Merland JJ, Hodes JE, et al. Aneurysms of spinal arteries associated with intramedullary arteriovenous malformations. I. Angiographic and clinical aspects. *AJNR* 1992; 13:913–922.

96. Osborn AG. Diagnostic neuroradiology. St. Louis: Mosby Year Book, 1994:830–836.
97. Anson JA, Spetzler RF. Classification of spinal arteriovenous malformations and implications for treatment. *BNI Quarterly* 1992; 8:2–8.
98. Mourier KL, Gobin YP, George B, Lot G, Merland JJ. Intradural perimedullary arteriovenous fistulae: results of surgical and endovascular treatment in a series of 35 cases. *Neurosurgery* 1993; 32:885–891.
99. Gilbertson JR, Miller GM, Goldman MS, Marsh WR. Spinal dural arteriovenous fistulas: MR and myelographic findings. *AJNR* 1995; 16:2049–2057.
100. Miller G. Spine. In: T. H. Berquist, (ed). MRI of the Musculoskeletal System. 3rd ed. Lippincott-Raven Publishers, 1996:111–195.
101. Merland JJ, Riche MC, Chiras J. Intraspinal extramedullary arteriovenous fistulae draining into the medullary veins. *J Neuroradiol* 1980; 7:271–320.
102. Naidich TP, McLone DG, Harwood-Nash DC. Vascular malformations. In: Newton TH, Potts DG, (eds). Modern Neuroradiology, vol 1: Computed Tomography of the Spine and Spinal Cord. 1983:397–400.
103. Larsen DW, Halbach VV. Diagnostic evaluation of spinal vascular malformations. Core Curriculum Course in Neuroradiology. Part I: vascular lesions and degenerative diseases. Reported at the Annual Scientific Meeting of the American Society of Neuroradiology. Chicago, Illinois, April 21–22, 1995.
104. Giegiem B, Merland JJ, Riche MC, Rey A. Vascular malformations of the spinal cord: intrathecal perimedullary arteriovenous fistulas fed by medullary arteries. *Neurology* 1987; 37:969–979.
105. Merland JJ, Riche MC, Chiras J. Les fistules arterioveineuses intracanalaires extramedullaires a drainage veineux medullaire. *J Neuroradiol* 1980; 7:271–320.
106. Merland JJ, Reizine D. Malformations vasculaires vertebro–medullaires. *Encylc Med Chir (Paris, France), Radiodiagnostic II*, 31671 G10, 5–1987:22.
107. Casazza M, Bracchi M, Girotti F. Spinal myoclonus and clinical worsening after intravenous contras medium in a patient with spinal arteriovenous malformations. *AJNR Am J Neuroradiol* 1985; 6:965.
108. Nichols DA, Rufenacht DA, Jack CR Jr, Forbes GS. Embolization of spinal dural arteriovenous fistula with polyvinyl alcohol particles: experience in 14 patients. *Am J Neuroradiol* 1992; 13:933–940.

11

Transcranial Doppler Applications

George W. Petty
Mayo Clinic and Mayo Medical School, Rochester, Minnesota

I. INTRODUCTION

Transcranial Doppler (TCD) ultrasonography is a noninvasive technique for assessing the intracerebral circulation in patients with cerebrovascular disease. The technique was introduced by Aaslid [1] and colleagues at the University of Bern in Switzerland in 1982. Since that time, neurologists, neurosurgeons, vascular surgeons, and anesthesiologists have found a variety of applications for TCD in the outpatient, inpatient, intensive care unit, and operating room setting [2].

II. TRANSCRANIAL DOPPLER TECHNOLOGY AND TECHNIQUE

The TCD technology permits the measurement of cerebral blood flow velocity in the major arteries at the base of the brain by utilizing ultrasound techniques and the Doppler shift principle. Commercially available TCD devices utilize a 2-MHz probe that emits ultrasound signals that are then bounced off the red blood cells and received by the same probe. The signal received by the probe is converted into an electrical signal and transmitted to a microcomputer and analyzed using fast Fourier techniques. Given the frequency of the emitted signal and the measured frequency of the received signal, the Doppler shift equa-

---

Reproduced in part from the syllabus of After Dinner Seminar Number 173 "Intensive Care Monitoring Techniques" presented at the 45th Annual Meeting of the American Academy of Neurology, April 25, 1993. Reproduced with permission of the American Academy of Neurology.

tion is used to calculate the blood-flow velocity in the artery being examined. The Doppler velocity spectrum is then presented on a video monitor (spectral analysis). Most devices measure the peak and mean blood-flow velocity as well as calculate an index of vascular resistance, usually the pulsatility index ([systolic velocity − diastolic velocity]/mean velocity).

Several features of TCD ultrasound devices permit detailed examination of the blood-flow velocities in the arteries at the base of the brain. Devices for TCD usually utilize a 2-MHz frequency which is somewhat lower than the 7–10-MHz frequencies used for carotid duplex ultrasound examination. The lower frequency used in TCD technology permits greater tissue penetration so that the arteries at the base of the brain may be examined. However, the TCD probe may not be placed anywhere over the skull. In fact, there are only three commonly used ultrasound "windows" that permit transmission and reception of signals from the intracranial arteries (Figure 1). The transtemporal approach is utilized by placing the probe just above the zygomatic arch anterior to the ear so that the ultrasound beam may be transmitted through the thin portion of the temporal bone. Via the transtemporal window, velocity can be measured in the middle cerebral artery M_1 segment, anterior cerebral artery A_1 segment, distal internal carotid artery siphon,

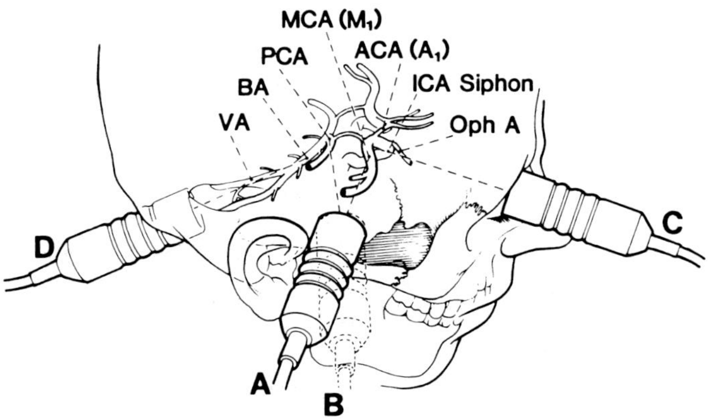

Figure 1 Transcranial ultrasound windows. The transtemporal approach (A and B) permits insonation of the middle cerebral artery M_1 segment (MCA-M_1), anterior cerebral artery A_1 segment (ACA-A_1), and the distal intracranial internal carotid artery siphon segment (ICA siphon). By directing the probe slightly posteriorly and inferiorly, the transtemporal window permits insonation of the posterior cerebral artery P_1 segment and occasionally the P_2 segment (PCA) as well as the posterior communicating artery in instances of abnormal collateral flow through this vessel. The transorbital ultrasound window (C) permits insonation of the ophthalmic artery (Oph A) and the internal carotid artery siphon (ICA siphon) in the region of the cavernous sinus. The suboccipital or transforaminal window (D) permits insonation of the distal intracranial segments of the vertebral arteries (VA) and the basilar artery (BA). (Reproduced with permission from Petty and Associates [2].)

and posterior cerebral artery P_1 segment as well as the posterior communicating artery when present. The transorbital approach is employed by placing the ultrasound probe directly over the eye (lids closed) and directing the ultrasound beam through the orbit to measure velocity in the ophthalmic artery and in the infraclinoid and supraclinoid and cavernous segments of the internal carotid artery siphon. Via the suboccipital window, the ultrasound beam may be directed through the foramen magnum to measure blood-flow velocity in the distal intracranial segments of the vertebral arteries and the basilar artery. A normal TCD study is illustrated in Figure 2. Most TCD devices use a pulsed, range-gated probe that permits the examiner to vary the depth at which the velocity is measured. In this way, the arteries can be examined over multiple segments.

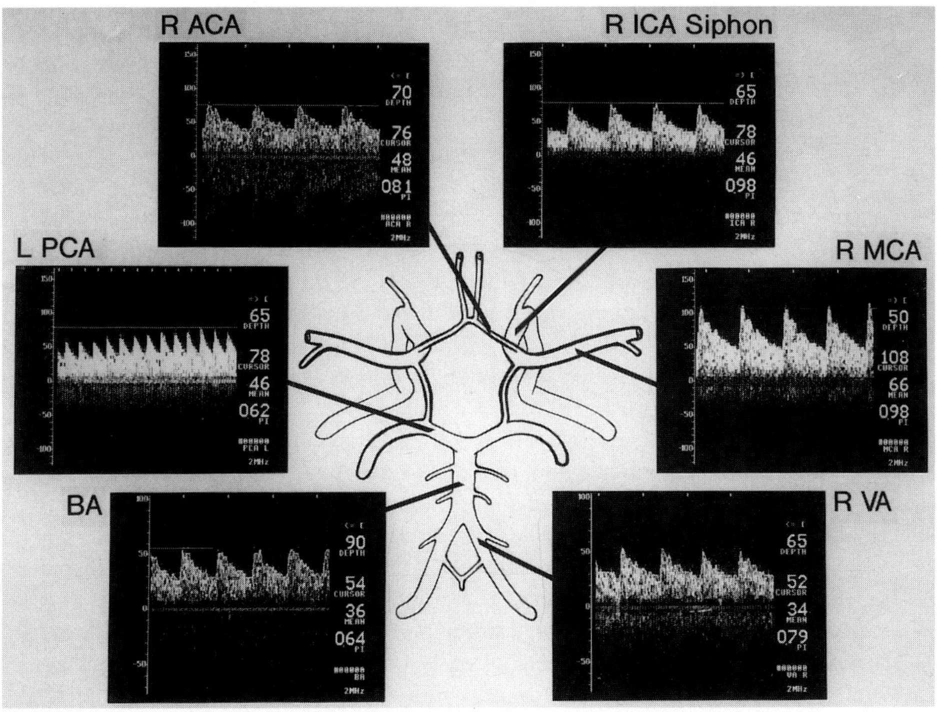

Figure 2 Normal transcranial Doppler examination. R = right, L = left, ICA = internal carotid artery, MCA = middle cerebral artery, VA = vertebral artery, BA = basilar artery, PCA = posterior cerebral artery, ACA = anterior cerebral artery, PI = pulsatility index. Depths are in millimeters. Notice direction of flow indicated by icon above depth measurement. In ICA, MCA, and PCA, flow is directed towards the probe. In ACA-A_1 segment, VA, and BA, flow is directed away from the probe. Note also augmentation of flow velocity in PCA as subject opens eyes and regards bright light. (Reproduced with permission from Petty and Associates [2].)

Normative reference data for mean velocity and pulsatility indices have been published [3,4]. A variety of factors may influence mean velocity. Mean velocities tend to decrease with age [5], increase with decreases in hematocrit [6], and increase with increases in arterial carbon dioxide content [5].

Inferences regarding intracranial arterial pathology can be made by analyzing mean velocity, pulsatility index, and direction of flow. Mean velocity is increased in conditions that reduce vessel lumen diameter (stenosis, vasospasm) or increase blood flow (arteriovenous malformation shunt systems). Velocities may be decreased in conditions that reduce cerebral perfusion (increased intracranial pressure, brain death) or in instances where there is a high-grade stenosis or occlusion distal or proximal to the segment of the artery being insonated. Pulsatility index, a measure of vascular resistance, is increased in conditions that result in increased vascular resistance (increased intracranial pressure, stenosis or occlusion distal to the segment of the vessel being insonated). The pulsatility index may be reduced in situations where vascular resistance is reduced (low-resistance arteriovenous malformation shunt systems or compensitory vasodilatation of cerebral resistance vessels in the setting of hemodynamically significant carotid occlusive disease in the neck).

Devices for TCD are light weight, portable, and ideally suited to applications in the intensive care unit. Studies can be performed rapidly at the bedside and can be easily repeated for serial monitoring. The TCD technique is relatively inexpensive compared to angiography. There are, however, a number of disadvantages and limitations that the clinician must be aware of in order to make clinical decisions based on TCD studies. First, the velocities that are measured using TCD are actually a function of the cosine of the angle that the ultrasound beam makes with the artery being studied. For most vessels of interest, such as the middle cerebral artery M_1 segment and the basilar artery, the angle of insonation is small, and the cosine effect is negligible. However for many intracranial vessels, such as the middle cerebral artery branches beyond the M_1 segment and the anterior cerebral artery A_2 segment, the angle of insonation approaches 90 degrees, and the cosine effect results in loss of the signal. The distal branches of the middle cerebral artery, posterior cerebral artery, and anterior cerebral artery, therefore, cannot be studied with TCD technology. A second drawback is that anywhere from 5 to 15 percent of patients may not have a technically adequate ultrasound window to permit an examination. This appears to be a function of variation in skull configuration as well as bone thickness and density. Failure to find an adequate ultrasound window is more common in women, blacks, and the elderly. Finally, TCD is not an imaging study (an obvious disadvantage compared to angiography). However, color-coded B-mode TCD ultrasound devices have recently been introduced [7].

Transcranial Doppler ultrasonography is a diagnostic tool of established clinical utility. The Therapeutics and Technology Assessment Subcommittee of the American Academy of Neurology issued a position statement regarding TCD

Table 1 Clinical Indications for Transcranial Doppler Testing

1. Assessment of patterns and extent of intracranial collateral circulation in patients with known regions of severe stenosis or occlusion in the internal carotid arteries, vertebral arteries, and subclavian arteries
2. Detection of hemodynamically significant stenosis in the major intracranial arteries at the base of the brain
3. Assessment and follow up of patients with vasoconstriction of any cause, especially vasospasm occurring after subarachnoid hemorrhage
4. Detection of arteriovenous malformations and study of their feeding arteries and the hemodynamic effects of treatment
5. Confirmation of the clinical diagnosis of brain death

Source: American Academy of Neurology, Therapeutics and Technology Assessment Subcommittee, Ref. 8.

ultrasonography in 1990 [8]. The panel found that TCD is "of established value" in the following clinical applications (see Table 1): 1. assessing intracranial collateral patterns in patients with occlusive disease of the cervical, carotid, or vertebral arteries; 2. detection of stenosis in the intracranial vessels at the base of the brain [9–12], 3. detection of vasospasm, particularly in the setting of subarachnoid hemorrhage [13,14], 4. detection of arteriovenous malformations and assessment of flow patterns in their feeding arteries, and 5. assessing patients with suspected cerebral death.

III. DIAGNOSIS OF VASOSPASM IN PATIENTS WITH SUBARACHNOID HEMORRHAGE

Perhaps the most useful clinical application of TCD technology in the intensive care unit setting is in the diagnosis of vasospasm in the setting of subarachnoid hemorrhage. Most TCD devices are light weight and portable, ideally suited to bedside examination of critically ill patients. The principle underlying the ability of transcranial Doppler to detect pathologic narrowing in arteries (stenosis, vasospasm, recanalized embolus) is that the velocity of blood flow increases in proportion to the decrease in residual arterial lumen radius. The increase in blood-flow velocity over narrowed arterial segments is frequently accompanied by abnormal acoustic properties of the signal corresponding to turbulence. Mean velocity threshold for diagnosis of vasospasm in the anterior circulation varies from laboratory to laboratory, but most communications have used a threshold of 120–150 cm/sec [12,14–16]. For the posterior circulation, Sloan et al. used mean flow velocities of 80 cm/sec and 95 cm/sec for the vertebral and basilar arteries respectively as criteria for diagnosis of vasospasm [16].

Figure 3 illustrates typical transcranial Doppler findings of velocity elevation and turbulence due to vasospasm in the middle cerebral artery M_1 segment

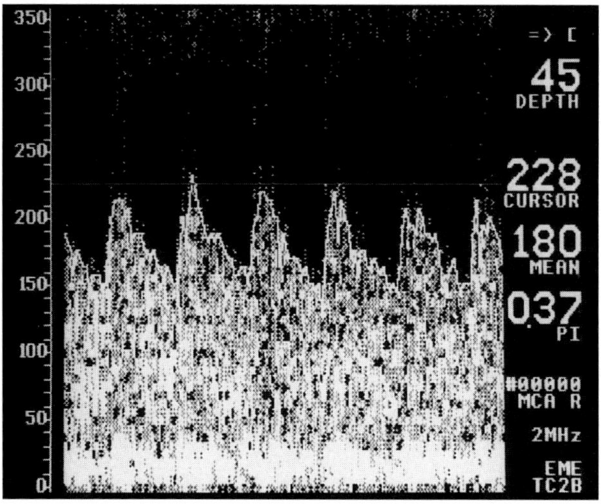

(a)

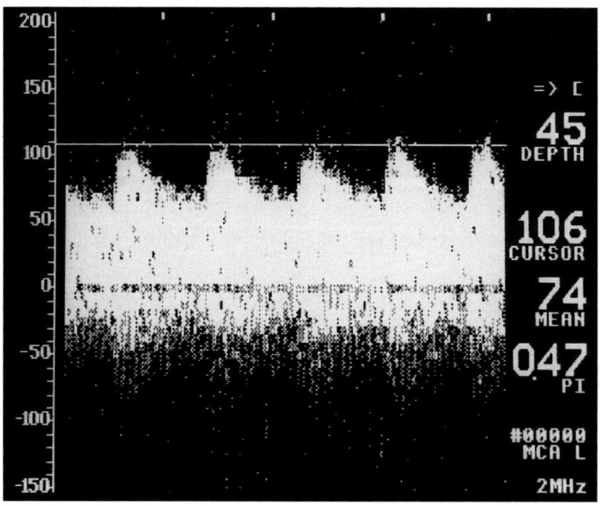

(b)

Figure 3 Transcranial Doppler detection of vasospasm in a 35-year-old man with subarachnoid hemorrhage. Transcranial Doppler ultrasonography demonstrated increased flow velocity and turbulence in the right middle cerebral artery M_1 segment (a) and normal to slightly increased velocities in the left middle cerebral artery M_1 segment (b). Angiography demonstrated vasospasm in the right middle cerebral artery M_1 segments and distal internal carotid artery siphon (c). A left carotid injection demonstrated an

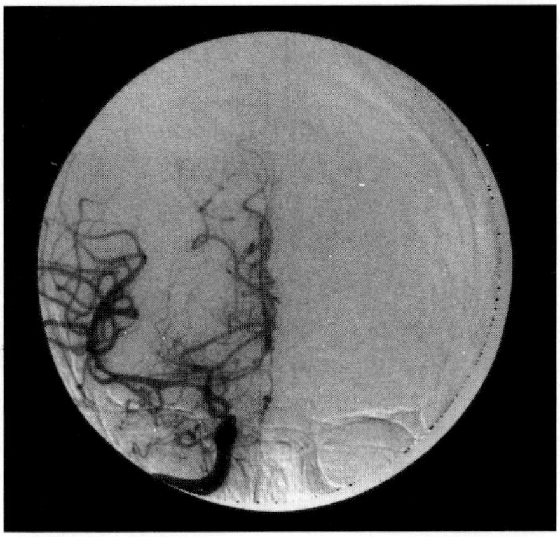

(c)

Figure 3 Continued.
anterior communicating artery aneurysm and no evidence of vasospasm in the left middle cerebral M_1 segment. Depth is in millimeters. Mean = mean velocity in centimeters per second. The number above "cursor" is peak velocity in centimeters per second. PI = pulsatility index. (Reproduced with permission from Petty and Associates [2].)

of a patient with subarachnoid hemorrhage due to an anterior communicating artery aneurysm.

The value of TCD in the setting of subarachnoid hemorrhage is that it is highly specific for the diagnosis of vasospasm. Specificities range from 82 to 100 percent in the detection of vasospasm in the posterior circulation (vertebral and basilar arteries) to 89 to 100 percent in detection of vasospasm in the anterior circulation (Tables 2 and 3) [12,14–16]. Therefore, when TCD detects findings of mean velocity elevation in the vasospasm range in patients with subarachnoid hemorrhage, clinical decisions regarding timing of surgery, institution of medical treatment for vasospasm (hypervolemic therapy, hypertensive therapy), and selection of patients for balloon angioplasty [17] can be made with confidence.

Table 2 Transcranial Doppler Diagnosis of Vasospasm Involving Middle Cerebral Artery M_1 Segment

	Sensitivity	Specificity
Lennihan, 1993 [13]	86%	98%
Sloan, 1989 [14]	84%	89%

Table 3 Transcranial Doppler Detection of Vasospasm in the Anterior Cerebral Artery

	Sensitivity	Specificity
Lennihan, 1993 [13]	13%	100%
Low sensitivity due to:		
Variable ACA anatomy		
Inability to insonate ACA A_2		
Behavioral disturbance due to frontal lobe ischemia		

Case Study (Figure 4): A 33-year-old woman six-weeks postpartum developed the sudden onset of loss of consciousness with subsequent symptoms of headache and vomiting. Admission examination demonstrated that she was somnolent but arousable and without language disturbance. There was mild nuchal rigidity. There were no cranial nerve abnormalities, and she moved all four extremities to pain. A CT scan demonstrated diffuse subarachnoid hemorrhage [Figure 4A]. The patient was admitted to the intensive care unit and treated with nimodipine, pain medication, sedatives, and anticonvulsants. Transfemoral cerebral angiogram demonstrated an anterior communicating artery aneurysm. A right frontotemporal craniotomy was performed, and the aneurysm was clipped. Postoperatively, the patient had a normal neurological examination. However, one day postoperatively a transcranial Doppler examination demonstrated an elevated mean velocity (152 cm/sec) in the distal right internal carotid artery siphon insonating via the transtemporal approach (Figure 4b). There was also evidence of vasospasm in both middle cerebral artery M_1 segments, the right and left anterior cerebral artery A_1 segments, and the left internal carotid artery siphon. She was treated with volume expansion, but during the hours following the transcranial Doppler examination, she became mute and developed a right hemiparesis. Angiography subsequently confirmed vasospasm and balloon dilatation was undertaken and successfully performed in both distal internal carotid artery siphon segments, both middle cerebral artery M_1 segments and the left anterior cerebral artery A_1 segment. Figures 4c and 4d illustrate the pre- (4c) and post- (4d) balloon dilatation appearances of the distal internal carotid artery siphon segment on the right. Transcranial Doppler examination subsequently documented resolution of vasospasm. Normal post-dilatation velocities in the right distal internal carotid artery siphon are depicted in Figure 4e, compared to predilatation transcranial Doppler velocities in waveforms over the same segment (Figure 4b). This case illustrates that transcranial Doppler may assist in selecting patients for medical and interventional neuroradiologic procedures for treatment of symptomatic vasospasm and may also provide a noninvasive method of following the hemodynamic effects of such treatments.

Unfortunately, negative TCD studies for vasospasm in the setting of subarachnoid hemorrhage are less helpful clinically. For the detection of vasospasm in the middle cerebral artery M_1 segment, sensitivity is high (84–86 percent) [13,14]. However, the sensitivity of detection of vasospasm in the anterior cerebral artery is disappointingly low, 13 percent in the study of Lennihan et al. [13]. There are a variety of reasons for this poor sensitivity in detection of anterior cerebral artery vasospasm. The A_1 segment of the anterior cerebral artery is quite variable in its course. Patients with anterior communicating artery aneurysms frequently have large deposits of subarachnoid blood in the region of the anterior cerebral artery A_2 segment (pericallosal). This segment may, therefore, be frequently subject to the development of vasospasm, yet the TCD cannot detect blood flow in the anterior cerebral artery A_2 segment because this vessel travels at a right angle to the ultrasound beam when the transtemporal window is used. Also, patients with anterior cerebral artery vasospasm and symptomatic ischemia in the frontal lobes frequently have behavioral abnormalities that render them less cooperative for detailed TCD examination. According to the studies of Sloan et al., the sensitivity of TCD in detection of vasospasm in the posterior circulation is only 44 percent in the vertebral arteries but 77 percent in the basilar artery [16]. The occasional development of vasospasm in the distal intracranial branch vessels only may also contribute to decreased TCD sensitivity for detection of vasospasm [18]. Also, patients with markedly increased intracranial pressure may have a low mean velocity in the face of vasospasm because of decreased cerebral perfusion pressure [19].

The TCD technique has provided some insights into the time course of the development of vasospasm and may also assist in identification of patients who are at greater risk for development of delayed ischemic deficits due to vasospasm. Studies have demonstrated a correlation between the rate of increase of TCD velocities in patients with subarachnoid hemorrhage and the development of delayed ischemic deficits (Figure 5) [20–22]. In the study of Fahmy and Smith, a TCD velocity increase of more than 25 percent per day for two consecutive days was highly specific (100 percent) and sensitive (90 percent) in identifying patients destined to become symptomatic from vasospasm [22]. This potential use of TCD in identifying patients destined for cerebral ischemia in the setting of vasospasm may have obvious implications in terms of selection of patients for presymptomatic medical and endovascular therapy for this condition.

The TCD technique has also provided some evidence on at least one aspect of the mechanism of action of nimodipine in the reduction of severe neurological ischemic deficits attributable to vasospasm. Although a neuronal protec-

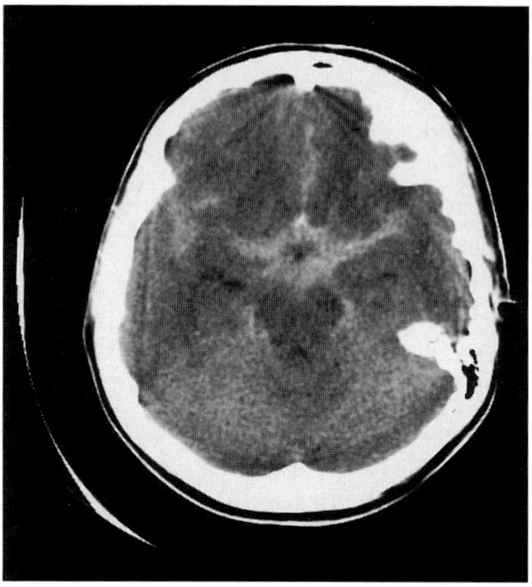

(a)

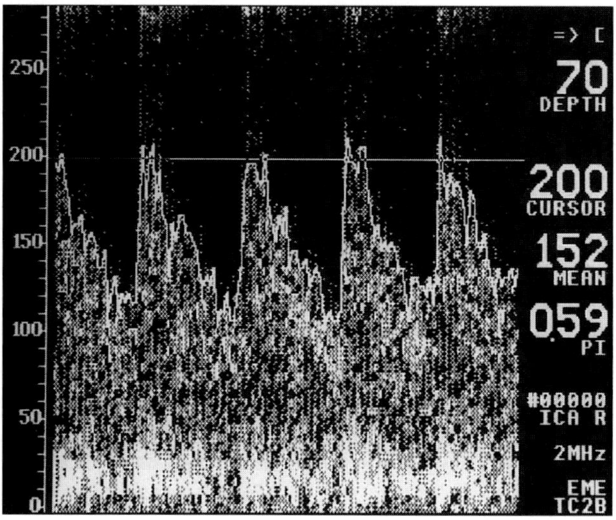

(b)

Figure 4 A 33-year-old woman presented with sudden loss of consciousness and subsequently experienced headache and vomiting. CT scan (a) demonstrated diffuse subarachnoid hemorrhage with concentration of blood in the intrahemispheric fissure and ambient cisterns. A cerebral angiogram subsequently documented an anterior communicating artery aneurysm. Craniotomy was performed and the aneurysm was clipped. One day postoperatively neurological examination was normal, but transcranial Doppler examination demonstrated vasospasm in both anterior cerebral artery A_1 segments, both distal internal carotid artery siphon segments, and both middle cerebral artery M_1 segments (see vasospasm documented on transcranial Doppler examination of right internal carotid artery siphon via transtemporal window), (b). Angiography documented vaso-

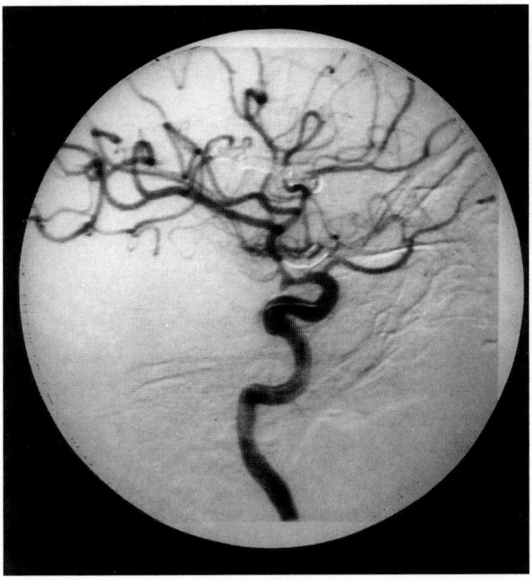

(c)

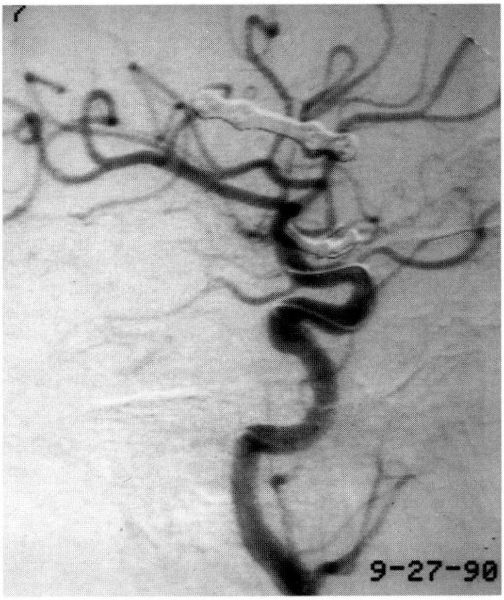

(d)

Figure 4 Continued.
spasm over these segments (c). Balloon dilatation was performed. Note predilatation angiographic appearance of right internal carotid artery siphon (c) compared to post-dilatation resolution of vasospastic narrowing (d). Transcranial Doppler examination demonstrated resolution of abnormally elevated vasospasm range velocities (e).

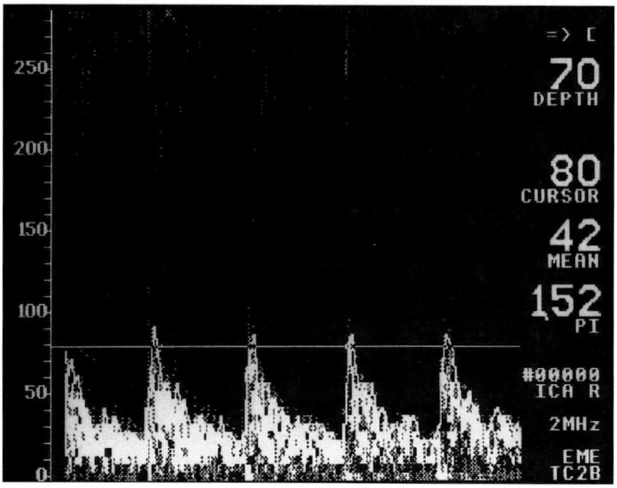

(e)

Figure 4 Continued. (Radiographs courtesy of Dr. Douglas A. Nichols and the Department of Diagnostic Radiology, Mayo Clinic, Rochester, Minnesota.)

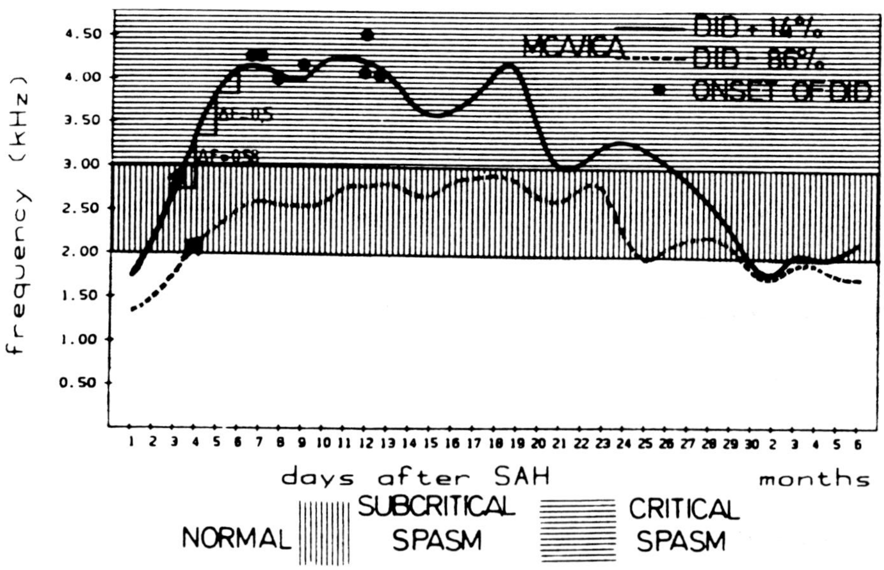

Figure 5 The time course of velocity increases following subarachnoid hemorrhage. Frequency is proportional to velocity. Note that patients with more rapid acceleration of velocity increase in the first six days following subarachnoid hemorrhage were more likely to develop delayed ischemic deficits (DID). (From Ref. 20. Reproduced with permission from the Journal of Neurosurgery.)

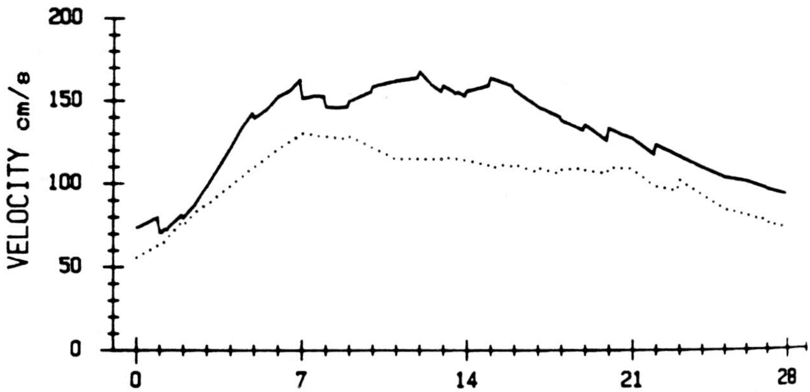

Figure 6 Mean blood flow velocity curves of patients with subarachnoid hemorrhage treated with nimodipine (. . .) compared to those not treated with nimodipine (———). Note lower mean velocities in the nimodipine-treated group. (From Ref. 23 with permission of ACTA Neurosurgica.)

tive effect likely plays a role, there is also TCD evidence that nimodipine may reduce the severity of vasospasm. For example, in the study of Seiler et al. [23], blood flow velocities were less increased in nimodipine-treated subarachnoid hemorrhage patients compared with control nontreated patients (Figure 6).

REFERENCES

1. Aaslid R, Markwalder TM, Nornes H. Noninvasive transcranial Doppler ultrasound recording of flow velocity in basal cerebral arteries. *J Neurosurg* 1982; 57:769–774.
2. Petty GW, Wiebers DO, Meissner I. Transcranial Doppler ultrasonography: clinical applications in cerebrovascular disease. *Mayo Clin Proc* 1990; 65:1350–1364.
3. Arnolds BJ, von Reutern GM. Transcranial Doppler sonography. Examination technique and normal reference values. *Ultrasound in Med and Biol* 1986; 2:115–123.
4. Hennerici M, Rautenberg W, Sitzer G, Schwartz A. Transcranial Doppler ultrasound for the assessment of intracranial arterial flow velocity—Part 1. *Surg Neurol* 1987; 27:439–448.
5. Vriens EM, Kraaier V, Musbach M, Wieneke GH, van Huffelen AC. Transcranial pulsed Doppler measurements of blood velocity in the middle cerebral artery: reference values at rest and during hyperventilation in healthy volunteers in relation to age and sex. *Ultrasound in Med and Biol* 1989; 15:1–8.

6. Brass LM, Pavlakis SG, DeVivo D, Piomelli S, Mohr JP. Transcranial Doppler measurements of the middle cerebral artery. Effect of hematocrit. *Stoke* 1988; 19:1466–1469.
7. Bogdahn U, Becker G, Winkler J, Greiner K, Perez J, Meurers B. Transcranial color–coded real–time sonography in adults. *Stroke* 1990; 21:1680–1688.
8. American Academy of Neurology, Therapeutics and Technology Assessment Subcommittee's report. Assessment: Trancranial Doppler. *Neurology* 1990; 40:680–681.
9. Ley-Pozo J, Ringelstein EB. Noninvasive detection of occlusive disease of the carotid siphon and middle cerebral artery. *Ann Neurol* 1990; 28:640–647.
10. de Bray JM, Maugin JD, Jeanvoine H, Emile J. Long–term study of 20 cases of proximal stenosis of the middle cerebral artery. *Rev Neurol (Paris)* 1989; 145:117–126.
11. Spencer MP, Whisler D. Transorbital Doppler diagnosis of intracranial arterial stenosis. *Stroke* 1986; 17:916–921.
12. Estol CJ, DeWitt LD, Tettenborn B, Kraemer G, Pessin MS, Caplan LR. Accuracy of transcranial Doppler in the verebrobasilar circulation (abstract). *Ann Neurol* 1990; 28:225–226.
13. Lennihan L, Petty GW, Fink ME, Soloman RA, Mohr JP. Transcranial Doppler detection of anterior cerebral artery vasospasm. *J Neurol Neurosurg Psychiatry* 1993; 56:906–909.
14. Sloan MA, Haley EC, Kassell NF, Henry ML, Stewart SR, Beskin RR, Sevilla EA, Torner JC. Sensitivity and specificity of transcranial Doppler ultrasonography in the diagnosis of vasospasm following subarachnoid hemorrhage. *Neurology* 1989; 39:1514–1518.
15. Sloan MA, Rigamonti D, Rothman M, Burch C, Permutt T, Bradstreet P, Numaguchi Y. Sensitivity and specificity of transcranial Doppler for detecting vertebral artery vasospasm (abstract). *Stroke* 1992; 23:469.
16. Sloan MA, Burch CM, Wozniak MA, Rothman MI, Rigamonti D, Permutt T, Numaguchi Y. Transcranial doppler detection of vertebrabasilar vasospasm following subarachnoid hemorrhage. *Stroke* 1994; 25:2187–2197.
17. Konishi Y, Maemura E, Sato E, Hara M, Takeuchi K. A therapy against vasospasm after subarachnoid haemorrhage: clinical experience of balloon angioplasty. *Neurol Res* 1990; 12:103–105.
18. Newell DW, Grady MS, Eskridge JM, Winn HR. Distribution of angiographic vasospasm after subarachnoid hemorrhage: implications for diagnosis by transcranial Doppler ultrasonography. *Neurosurgery* 1990; 27:574–577.
19. Klingelhofer J, Sander D, Holzgraefe M, Bischoff C, Conrad B. Cerebral vasospasm evaluated by transcranial Doppler ultrasonography at different intracranial pressures. *J Neurosurg* 1991; 75:752–758.
20. Harders AG, Gilsbach JM. Time course of blood velocity changes related to vasospasm in the circle of Willis measured by transcranial Doppler ultrasound. *J Neurosurg* 1987; 66:718–728.
21. Grosset DG, Straiton J, du Trevou M, Bullock R. Prediction of symptomatic vasospasm after subarachnoid hemorrhage by rapidly increasing transcranial Doppler velocity and cerebral blood flow changes. *Stroke* 1992; 23:674–679.

22. Fahmy MA, Smith RR. Identification of presymptomatic cerebral vasospasm by transcranial Doppler sonography (abstract). *Stroke* 1992; 23:156.
23. Seiler RW, Grolimund P, Zurbruegg HR. Evaluation of the calciumantagonist nimodipine for the prevention of vasospasm after aneurysmal subarachnoid haemorrhage: a prospective transcranial Doppler ultrasound study. *Acta Neurochir* (*Wein*) 1987; 85:7–16.

12

Medical Management of Subarachnoid Hemorrhage

J. R. Fulgham
Mayo Clinic, Rochester, Minnesota

I. INTRODUCTION

Following aneurysmal subarachnoid hemorrhage (SAH) 30% to 40% of the patients will die in the first month [1,2] and in survivors, motor and cognitive deficits may preclude a return to their previous level of functioning [3–5]. Subarachnoid hemorrhage from the rupture of an intracranial aneurysm is a major public health problem; however, there are other etiologies for nontraumatic subarachnoid bleeding that need to be considered. Other sources include cerebral arterial venous malformations, rupture of a superficial cortical artery, spinal cord aneurysm or spinal cord vascular malformation, and SAH without any identifiable source [6–9].

The goals of medical management of SAH, stated simply, are to prevent secondary deterioration after the ictus and to treat medical complications that may result from the initial hemorrhage. Anticipation, prophylactic therapies, and timely intervention are the keys to success and require a dedicated team of neurologists, neurosurgeons, and nurses. Although there is no universal consensus regarding the correct medical management of SAH there are specific medical issues that frequently complicate subarachnoid hemorrhage, and an understanding of these issues are necessary for anyone involved in the care and management of patients following subarachnoid hemorrhage (Table 1).

II. INITIAL ASSESSMENT AND INVESTIGATIONS

The sine quo non of aneurysmal SAH is the sudden onset of a severe headache without neurologic deficit. Sudden loss of consciousness may preceed the head-

Table 1 Complications that May Occur After Subarachnoid Hemorrhage

Rebleeding
Disturbances of sodium and water balance
Vasospasm
Seizures
Hydrocephalus
Cardiac arrhythmias

ache and focal deficits such as hemiparesis, aphasia, or cranial nerve palsies may be noted at presentation (Figure 1) [10,11]. Seizures at the onset of the ictus have been reported in 20% of patients [12]. The initial examination is therefore crucial to document the presence or absence of focal neurological deficits and to establish a baseline to which subsequent examinations can be compared.

Several scales have been developed to aid in assessing patients following SAH. The Hunt and Hess scale [13] and the scale developed by the World Federation of Neurological Surgeons (WFNS) [14] are two that are commonly used (Table 2). The latter places a premium on the level of consciousness by incorporating the Glascow Coma Score. The WFNS scale has proven useful in our practice but one must be aware that the increasing use of short-acting benzodiazepines in intensive care units makes the accurate assessment of mental status difficult. No scale or grading system can be a substitute for serial bedside evaluations by physicians and the nursing staff.

Head computerized tomography (CT) has become indespensible in the diagnosis of SAH and should be performed in all suspect patients. Within twenty-four hours of the ictus a head CT will be positive for subarachnoid bleeding in 90% of patients; however, the sensitivity of the CT scan decreases rapidly and it will be positive in only 50% of patients on day seven [15]. The disappearence of the blood can be either through diffusion, reabsorption, or both. An early head CT scan is useful in the diagnosis of SAH and also for predicting the risk of vasospasm (VSP) following subarachnoid hemorrhage [16–18].

If SAH is clinically suspected and the initial head CT is negative for subarachnoid blood then analysis of the spinal fluid is necessary. The cerebrospinal fluid (CSF) sample should be sent for a red blood cell count and to look for the presence of xanthochromia. Xanthochromia is a yellow discoloration of the normally clear CSF and may be found in patients with an elevated CSF protein or in patients with jaundice. Xanthochromia also results from the lysis of red blood cells and it is therefore a sensitive indicator of subarachnoid blood. Unfortunately many laboratories report xanthochromia as being positive or nega-

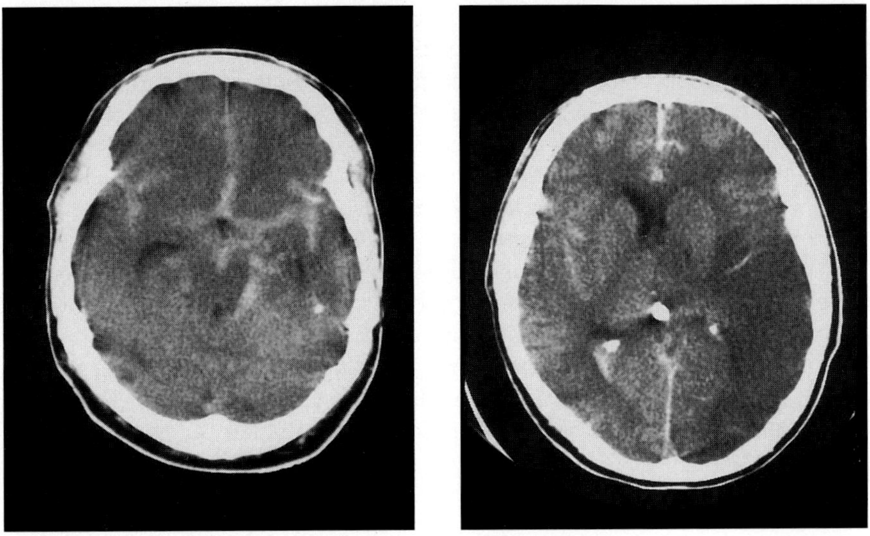

(a) (b)

Figure 1 A head CT scan with extensive subarachnoid blood in the right sylvian fissure and the basal cisterns. The hemorrhage extends into the frontal lobe and the ventricular system. There is mild to moderate mass effect with midline shift. A right middle cerebral artery aneurysm was found at angiography.

Table 2 Clinical Grading Scales for the Assessment of Patients After Subarachnoid Hemorrhage

	Scale of Hunt and Hess
Grade	Clinical description
i	Asymptomatic or mild headache
ii	Moderate to severe headache, nuchal rigidity, +/− oculomotor palsy
iii	Confusion, drowsiness, or mild focal signs
iv	Stupor or hemiparesis

Scale of the World Federation of Neurological Surgeons

Grade	Glascow coma score	Neurological deficit
i	15	−
ii	13–14	−
iii	13–14	+
iv	8–12	+/−
v	3–7	+/−

tive upon visually inspecting a centrifuged sample of spinal fluid. Visual inspection for xanthochromia is not acceptable practice. In patients suspected of having SAH, a report positive for xanthochromia requires spectrophotometric analysis of the CSF sample to be valid [19].

In an SAH suspect a lumbar puncture prior to CT scanning of the head should be performed with caution. Lumbar puncture should be deferred if there is papilledema or a focal neurological deficit and the patient should be transferred to a facility where CT scanning is available.

All patients will require cerebral angiography to document the source of the bleeding and to ascertain whether there are multiple aneurysms. A baseline electrocardiogram, electrolytes, and complete blood-cell count to include platelets should be obtained. Other testing will be dictated by preexisting medical conditions. A chest roentgenogram should be done, particularly if there is loss of consciousness with the ictus since pulmonary aspiration is common in these situations.

III. REBLEEDING

The early surgical obliteration of an aneurysm is the most effective means of preventing rehemorrhage. Rebleeding is a major complication following SAH and it is associated with significant morbidity and mortality [20–23]. Following an aneurysmal SAH the peak incidence of rebleeding is in the first week [20]. Inagawa et al. [22] reported aneurysmal rebleeding in 33 of 150 consecutive patients with most occurring in the first 24 hours. The mortality after rehemorrhage is high and ranges from 50% to 75% [21,22] and the prognosis for an alert patient following a second hemorrhage is the same as for the patient admitted in coma after the initial hemorrhage [23].

The fibrinolytic activity of the CSF is increased after SAH, and theoretically treatment aimed at preserving the clot over the dome of a ruptured aneurysm would be beneficial in preventing rebleeding. The first clinical experience using antifibrinolytic agents in SAH occurred in the sixties [24,25], and two agents, tranexamic acid (TXA) and epsilon-aminocaproic acid (EACA), with antifibrinolytic activity have been through extensive trials testing this hypothesis. Although there are reports that the rate of rebleeding with antifibrinolytic therapy is unchanged [26] the majority of studies found a significant decrease in the incidence of rebleeding using either agent [27–32].

Although antifibrinolytic therapy decreases the incidence of rebleeding it does not decrease the overall mortality or morbidity in patients [30–32]. In a double-blind placebo-controlled multicenter trial, Vermeulen et al. [30] found rebleeding reduced from 24% in the controls to 9% in the group treated with TXA but at three months there was no statistical difference in outcome in the controls verses patients receiving TXA. Similar findings were reported by Kassell et al. [31] with EACA. The increased morbidity and mortality with antifibrinolytic therapy was not due to an increased number of systemic embolic or thrombotic events as one might anticipate [30]. There was, however, a dramatic increase in the incidence of delayed cerebral ischemic events despite decreased rebleeding from the aneurysm in those patients receiving antifibrinolytic therapy. A shorter duration of antifibrinolytic treatment using TXA has similarly resulted in a high incidence of ischemic complications [32].

Recommendations

Urgent head CT scan if rebleeding suspected; early surgical obliteration of the source of subarachnoid bleeding; no role for antifibrinolytic therapy.

IV. DISTURBANCES OF SODIUM AND WATER BALANCE

Hyponatremia with serum sodium less than 135 mEq/L occurs in 9% to 30% of patients after SAH [33–35]. Although the hyponatremia is not often severe, patients may have complaints of nausea with emesis, muscle weakness, confusion, and seizures. If serum sodium is less than 120 mEq/L a patient may lapse into coma. The cause of the low serum sodium in these patients is inappropriate natriuresis, and although it resembles the hyponatremia of inappropriate secretion of antidiuretic hormone (SIADH) [36] it is actually the cerebral salt-wasting syndrome following acute head injury, first described by Cort [37]. The distinction between SIADH and cerebral salt-wasting syndrome is important as the treatments are diametrically opposed: SIADH results in volume expansion with dilutional hyponatremia and the appropriate treatment is fluid restriction, whereas cerebral salt wasting is a true natriuresis with the loss of sodium in excess of water. Appropriate treatments for the latter are salt and water repletion. The precise mechanism for the natriuresis in cerebral salt wasting is unclear; however, a prime candidate is the atrial natriuretic factor (ANF) or some similar substance [34,38–40]. Atrial natriuretic factor levels are elevated following SAH when compared to ill-patient controls and this elevation is associated with natriuresis and a negative sodium balance [39].

Hypovolemia with a decreased plasma volume is common in patients after a SAH [41,42]. The causes of decreased plasma volume are multifactorial and include iatrogenic blood loss, diuresis associated with bed rest, cerebral salt wasting, and decreased erythropoeisis [41]. The activity of the sympathetic nervous system is also increased in these patients and increased sympathetic activity has been associated with diminished total blood volume [43]. All of these factors may contribute in varying degrees to water loss and dehydration after SAH. Symptoms exhibited by patients suffering hypovolemia are similar to those of hyponatremia and include confusion, agitation, nausea and vomiting, and may progress to coma.

In any patient with SAH, hypovolemia is to be avoided and fluid management should be directed toward restoring plasma volume and sodium balance. A reasonable approach to fluid management is to provide 2.5 to 3.5 L/day of normal saline often with 20 mEq of potassium added per liter. Albumin may be used in addition to saline. The precise fluid volume required in 24 hours is impossible to predict for every patient as requirements are influenced by hydration on admission, enteral intake, fever, and the presence of inappropriate natriuresis. Sodium correction requires both salt and water repletion. Intravenous normal saline or albumin will restore volume; however, additional sodium supplementation may be necessary. Pharmacologic treatment with fludrocortisone acetate has proven effective in restoring sodium balance after aneurysmal SAH [44,45]. Doses of fludrocortisone acetate of 0.4 mg/day intravenously or orally have been effective [45]. Whenever correcting volume and sodium balance, the central venous pressure should be monitored to prevent untoward side effects such as congestive heart failure. In some patients the pulmonary capillary wedge pressure may need to be monitored (Table 3). Other measures to monitor overall hydration include strict recording of fluid input and output and daily

Table 3 General Care of Patients After Subarachnoid Hemorrhage

Initial evaluation: Clinical assessment
Head CT Scan +/− CSF examination
CBC, Electrolytes, ECG, Chest x-ray
Nursing care
Step-down bed or ICU bed
Deep venous thrombosis prophylaxis
Stool softener
+/− bladder catheterization
Analgesia
Supplemental oxygen by nasal cannula or face mask
Monitoring
Cardiac monitoring
Frequent neurological checks
Daily weights
Daily serum sodium
Strict measurement of fluid input and output
CVP or PCWP

weights. The temperature chart should be watched closely and intravenous or oral fluid intake adjusted for insensible losses associated with fever.

Recommendations

Maintain euvolemia; monitor daily weight and serum sodium; strict input and output records; volume replacement with normal saline 2.5 to 3.5 L/day and consider 5% albumin for volume replacement; fludrocortisone acetate, 0.4 mg/day for hyponatremia.

V. PREVENTION OF VASOSPASM

Vasospasm after aneurysmal SAH occurs in 20% to 30% of patients [46,47] and persistant deficits are found in up to 14% of those afflicted. This is most appropriately defined as symptomatic VSP, as some degree of arterial narrowing can be seen with cerebral angiography but it is not associated with clinical symptoms [48]. The incidence of delayed ischemic neurological deficit (DIND) from VSP is similar to the incidence of aneurysmal rebleeding [20] and is an important cause of secondary morbidity and mortality. It is encumbent upon those who manage patients after SAH to initiate treatments that will prevent symptomatic VSP and delayed neurologic deficits.

Vasospasm can occur at anytime following the ictus although the onset of symptoms is most often between day 2 and day seventeen [49]. Spasm of the cerebral arteries is almost never seen with SAH due to other causes (such as bleeding from a vascular malformation) and it is present rarely after traumatic SAH [46]. The lack of VSP in these latter situations may be related to the volume of blood clot lying in the subarachnoid space. Because of these observations, efforts have been made to develop predictors of patients at greatest risk of developing VSP. A cooperative study showed an increased incidence of VSP in patients with a high clinical grade on admission to the hospital as compared to those with a low grade [50]. Perhaps one of the most reliable predictors of the occurrence and distribution of VSP has been the amount and localization of subarachnoid blood seen on head CT scan [16–18]. Reproduced head CT images demonstrating subarachnoid clot measuring 3×5 mm correlated with a high incidence of symptomatic VSP and the VSP occurred in the territory of the artery or arteries surrounded by the clot [18]. The prediction of the vascular territory in which VSP will occur based on CT evidence has been questioned; however, the volume of clot does correlate with the occurrence of vasospasm [51].

The technique of transcranial Doppler (TCD) sonography of the basal cerebral arteries developed by Aaslid et al. [52] is an established noninvasive method to study cerebral hemodynamics. The TCD technique finds its greatest clinical utility in predicting and monitoring cerebral VSP after SAH [53,54]. An increase in blood flow velocity greater than 50 cm/sec in a 24-hour period is associated with the onset of DIND, as well as decreased cerebral blood flow in the appropriate arterial territory [54].

The symptoms of VSP are often subtle. Mild changes in the sensorium, agitation, or confusion are often present early. Mild pronator drift or a decrease in the alternating motions rate may be the first focal signs to appear [55]. These minor motor deficits may persist, fluctuate, or progress to significant motor impairment, coma, or death. It is therefore important to initiate therapy early to prevent VSP and its sequelae.

One of the primary management strategies to prevent VSP is the maintainence of the normal circulating blood volume. Often the expansion of the blood volume is necessary if VSP is symptomatic and then treatment should be titrated to the clinical response [33,42,56]. Volume expansion with normal saline and periodic infusion of 250 cc of 5% albumin to a central venous pressure (CVP) of 10–12 mm Hg or pulmonary capillary wedge pressue (PCWP) of 12–16 mm Hg should be the goal of therapy [56]. These steps will often increase the mean arterial blood pressure by 10 mm above the patients baseline. If the use of volume alone is not effective at elevating the blood pressure, then pressor agents, dopamine, or phenylephrine hydrochloride may be added [56]. All patients should remain euvolemic and if the patient is hyponatremic this should be corrected.

Those patients judged to be at considerable risk for the development of symptomatic VSP based on head CT scan criteria or increasing TCD velocities should be aggressively managed with volume expansion and blood pressure elevation. Patients should be cared for in a neurological/neurosurgical intensive care unit for close clinical and hemodynamic monitoring.

The use of the calcium channel antagonist, nimodipine, has become part of the standard practice in the care of patients after aneurysmal SAH. Allen et al. [57] demonstrated a clear benefit in the prevention of DIND in patients receiving nimodipine. Similar benefits have been demonstrated in other trials using nimodipine including large multicenter randomized placebo-controlled trials [58–60]. The Canadian multicenter trial documented benefit from nimodipine in patients of unfavorable grade, Hunt and Hess grades 3 to 5 [59]. The British trial enrolled patients of all grade and demonstrated a 34% reduction in cerebral infarction and a 40% reduction in poor outcome with oral nimodipine [60]. Although nimodipine was initially felt to prevent spasm of the conducting cerebral arteries [57] this appears not to be the case. Nimodipine may prevent delayed cerebral ischemia by improving collateral flow via pial vessels and it may have a direct neuronal protective effect [61,62].

Nimodipine is administered as a test dose of 30 mg, either orally or via a nasogastric tube. If there is not a significant decrease in the blood pressure with a test dose then 60 mg is administered every four hours for 21 consecutive days. Hypotension is usually not a problem if euvolemia is maintained.

Other therapies have been tried in an effort to prevent delayed ischemic deficits secondary to vasospasm. The calcium channel blockers flunarizine and nicardipine have met with success [63,64]. The 21-aminosteroid tirilazad mesylate, a lipid peroxidation inhibitor, has demonstrated a significant protective effect on neuronal ischemia including ischemia due to vasospasm [65,66]. Clinical trials using tirilizad mesylate are ongoing.

Two approaches to prevent VSP are designed to directly affect the presumed cause or causes of vasospasm. Vasospasm after subarachnoid hemorrhage is a complex phenomena and is most probably due to breakdown products of hemoglobin in the subarachnoid space. Perivascular inflammation may also play a role. Methylprednisolone in high doses has reduced the incidence of DIND and death in patients treated as compared to controls [67], and cyclosporine A has similarly been effective in animal studies and in a limited number of patients [68,69]. Steroids and cyclosporine A would presumably have an effect on perivascular inflammation that may be contributing to or initiating vasospasm. Perhaps one of the most exciting new additions to the therapeutic arsenal is the use of thrombolytic agents to lyse subarachnoid clot and to facilitate its removal [70,71].

Recommendations

Frequent neurological checks; baseline transcranial doppler; nimodipine 60 mg every four hours orally; euvolemia maintained with normal saline and albumin; volume expansion may be necessary if symptomatic VSP; MAP elevation to 10–15 mm Hg above baseline; CVP or PCWP monitoring.

VI. SEIZURES

Seizures after SAH are present in 4% to 28% of patients [12,72–74]. Hart reported seizures in 19% of patients with SAH and 20% of patients with recurrent hemorrhage had a seizure within 12 hours [12]. Temporally, the onset of seizures can be divided into early isolated seizures or late recurrent seizures or epilepsy. An isolated seizure associated with the initial hemorrhage or with rebleeding is related to the injury resulting from the hemorrhage and is an epiphenomenon. Late seizures and recurrent seizures are less frequent; they had an incidence of 10% in a large Scandinavian series [74]. In the latter study seizures occurred on average 6.7 months from the ictus. It is often difficult to define those patients at risk for recurrent seizures. Neurological deficits on examination, intraparenchymal extension of the hemorrhage, cerebral infarction on delayed head CT scan, prolonged coma, and middle cerebral artery aneurysm are features identified as increasing the risk of epilepsy [72]. The presence of antecedent hypertension has been noted to be an independent risk factor for late seizures [74].

Because of the relatively high incidence and the potential adverse affects of a generalized seizure on a patient with an unclipped aneurysm, prophylactic treatment with an antiepileptic drug is warrented. Phenytoin, loaded either intravenously or orally, is the antiepileptic drug of first choice. A loading dose of 20 mg/kg should be given and then a maintainence dose of 5 mg/kg to 7 mg/kg per day, divided into twice a day. If the patient has an allergy to phenytoin, then phenobarbitol may be substituted. Because of the sedation associated with phenobarbitol it may mask the early signs of secondary neurologic deterioration.

Due to the risk of delayed seizures in those patients in whom antiepileptic medications are continued after dismissal from the hospital, an electroencephalogram may be helpful in making the decision to continue or stop the antiseizure medications.

Recommendations

Prophylaxis with phenytoin; loading dose of 20 mg/kg and maintenance dose of 5 to 7 mg/kg/day.

VII. HYDROCEPHALUS

Hydrocephalus after SAH is not unusual and is reported in up to 20% or more of cases and it is one cause of secondary deterioration [75,76]. Hydrocephalus can develop suddenly, particularly if there is intraventicular hemorrhage, and may cause stupor or coma. Symptoms are most often gradual in onset and include increase in headache followed by a progressive deterioration in the level of consciousness.

Some have advocated delay in the treatment of hydrocephalus for 24 hours and this approach is warranted in the patient who has headache but is otherwise alert [77]. Head CT scanning offers a method to serially follow patients, especially those with hydrocephalus on the admission CT scan. If an increase in the size of lateral ventricles correlates with progressive obtundation in the previously alert patient, then specific therapy can be initiated. In some cases it is unclear whether the level of consciousness is a reflection of the initial hemorrhage or from secondary obstruction of CSF flow. This is particularly true in the patient who presents in coma after SAH and a CT scan demonstrates intraventricular blood and some degree of ventricular enlargement. Intervention is indicated in the patient presenting in coma or the patient who becomes progressively obtunded.

Removal of CSF lowers the intracranial pressure resulting in an increased transmural pressure gradient across an aneurysm. Nornes [78] measured epidural pressure in 29 patients and found an increased risk of rerupture of an aneurysm as the intracranial pressure decreased towards normal. An external ventricular drain (EVD) would hasten this pressure normalization and increase the risk of rebleeding in the unclipped aneurysm [76]. In those patients who had early surgical obliteration of an aneurysm, EVD and the removal of large volumes of CSF was associated with a high incidence of delayed ischemic deficits [79]. Meningitis or ventriculitis may complicate the use of an EVD in up to 10% of patients if the drain is in place for 4 days or longer [76].

Patients with obstructive hydrocephalus with secondary deterioration in their level of consciousness or who are in coma on admission should be considered for an external ventricular drain. If there is no improvement in the level of consciousness in 24 hours in a comatose patient then there is little to be gained from prolonged drainage [76]. If there is nonobstructive hydrocephalus then lumbar puncture is a safe method to assess the clinical response to the removal of spinal fluid [77].

Recommendations

Head CT scan; if hydrocephalus then EVD (consider lumbar puncture if nonobstructive hydrocephalus); if no improvement in 24 hours removal of the drain may be warranted.

VIII. CARDIAC ARRHYTHMIAS

Changes on the electrocardiogram (ECG) are not uncommon after subarachnoid hemorrhage. The changes most often found are repolarization abnormalities with T-wave inversions and nonspecific S-T wave changes [80–82]. In a series of patients reported by Brouwers et al. the ECG abnormalities in individual patients were found to change with serial tracings [82]. Prolonged recording utilizing Holter monitoring has detected arrhythmias in 64 out of 70 patients after SAH and the arrhythmias were life threatening in 41% [83]. Ventricular fibrillation, ventricular flutter, and torsades de pointe have been documented after subarachnoid hemorrhage [82–84]. Despite the frequency of ECG abnormalties there is no good correlation between ECG changes and abnormal 2-D echocardiograms or thallium perfusion studies [85,86].

The cause of arrhythmias after SAH is unclear but is most likely due to increased sympathetic tone [81,87]. Subendocardial necrosis and other evidence of myocardial ischemia/injury have been documented at postmortem [81,82] and may be the result of increased sympathetic tone or adrenergic storm. Functional compromise of myocardial performance on echocardiography correlates with the clinical grade of the patient [83]; however, abnormal myocardial perfusion does not [86].

All patients are at risk for potentially fatal cardiac arrhythmias following SAH and prudent management requires close observation. Cardiac monitoring either in an intensive care unit or a step-down bed with portable cardiac monitoring equipment is a reasonable management approach. Prophylactic treatment for tachyarrhythmias with beta-blockade is not warranted; however, if tachyarrhythmias develop, then treatment with propranolol or esmolol is appropriate. Cardiac monitoring allows early detection and treatment of malignant arrhythmias that may occur, and prompt response and treatment may prevent episodes of sudden death.

Recommendations

Baseline ECG; cardiac monitoring in a step-down unit or ICU; treat arrhythmias as they occur (Advanced Cardiac Life Support protocols).

IX. OTHER MANAGEMENT ISSUES

A. Blood Pressure

There is no concensus on the appropriate blood pressure for a patient following aneurysmal subarachnoid hemorrhage. Of concern is that elevation of the blood pressure may precipitate rebleeding; whereas, cerebral ischemia may result from inadequate perfusion pressure if blood pressure is tightly controlled [88,89]. In general maintaining the mean arterial blood pressure at 105 to 110 mm Hg is well tolerated by patients. Significant elevations to systolic pressures of greater than 180 mm Hg or diastolic pressures of 100 to 105 mm Hg in unclipped aneurysms may require treatment to prevent the risk of rebleeding.

Often the increased blood pressure is a response to pain or bladder distension and analgesics or bladder drainage may be all that is required. If pharmacologic treatment is needed then labatolol as a bolus of 5 to 10 mg or an infusion of 0.5–2 mg/min should be instituted. The short-acting beta-blocker esmolol, is an alternative therapy. To mitigate against the risk of cerebral infarction, patients should be euvolemic if blood pressure is treated.

B. Pulmonary Complications

Pulmonary complications with the ictus caused by aspiration of oral secretions or gastric contents are not uncommon. Patients may be intubated or drowsy thereby compromising the natural respiratory defense mechanisms that normally prevent aspiration pneumonia. A chest roentgenogram should be standard for all patients admitted to the hospital. If fever develops or infiltrates appear on the chest film then antibiotics should be initiated after appropriate cultures.

In most cases of community-acquired aspiration pneumonitis, penicillin is the drug of first choice. Clindamycin is an appropriate alternative. The culture results, bacterial sensitivities, and the patient's response will subsequently guide selection of antibiotics.

Because of enforced bedrest, patients are at risk for deep venous thrombosis and pulmonary emboli. Sequential compression garments for the lower extremities and support hose should be standard care for these patients. Nusing care should incorporate passive range of motion for the upper and lower extremities every nursing shift.

C. Nutrition

Critically ill patients have increased caloric demands. Nutritional requirements should be assessed early and appropriate nutritional support instituted. Awake and alert patients with little risk for aspiration are able to take food orally. Obtunded patients and those in coma should receive nutrition preferably by way of a soft enteral feeding tube passed beyond the gastric pylorus. Parenteral nutrition is an alternative, but in most patients this form of nutrition is not necessary.

D. Pain Control and Patient Comfort

It is essential to manage pain in patients after subarachnoid hemorrhage. In some cases this is not the elimination of pain but rather the control of pain. Simple measures, such as frequent turning and position changes while in bed and providing analgesics, should be part of the overall patient care plan. Acetaminophen, 325 mg; codeine, 30 mg orally or intravenously; or a combination tablet of acetaminophen/codeine may be given every four to six hours. In some cases morphine sulfate, 2 mg intravenously, is necessary. If patients complain of pain then scheduled medication is preferable to an as-needed order.

Often pain control will eliminate surges in the blood pressure and reduce anxiety and patient agitation. If the patient remains agitated or has labile blood pressure after medication, then causes other than pain should be investigated (VSP, hyponatremia, hydrocephalus, rebleeding).

Efforts should be made to provide a restful environment for patients. Visits from family members should be brief and limited to two at a time. Stool softeners, antacids, and possibly H_2 blockers should be provided. If patients complain of photophobia with their headache then a darkened room is appropriate. Patients may require supplemental oxygen, which can be delivered by nasal cannula or face mask. If there are symptoms of cerebral ischemia then supplemental oxygen is mandatory with the goal of maintaining the partial pressure of oxygen greater or equal to 100 mm Hg.

X. CONCLUSION

Experimental research and clinical investigations will continue to advance our understanding of the complex pathophysiology of subarachnoid hemorrhage. These endeavors will provide new therapies, and perhaps in the future current practices will be discarded as detrimental or ineffective and they will be replaced by new innovative techniques that will provide improved neurological outcomes. Patients surviving SAH have the potential to return to productive activity and the medical management of these patients must be constantly reassessed and refined to provide that opportunity.

REFERENCES

1. Phillips LH, Whisnant JP, O'Fallon WM, Sundt TM Jr. The unchanging pattern of subarachnoid hemorrhage in a community. *Neurol* 1980; 30:1034–1040.
2. Pakarinen S. Incidence aetiology and prognosis of primary subarachnoid hemorrhage: a study based on 589 cases diagnosed in a defined urban population during a defined period. *ACTA Neurol Scand (Suppl)* 1967; 29:1–28.
3. Ropper AH, Zervas NT. Outcome one year after subarachnoid hemorrhage from cerebral aneurysm. Management, morbidity, mortality and functional status in 112 consecutive good–risk patients. *J Neurosurgery* 1984; 60:909–915.
4. Deruty R, Patet GD, Mottolese C, Portilla F. Long–term outcome of the management of ruptured intracranial aneurysm. *Neurol Res* 1988; 10:217–220.
5. Stenhouse LM, Knight RG, Longmore BF, Bishara SN. Long–term cognitive deficits in patients after surgery on aneurysms of the anterior communicating artery. *J Neurol Neurosurg Psychiatry* 1991; 54:909–914.
6. Shepard RH. Prognosis of spontaneous (nontraumatic) subarachnoid hemorrhage of unknown cause. A personal series 1958–1980. *Lancet* 1984; 1:777–779.
7. Hopkins CA, Wilke FL, Voris DC. Extramedullary aneurysm of the spinal cord. *J Neurosurgery* 1966; 24:1021–1023.
8. Hochberg FH, Fischer CM, Roberson GH. Subarachnoid hemorrhage caused by rupture of of a small superficial artery. *Neurol* 1974; 24:319–321.
9. Garun CA, Dulcey S, Dulcey J. Ruptured aneurysm of the spinal artery of Adamkiewicz during pregnancy. *Neurol* 1979; 29:394–398.
10. Sarnes M, Rose GC. Clinical presentation of ruptured intracranial aneurysm. *J Neurol Neurosurg Psychiatry* 1967; 30:67–70.
11. Fischer CM. Clinical syndromes in cerebral thrombisis, hypertensive hemorrhage and ruptured sacular aneurysm. *Clin Neurosurgery* 1975; 22:117–147.
12. Hart RC, Byer JA, Slaughter JL, Hewett JE, Easton JD. Occurrence and implication of seizures in subarachnoid hemorrhage due to ruptured intracranial aneurysm. *Neurosurgery* 1981; 8:417–421.
13. Hunt WE, Hess RM. Surgical risk as related to time of intervention in the repair of intracranial aneurysms. *J Neurosurgery* 1968; 28:14–20.

14. Drake CG, Hunt WE, Sano K, Kassell N, Teasdale G, Pertuiset B, Devillers JC. Report of the World Federation of Neurological Surgeons comittee on a universal subarachnoid hemorrhage grading scale. *J Neurosurgery* 1988; 68:985–986.
15. van Gijn J, van Dongen KJ. The time course of aneurysmal hemorrhage on computed tomograms. *Neuroradiol* 1982; 23:153–156.
16. Fischer CM, Kistler JP, Davis JM. Relation of cerebral vasospasm to subarachnoid hemorrhage visualized by computed tomographic scanning. *Neurosurgery* 1980; 6:1–9.
17. Mizukami M, Takemae T, Tazawa T, Kawase T, Matsuzuki T. Value of computed tomography in the prediction of cerebral vasospasm after aneurysm rupture. *Neurosurgery* 1980; 7:583–586.
18. Kistler JP, Crowell RM, Davis KR, Heros R, Ojemann RG, Zervas T, Fischer CM. The relation of cerebral vaspasm to the extent and location of subarachnoid blood visualized by CT scan: a prospective study. *Neurol* 1983; 33:424–436.
19. Soderstrom CE. Diagnostic significance of CSF spectrophotometry and compute tomography in cerebrovascular disease. A comparative study in 231 cases. *Stroke* 1977; 5:606–612.
20. Kassell NF, Torner JC. Aneurysmal rebleeding: a preliminary report from the Cooperative Aneurysm Study. *Neurosurgery* 1983; 13:479–481.
21. Hikdra A, Verneulen M, van Gijn J, van Creval H. Rerupture of intracranial aneurysm: a clinical pathological study. *J Neurosurgery* 1987; 67:29–33.
22. Inagawa T, Kamiya K, Ogasawara H, Yano T. Rebleeding of ruptured intracranial aneurysm in the acute stage. *Surg Neurol* 1987; 28:93–99.
23. Aoyagi N, Hayakawa I. Analysis of 223 ruptured intracranial aneurysms with special referince to rerupture. *Surg Neurol* 1984; 21:455–462.
24. Mullan S, Dawkey J. Antifibrinolytic therapy for intracranial aneurysm. *J Neurosurgery* 1968; 28:21–23.
25. Norlen G, Thulin CA. The use of antifibrinolytic substance on ruptured intracranial aneurysms. *Neurochirurgia* 1969; 12:100–102.
26. Ramirez-Lassepas M. Antifibrinolytic therapy in subarachnoid hemorrhage caused by ruptured intracranial aneurysm. *Neurol* 1981; 31:316–322.
27. Sengupta RP, So SC, Villarejo-Ortega FJ. Use of epsilon aminocaprocic acid (EACA) in the preoperative management of ruptured intracranial aneurysms. *J Neurosurgery* 1976; 44:479–484.
28. Shucurt WA, Hussain DK, Cooper PR. Epsilon–aminocaproic acid and recurrent subarachnoid hemorrhage. A clinical trial. *J Neurosurgery* 1980; 53:28–31.
29. Nibbelink DQ, Torner JC, Henderson WG. Intracranial aneurysms and subarachnoid hemorrhage. A cooperative study in recent onset subarachnoid hemorrhage. *Stroke* 1975; 6:622–629.
30. Vermeulen M, Lindsay KW, Murray GD, Cheah F, Hijdra A, Muizelar JP, Schcnong M, Teasdale GM, van Creval H, van Gijn J. Antifibrinolytic therapy in subarachnoid hemorrhage. *N Eng J Med* 1984; 311:432–437.
31. Kassell NF, Torner JC, Adams HP Jr. Antifibrinolytic therapy in the acute period following aneurysmal subarachnoid hemorrhage. Preliminary observation from the Cooperative Aneurysm Study. *J Neurosurgery* 1984; 61:225–230.

32. Wijdicks EFM, Hason D, Lindsay KW, Brouwers PSAM, Hatfield R, Murray GD, van Gijn J, Vermeulen M. Short–term tranexamic acid in aneurysmal subarachnoid heorrhage. *Stroke* 1989; 20:1674–1679.
33. Wijdicks EFM, Verneulen M, Hijdra A, van Gijn J. Hyponatremia and cerebral infarction in patients with ruptured intracranial aneurysms: is fluid restriction harmful. *Ann Neurol* 1985; 17:137–140.
34. Diringer M, Ladenson PW, Stern BJ, Schleiner J, Hanley DF. Plasma atrial natriuretic factor and subarachnoid hemorrhage. *Stroke* 1988; 19:1119–1124.
35. Heros RC, Kistler JP. Intracranial aneurysm: an update. *Stroke* 1983; 14:628–631.
36. Lester M, Nelson PB. Neurological aspects of vasopressin release and syndrome of inappropriate secretion of antidiuretic hormone. *Neurosurgery* 1981; 8:735–740.
37. Cort JH. Cerebral salt wasting. *Lancet* 1954; 1:752–754.
38. Rosenfeld JV, Barnett GH, Sila CA, Little JR, Bravo EL, Beck GJ. The effects of subarachnoid hemorrhage on blood and CSF atrial natriuretic factor. *J Neurosurgery* 1989; 71:32–37.
39. Wijdicks EFM, Ropper AH, Hunnicutt EJ, Richardson HS, Nathanson JA. Atrial natriuretic factor and salt wastin after aneurysmal subarachnoid hemorrhage. *Stroke* 1991; 22:1519–1524.
40. Wijdicks EFM, Vermeulen M, van Brummelen P, Den Boer NC, van Gijn J. Digoxin–like immunoreactive substance in patients with aneurysmal subarachnoid hemorrhage. *Br Med J* 1987; 294:729–732.
41. Maroon JC, Nelson PB. Hypovolemia in patients with subarachnoid hemorrhage. Therapeutic implications. *Neurosurgery* 1979; 4:223–226.
42. Solomon RA, Post KD, McMurtry JC III. Depression of circulating blood volume in patients after subarachnoid hemorrhage: implication for the managenent of symptomatic vasospasm. *Neurosurgery* 1983; 15:354–361.
43. Mason DT, Bartles FC. Autonomic regulation of blood volume. *Anesthesiology* 1968; 29:681–692.
44. Wijdicks EFM, Vermeulen M, van Brummelen P, van Gijn J. The effects of fludrocortisone acetate on plasma volume and natriuresis in patients with aneurysmal subarachnoid hemorrhage. Clin Neurol Neurosurgery 1988; 90:209–214.
45. Hasan D, Lindsay KW, Wijdicks EFM, Murray GD, Brouwers PJAM, Bakker WH, van Gijn J, Vermeulen M. Effects of fludrocortisone acetate in patients with subarachnoid hemorrhage. *Stroke* 1989; 20:1156–1161.
46. Heros RC, Zerval NT, Varsos V. Cerebral vasospasm after subarachnoid hemorrhage: an update. *Annals Neurol* 1983; 14:599–608.
47. Kassell NF, Sasaki T, Colohan ART, Nazar G. Cerebral vasospasm following aneurysmal subarachnoid hemorrhage. *Stroke* 1985; 16:562–572.
48. Fletcher TM, Taveras JM, Pool JL. Cerebral vasospasm in angiography for intracranial aneurysm: incidence and significance in one hundred consecutive angiograms. *Arch Neurol* 1959; 1:38–47.
49. Weir B, Grace M, Hansen J, Rothberg C. Time course of vasospasm in man. *J Neurosurgery* 1978; 48:173–179.
50. Graf CJ, Nibblelink DW. Cooperative study of intracranial aneurysms and subarachnoid hemorrhage. *Stroke* 1974; 5:559–601.

51. Hijdra A, van Gijn J, Nugelkerke NJD, Vermeulen M, van Creval H. Prediction of delayed cerebral ischemia, rebleeding and outcome after aneurysmal subarachnoid hemorrhage. *Stroke* 1988; 19:1250–1256.
52. Aaslid R, Markwalder TM, Nornes H. Noninvasive transcranial Doppler ultrasound recording of flow velocity in basal cerebral arteries. *J Neurosurgery* 1982; 57:769–774.
53. Seiler RW, Grolimund P, Aaslid R, Huber P, Nornes H. Cerebral vasospasm evaluated by transcranial ultrasound with clinical grade and CT–visualized subarachnoid hemorrhage. *J Neurosurgery* 1986; 64:594–600.
54. Grosset DG, Straiton J, du Trevou M, Bullock R. Prediction of symptomatic vasospasm after subarachnoid hemorrhage by rapidly increasing trascranial Doppler velocity and cerebral blood flow changes. *Stroke* 1992; 23:674–679.
55. Fischer CM, Robertson GH, Ojemann RG. Cerebral vasospasm with ruptured saccular aneurysm: the clinical manifestations. *Neurosurgery* 1977; 1:245–248.
56. Soloman RA, Fink ME, Lennihan L. Prophylactic volume expansion therapy for the prevention of delayed cerebral ischemia following early aneurysm surgery: results of a preliminary trial. *Arch Neurol* 1988; 45:325–332.
57. Allen GS, Ahn HS, Preziosi TJ, Battye R, Boone SC, Chou SN, Kelly DC, Weir BK, Crabbe RA, Lavik PJ, Rosenbloom SB, Dorsey FC, Ingram CR, Mellits DE, Bertsch LA, Boisevert DPJ, Hundby MB, Johnson RK, Strom JA, Transon CR. Cerebral arterial spasm: a controlled trial of nimodipine in patients with subarachnoid hemorrhage. *N Eng J Med* 1983; 308:619–624.
58. Ohman J, Servo A, Heiskanen. Long–term effects of nimodipine on cerebral infarcts and outcome after aneurysmal subarachnoid hemorrhage and surgery. *J Neurosurgery* 1991; 74:8–13.
59. Petruk KC, West M, Mohr G, Weir BKA, Benoit BG, Gentili F, Disney LB, Khan MI, Grace M, Holness RO, Karwon MS, Ford RM, Cameron GS, Tucker WS, Purves GB, Miller JDR, Hunter KM, Richard MT, Durity FA, Chan R, Clein LJ, Maroon FB, Gordon A. Nimodipine treatment in poor–grade aneurysm patients. Results of a multicenter double–blind placebo–controlled trial. *J Neurosurgery* 1988; 68:505–517.
60. Pickard JD, Murray GD, Illingworth R, Shaw MDM, Teasdale GM, Foy PM, Humphrey PRD, Lang DA, Nelson R, Richards P, Sinar J, Barley S, Skene A. Effect of oral nimodipine on cerebral infarction and outcome after subarachnoid hemorrhage: British aneurysm nimodipine trial. *Br Med J* 1989; 298:636–642.
61. Auer LM, Oberbauer RW, Schalk HV. Human pial vascular reaction to intravenous nimodipine infusion during EC–IC bypass surgery. *Stroke* 1983; 114:210–213.
62. Dorsch NWC, Branston NM, Harris RJ. An experimental study of the effects of nimodipine in primate subarachnoid hemorrhage. *ACTA Neurchir* 1989; 99:65–75.
63. Fujita S, Kawaguchi T, Shose Y, Urui S. Flunarizine treatment in poor–grade aneurysm patients. *ACTA Neurochir* 1990; 103:11–17.
64. Beck DW, Adams HP, Flamm ES, Godashy HC, Loftus CM. Combination of aminocarrocic acid and nicardipine in the treatment of aneurysmal subarachnoid hemorrhage. *Stroke* 1988; 19:63–67.

65. Vollar DG, Kassell NF, Hongok, Ogawa N, Tsakahura T. Effect of the nonglicocorticoid 21–aminosteroid U74006F on experimental cerebral vasospasm. *Surg Neurol* 1989; 31:190–193.
66. Zuccarello M, Marsch J, Schmitt G, Woodward J, Anderson DK. Effect of the 21 aminosteroid U–74006F on cerebral vasospasm following subarachnoid hemorrhage. *J Neurosurgery* 1989; 71:98–104.
67. Chyatte D, Fode NC, Nichols DA, Sundt TM Jr. Preliminary report: effects of high dose methylprednisolone on delayed cerebral ischemia in patients at high risk for vasospasm after aneurysmal subarachnoid hemorrhage. *Neurosurgery* 1987; 21:157–160.
68. Peterson JW, Nischizawa S, Hackett JD, Bun T, Teramura A, Zervas NT. Cyclosporine A reduces vasospasm after subarachnoid hemorrhage in dogs. *Stroke* 1990; 21:133–137.
69. Ruba M, Pastuszko M, Iwarska K, Bidzinski J, Dziewiecki C. Cyclosporine A prevents neurological deterioration of patients with SAH: a preliminary report. *ACTA Neurochir* 1991; 112:25–27.
70. Zabramski JM, Spetzler RF, Belerson JB. Phase I trial of tissue plasminogen activator for the prevention of vasospasm in patients with aneurysmal subarachnoid hemorrhage. *J Neurosurgery* 1991; 75:189–196.
71. Ohman J, Servo A, Heiskanen O. Effects of intrathecal fibrinolytic therapy on clot lysis and vasospasm in patients with aneurysmal subarachnoid hemorrahge. *J Neurosurgery* 1991; 75:197–210.
72. Keranen T, Tapaninaho A, Hernesniemi J, Vapalahti M. Late epilepsy after aneurysm operation. *Neurosurgery* 1985; 17:897–900.
73. Sbeih I, Tamar LB, O'Laoine SA. Epilepsy after operation for aneurysm. *Neurosurgery* 1986; 19:784–788.
74. Ohman J. Hypertension as a risk factor for epilepsy after aneurysmal subarachnoid hemorrhage and surgery. *Neurosurgery* 1990; 27:578–581.
75. van Gijn J, Hijdra A, Widdicks EFM, Vermeulen M, van Creval H. Acute hydrocephalus after aneurysml subarachnoid hemorrhage. *J Neurosurgery* 1985; 63:355–362.
76. Rajshekhan V, Harbaugh RE. Results of routine ventriculostomy with external ventricular drainage for acute hydrocephalus following subarachnoid hemorrhage. *ACTA Neurochir* 1992; 115:8–15.
77. Hasan D, Verneulen M, Wijdicks EFM, Hijdra A, van Gijn J. Management problems in acute hydrocephalus after subarachnoid hemorrhage. *Stroke* 1985; 20:747–755.
78. Nornes H. The role of intracranial pressure in arrest of hemorrhage in patients with ruptured intracranial aneurysms. *J Neurosurgery* 1973; 39:226–234.
79. Kasuya H, Shimizu T, Kagawa M. The effects of continous drainage of cerebral spinal fluid in patients with subarachnoid hemorrhage: a retrospective analysis of 108 patients. *Neurosurgery* 1991; 28:56–59.
80. Galloon S, Rees GAD, Briscoe CE, Davis S, Kilpatrick GS. Prospective study of electrocardiographic changes associated with subarachnoid hemorrhage. *Brit J Anaesthesia* 1972; 44:511–517.

81. Marion DW, Segal R, Thompson ME. Subarachnoid hemorrhage and the heart *Neurosurgery* 1986; 18:101–106.
82. Brouwers PJAM, Wijdicks EFM, Hasan D, Vermeulen M, Wever EFD, Frericks H, van Gijn J. Serial electrocardiographic recording in aneurysmal subarachnoid hemorrhage. *Stroke* 1989; 20:1162–1167.
83. Andreoli A, diPasquale G, Pinelli G, Grazi P, Tognetti F, Testa C. Subarachnoid hemorrhage: frequency and severity of cardiac arrhythmias. A survey of 70 cases studied in the acute phase. *Stroke* 1987; 18:558–564.
84. Estanol BV, Badui Degal E, CAserman E, Marin OSM, Coyo M, Vargas-Lugo B, Pertez-Ortega R. Cardiac arrhythmia associated with subarachnoid hemorrhage: prospective study. *Neurosurgery* 1979; 5:657–679.
85. Davies KR, Gelb AW, Manninen PH, Boughner DR, Bisnaire D. Cardiac function in aneurysmal subarachnoid hemorrhage: A prospective study of electrocardiographic and echocardiographic abnormalities. *Brit J Anaesthesia* 1991; 67:58–63.
86. Szabe MD, Crosby G, Hurfod WE, Strauss HW. Myocardial perfusion following acute subarachnoid in patients with abnormal electrocardiograms. *Anesth Analg* 1993; 76:253–258.
87. Cruickshank JM, Neil-Dwyer G, Degaute JP, Hayes Y, Kuurne T, Kytta J, Vincent JL, Carruthers ME, Patel S. Reduction of stress catecholamine–induced cardiac necrosis by beta–selective blockade. *Lancet* 1987; 2:585–589.
88. Wijdicks EFM, Vermeulen M, Murray GD, Hijdra A, van Gijn J. The effects of treating hypertension following aneurysmal subarachnoid haemorrhage. *Clin Neurol Neurosurgery* 1990; 92:111–117.
89. Britton M, deFaire U, Helmers C. Hazards of therapy for excessive hypertension in acute stroke. *ACTA Med Scand* 1980; 207:253–257.

13
Medical Management of Vasospasm

J. R. Fulgham
Mayo Clinic, Rochester, Minnesota

I. INTRODUCTION

A dreaded complication after a subarachnoid hemorrhage (SAH) is delayed neurologic deterioration from focal or diffuse narrowing of the major intracranial arteries. This phenomenon, vasospasm (VSP), affects one third of the patients following SAH and results in death or permanent disability in up to 14% of those afflicted [1,2]. Vasospasm may be defined as neurological deterioration that is not due to hydrocephalus, hyponatremia, or rebleeding; vasospasm is neurological deterioration in the presence of angiographically demonstrated narrowing of the intracranial arteries after the exclusion of other causes of delayed neurological decline. This chapter will discuss the medical management of VSP in patients after subarachnoid hemorrhage, first identifying patients who may be at increased risk of developing arterial spasm and second proposing an approach toward medical therapy.

II. PREDICTING AND MONITORING THE AT-RISK PATIENT

Vasospasm occurs most often between days 2 to 17 following the ictus with the peak incidence on days 7 to 12 [3]. The signs and symptoms exhibited by patients are often subtle and nonspecific. Initially there may be confusion, agitation, and altered sensorium. Mild motor deficits such as pronator drift and a decrease in the alternating motion rate may be noted. These deficits may fluctuate, persist, or progress to paralysis, coma, or death [4]. The common usage of short-acting benzodiazepines and anesthetics in the intensive care unit may mask early cognitive difficulties, and anesthetic agents, such as propofol, may obscure the neurological examination entirely. In these situations little confidence can be placed on the physical examination to detect early VSP and other techniques must be relied upon.

Because of the presence of subarachnoid blood, all patients are at risk for VSP after a subarachnoid hemorrhage; however, this risk is not shared equally among patients. Due to the significant morbidity associated with VSP it is extremely important to identify those patients at high risk for developing symptomatic vasospasm. The admission head computerized tomography (CT) scan, invaluable in diagnosing SAH, has proven useful in predicting patients who are at highest risk for the development of vasospasm [5–7]. In a retrospective study, Fisher et al. [5] found a high correlation between the onset of severe VSP and the presence of subarachnoid clot greater than 5×3 mm in area in the cisterns and fissures in the horizontal plane or clots greater than 1 mm thick in the vertical plane. Application of these criteria in a prospective study of 41 patients with verified aneurysmal SAH successfully predicted VSP in 20 of 22 patients felt to be at high risk based on clot thickness [7]. Using CT critera, patients can be placed into groups (Table 1) with those in group 3 at highest risk for vasospasm (Figure 1).

Transcranial Doppler (TCD) ultrasonography, developed by Aaslid et al. [8], is a noninvasive method for measuring the flow velocities in the basal cerebral arteries, which perhaps finds its greatest utility in monitoring patients for VSP after subarachnoid hemorrhage [9].

Blood flow velocities increase in areas of stenosis and this phenomenon is characteristic of stenosis whether from atherosclerosis or from spasm of the artery. In a study of 34 consecutive patients by Sloan et al. [10], the specificity of TCD in the detection of VSP was 100%, whereas the sensitivity for detection of VSP in the same study was significantly lower at 59%. There are a number of reasons for the false negative results, such as operator skill, suboptimal acoustic

Table 1 Localization of Blood on the CT Scan After Subarachnoid Hemorrhage and the Prediction of Vasospasm

Group	Subarachnoid blood	Risk of VSP
1	None	−
2	Diffuse only	−
3	Clot or thick layer	+
4	Blood in lateral ventricles	−

Source: Ref. 7.

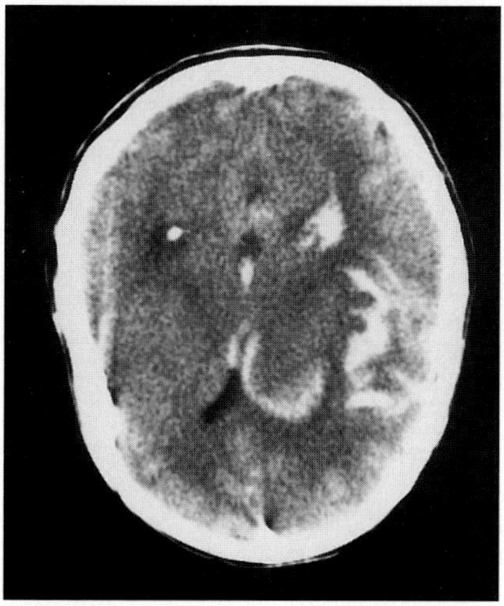

Figure 1 A 51-year-old man was found unconscious at home. A head CT scan on admission to hospital demonstrated a subarachnoid hemorrhage with thick clot in the cisterns, interhemispheric fissure, and the left sylvian fissure (Group 3, Table 1). The patient regained consciousness and a dense right pareisis present on admission improved. Five days later his neurological status deteriorated and a second head CT scan was done. This study demonstrated ischemic infarction from vasospasm. The patient expired.

windows, increased intracranial pressure, and VSP in arteries that can not be insonnated with transcranial Doppler [9].

Predicting vasospasm based on increasing velocites over time is also possible. Grosset et al. [11] found that an increase in the mean flow velocity of 50 cm/sec in a 24-hour period would reliably foretell the occurrence of VSP, and the velocity change correlated with decreased blood flow in the appropriate vascular territory.

Despite the limitations of TCD, this method is an important adjunct for identifying VSP noninvasively and making management decisions in patients after subarachnoid hemorrhage.

Clinically suspected vasospasm in the absence of Doppler verification requires a cerebral angiogram. A grading system for the severity of VSP based on the presence of luminal narrowing in the middle cerebral artery present at angiography (Table 2) has been devised by Fisher et al. [4].

Recommendations

Admission head CT scan; if neurological deterioration then a repeat CT is urgent; TCD as a baseline and then daily during the period of greatest risk

Table 2 Grading of Vasospasm on the Basis of Angiographic Criteria

Fisher grade	MCA diameter	Severity of VSP
0	3–5 mm	—
1	minimal vessel changes	mild
2	lumen narrowed; ≥1.0 mm	mild
3	lumen 0.5–1.0 mm; delayed flow	moderate
4	lumen <0.5 mm; flow almost halted	severe

Source: Ref. 4.

for VSP; cerebral angiography if vasospasm is suspected and TCD is negative; bed in an intensive care unit; frequent neurological examinations.

III. HYPERVOLEMIA-HYPERTENSION-HEMODILUTION

When symptomatic VSP develops, the therapeutic goal is to maintain cerebral perfusion and hopefully prevent infarction. Adequate blood flow to the brain depends on cerebral perfusion pressure (CPP), which is directly related to the mean arterial blood pressure (MAP) and the intracranial pressure (ICP).

$$\text{CPP} = \text{MAP} - \text{ICP}$$

Cerebral perfusion can be improved by manipulating the variables in the above equation. Lowering the ICP does improve cerebral perfusion pressure and blood flow; however, in patients with SAH the drainage of large volumes of spinal fluid to improve cerebral perfusion has been asociated with an increased incidence of delayed ischemic deficits [12]. This can not, therefore, be recommended as standard practice.

The most successful therapy currently available for maintaining cerebral perfusion is to increase cardiac output with volume expansion and blood pressure elevation. Hypervolemia, hypertension, and hemodilution—Triple-H therapy—has become the mainstay for the treatment of symptomatic vasospasm. This approach theoretically improves blood flow to ischemic brain tissue and prevents infarction. Although there is animal and human data that would dispute that this therapy increases blood flow [13,14], nevertheless Triple-H therapy has been effective in improving outcome in patients with VSP after subarachnoid hemorrhage [15–17].

Triple-H therapy should be initiated with specific measurable goals in mind. The obvious goal is amelioration of neurological symptoms; however, based on risk for the development of VSP predicted from the CT scan, TCD, and the presence of symptoms, a specific blood pressure or central venous pressure may be the appropriate therapeutic goal. These parameters must be individually decided for each patient.

Volume expansion should be the initial step in this protocol. Periodic infusions of 5% albumin is an excellent volume expander and avoids excessive free water from crystalloid solutions, which may exacerbate cerebral edema [18]. Other colloid agents that may be used are Plasmanate, dextran, or Hetastarch [19]. To meet daily fluid requirements crystalloid solutions will be necessary and normal saline with 20 mEq of potassium per liter should be used. With volume expansion the central venous pressure may be increased to 10 to 12 mm Hg but should be titrated to the clinical response.

Volume expansion alone is often sufficient to increase the MAP from 10 to 15 mm Hg above the patient's baseline. Symptomatic patients can be exquisitely sensitive to blood pressure and deficits may resolve with increased blood pressure only to recur if the blood pressure decreases. If neurologic deficits persist after addition of volume or the blood pressure does not increase, then vasopressor agents such as phenylepherine hydrochloride or dopamine should be used. The blood pressure can then be titrated upward to ameliorate the symptoms of cerebral ischemia. In a patient with an unclipped aneurysm, increasing the systolic blood pressure beyond 150 mm Hg may increase the risk of rebleeding. This risk of rebleeding must be weighed in face of the present danger of ischemic infarction due to vasospasm.

Hematocrit will decline with volume expansion. The hematocrit that has been felt to be optimum is in the range of 33% to 37% [20,21] and some have advocated venesection if the hematocrit is not at the prescribed range in the first 12 to 24 hours of Triple-H therapy [22]. The advantage of decreasing the hematocrit as a treatment for cerebral ischemia has not been proven [23]; however, blood rheology and oxygen delivery is improved with the hematocrit in the 33% to 37% range [21]. A hematocrit of less than 33% diminishes oxygen delivery and may exacerbate cerebral ischemia [20]. If the hematocrit is below 33% then transfusion of packed red blood cells is indicated.

Constant monitoring of the electrocardiogram, blood pressure, and central venous pressure are mandatory during Triple-H therapy. In patients with cardiopulmonary disorders, a pulmonary artery catheter should be placed with the goal of a pulmonary capillary wedge pressure of 12 to 16 mm Hg. Supplemental oxygen by nasal cannula or face mask should be provided to all patients to maintain the partial pressure of oxygen at 100 mm Hg. Patients unable to protect their airway should be intubated. Bedside pulse oximetry should be available for monitoring oxygen saturation. Daily weights and strict monitoring of fluid input and output are necessary to facilitate monitoring of the patient's fluid status.

The results of treatment protocols employing Triple-H therapy have been impressive. Kassell et al. [24] treated 58 patients with symptomatic VSP (verified on a cerebral angiogram) and had permanent improvement in 43. Failure to improve was felt to be due to initiation of treatment after infarction had occurred, relentless progression of VSP, or failure of the blood pressure to increase. In the series reported by Awad et al. [19], sustained improvement of symptoms from delayed cerebral ischemia was obtained in 60% of the patients. In the latter series, as in that reported by Kassell [24], patients began Triple-H therapy only after the onset of ischemic symptoms.

Solomon et al. [17] and Origitano et al. [22] intiated treatment, prophylactically, prior to the onset of symptoms in all patients with subarachnoid hemorrhage. Solomon reported on 56 patients treated on a protocol that required initiation of volume expansion and blood pressure elevation early on. Ten of the patients developed delayed cerebral ischemia from VSP; however the symptoms were totally reversed in six [17]. Of the 43 patients reported by Origitano [22], cerebral infarcts due to vasospasm were present in two patients.

When to initiate Triple-H therapy is problematic as the treatment is not without possible morbidity. Pulmonary edema is not uncommon [24] and may precipitate respiratory failure. Strict monitoring of the hemodynamic parameters and pulmonary artery catheterization in patients with prexisting cardiac or pulmonary disease should substantially reduce this complication [19]. Hemothorax, pneumothorax, and line infection [22,24] are other complications that are the direct result of the necessary invasive monitoring required for successful Triple-H therapy. Other complications attributed to Triple-H therapy are dilutional hyponatremia, coagulopathy, myocardial infarction, and aneurysmal rebleeding [22,24].

A rational approach to managing a patient after SAH is given in Figure 2. Maintaining euvolemia is essential in all patients, however those considered to be at high risk for VSP may benefit from gentle volume expansion while monitoring closely for signs and symptoms of delayed cerebral ischemia. If such symptoms develop, then escalation of therapy is appropriate. Obliteration of the aneurysm allows greater latitude for aggressively treating patients with Triple-H therapy [19]. Transcranial Doppler and the amount of blood on the head CT scan can be useful in anticipating which patients may require more aggressive management.

Ischemia from VSP may damage the blood–brain barrier, which can result in increased intracranial pressure, and volume expansion may further exacerbate intracranial hypertension and promote ischemic cerebral injury [25]. Intracranial pressure monitoring should therefore be performed in patients for whom intracranial hypertension is considered to be an issue. If the intracranial pressure is increased, treatment with an osmotic agent such as mannitol should begin [24].

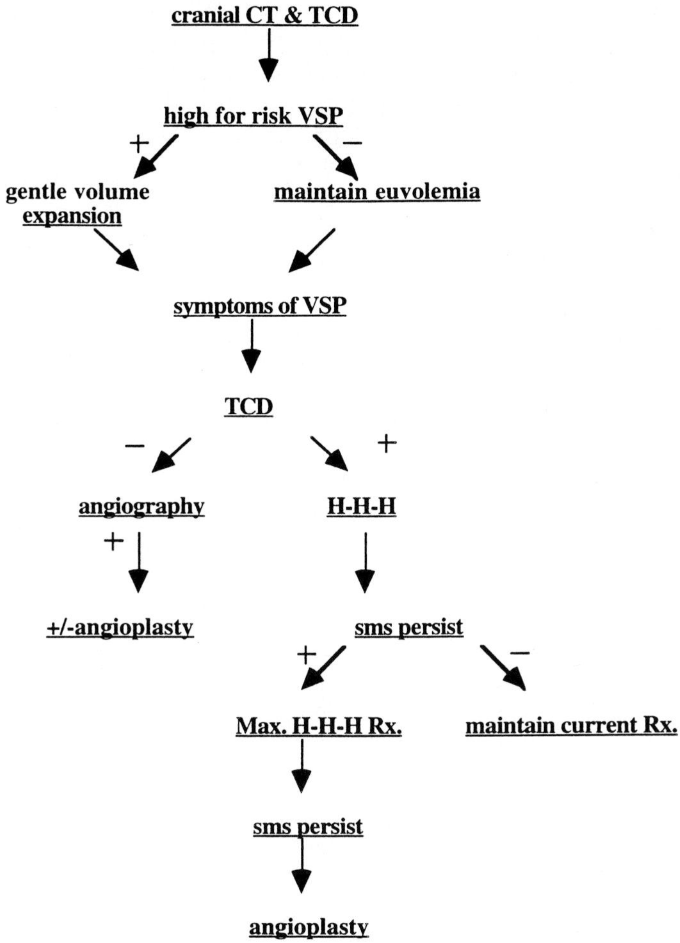

FIGURE 2 Approach to the management of a patient after subarachnoid hemorrhage.

IV. ENDOVASCULAR TREATMENT OF VASOSPASM

Despite the effectiveness of volume expansion, hypertension, and hemodilution for the treatment of sympatomatic vasospasm, there are patients in whom the neurologic deficits progress relentlessly despite maximum medial therapy. In those patients, mechanical dilitation of the stenotic arterial segment is an option.

Translumal angioplasty as an effective treatment for VSP after aneurysmal SAH was first reported in 1984 by Zubov et al. [26]. In 33 patients with symptomatic VSP they found long-lasting restoration of neurologic function. Other centers have reported improved neurologic function in approximately 70% of treated patients [27,28]. This technique holds great promise in the treatment of medically refractory VSP but clearly requires centers with specialists proficient in endovascular techniques.

V. CONCLUSION

Patients who have survived the initial insult from a ruptured cerebral aneurysm are a select group of patients. Unfortunately approximately one-third will develop symptomatic vasospasm and delayed neurologic deficits. All who care for these patients have known bitter disappointment when all efforts to reverse the effects of VSP are unsuccessful. It is hoped that early recognition of patients at particularly high risk for vasospasm, early intervention, and continued research into the pathophysiology of cerebral arterial vasospasm will result in improved clinical outcomes.

REFERENCES

1. Heros RC, Zervas NT, Varsos V. Cerebral vasospasm after subarachnoid hemorrhage: an update. *Annals Neurol* 1983; 14:599–608.
2. Kassel NF, Sasaki T, Colohan ART, Nazar G. Cerebral vasospasm following aneurysmal subarachnoid hemorrhage. *Sroke* 1985; 16:562–572.
3. Weir B, Grace M, Hansen J, Rothberg C. Time course of vasospasm in man. *J Neurosurgery* 1978; 48:173–179.
4. Fisher CM, Robertson GH, Ojemann RG. Cerebral vasospasm with ruptured saccular aneurysm: the clinical manifestations. *Neurosurgery* 1977; 1:245–248.
5. Fisher CM, Kistler JP, Davis JM. Relation of cerebral vasospasm to subarachnoid hemorrhage visualized by computed tomographic scanning. *Neurosurgery* 1980; 6:1–9.
6. Mizukami M, Takemae T, Tazawa K, Kawase T, Matsuzuki T. Value of computed tomography in the prediction of cerebral vasospasm after aneurysm rupture. *Neurosurgery* 1980; 7:583–586.
7. Kistler JP, Crowell RM, Davis KR, Heros R, Okemann RG, Zervas NT, Fisher CM. The relation of cerebral vasospasm to the extent and localization of subarachnoid blood visualized by CT scan: a prospective study. *Neurol* 1983; 33:424–436.
8. Aaslid R, Markwalder TM, Nornes H. Noninvasive transcranial Doppler ultrasound recording of flow velocity in basal cerebral arteries. *J Neurosurgery* 1982; 57:769–774.

9. Seiler RW, Grolimund P, Asslid R, Huber P, Nornes H. Cerebral vasospasm evaluated by trascranial ultrasound with clinical grade and CT–visualized subarachnoid hemorrhage. *J Neurosurgery* 1986; 64:594–600.
10. Sloan MA, Haley EC Jr, Kassell NF, Henry ML, Stewart SR, Beskin RR, Sevilla EA, Torner JC. Sensitivity and specificity of transcranial Doppler ultrasonography in the diagnosis of vasospasm following subarachnoid hemorrhage. *Neurol* 1989; 39:1514–1518.
11. Grosset DG, Straiton J, du Trevou M, Bullock R. Prediction of symptomatic vasospasm after subarachnoid hemorrhage by rapidly increasing trascranial Doppler velocity and cerebral blood flow changes. *Stroke* 1992; 23:674–679.
12. Kasuya H, Shimizu T, Kagawa M. The effects of continuous drainage of cerebral spinal fluid in patient with subarachnoid hemorrhage: a retrospectove analysis of 108 patients. *Neurosurgery* 1991; 28:56–59.
13. Yanakami I, Isobek K, Yamaura A. Effects of intravascular volume expanison on cerebral blood flow in patients with ruptured cerebral aneurysm. *Neurosurgery* 1987; 21:303–309.
14. Davis DH, Sundt TM. Relationship of cerebral blood flow to cardiac output, mean arterioa blood pressure, blood volume, and alpha and beta blockade in cats. *J Neurosurgery* 1980; 52:745–754.
15. Giannotta SL, McGillicudy JE, Kindt GW. Diagnosis and treatment of postoperative vasospasm. *Surg Neurol* 1977; 8:286–290.
16. Tanabe T, Saitoh T, Tachibana S, Tukagi H, Yada K. Effect of hyperdynamic therapy on cerebral ischemia caused by vasospasm associated with subarachnoid hemorrhage. *ACTA Neurchir* 1982; 63:291–296.
17. Solomon RA, Fink ME, Lennihan L. Early aneurysm surgery and prophylactic hypervolemic hypertensive therapy for the treatment of aneurysmal subarachnoid hemorrhage. *Neurosurgery* 1988; 23:699–704.
18. Heros RC, Korosue K. Hemodilution for cerebral ischemia. *Stroke* 1989; 20:423–427.
19. Awad IA, Carter P, Spetzler RF, Medina M, Williams FW Jr. Clinical vasospasm after subarachnoid hemorrhage: response to hypervolemia hemodilution and arterial hypertension. *Stroke* 1987; 18:365–372.
20. Kee DB, Wood JH. Rheology of the cerebral circulation. *J Neurosurgery* 1984; 15:125–131.
21. Wood JH, Kee DB. Hemorheology of the cerebral circulation in stroke. *Stroke* 1985; 16:765–762.
22. Origitano TC, Wascher TM, Reichman H, Anderson D. Sustain increased cerebral blood flow with prophylactic hypertensive hypervolemic hemodilution ("Triple–H Therapy") after subaracnnoid hemorrhage. *Neurosurgery* 1990; 27:729–740.
23. Italina Stroke Study Group. Haemodilution in acute stroke: results of the Italian haemodilution trial. *Lancet* 1988; 13:318–321.
24. Kassell NF, Peerless SJ, Durwood QJ, Beck DW, Drake CG, Adams HP. Treatment of ischemic deficits from vasospasm with intravascular volume expansion and induced arterial hypertension. *Neurosurgery* 1982; 11:337–342.
25. Voldby B, Enevoldsen EM, Jensen FT. Regional CBF, intraventricular pressure, and cerebral metabolism in patients with ruptured intracranial aneurysms. *J Neurosurgery* 1985; 62:48–58.

26. Zubov YN, Nikiforov VM, Shustin VA. Balloon catheter technique for dilatation of constricted cerebral arteries after aneurysmal SAH. *ACTA Neurochir* 1984; 70:65–79.
27. Barnwell SL, Higashida RT, Halbach VV, Dowd CF, Wolson CV, Hieshima GB. Transluminal angioplasty of intracerebral vessels for cerebral arterial spasm: reversal of neurological deficits after delayed treatment. *Neurosugery* 1989; 25:424–429.
28. Eskridge JM, Newell DW, Pendleton GA. Transluminal angioplasty for treatment of vasospasm. *Neurosurg Clin North Am* 1990; 1:387–395.

14
Surgery of Intracranial Aneurysms

Akio Morita
George Washington University, Washington, D. C.

Michael R. Puumala, Fredric B. Meyer, and Nicolee C. Fode
Mayo Clinic, Rochester, Minnesota

I. INTRODUCTION

Early descriptions of intracranial aneurysms can be found in ancient Egyptian, Greek, and Arabic literature [1–3]. Although the first successful treatment of a cerebral aneurysm was reported in the early 1800s [3,4], good systematic treatment could not be achieved until the advent of modern neurosurgical techniques, which first evolved in Dandy's era [5]. Perhaps the greatest advance in the treatment of intracranial aneurysms was the introduction of the operating microscope and microneurosurgical techniques [6,7]. More recently, understanding the pathophysiology of these lesions along with their potential complications including posthemorrhage vasospasm and hydrocephalus had led to significant improvements in surgical results. Currently, there are multiple modalities to treat cerebral aneurysms including various surgical approaches, different types of aneurysm clips, bypass surgery, and more recently endovascular techniques.

The incidence of intracranial aneurysms is estimated at 1–8% of the general population according to autopsy and angiographic series [8–12]. The most common presentation is subarachnoid hemorrhage (SAH) with an incidence of 10–15 per 100,000 population each year [10,13] or 1–1.5% per year of known aneurysm patients [14,15]. The outcome from a subarachnoid hemorrhage is disappointing with 8–60% of patients dying before reaching the hospital [10,13,16,17]. After admission to the hospital, the mortality is 37% and the severe disability is 17% with a favorable outcome achieved in only 47% of patients assessed 3 months postoperatively according to the Cooperative Study

[18]. In addition, two-thirds of patients who are treated successfully never return to the same quality of life as prior to the SAH [19]. Despite tremendous effort to improve the outcome following SAH, the overall mortality has not been significantly reduced over the last 30 years because of the difficulty in reducing both the number of deaths prior to hospitalization and the number of poor-grade patients who have suffered severe brain injury from the initial hemorrhage [13]. Despite these pessimistic facts, aggressive management can salvage many patients with severe neurological injury following the SAH by preventing rerupture of the aneurysm, attenuating the severity and sequela of vasospasm, and reducing surgical complications [20,21].

II. PATHOGENESIS

Since the incidence of idiopathic intracranial aneurysms is age dependent [22] and there are reports of de novo development of aneurysms and growth of aneurysms [23–27], intracranial aneurysms can be considered acquired lesions [12,15,28]. Supporting this acquired theory is the observation that aneurysms typically develop at branching points of major arteries where the hemodynamic stress forces are greatest. It is also probable that there are genetic influences that contribute to the development of intracranial aneurysms, as evidenced by some familial cases of intracranial aneurysms [29,30], and associations with certain pathologies such as polycystic kidney disease [31]. In addition, Type III collagen deficiency is noted to have a strong relationship with aneurysm formation [32]. Therefore, the etiology of idiopathic aneurysms should be considered multifactorial with the following factors contributing to their evolution: 1. developmental defects of the arterial wall that may be affected by genetic factors; 2. hypertension or hemodynamic stress; and 3. atherosclerosis, especially in the development of fusiform or giant ectatic aneurysms [33].

There are several medical conditions that are associated with intracranial aneurysms. Approximately 10–30% of patients with polycystic kidney disease have an intracranial aneurysm [31]. Abnormalities in the arterial wall are known to accompany this disease, along with a high incidence of hypertension. Fibromuscular dysplasia is also associated with intracerebral aneurysms. Hemodynamic stress can be a major etiology of aneurysms in cases with intracranial arteriovenous malformations, moyamoya disease [34,35], unilateral carotid occlusion or agenesis [36], or coarctation of the aorta. Diseases that have defects in the arterial wall may also have cerebral aneurysms such as Ehlers-Danlos, Marfans' syndrome, and pseudoxanthoma elasticum [37].

Other acquired pathologies that damage the arterial wall such as infection, neoplasm, or trauma can lead to the development of cerebral aneurysms. These etiologies usually result in aneurysms in the periphery of a major cerebral artery as opposed to the typical location along the circle of Willis. Though rare, severe trauma associated with a skull-base fracture can result in development of an aneurysm in the petrous segment of the internal carotid artery [38].

III. CLINICAL PRESENTATIONS AND PATHOPHYSIOLOGY

Intracranial aneurysms can present in many different ways. Aneurysms without any presenting symptoms are termed asymptomatic aneurysms. Notably, asymptomatic aneurysms should be differentiated from unruptured aneurysms, since aneurysms can cause symptoms without rupture and these symptoms are important warning signs that can be useful in the detection of an aneurysm prior to a disastrous hemorrhage. The rate of rupture is higher in aneurysms that are symptomatic. In one study with a 5-year follow-up, 26% of patients with symptomatic unruptured aneurysms died of SAH, compared to 2.6% of patients with asymptomatic aneurysms [18]. The clinical presentations of cerebral aneurysms are summarized as follows.

A. Subarachnoid Hemorrhage or Other Intracranial Hemorrhage

The most common presentation of an intracranial aneurysm is subarachnoid hemorrhage, which is the first manifestation in 90% of cases [39]. In addition, most (>80%) nontraumatic subarachnoid hemorrhage is caused by aneurysmal rupture. Patients typically complain of "the worst headache of my life," which may or may not be associated with nausea and vomiting. Patients with a severe SAH rapidly deteriorate to a comatose state or have a respiratory arrest from extremely high intracranial pressure, which induces a profound reduction in cerebral perfusion pressure. Of note, approximately 40–50% of patients have been reported to experience warning signs caused by a minor leak or expansion of the aneurysm prior to rupture [40,41]. These warning signs are often followed by aneurysm rupture in 10–20 days.

The prognosis of subarachnoid hemorrhage is quite dependent on the presenting clinical status (consciousness and neurological deficit), which is a good indicator of the severity of the initial brain injury. Damage to the brain by subarachnoid hemorrhage is not caused by mass effect but rather by the initial impact of high intracranial pressure. Therefore, dramatic improvement after removing pure subarachnoid clot or decompression is rare. There have been many approaches to grading the severity of SAH on a clinical basis. For exam-

Table 1 Subarachnoid Hemorrhage Grading Systems

Clinical grade (modified Botterell)	
0	Nonruptured or no SAH in past 30 days.
1	With or without mild headache, alert, oriented, no motor or sensory deficits.
2	Severe headache and major meningeal signs, mild alteration in sensorium or focal deficits.
3	Major alteration in sensorium or a major focal deficit.
4	Semicomatose or comatose, with or without major lateralizing findings

Clinical grade (Hunt and Hess)	
0	Nonruptured.
1	Asymptomatic or minimal headache and slight nuchal rigidity.
2	Moderate to severe headache, nuchal rigidity, no neurologic deficit (other than cranial nerve palsy).
3	Drowsiness, confusion, or mild focal deficit.
4	Stupor, moderate to severe hemiparesis, possibly early decerebrate rigidity and vegetative disturbances.
5	Deep coma, decerebrate rigidity, moribund appearance.

Clinical Grade (WFNS)	Glasgow coma scale	Motor deficit
1	15	Absent
2	13–14	Absent
3	13–14	Present
4	7–12	Absent or present
5	3–6	Absent or present

ple, grading systems such as the World Federation of Neurologic Surgeons (WFNS) [42], Hunt and Hess [43], or Botterell system [44] have correlated well with outcome (Table 1). According to Phillips [13] in the Olmsted County, Rochester, Minnesota, group of patients who present to the Mayo Clinic, approximately 48% will be clinical grade Hunt and Hess 1 and 2, 20% will be Grade 3, and 30% will be Grade 4 and 5. Each hospital or referral center may have a different percentage of clinical grades depending on that institution's referral pattern [45].

Other factors that influence the outcome following SAH include delayed cerebral arterial vasospasm, hydrocephalus, and aneurysm rerupture. There have been several reports that have classified SAH on computerized tomography (CT) appearance in an attempt to predict the incidence of cerebral vasospasm

Table 2 Fisher CT Scan Classification for SAH

Group 1	No blood detected
Group 2	Diffuse deposition on thin layer with all vertical layers of blood (interhemispheric fissure, insular cistern, ambient cistern) less than 1 mm
Group 3	Localized clot and/or vertical layers of blood 1 mm or greater in thickness
Group 4	Diffuse or no subarachnoid blood, but with intracerebral or intraventricular clots

Source: Ref. 46.

(Table 2) [46]. The Fisher Group 3 patients have a statistically significant higher risk (96%) of developing symptomatic vasospasm compared to the other groups.

These clinical and CT grading systems are useful in the decision as to the indications and timing of surgery. Other factors that are considered in this decision include the location and size of the aneurysm and the patient's overall general medical condition.

Other types of hemorrhage associated with aneurysms include intracerebral or intraventricular hemorrhage. These hemorrhages can be decompressed by surgery, ventricular drainage and the use of tissue plasmin activator (tPA), or urokinase irrigation [47] with greater ease than a pure subarachnoid hemorrhage. The damage to the brain from a cerebral hemorrhage may be reversible depending on its location and size. In fact, surgical removal of an intracerebral clot or placement of an external ventricular drain may lead to dramatic improvement in the clinical grade.

B. Post-SAH Complications

Post SAH complications include 1. rerupture, 2. hydrocephalus, and 3. delayed cerebral arterial vasospasm with ischemic neurological deficits. These complications are discussed extensively in other chapters but will be mentioned here for completeness.

1. Rerupture

This is the most dreaded complication in the early phase of SAH management. The greatest risk for rerupture is in the first 24 hours (4.1%) and then decreases to 1.5% per day for the next 13 days. The cumulative risk of rerupture is 19% in 14 days, 40–50% overall at 6 months, and then 3% per year thereafter [14,48]. The reported mortality from rerupture is as high as 78% [39,49]. The fear of early rerupture is the primary motivation for considering early surgical intervention.

2. Hydrocephalus

This problem occurs in the acute phase as well as in the chronic phase following SAH. Hydrocephalus in the acute phase is caused by blockage of the ventricular system or cisterns by blood clot [50]. It is seen in 10–30% of patients with SAH by CT scan; 30–40% of those are symptomatic [51,52]. In symptomatic cases, external ventricular drainage should be performed to prevent further neurological deterioration. In general terms, patients with acute hydrocephalus have a poor prognosis compared to those without enlarged ventricles [51]. When placing an external ventricular drain prior to repair of the aneurysm, the surgeon must be careful not to drain too much cerebrospinal fluid (CSF) for fear of removing a tamponade effect and leading to a risk of aneurysm rerupture.

Hydrocephalus in the chronic phase following SAH is caused by scarring of the arachnoid granules with disturbances in CSF absorption. It is seen in 10–15% of post-SAH patients [52–54]. These patients may present with a normal-pressure hydrocephalus syndrome including incontinence, gait instability, and cognitive deterioration. The CT or magnetic resonance imaging (MRI) scan will typically show enlarged ventricles including the 4th ventricle and probable transependymal CSF absorption. The treatment for chronic post-SAH hydrocephalus is placement of a permanent ventricular shunt [53,55].

3. Delayed Cerebral Arterial Vasospasm

This is the phenomenon in which major cerebral vessels constrict 3–9 days after the SAH [56,57]. The pathophysiology of post-SAH vasospasm is still not well defined despite intensive investigation for over three decades [58–61]. The instigators of vasospasm are the products of blood-clot lysis in the subarachnoid space including oxyhemoglobin, leukotrienes, and arachidonic acid. Nutritional deficits of the arterial wall in the basal cisterns have also been proposed to be a cause of vasospasm. From the surgical perspective, the incidence and severity of vasospasm is clearly related to the amount of subarachnoid or periarterial blood as demonstrated by Fisher [46,62].

The incidence of this phenomenon by angiogram is reported to be 30–70% and is symptomatic in 20–30% with a permanent morbidity of 10–20% (mortality 7%, severe morbidity 7%) [58].

C. Mass Effect

A secondary common presentation of intracranial aneurysms is mass effect, which occurs in approximately 10% of patients. The aneurysm that presents with mass effect is typically large; however, even small aneurysms can exert pressure against the adjacent neural structures [18]. The symptoms may include retro-orbital pain, a third-nerve palsy, cavernous sinus syndromes, hydrocephalus, visual-field deficits, mild to moderate hemiparesis, or hypothalamic-pituitary dysfunction. If the aneurysm enlarges rapidly over a short period of time, it can cause pain by stretching the arterial wall or adjacent dura. Although these signs can be a significant problem in themselves for the patient, they also forewarn that there is an increased risk for rupture in the near future [3]. Accordingly, immediate surgical intervention is indicated.

D. Embolus

Intracranial aneurysms, especially partially thrombosed giant or fusiform aneurysms, can occasionally be the source of a cerebral embolus [63,64]. The treatment in this situation is difficult since anticoagulation, although the primary treatment for a cerebral embolus, is contraindicated in a cerebral aneurysm. In addition, treatment of a fusiform or partially thrombosed giant aneurysm is often difficult. Often these aneurysms require bypass surgery with trapping of the aneurysm.

IV. CLASSIFICATION OF INTRACRANIAL ANEURYSMS

Intracranial aneurysms are classified by 1. etiology, 2. size, 3. location, and 4. shape. All of these factors are important in deciding the appropriate treatment.

A. Etiological Classification of Aneurysms

As reviewed in the preceding paragraphs on pathogenesis, aneurysms can be caused by multiple etiologies and classified accordingly.

1. Idiopathic

These aneurysms are related in some way to a combination of abnormalities in the arterial wall, perhaps influenced by both genetic factors and hemodynamic stresses. Advanced age, hypertension, and smoking can be risk factors for the development of aneurysms.

2. Aneurysms Associated with Specific Medical Conditions

Polycystic kidney disease, fibromuscular dysplasia, coarctation of aorta, connective tissue diseases, arteriovenous malformations, moyamoya disease, and unilateral carotid or vertebral occlusion or agenesis can be associated with intracranial aneurysms. These aneurysms are at similar locations to those of idiopathic aneurysms.

3. Miscellaneous Causes that Affect the Arterial Wall

Trauma, metastatic neoplasms, or septicemia can induce aneurysm formation. These aneurysms are typically located in peripheral arteries and are fusiform in shape. At surgery, there is often no neck that can be clipped and therefore the diseased segment of artery with aneurysm must be resected and possibly reconstructed.

B. Aneurysm Size

Aneurysm size is categorized by the largest diameter of the dome as 1. saccular—less than 1.5 cm, 2. globular—1.5–2.5cm, and 3. giant—greater than 2.5 cm [3]. The size of an aneurysm is important in the decision to consider treatment of unruptured aneurysms since there is some evidence that small aneurysms are at decreased risk for hemorrhage. Alternatively, giant aneurysms require special surgical considerations due to factors such as the presence of a calcified neck, thrombus, and the location of major arteries and perforators in relationship to the aneurysm neck.

C. Location of Aneurysms

Intracranial aneurysms are usually located at the bifurcation of major circle of Willis arteries because of hemodynamic stresses. The location of aneurysms from major cooperative studies are as follows: internal carotid artery (ICA) in 41%, anterior communicating/anterior cerebral artery (AComA/ACA) in 34%, middle cerebral artery (MCA) in 20%, vertebrobasilar artery (VBA) in 4%, and other locations in 1% [18]. Autopsy studies have noted locations as ICA in 24%, ACA/AComA in 30%, MCA in 33%, and VBA in 12% [12]. Multiple cerebral aneurysms are seen in approximately 20% of patients [12,65].

D. Shape of Aneurysms

This classification is strongly related to the etiology of the aneurysm and has important implications regarding surgical accessibility.

1. Saccular Aneurysm

This shape is the most common observed in clinical practice. By definition, this type of aneurysm should have a well-defined neck and aneurysm dome. However, in some situations, especially with giant aneurysms, the neck may be obscured and sometimes involve the parent artery [3,66]. Most idiopathic aneurysms are of the saccular type.

2. Fusiform Aneurysm

These are primarily caused by atherosclerosis similar to that observed in aortic aneurysms. Trauma, infection, or tumor can occasionally result in the development of a fusiform aneurysm.

These two categories above make up the majority of aneurysms that are approached surgically. However, the following two categories below may also occur and have important surgical implications.

3. Dissecting Aneurysms

These are intraluminal dissections of arteries and are quite rare in the intracranial vasculature. Typically, dissecting aneurysms are seen in the extracranial internal carotid or vertebral arteries and usually present with ischemic events. There are some rare reports of intracranial dissecting aneurysms. They appear to be more common in the posterior circulation as opposed to the anterior circulation. They often present with hemorrhage. At surgery, these aneurysms are a purplish, fusiform dilatation of the parent artery [67].

4. False Aneurysm

Although this is not a category by shape, it may be included in this classification. Except for some dissecting aneurysms, the three shapes mentioned above are usually true aneurysms that involve some component of the arterial wall in the aneurysm dome. However in false aneurysms, there is no definite wall except for reactive connective tissue or blood clot. False aneurysms are usually due to trauma but occasionally occur from infection or a tumor. Special care is required at surgery since these aneurysms can rupture easily and also are difficult to repair without sacrificing or reconstructing the parent artery (see Illustrative Case 4 below).

V. PRESURGICAL ASSESSMENT

A. General Assessment

Since cardiac and pulmonary function can be altered by a subarachnoid hemorrhage [68–70], all patients should have electrocardiogram and arterial blood-gas monitoring. In many patients, it may be necessary to monitor parameters such as pulmonary-wedge pressure, central venous pressure, and cardiac output through a Swan–Ganz catheter. The optic fundi should be examined for the existence of subretinal hemorrhage, which occurs in 10% of patients and may require ophthalmological care to prevent vision loss [71].

B. Neurological Assessment

A full neurological baseline examination is mandatory, along with close follow-up examinations, to detect early evidence of complications such as the development of hydrocephalus, vasospasm, or rerupture of the aneurysm. The current SAH grading scales are listed in Table 1. However, minor neurological changes such as mood, mentation, psychological alterations (euphoria or depression), or very subtle weakness are important findings to detect early development of arterial vasospasm. Prompt response to these findings may be a key factor to improve the outcome from SAH induced vasospasm [58,72,73].

A lumbar puncture to examine the cerebrospinal fluid is still a useful method to diagnose SAH especially in those patients in which a CT scan is negative. Accordingly, in a patient who presents with symptoms that suggest a warning leak, CSF examination may be fruitful.

C. Radiological Assessment

A transfemoral cerebral angiogram is currently the gold standard for the diagnosis of intracranial aneurysms. The angiogram provides important information regarding location, size, direction of the aneurysm dome and neck and relationship with the parent vessel and perforators. To visualize the aneurysm neck, multiple-angle views are helpful. Furthermore, a follow-up angiogram after surgical intervention is useful to detect and evaluate for possible delayed arterial vasospasm and to confirm that the aneurysm has been obliterated with good clip placement.

Transcranial doppler is useful in detecting the development of arterial vasospasm. It may also be a helpful monitoring therapy once vasospasm has developed [74].

A CT scan is important to establish the diagnosis of SAH. The amount of subarachnoid blood in the basal cisterns is a good predictor of the risk for development of delayed arterial spasm (Table 2). A CT scan will disclose intracerebral hemorrhage or early hydrocephalus if present. The CT scan may also detect calcification of the aneurysm neck and thrombus, both of which have important surgical implications.

The magnetic resonance imaging (MRI) scan is evolving into an important diagnostic tool for the patient with a cerebral aneurysm. Currently, it will detect with a high reliability aneurysms that are greater than 5 mm in size. This may be especially useful for following a patient who has a small, unruptured aneurysm. The MRI scan is also helpful in demonstrating the degree of intramural thrombus in giant aneurysms [75].

A trial balloon occlusion of the parent artery during the diagnostic angiogram can be quite important in the preoperative surgical planning, especially in giant or fusiform aneurysms. It may be necessary to trap these aneurysms since a neck may not be accessible for clipping. A trial balloon occlusion is a good assessment of the potential for collateral blood flow. If the trial balloon occlusion suggests that the patient will not tolerate parent vessel occlusion, then a bypass procedure during aneurysm treatment will be necessary.

VI. SURGICAL INDICATIONS

There are many factors that are important to consider when determining if an aneurysm should be surgically treated. Currently, the most important issue is whether the aneurysm has ruptured or whether it is asymptomatic. Other important factors include accessibility of the aneurysm for surgical repair, configuration and size of the aneurysm neck, the presence of thrombus, and the relationship of the neck of the aneurysm to the parent artery and perforators. The patient's age and general medical condition are also important considerations.

A. Ruptured Aneurysms

In the better grade patients such as WFNS Grade 1–3, surgery is strongly indicated since the risk of rebleed with associated morbidity and mortality is exceedingly high compared to the surgical risk. In poor-grade patients, some clinicians question the value of surgical intervention since the patient's outcome is poor regardless of treatment. In our institution, poor-grade patients are not excluded from surgery unless they are brain dead. It is important to emphasize that although a patient may arrive in the emergency room in a comatose, moribund state, they may benefit dramatically, with significant improvement in their clinical grade, after placement of an external ventricular drain if the CT scan shows acute hydrocephalus.

B. Unruptured Symptomatic Aneurysms

Surgery for this type of aneurysm is typically recommended since, as mentioned earlier, these symptoms are often disabling and are a warning sign for rupture in the near future. However, most of these aneurysms are large or giant in size and the risk of surgery is accordingly higher than that for a small saccular aneurysm. This increased surgical risk needs to be recognized both by the surgeon and the patient in order to make the appropriate therapeutic decision.

C. Asymptomatic Aneurysms

Surgery for this group of patients has been controversial for decades [15,76,77]. The comparison between risks of surgery versus the natural history of unruptured aneurysms is critical in making the appropriate decision for this group. Unruptured aneurysms are reported to rupture at approximately 1–1.4% rate per year [14,15]. The risk of aneurysm rupture also increases with size, although a critical size in relationship to increased risk of rupture is still unknown. The consensus thus far is that the risk of rupture for aneurysms larger than 1.0 cm is greater than the risk of surgery, if the surgery is performed in patients under the age of 65 [77]. Although some natural history studies suggest that the risk for rupture of an aneurysm under 1.0 cm is small, many surgeons do operate on small aneurysms based on the intraoperative observation that most aneurysms that have ruptured are under 1.0 cm in size.

VII. TIMING OF SURGERY FOR RUPTURED INTRACRANIAL ANEURYSMS

The timing of surgery after subarachnoid hemorrhage has been a debated issue over the last three decades [72,73,78,79]. Currently, the decision to operate should be based on the clinical grade of subarachnoid hemorrhage, the location of the aneurysm, and the patient's medical condition. The advantages and disadvantages of early versus delayed surgery are listed in Table 3.

For better grade patients (WFNS Grade 1–2), several early cooperative studies demonstrated a superior outcome for delayed surgery [18]. Although the surgical outcome in these preceding studies was better with late surgery, approximately 30% of patients did not survive until surgery [78,79]. In prospective studies from Sweden, early surgery offered the best opportunity for a good recovery (81%) in better grade patients (Hunt and Hess Grades 1–3 [80]. Although some data suggests that surgery performed between the 4th and 7th days has a poor outcome, thought to be due to an aggravation of cerebral vasospasm, data from the Mayo Clinic did not confirm this finding (Table 4). Therefore, our current approach is to operate on all patients in good grade as soon as possible, irrespective of the date from hemorrhage, in the hope of decreasing the risk of rerupture since rehemorrhage is associated with a high mortality. The one exception to this general rule is posterior circulation aneurysms, especially those of the basilar tip. Surgery for aneurysms in this location often requires significant brain retraction for exposure. It may be advantageous to delay surgery for several days to allow for the initial edema after the SAH to decrease.

Table 3 Timing of Surgery: Advantage and Disadvantages

Early Operation (within 3 days)
Advantage
Prevention of rebleeding
Amelioration of vasospasm by removal of subarachnoid clot
Prevention and treatment of ischemic complications
Prevention of medical complication
Psychological factors
Shorter hospitalization
Disadvantage
Brain is tight & swollen
High risk for intraoperative rupture
Delayed Operation (after 11 days)
Advantage
Brain slackness
Ease of dissection
Opportunity to monitor patients
Flexibility of scheduling
Disadvantage
Rerupture
Difficult to manage if spasm developed
Adhesions around aneurysm

For intermediate grade patients (WFNS Grade 3) the timing of surgery is controversial. Data from our institution did not show any difference in mortality or morbidity between early or delayed surgery for this group of patients. A recent report from a group in Japan demonstrated a benefit of early surgery in grade 3–4 patients [81].

For poor grade patients (WFNS Grade 4–5), it is difficult to decide if and when surgery should be performed since the overall outcome is poor, with or without surgical intervention. If a patient in a poor grade improves with conservative treatment, then a more aggressive approach would be pursued. In addition, if the patient has an intraparenchymal or intraventricular hemorrhage that is causing mass effect, then early surgical decompression, aneurysm clipping, and placement of a ventricular drain should be considered. Although the overall prognosis for this group of patients is poor, surgery does appear to salvage some patients and therefore, until proved otherwise, an aggressive approach should be adopted. In our experience with poor-grade patients, although there is a significant mortality, approximately 10–30% of patients have a good outcome (Table 5).

Table 4 Surgical Timing and Outcome

Grade	Grade 1				Grade 2				Grade 3				Grade 4			
timing[a]	A	B	C	D	A	B	C	D	A	B	C	D	A	B	C	D
Excellent	87%	81%	92%	85%	75%	71%	66%	65%	38%	29%	50%	30%	10%	29%	17%	8%
Good	9%	8%	5%	10%	14%	17%	17%	21%	18%	36%	20%	25%	23%	0%	25%	0%
Poor	2%	4%	2%	4%	6%	5%	9%	13%	31%	18%	24%	39%	36%	14%	42%	54%
Dead	2%	6%	1%	2%	6%	7%	8%	1%	13%	18%	7%	6%	32%	57%	17%	39%

SAH cases; Total of 1196 patients

[a] Timing A: day 0–3; B: day 4–7, C: day 8–11, D: day 12–.

Table 5 Admission Grade and Surgical Result

Admission grade (modified Botterell)	0	1	2	3	4
Hunt and Hess grade	0	1 and 2	3	4	5
Result					
Excellent	623 (83%)	534 (86%)	221 (64%)	58 (35%)	9 (14%)
Good	69 (9%)	52 (8%)	57 (17%)	41 (25%)	12 (19%)
Poor	31 (4%)	25 (4%)	47 (14%)	40 (24%)	28 (44%)
Death	28 (4%)	14 (2%)	18 (5%)	26 (16%)	14 (22%)
Total	751	625	343	165	63

VIII. SURGICAL OPTIONS: GENERAL REVIEW

Surgical techniques for the repair of intracranial aneurysms have improved tremendously with the introduction of the operating microscope, microsurgical techniques, and—more recently—interventional radiology. However, difficult cases still exist that challenge the surgical and radiological team. The current surgical options for the treatment of intracranial aneurysms are summarized as follows.

A. Direct Clipping

Currently, this is the most routine and definitive treatment for an intracranial aneurysm. With direct clipping, the aneurysm neck is obliterated by application of a aneurysm clip whose strength, shape, and size prevents blood flow into the aneurysm dome but preserves the parent artery. There are many aneurysm clips available that are reliable and have sufficient strength to achieve this goal for most aneurysms. However, when treating giant aneurysms or aneurysms that have an atherosclerotic or calcified neck, especially strong aneurysm clips are required and tandem clips or the use of booster clips are necessary. All aneurysm clips come in various sizes and shapes to allow for placement of the clip without compromise of the parent artery and perforating vessels. Since aneurysm surgery is performed in small spaces, visualization of the relationship of the clip blades and aneurysm with the perforating and parent vessel is important. To achieve this goal, curved, angled, or cut-out clips are manufactured for the surgeon's use. For giant aneurysms, it is often necessary to decompress the aneurysm sac, including thrombectomy, prior to placement of clips. Otherwise, retained thrombus in the dome may force the clip down onto the parent vessel. In cases with atherosclerotic changes in the parent vessel, preservation of these arteries may be challenging since the clip may lead to kinking of the parent vessel if applied too closely to the base of the neck of the aneurysm [82].

B. Interventional Neuroradiological Treatment

This type of treatment is evolving rapidly and over the next several years the indications for this procedure will become more clear-cut. It is reasonable to predict that endovascular treatment will play an important role in the treatment of cerebral aneurysms [83]. Since the development by Romodanov [84] and Serbinenko [85] of balloons to obliterate aneurysms, there has been a rapid evolution in techniques including the placement of platinum coils into the aneurysm dome (Guglielmi coil). Higashida [86] recently reported the outcome in 215 cerebral aneurysm cases treated by detachable balloon. Parent-vessel occlusion was performed in 59.1% and primary-aneurysm obliteration was achieved in 40.9%. The mortality was 9.8% and the stroke rate was 7.4%. More recently, Guglielmi [87,88] introduced a platinum coil electrothermocoagulation method. Although the clinical results with these Guglielmi detachable coils (GDC) are still preliminary, our clinical experience suggests that they will have a significant impact on the treatment of aneurysms. Balloons have the disadvantage of deflation, rupture, parent-artery compromise, and a water hammer effect [86,89–92]. Alternatively, Guglielmi coils eliminate some of these problems since they are soft, flexible, and induce thrombosis within the aneurysm dome. These coils can be applied or contoured to fit the configuration of the aneurysm. They have proved to be effective in the treatment of small- to large-size aneurysms with a definitive neck [93]. A recent report on coil (non-Guglielmi type) embolization of aneurysms showed an excellent outcome in 84.5% of cases at 1-year followup with a morbidity of 4.2% and mortality of 11.3% [94]. The introduction of these new treatments may affect the decision for treatment irrespective of the timing or grade of the patient. Disadvantages of endovascular treatment include the risk of stroke or hemorrhage [89,91,95]. Also, endovascular therapy may have a limited role in giant aneurysms or aneurysms with a wide neck for fear of embolization of coils and thrombus out of the aneurysm into the parent artery [96]. Since endovascular treatment with detachable coils is a relatively new technique, it will be necessary to await long-term followup before a decision can be made regarding its role for the treatment of cerebral aneurysms [97,98].

Occasionally the combination of endovascular and surgical approaches are useful in achieving the optimum results in complex cases. Accordingly, the future treatment of cerebral aneurysms will evolve into a team approach in which the surgeon and interventional neuroradiologist analyze each case to determine the optimum treatment.

Another indication for endovascular treatment is planned occlusion of the parent vessel, which can be useful in cases such as fusiform carotid cavernous aneurysms [99]. Prior to the occlusion, a trial balloon occlusion is performed to determine whether parent vessel occlusion will be tolerated. During this trial balloon occlusion, in addition to a neurological examination, blood-flow studies including SPECT scan [100] can be performed to provide useful data. In complex aneurysms in which a temporary parent-vessel occlusion is anticipated, a preoperative trial balloon occlusion provides important data.

One further radiological technique useful in the management of cerebral aneurysm patients is balloon dilatation of spastic arteries [101]. This technique can produce dramatic improvement in a patient suffering from ischemic deficits. Higashida reported neurological improvement in 69% of cases who were deteriorating [102]. Balloon dilatation of a spastic artery should be performed with caution since it can cause rupture of a vessel or embolic stroke [103]. Currently, therefore, balloon dilatation should not be performed for *asymptomatic* angiographic vasospasm.

C. Proximal Ligation or Trapping of Aneurysms With or Without Bypass

If the neck of an aneurysm is poorly defined, one option is proximal ligation of the parent vessel or trapping of the aneurysm either with surgery or through endovascular techniques. Proximal ligation has been used since the 1800s [3]. A cooperative study demonstrated a failure rate of 6–8% [18] in ruptured aneurysms. However, proximal ligation, by facilitating thrombosis, appears to be an effective treatment for giant aneurysms in the cavernous sinus and possibly other locations [104–106]. Drake has successfully treated giant basilar artery aneurysms with a tourniquet technique [107,108].

Trapping is a relatively definitive treatment for aneurysms since there is minimal perfusion to the vessel that has been trapped. In cases with cavernous or ophthalmic aneurysms, there can be collateral blood flow to the aneurysm through the ophthalmic artery. Rarely, aneurysms in other locations recruit retrograde blood supply from back flow through perforators. Failure of trapping can occur through this collateral blood flow.

In performing a trapping procedure, the major concern is the risk of ischemia to the territory of the parent vessels that will be occluded. Ligation of the internal carotid artery has been reported to cause ischemic complications in 49% of patients and 28% in common carotid ligation (30% overall) [49]. Hashi [109] reported that extracranial–intracranial (EC–IC) bypass using the superficial temporal artery did not improve this rate of ischemic complications (25% in their experience). They also found that gradual ligation using the Selverstone clamp or other techniques had an ischemic complication rate as great as that with abrupt ligation. Currently endovascular techniques allow a trial balloon occlusion to predict the risk of early ischemic complications. By using preoperative trial balloon occlusion for assessment, the surgeon can determine which patient might need a bypass graft to prevent ischemic complications. If a patient successfully passes a trial balloon occlusion, the requirement for a bypass during the trapping procedure is unlikely, although this decision must be based on each individual case. For example, if there is a small aneurysm on the contralateral side or other vessel territory that may have increased hemodynamic stress by occlusion of one vessel, bypass might be indicated to prevent enlargement or rupture of this aneurysm [23]. In addition, despite a successful trial balloon occlusion, there is the risk of late ischemic complications [110]. The ischemic complication rate by balloon occlusion after a negative trial occlusion test has been reported to be 4–5% [111,112].

When trapping an aneurysm, the surgeon must be meticulous to ensure that there is no entrapment of perforating vessels. One limitation of the balloon occlusion is that a minimum of 3–5 mm of parent artery is obliterated. Depending on the location, there may be important perforators originating from that parent artery that cannot be visualized on the angiogram. In that situation, such as that which might occur with a proximal posterior cerebral artery aneurysm, balloon occlusion would be contraindicated.

In some cases, the patient presents with deterioration due to mass effect from thrombosis of a giant aneurysm [106]. In that circumstance, after trapping of the aneurysm, decompression is performed to relieve mass effect against critical neuronal structures.

The selection for the technique of vessel obliteration depends on the skills of both the neurosurgeon and interventional radiologists. Both techniques have some risk of embolus from the stump of the artery distal to the clip or balloon. It can be difficult to differentiate between an embolus and a retrograde thrombus forming from the stump of the ligated artery [113]. It may be necessary to place a patient on heparin for the first few days after a trapping procedure if a transient neurological deficit develops. For intracranial trapping procedures, direct surgical obliteration with clips and ligatures may be preferable to ensure that no perforators are involved [107,108,114].

Fox et al. [99] reported their results of balloon occlusion of proximal vessels after a trial balloon occlusion test. In 18 cases, an EC–IC bypass was performed prior to permanent occlusion. Delayed ischemia was seen in 13.2% and permanent morbidity (major stroke) was seen in only one case. Eighty-five percent of internal carotid and 65% of VB aneurysms were thrombosed following the balloon occlusion.

With regard to bypass surgery during balloon occlusion, we typically prefer a saphenous vein interposition graft and rarely use a superficial temporal artery bypass pedicle because of its insufficient blood supply [115]. However, the superior temporal artery–middle cerebral artery bypass still has use in cases of marginal ischemia secondary to the loss of a single arterial branch. Currently, our results with vein bypass have been satisfactory in preventing ischemia with good long-term patency rates. Specifically, the patency rate at a followup of one year has been 86% in a total of 132 grafts. The long-term followup patency rate at five years was 82% and at 13 years was 73% (L. Regli and D. Piepgras, personal communication). An excellent or good result was achieved in 80% of patients with anterior circulation giant aneurysms and in 44% of patients with posterior circulation giant aneurysms. Some problems associated with a vein bypass include multiple incisions and the length of surgery, which is approximately 7–8 hours compared to an STA–MCA bypass which requires only about 3–4 hours. The complication rate is higher in a vein bypass; however, this reflects the fact that these are difficult, complicated problems. Some of the specific complications associated with a vein bypass compared to STA–MCA bypass include thrombosis at either the proximal or distal anastomosis or hemorrhage from a high-flow bypass graft. Internal carotid artery aneurysms can be bypassed from either the cervical or petrous carotid artery distal to the aneurysm in the supraclinoid carotid artery (Figure 1) [3,116,117]. If the aneurysm involves the C_2 segment of the internal carotid artery, our current choice is to perform an EC–MCA bypass to the proximal MCA-M_2 segment. In some cases, multiple bypasses are necessary to supply all major branches of the MCA. In these circumstances, the STA can be an important donor vessel. In the posterior circulation, the surgical options are more limited since there are only three vessels that are available for bypass. The occipital artery to posterior inferior cerebral artery bypass is an option for vertebral artery aneurysms although the blood supply is comparable to that achieved through an STA–MCA bypass. More often, we will perform vein bypass from the external carotid to either the posterior cerebral artery (PCA) or a superior cerebral artery as a treatment for giant basilar, vertebral, or PCA aneurysms [3,116].

D. Wrapping or Coating of Aneurysm

In some rare cases with fusiform or dissecting aneurysms, wrapping or coating might be the only option available. Coating of an aneurysm will not prevent enlargement of the aneurysm or eventual rerupture. In addition, it makes exploration of the aneurysm extremely difficult by obscuring planes and perforators as indicated in Illustrative Case 12 below.

Occasionally, when there is a small remnant of aneurysm neck after clipping, placement of some cotton or teflon around the neck will induce fibrosis and decrease enlargement of the neck of the aneurysm [82].

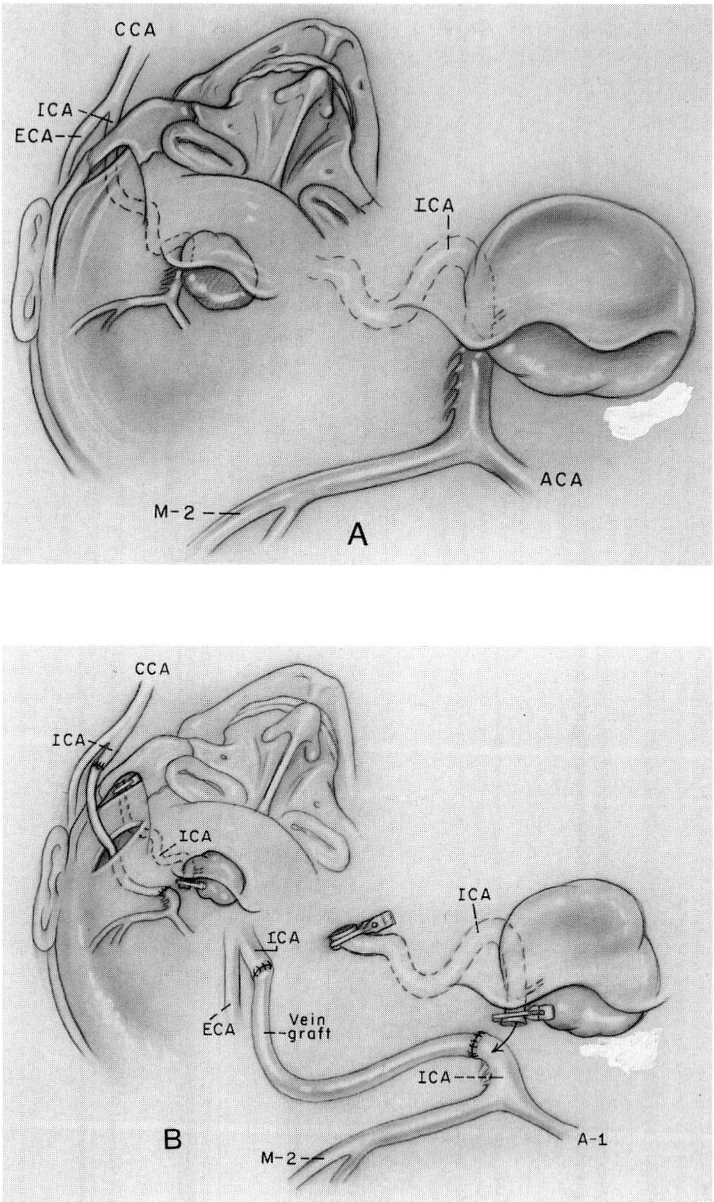

Figure 1 Saphenous vein bypass graft for a medially projecting internal carotid artery aneurysm. a) This aneurysm was arising from the ICA just distal to its anterior loop and

E. Cerebral Protection During Aneurysm Surgery

During aneurysm surgery, temporary occlusion of parent vessels is often required to decompress the aneurysm, perform a thrombectomy, or to prevent premature aneurysm rupture. Methods of protecting the brain from focal ischemia include a variety of pharmacological manipulations such as the administration of barbiturates, etomidate, and/or using mild to profound hypothermia. Some surgeons also routinely administer mannitol and vitamin E for the potential free-radical scavenging effects [118]. Most potentially neuroprotective agents that work by metabolic suppression must be administered prior to the onset of ischemia. We also utilize anesthetics to induce EEG isoelectricity as a means of providing brain protection. Another useful measure during aneurysm surgery is to combine temporary parent-vessel occlusion with hypertension and brief periods of reperfusion. This is opposite the older practice of using induced hypotension during dissection of the aneurysm [119,120]. For cases in which the aneurysm is giant and prolonged ischemia is anticipated, cardiac arrest under profound hypothermia may be beneficial [121,122].

IX. SURGICAL APPROACH AND PITFALLS FOR SPECIFIC ANEURYSMS

A. General Considerations

Details regarding surgical technique can be obtained in many superb neurosurgical textbooks [3,66,123,124]. At our institution, surgery for the routine anterior circulation aneurysm is performed via a pterional craniotomy. In rare occasions an interhemispheric approach is used in cases of an anterior communicating artery aneurysm; it is commonly used for an anterior cerebral artery-A_2 aneurysm. For posterior circulation aneurysms, the basilar caput and some basilar trunk aneurysms are approached via a modified pterional craniotomy or through a subtemporal approach. Vertebral or low basilar artery aneurysms are approached through a suboccipital route. Occasionally, we will utilize a presigmoid or transpetrous approach to the basilar trunk. In cases without

---

presented as a mass lesion in the sella. b) A saphenous vein bypass graft was placed between the intracranial internal carotid artery and the cervical internal carotid artery, and the aneurysm was treated by trapping. The intracranial anastomosis was accomplished with multiple interrupted 8–0 prolene sutures, with both the recipient and donor vessels being fishmouthed. This bypass is preferable to a bypass with one of the M_2 segments as a recipient vessel, but it is more difficult to perform because of the depth of the wound and the short segment of internal carotid artery available to the surgeon for mobilization.

intracranial hemorrhage or mass effect, a lumbar drain is placed to remove cerebrospinal fluid during surgery and to facilitate brain relaxation and dissection. Intraventricular drains can also be another option in cases of acute hydrocephalus. If there is massive intracerebral clot, then placement of a lumbar drain is contraindicated because of the risk of uncal or tonsilar herniation. Intracranial pressure can be managed by removing clot during surgery for aneurysm repair.

Dissection of the aneurysm should be performed with meticulous microsurgical techniques. Anatomical knowledge is critical for dissecting in the appropriate planes to help preserve important perforators and the surrounding neurovascular structures [125–131]. After SAH, anatomic planes are often difficult to delineate and frequent irrigation with normal saline may be useful. This use of small microdissectors, teardrop suction tips, and various retraction systems are helpful. However, brain retraction should be kept to a minimum [132]. Frequent repositioning and resting of the retractor is important to prevent retraction related injury. Intraoperative aneurysm rupture is a dreaded complication during surgery with a reported incidence of 15–30% [66,79]. Although it was usually thought to contribute to a poor prognosis, in the hands of experienced surgeons, the outcome was no different than without this complication. Newer and finer microsurgical techniques have helped decrease the risk of intraoperative rupture [66].

The most important points in the surgical repair of a cerebral aneurysm include 1. complete obliteration of the aneurysm, 2. preservation of the parent and distal vessels, and 3. preservation of perforating vessels.

B. Anterior Circulation Aneurysms

1. Aneurysms of the Internal Carotid Artery

Aneurysms of the internal carotid artery occur in 40% of patients with cerebral aneurysms. The most common location is at the junction of the internal carotid artery and posterior communicating arteries (IC-PCom). Aneurysms here are routinely approached through a pterional craniotomy with separation of the proximal Sylvian fissure. The two important perforating arteries in this region are the posterior communicating and anterior choroidal arteries. Injury to the anterior choroidal artery is unforgiving and will lead to a significant perioperative ischemic stroke. Other important arteries in this general location are the recurrent artery of Heubner, which can originate from the anterior cerebral artery, and lenticulostriates, which can originate off the proximal anterior cerebral and middle cerebral arteries.

Illustrative Case 1

This 58-year-old lady was in good health until March 7, 1992, when she developed the acute onset of a severe headache and left-eye blurred vision.

The neurological exam was normal except for mild meningismus. A CT scan showed diffuse SAH. An angiogram performed the next day demonstrated both a left intracavernous fusiform aneurysm and a supraclinoid internal carotid artery globular aneurysm (Figure 2A and B). Surgery was performed on day 4 after SAH. The cervical carotid arteries were exposed and a left pterional craniotomy performed. The intracavernous aneurysm was intradural and the supraclinoid aneurysm was found to be the source of SAH. A direct clipping of the supraclinoid aneurysm was attempted but because of tension of the aneurysmal sac, the clip slipped down onto the internal carotid artery narrowing the lumen. Therefore, a modified Tamaki's suction evacuation (Figure 3) procedure was used to decompress the aneurysm. The external carotid artery was catheterized with a small carotid shunt. After temporarily occluding the distal intracranial internal carotid artery and common carotid artery in the neck, the aneurysm was decompressed by suctioning blood through the external carotid artery shunt. By decompressing the aneurysm, a clip could be successfully placed across the neck of aneurysm without compromising the parent artery. The postoperative angiogram showed satisfactory clipping of the supraclinoid aneurysm and the patient recovered well from surgery (Figure 2C). A follow-up MRI angiogram 9 months later showed no change in the intracavernous aneurysm.

2. Aneurysms of the Intracavernous and Ophthalmic Internal Carotid Artery

Until recently, direct surgical repair of aneurysms in this location was thought to be associated with high risk. However, the contributions of surgeons like Parkinson [133,134] and Dolenc [135,136] along with other pioneer skull-base surgeons [117,137], increased knowledge of surgical anatomy in this region, and improvement in technical skills has led to a dramatic decrease in the surgical risk for intracavernous aneurysms. Currently, in experienced hands the risk of permanent injury to the cranial nerves during direct cavernous sinus surgery is only approximately 10% [117]. Some of the aneurysms in this region are giant in size and require an intracranial bypass procedure (Fukushima bypass). In our experience, about half of the aneurysms in this location have an acceptable neck and can be directly clipped, with a good result achieved in approximately 90% of patients [138].

Endovascular treatment of these aneurysms may be a good alternative to surgery. Specifically, in one report of 87 cases, endovascular detachable balloon occlusion of the parent carotid artery was performed in 78%, and primary aneurysm obliteration was achieved in 22%. Bypass surgery was required in only 2% of patients. Transient ischemia was seen in 10.3% and permanent morbidity (stroke) was seen in only 4.6% of cases [111]. By comparison, Fukushima et al. [117] reported their experience in 79 cases, which included cranial nerve

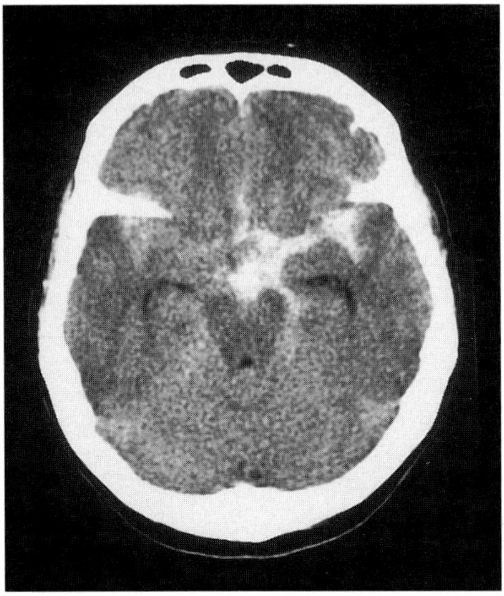

(a)

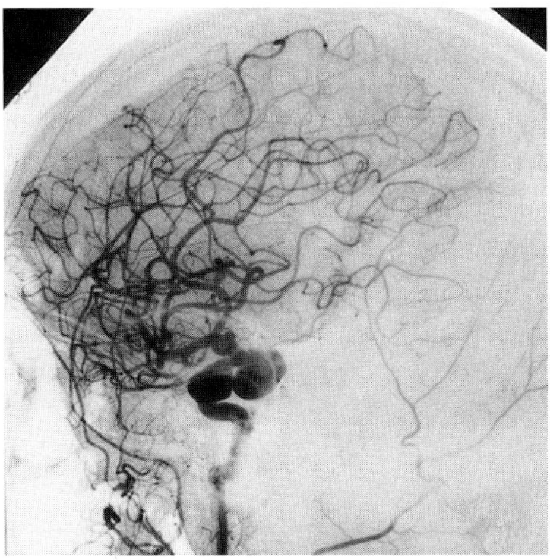

(b)

Figure 2 A 58-year-old lady presented with a subarachnoid hemorrhage. a) CT scan confirms subarachnoid hemorrhage mainly in the left basal cistern. b) (Oblique) Preoperative left carotid angiogram including anteroposterior, lateral, oblique views disclosed two aneurysms in close proximity. One is just above the clinoid and the other in the cavernous sinus and thus not the cause of SAH. Hence, only the intradural aneurysm was clipped with the help of Tamaki's suction method. c) Postoperative angiogram demonstrates successful clipping of the supraclinoid aneurysm.

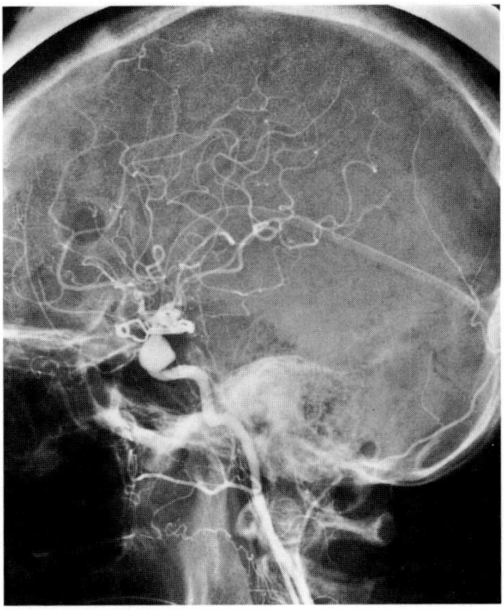

(c)

Figure 2 Continued

deficits in 6, optic nerve injury in 5, cochlear damage in 2, temporary hemiparesis or hemiplegia in 3, and CSF leak in 2 patients. Their overall morbidity was 17% with a mortality of 0%. It should be noted that the case material between these two series was different and therefore not directly comparable.

The natural history of aneurysms of the cavernous carotid artery that are completely within the cavernous sinus is relatively benign [139]. Since both surgical and endovascular treatments have a high complication rate, they should be reserved for cavernous carotid aneurysms that extend into the subarachnoid space or present with significant mass effect including pain or ophthalmoplegia. The small asymptomatic cavernous carotid artery aneurysm should be observed only.

Illustrative Case 2

This 79-year-old female presented with progressive visual loss in her right eye over 3–4 years. A CT scan and angiogram revealed a giant right internal carotid artery aneurysm originating in the intracavernous portion of the ICA and projecting intradurally. Preoperatively, the patient had a bitemporal hemianopsia and loss of visual acuity on the right (Figure 4A). This aneurysm was approached through a right pterional craniotomy. By splitting the medial Sylvian fissure, the aneurysm dome was exposed. It was necessary

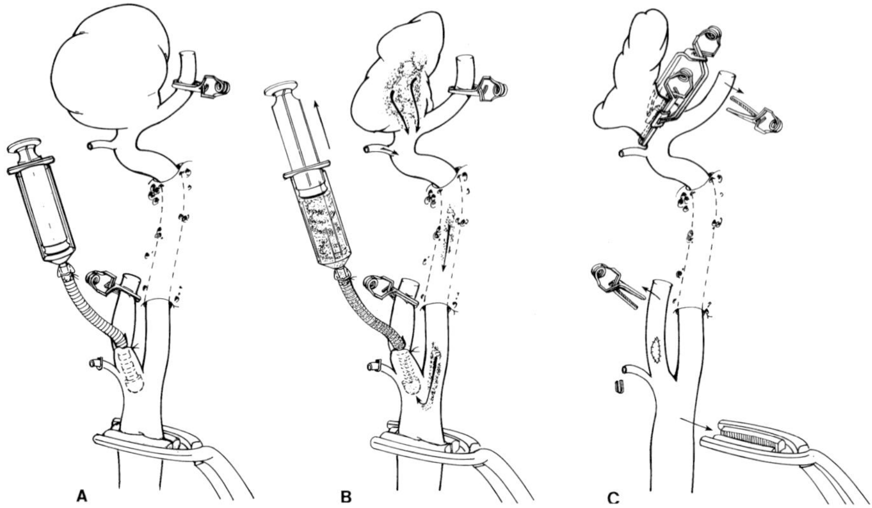

Figure 3 Modified Tamaki's suction method for internal decompression of a giant carotid artery aneurysm without thrombus or calcified wall. (A) The cervical external carotid is cannulated with a small Sundt shunt and then the proximal common carotid and distal intracranial internal carotid artery are temporarily occluded. By this procedure, the internal carotid artery system including the aneurysm is trapped with the suction tube exiting from the external carotid artery. (B) The second assistant now suctions blood from the catheter in the external carotid artery which decompresses the giant aneurysm. (C) A clip is then placed across the aneurysm neck and often reinforced with a second clip. The temporary clips on the distal internal and proximal common carotid arteries are then removed. The catheter is then removed from the external carotid artery which is then repaired. This technique of collapsing a giant aneurysm is useful if there is no thrombus within the aneurysm. It avoids using a suction apparatus in the aneurysm dome and a narrow operative field. By catheterization of the external carotid artery, there is less risk of injury to the cervical internal or common carotid artery. A large catheter must be used in this technique; approximately 60–100 mL of blood is suctioned over a 30-second period of time.

to remove the anterior clinoid and trace the carotid artery into the cavernous sinus. The neck originated from the cavernous sinus carotid artery at its C_3 segment. After isolation, the neck was clipped with the preservation of the parent artery. Postoperatively the patient had a partial right third-nerve palsy that resolved within six months. The preoperative visual-field deficits improved but visual acuity in the right eye remained unchanged. A postoperative angiogram demonstrated satisfactory repair of the aneurysm (Figure 4b). This case demonstrates the usefulness of skull-base surgical techniques to expose the cavernous carotid artery.

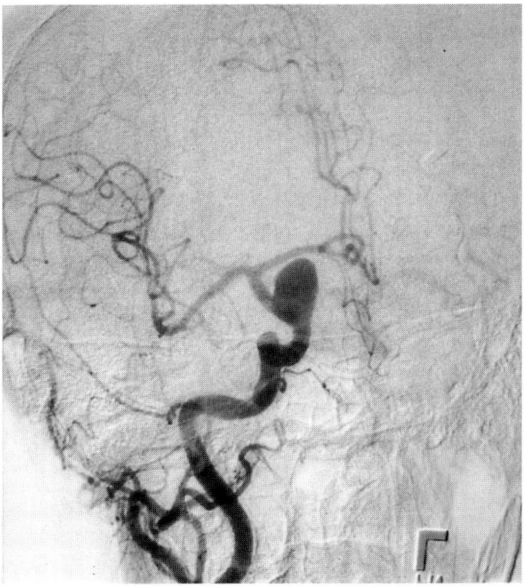

(a)

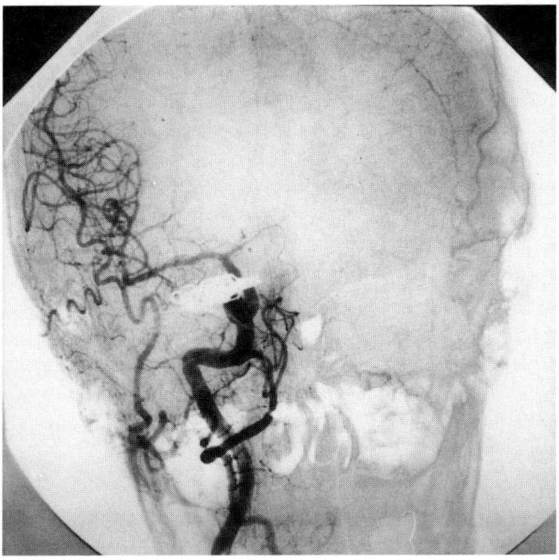

(b)

Figure 4 A 79-year-old male had a 3–4 year history of right visual loss. The CT scan showed a giant aneurysm in the right subfrontal area. (a) Pre-operative right carotid angiogram demonstrates an aneurysm originating from the intracavernous C_3 portion of the carotid artery. The dome is projecting mediosuperiorly and was actually intradural. (b) Postoperative angiogram confirms successful clipping of the aneurysm.

3. Aneurysms of the Anterior Cerebral Artery

Anterior communicating artery aneurysms are the most common aneurysms at a single site and are seen in approximately 34% of patients. At our institution, aneurysms in this location are approached through a pterional craniotomy, which is more suitable for Caucasians who have a scaphocephalic skull compared to Asians. In Asia, the interhemispheric approach is favored since the Asian skull is more brachycephalic. Aneurysms in this location are often associated with various anomalies of the circle of Willis, which can result in hemodynamic stress. The aneurysm dome can be in any direction. Aneurysms directed posteriorly are typically the most difficult in this location because of the relationship of the aneurysm dome to the adjacent perforators that are supplying the hypothalamus (Figure 5). Injury to any of these perforators can result in significant hypothalamic dysfunction. It is often necessary to resect part of the unilateral rectus gyrus to expose the neck of the aneurysm. Rupture of some ACom aneurysms can result in massive intraventricular hemorrhage with acute hydrocephalus. Ventricular drainage and the intraventricular application of tPA or urokinase may be helpful in dissolving these clots [47].

Aneurysms in the A_2 segment of the anterior cerebral artery, pericallosal artery, or callosal marginal artery are accessed via the interhemispheric approach. Aneurysms in the distal A_2 segment have been reported to have an increased tendency for premature rupture during the initial dissection.

Illustrative Case 3

This 70-year-old woman presented with several episodes of drop attack. A CT scan and angiogram demonstrated a 2.5 cm anterior communicating artery aneurysm (Figure 6a). This aneurysm was approached through a left pterional craniotomy. After exposing both proximal anterior cerebrals, the left A_2 segment of the anterior cerebral artery, and the recurrent artery of Heubner, the patient's systolic blood pressure was increased to 150 mmHg and temporary clips were placed on these vessels. The aneurysm was incised and suction was used to decompress the lesion. This allowed identification of the right A_2 segment. Subsequently, a long straight clip was placed across the neck of the aneurysm with preservation of the anterior communicating artery complex. Postoperatively the patient awoke without any neurological deficits and an angiogram demonstrated satisfactory clip placement (Figure 6b).

4. Aneurysms of the Middle Cerebral Artery

Middle cerebral artery aneurysms are seen in approximately 20% of patients. These aneurysms are routinely approached through an enlarged pterional craniotomy. The Sylvian fissure is widely separated. In situations in which there is a

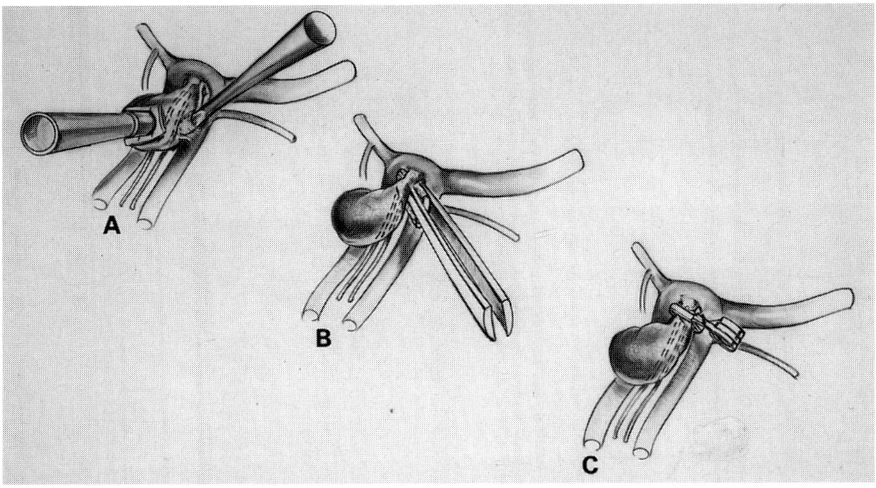

Figure 5 Clipping of saccular anterior communicating artery (Acom A) aneurysm. After the anterior cerebral ACom A complex is exposed, arachnoid, cerebral tissue, and blood clot over the aneurysm and parent vessels are dissected away. (A) Posteriorly projecting aneurysm is often adherent to A_2 segment of ACA and perforators in back of aneurysm. The walls and aneurysm neck need to be carefully dissected away via a small dissector or spatula. Aneurysm dome can be cautiously mobilized or compressed with a sucker tip and cottonoid. (B) Separated perforators are protected from harm's way by placing a small piece of gelfoam betweeen the aneurysm neck and perforators. (C) Clip should be placed across the aneurysm neck as close to the base as possible. Essential goals of clipping are not only obliterating the aneurysm, but maintaining patency of parent and perforating vessels. Size, type and shape of aneurysm clip used is based on the size of the aneurysm neck, wall thickness, and angle of approach. Inappropriate size or type of aneurysm clip can introduce failure of clipping or occlusion of perianeurysmal vessels.

fused fissure or the Sylvian fissure is absent, a trans-superior temporal gyrus approach can be quite useful [140]. These aneurysms occasionally present with an intracerebral hemorrhage that mimics a basal ganglia hypertensive hemorrhage. However, a distinguishing characteristic between the two is typically blood in the subarachnoid space as visualized by CT scan. Although MCA aneurysms are located relatively superficial, surgical repair can be difficult due to risk of injury to both the major vessels and perforators surrounding the aneurysm. Specifically, perforators originating off the proximal M_2 segment can be injured during clipping. Therefore, surgeons must be meticulous in their dissections and be exact in clip placements.

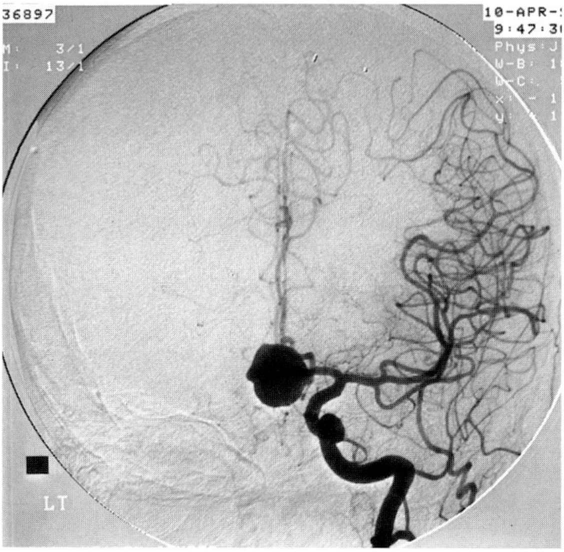

(a)

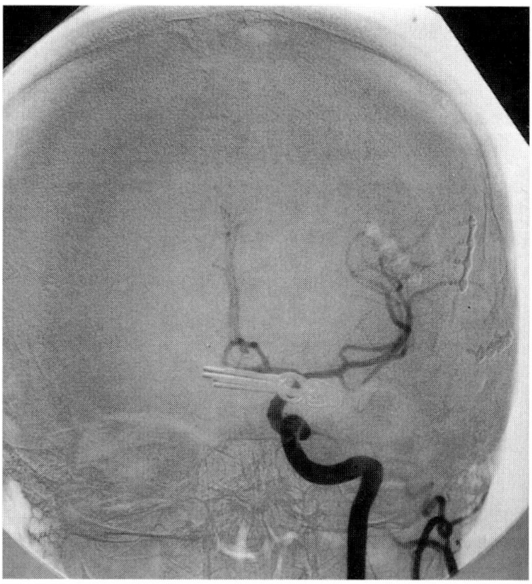

(b)

Figure 6 A 70-year-old lady suffered several episodes of drop attack. (a) Preoperative left carotid angiogram showed a giant anterior communicating artery aneurysm. (b) Postoperative angiogram proved successful clipping.

C. Posterior Circulation Aneurysms

1. Aneurysms of the Posterior Cerebral Artery

These are relatively rare aneurysms that can be exposed either through a modified pterional craniotomy or subtemporal approach depending on the location of the aneurysm in relation to the posterior cerebral artery. Typically, proximal posterior cerebral artery aneurysms are exposed through a modified pterional or subtemporal craniotomy. More distal P_2 and P_3 located aneurysms are approached primarily through a subtemporal opening. In some cases, it is difficult to locate the aneurysm especially in the distal P_3 segment and stereotaxis may have a useful role. Aneurysms of the proximal posterior cerebral artery are often fusiform or giant in 20% of cases and impossible to clip directly. Therefore, trapping may be necessary. Ischemic events related to proximal trapping of the posterior cerebral artery occur in approximately 10%. A major difficulty with proximal posterior cerebral artery aneurysms is the relationship between the aneurysm and the important thalmostriate perforators originating off this segment of artery. These perforators must be preserved, otherwise ischemic injury to the thalmus will occur. Trapping of the artery distal to these perforators will often lead to a homonymous hemianopsia. Techniques to preserve the posterior cerebral artery have included an STA–PCA end-to-end anastomosis, a saphenous vein bypass graft to the P_2 segment of the posterior cerebral artery, a direct end-to-end anastomosis of the posterior cerebral artery, and a PCA to SCA end-to-side anastomosis. The majority of these anastomoses are technically difficult and controversial [141].

Illustrative Case 4

This 27-year-old football player presented with increasing headaches over a 2–3 week period. An MRI scan demonstrated an aneurysmal lesion adjacent to the left midbrain. An angiogram revealed a left PCA aneurysm involving the P_1 segment (Figure 7a and b). It was fusiform in configuration. This aneurysm was approached through a left modified pterional craniotomy and found to be a false aneurysm. Temporary clips were placed proximal and distal to the false aneurysm and it was resected. The stumps of the posterior cerebral artery were then reanastomosed end-to-end using 8-0 Nylon sutures. Postoperatively, the patient had a temporary third-nerve palsy and dysnomia, which improved significantly over 3 months. A postoperative angiogram demonstrated a patent anastomosis, however with some mild stenosis (Figure 7c).

2. Aneurysms of the Basilar Caput

Vertebrobasilar aneurysms are seen in 5–10% of patients who harbor intracranial aneurysms. At our institution, this percentage is higher because of referral

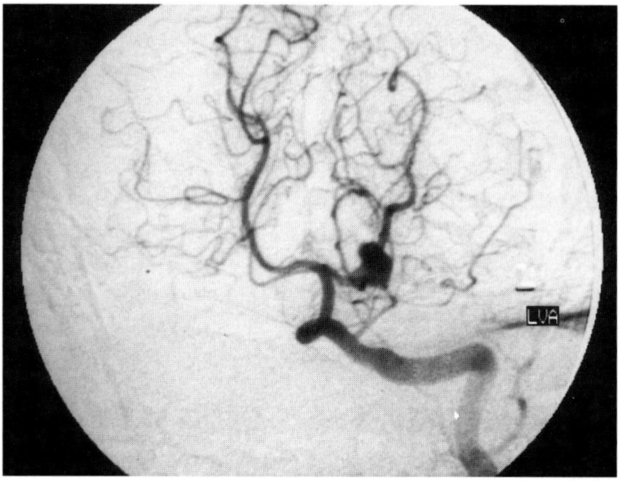

(a)

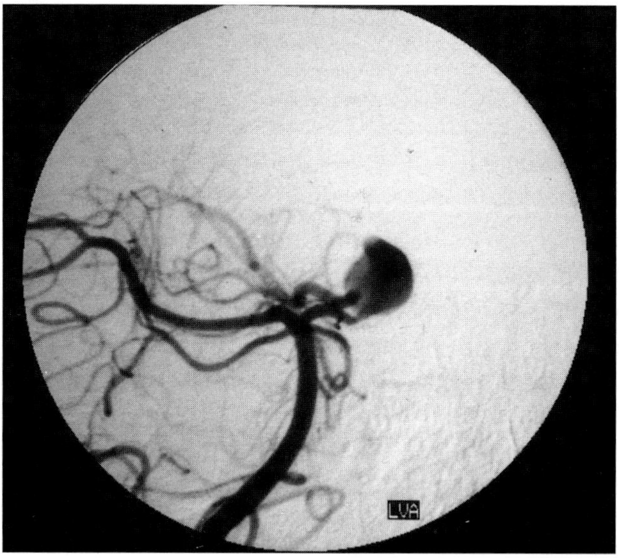

(b)

Figure 7 A 27-year-old professional football player diagnosed after increasing headache over 2–3 week period. a(A-P), b(Oblique) Vertebral angiogram disclosed left P_1–P_2 junction fusiform aneurysm. This aneurysm was approached through modified pterional craniotomy. Intraoperatively this was found to be a false aneurysm without wall. The aneurysm was resected and proximal distal PCA was anastomosed in end to end fashion. (c) Postoperative angiogram ascertains patency of anastomosis with some narrowing.

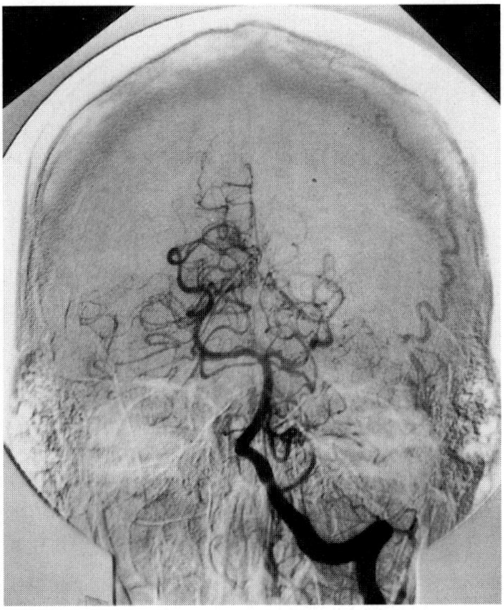

(c)

Figure 7 Continued

patterns. It is our preference to approach basilar caput aneurysms through a modified pterional craniotomy [3]. After widely exposing the Sylvian fissure, the temporal lobe is retracted in an anterior to posterior direction. From our experience, this retraction of the temporal lobe is better tolerated than upward retraction through a subtemporal approach. The free edge of the tentorium is then tacked lateral to expose the third nerve and prepontine cistern. The basilar trunk and basilar caput are then exposed by dissecting off arachnoid both above and below the third nerve. This approach gives a wide exposure with good visualization of the basilar trunk and both posterior cerebral arteries. Typically there is a mesh of perforators originating off the proximal posterior cerebral arteries and basilar caput and these are dissected in an arachnoid plane behind the neck of the aneurysm. One disadvantage of this modified pterional approach is that most patients have a postoperative third-nerve palsy but they usually recover in 3–6 months.

The subtemporal approach is preferred by many experienced surgeons [108,114,142]. The benefits of the subtemporal approach is good visualization of proximal basilar trunk and the posterior wall of the aneurysm and perforators. The disadvantages are that it is difficult to see the opposite posterior cerebral artery and it is poorly suited for high-bifurcation aneurysms. Other difficulties for the subtemporal approach include temporal lobe contusion and injury to the vein of Labbe.

Basilar caput aneurysms are quite difficult and should be operated on by experienced aneurysm surgeons only. Damage to a single perforator in this region can be devastating to the patient [143]. Large aneurysms in this location require special considerations including the need for temporary basilar-artery occlusion and methods to increase brain relaxation and protection.

Special concern should be noted to the relationship of the aneurysm neck with the posterior clinoid. If the neck is located higher than 1.5 cm above the posterior clinoid, it will be difficult to expose through a subtemporal craniotomy. The transzygomatic approach has been reported to be useful to visualize the aneurysm neck in these cases [144]. For high-bifurcation aneurysms, the authors have found that an anterior temporal lobectomy including uncal resection is helpful in visualizing the aneurysm neck in conjunction with removal of CSF through a lumbar drain. Often with significant removal of CSF through the lumbar drain, the basilar caput will descend downward along the clivus exposing the aneurysm neck. There has been a report of clipping of a basilar caput aneurysm that was 24 mm above the clinoid via a translamina terminalis through the 3rd ventricular floor. If the bifurcation is more than 1 cm below the posterior clinoid, then the subtemporal approach with or without removal of the posterior clinoid and petrous ridge is best. A similar subtemporal craniotomy can be useful for aneurysms of the upper and basilar trunk. Aneurysms above the level of 25 mm below the posterior clinoid are accessible via a subtemporal, transtentorial opening [145]. By removing anterior pyramidal bone, even lower basilar artery trunk aneurysms can be accessible [146].

Proximal control during basilar aneurysm surgery is a critical issue for the neurosurgeon. It is a difficult task and is one reason why basilar artery aneurysms are the most challenging of all cerebral aneurysms. Even in apparently straightforward cases, proximal control is difficult because of the posterior clinoid and petrous ridge. In cases of giant aneurysms or thrombosed aneurysms in which temporary occlusion and decompression are required, cardiac arrest under profound hypothermia may be a good alternative [122].

One other major difficulty with aneurysms is this location, especially those which are giant, is that perforating branches and the posterior cerebral and superior cerebral arteries may originate from the neck of the aneurysm. In some circumstances, giant basilar caput aneurysms are unclippable for fear of injury to these vessels. In that rare circumstance, a proximal ligation or balloon occlusion may be the only alternative [106–108,114].

Illustrative Case 5

This patient was a 53-year-old man who presented with SAH (Boterrell Grade 1). A CT scan demonstrated hemorrhage around the basilar tip with a thrombosed aneurysm (Figure 8a). Notably, there was calcification in the aneurysm wall. A follow-up angiogram demonstrated that this was a partially thrombosed lesion. On the MRI scan, the aneurysm measured 2.5 cm in size (Figure 8b). A modified pterional craniotomy was performed (Figure 8c). The primary difficulty with surgery was the calcified aneurysm neck, which did not easily accept a clip. This case was also complicated by the thrombus within the aneurysm. It was therefore necessary to perform a thrombectomy. The patient's blood pressure was increased to 155 mm Hg and EEG isoelectricity was induced by increasing the inspired concentration of isoflurane and administering thiopental (3.0 mg/kg IV). Thereafter, the basilar artery was temporarily occluded and the aneurysm was opened. Temporary occlusion was discontinued every 5–10 minutes to allow periods of reperfusion. The total time of basilar artery occlusion was 31 minutes. After an adequate thrombectomy and decompression, the aneurysm neck was manipulated to allow placement of three aneurysm clips (Figure 8d). Postoperatively, the patient had a third-nerve palsy, which resolved over 3 months. He also developed some transient ischemic deficits on the 4th day after hemorrhage that resolved with aggressive volume expansion.

3. Aneurysms of the Lower Basilar Trunk

These aneurysms are the most difficult to obtain direct access to, but fortunately are quite rare. They can be attacked through a subtemporal–transtentorial approach, a lateral suboccipital approach, or transclival approach [3,66,147]. A combined supra- and infratentorial approach—termed a petroclival approach—is also a possible alternative exposure [148,149]. These aneurysms also appear to be good candidates for endovascular treatment [93].

Illustrative Case 6

This 42-year-old woman presented with a history of subarachnoid hemorrhage twice over a six-month interval. The patient was left with bilateral blurred vision because of subretinal hemorrhages. No other neurological deficits were present except for a previous Bell's palsy. Two prior 3-vessel angiograms had been performed at other institutions and were nondiagnostic. However, only one vertebral artery had been injected. A third angiogram performed at our institution demonstrated a broad-based saccular aneurysm at the vertebrobasilar junction that filled from the right vertebral artery (Figure 9a and b). A right suboccipital craniectomy was performed and the aneurysm was found to be projecting anteriorly into the clivus. Although the aneurysm base was relatively broad and atherosclerotic, a straight clip was used to obliterate the majority of the lesion (Figure 9c and d). This case emphasizes the importance of performing a complete 4-vessel cerebral angiogram on any patient who presents with subarachnoid hemorrhage.

4. Vertebral Artery Aneurysms

The most common location for aneurysms of the vertebral artery are at the takeoff of the posterior inferior cerebellar artery (PICA). This aneurysm has a

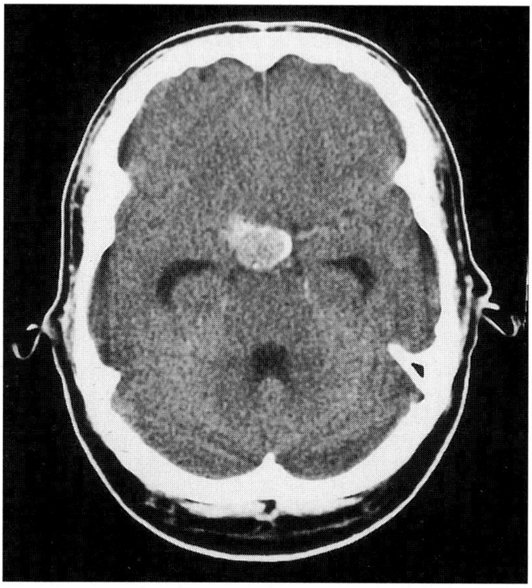

(a)

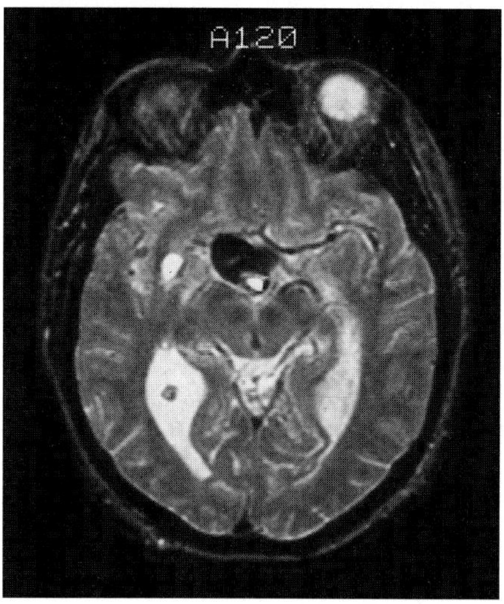

(b)

Figure 8 A 53-year-old man suffered SAH. CT scan (a) and MRI (b) diagnosed mild SAH in basal cistern and a giant basilar aneurysm with intraluminal thrombus and calcification in the aneurysmal wall. (c) Vertebral angiogram confirms giant aneurysm at the top of basilar artery. The posterior cerebral artery was involved in the aneurysm wall. With temporary proximal occlusion, the aneurysm was fully decompressed with throm-

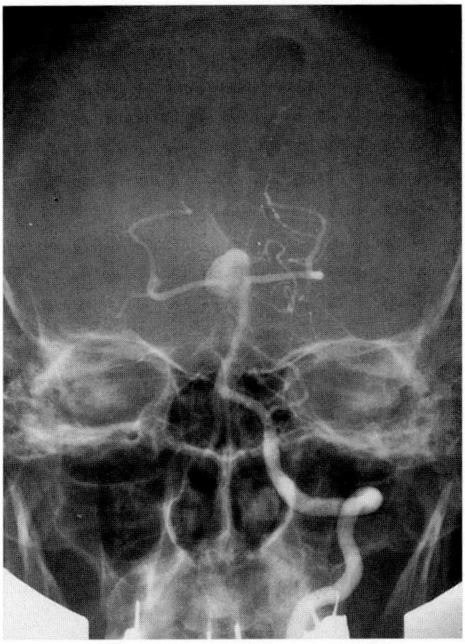

(c)

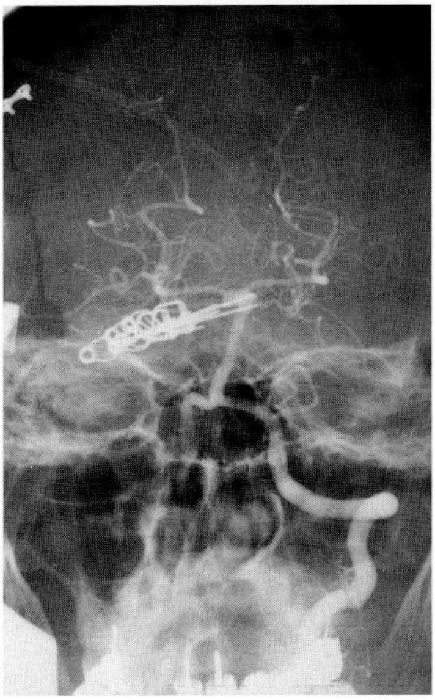

(d)

bectomy and a clip was placed above the origin of PCA. (d) Postoperative angiogram showed successful clipping of the aneurysm and preservation of PCA.

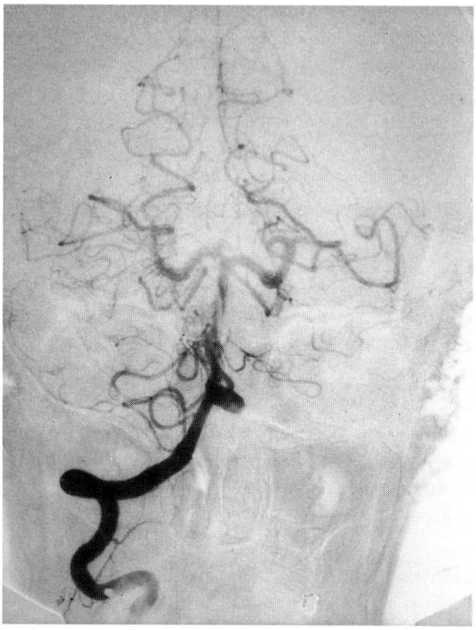

(a)

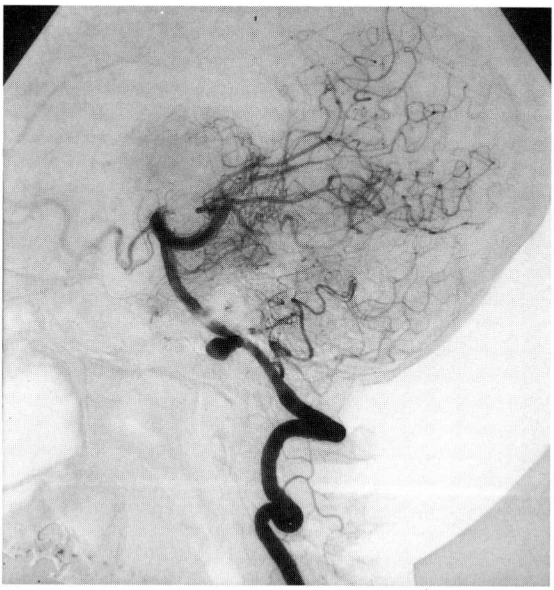

(b)

Figure 9 A 42-year-old lady had a history of two subarachnoid hemorrhages. Right vertebral angiogram visualized vertebrobasilar junction aneurysm (a, b). This was ac-

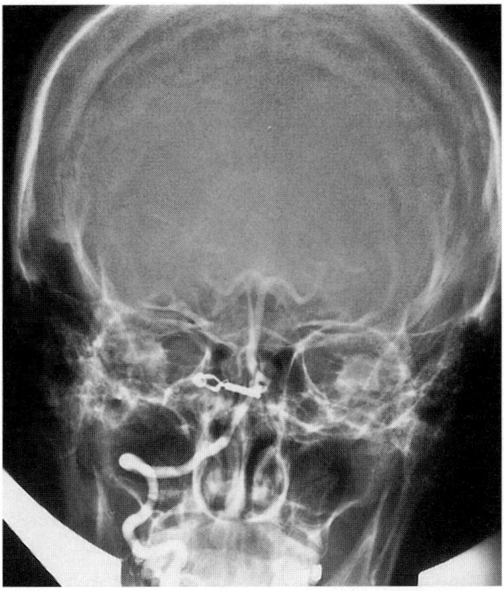

(c)

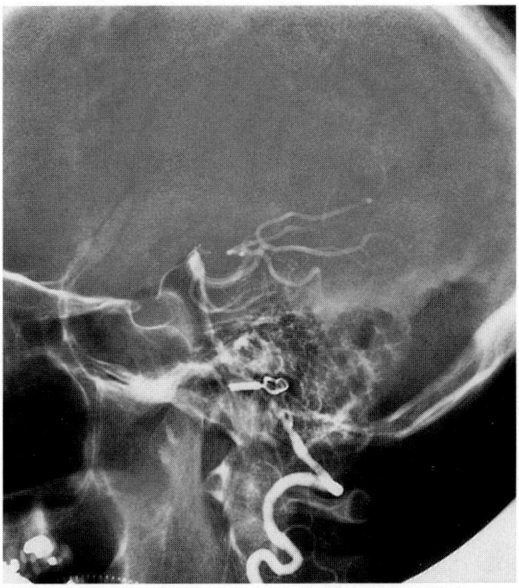

(d)

cessed by suboccipital approach. This aneurysm was very sclerotic, but the majority of the aneurysm was obliterated with straight clip (c, d).

close association with the lower cranial nerves. If approached by an extreme lateral or trans-condylar approach [150], the vagus and glossopharyngeal nerve are above the aneurysm. If approached through a routine suboccipital craniectomy, it should be approached above the 9th nerve. The 9th nerve then serves as a buffer to decrease injury to the 10th nerve. In cases of vertebrobasilar junction aneurysms, an extreme lateral approach may be best to expose this region.

5. Other Posterior Circulation Aneurysms

Distal posterior inferior cerebral artery (PICA), anterior inferior cerebral artery (AICA), and superior cerebral artery (SCA) aneurysms are rare causes of SAH or cerebellar hemorrhage. Intraoperative localization of these aneurysms can sometimes be difficult. The PICA and AICA aneurysms are usually approached through a suboccipital craniotomy whereas an SCA aneurysm is often exposed through a subtemporal approach similar to that used for a proximal posterior cerebral artery aneurysms.

The largest surgical series of posterior circulation aneurysms has been reported by Drake and Peerless [142]. In 1055 aneurysms, 82% had an excellent or good outcome, while 18% had a poor result and 6% died. Giant aneurysms had an especially poor outcome [142]. At our institution, comparable surgical results for posterior circulation aneurysms have been achieved with the same observation regarding giant lesions. The results of proximal basilar or vertebral artery ligation for the treatment of 201 unclippable posterior circulation aneurysms was recently reported from Drake's group [106]. In 78%, successful aneurysm thrombosis was induced. The overall outcome was excellent in 68%, good in 5%, poor in 3%, and 24% died. Partial thrombosis of the aneurysm was associated with early or late neurological deterioration by either SAH or thromboembolic complications in 67% of cases. Both of these resulted in a high mortality rate. Considering the high complexity of these selected cases, reported results for proximal arterial ligation are quite good and emphasize that the surgeon should consider this treatment if an aneurysm of the posterior circulation appears to be unclippable.

Endovascular treatment of 25 posterior circulation aneurysms using a detachable balloon technique was recently reported by Higashida et al. [151]. They achieved primary aneurysm obliteration in 65% and parent vessel occlusion in 35% of patients. Three patients had strokes and five patients died (20%) of immediate or delayed rupture of the aneurysm. Treatment of 43 vertebrobasilar aneurysms by GDC coils with good results was reported by Guglielmi [93,96]. Complete occlusion of the aneurysm was achieved in 81% of those with a small neck but in only 15% with a wide neck. The overall morbidity was 4.8% and the mortality was 2.4% including ischemia and rupture of the aneurysm during the procedure. Therefore, in posterior circulation aneurysms that have a well-defined small neck, GDC coils may prove to be a good alternative treatment to direct surgical repair.

D. Special Types of Aneurysms

1. Giant Aneurysms

Giant aneurysms are seen in approximately 5% of patients. At our institution, the incidence is approximately 20% because of referral patterns. These aneurysms often present with mass effect, although SAH occurs in 35% [152]. Giant aneurysms are quite difficult, not only because of their size but also because of their different pathogenesis. Some of these aneurysms are comparable to atherosclerotic aneurysms that occur in the aorta or extracranial carotid artery in that they have a thick calcified wall, intraluminal thrombus, and a poorly defined neck [153].

If the aneurysm has a well-defined neck and there is no thrombus in the sac or calcification in the wall, it can usually be directly repaired with clipping. It is usually necessary to decompress the aneurysm prior to clip placement. Collapsing the aneurysm prior to clip placement facilitates exposure to ensure that the adjacent arteries and perforators are not compromised. There are several techniques to decompress the aneurysm such as temporary vessel occlusion with puncture and suction. More recently, for giant carotid artery aneurysms without intramural thrombus or calcified wall, we have used the modified Tamaki method [154], which involves withdrawal of blood through the external carotid artery in the neck with temporary occlusion of the proximal common carotid, distal external carotid, and distal intracranial internal carotid arteries (Figure 3). For aneurysms in the posterior circulation, decompression can only be achieved by temporarily occluding the basilar artery. Often, upon exposing a giant aneurysm, it becomes apparent that the parent artery is merged with aneurysm wall. In that situation, it is necessary to apply clips in such a way that the parent artery is preserved. Typically, multiple clips are applied in sequence [123].

If the aneurysm is thrombosed or the wall is calcified but still has a well-defined neck, a direct surgical clipping should be attempted. In these situations, the parent vessels must be temporarily occluded and an incision made within the aneurysm. Thereafter, a thrombectomy is performed with currettes and occasionally an ultrasonic aspirator (Figure 10). Since thrombectomy does take some time, measures to provide brain protection must be instituted. If it appears on preoperative planning that prolonged parent vessel occlusion will be necessary or that clipping of the aneurysm might be impossible after the thrombectomy, it may be prudent to perform a preocclusion bypass distal to the

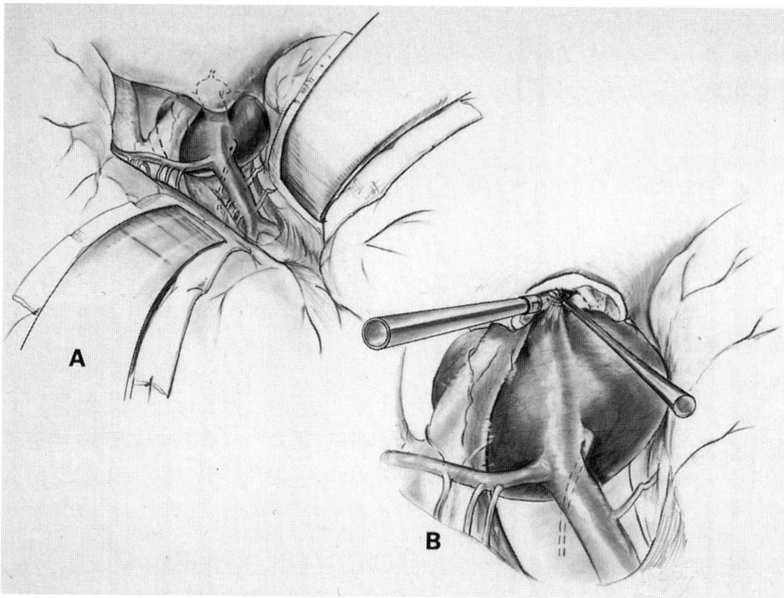
A
B

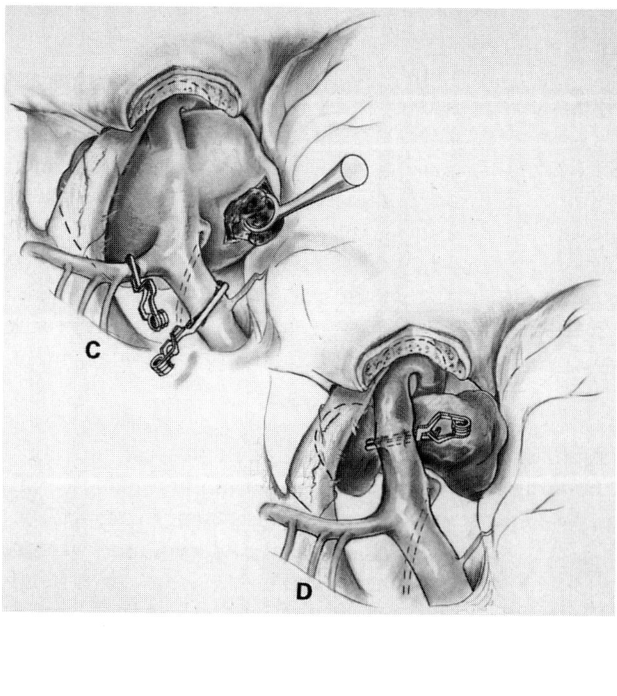
C
D

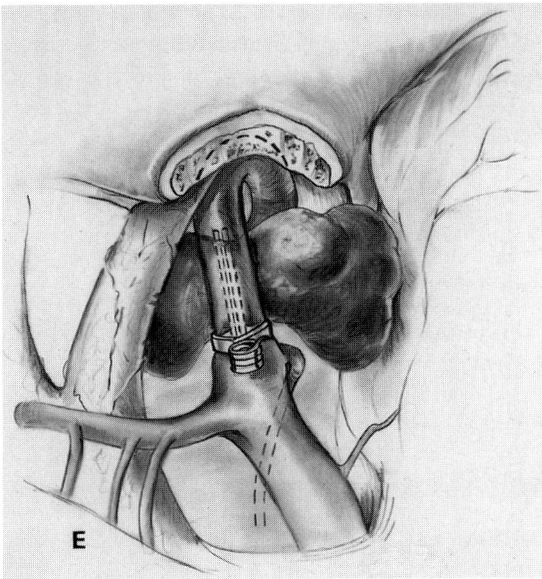

Figure 10 Clipping of a giant supraclinoid internal carotid artery aneurysm. (A) Via pterional approach, sylvian fissure is widely opened to expose carotid, posterior communicating, and anterior choroidal arteries, and optic nerves. (B) Anterior clinoid is removed using high speed drill epidurally or intradurally. (C) Using temporary occlusion of cervical carotid artery and distal vessels, aneurysmal dome is opened and thrombectomy is performed. As shown in Case 2, decompression is an extremely important part of giant aneurysm surgery. (D, E) Clip can be placed across the base of the aneurysm in several ways as long as parent vessel patency is maintained.

aneurysm. The risk of ischemic injury during parent vessel occlusion is then minimized and in cases where the aneurysm cannot be clipped, trapping can be performed with a decreased risk of ischemic injury.

In cases with a poorly defined aneurysm neck, bypass surgery should be considered. If the patient tolerates a trial balloon occlusion, a simple proximal ligation or trapping can be performed using endovascular techniques. As mentioned earlier, Drake's group has successfully ligated the proximal basilar trunk for the treatment of giant basilar aneurysms with good results [106]. The outcome of our surgical experience with giant aneurysms is depicted in Table 6.

Interventional endovascular treatment may have a role in the treatment of giant aneurysms [155,156]. However, because of the irregular shape and poorly defined aneurysm neck in many of these cases, successful obliteration is difficult to achieve [156]. As illustrated in Case 9 below, we have had two cases in which there was significant morbidity due to partial occlusion of a giant aneurysm with GDC coils. Following treatment, the aneurysms continued to enlarge possibly due to a water-hammer effect, necessitating surgical resection of the coils followed by aneurysm clipping. Removing the GDC coils can be extremely difficult since they become entangled in a thick fibrotic mass within the aneurysm. During removal, these coils become miniature gigli saws and can easily sever any adjacent neurovascular structures. At this point, the use of GDC coils for giant aneurysms needs further clinical investigation before their use can be confirmed.

Illustrative Case 7

This 61-year-old woman presented with a 6-month history of bifrontal headaches and 4 months of blurred vision. On ophthalmological examination there was a bitemporal hemianopsia. A CT scan and angiogram demonstrated a giant left ophthalmic artery aneurysm (Figure 11a). This was approached through a left pterional craniotomy. The aneurysm was exposed by drilling off the anterior clinoid through an intradural approach. The aneurysm extended underneath the optic nerve and chiasm explaining her preoperative visual deficits. The aneurysm neck was obliterated with two clips. An immediate postoperative angiogram demonstrated significant compromise of the internal carotid artery by the aneurysm clips (Figure 11b). The patient was therefore taken back to surgery and reexplored. During the second surgery, the proximal carotid artery in the neck and the carotid artery distal to the aneurysm were temporarily occluded. The aneurysm was incised and a thrombectomy and complete decompression were performed. An aneurysm clip was then reapplied in a way that reconstructed the parent vessel. The patient awoke with a mild right hemiparesis that was resolved at 3-month followup. A second postoperative angiogram demonstrated successful clipping without any carotid artery stenosis. This case emphasizes the importance of an immediate postoperative angiogram for difficult aneurysms (Figure 11c). Preferably, it is best to perform the angiogram in the operating room suite prior to closure of the craniotomy. In that way, the aneurysm clip can be repositioned immediately if there is some abnormality detected on the intraoperative angiogram. This case also emphasizes that with giant aneurysms it is mandatory to obtain adequate decompression prior to clip placement to prevent parent artery compromise.

Illustrative Case 8

This 31-year-old man presented with diplopia. A neurological examination demonstrated a right sixth-nerve palsy. A subsequent CT scan and angiogram demonstrated a giant intracavernous carotid artery aneurysm (Figure 12a and b). An extracranial to intracranial saphenous-vein bypass graft was performed and the aneurysm was then trapped (Figures 1 and 12c and d). The patient recovered well and the preoperative sixth nerve palsy resolved.

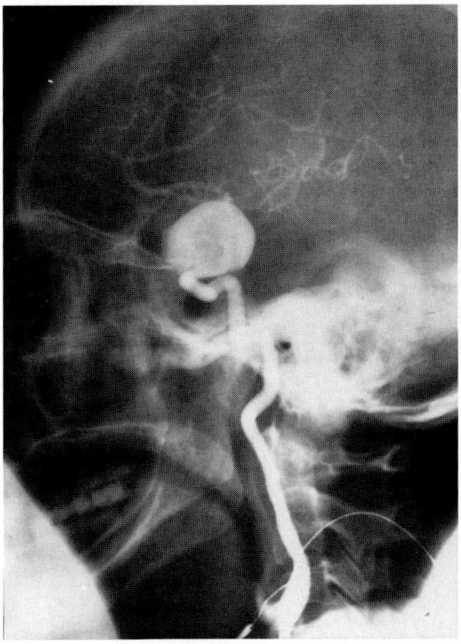

(a)

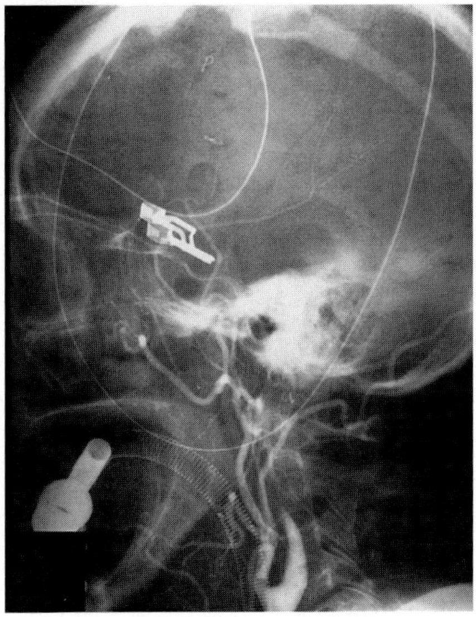

(b)

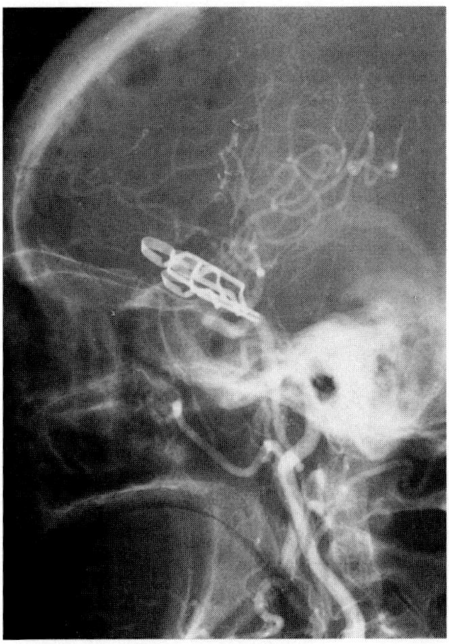

(c)

Figure 11 A 61-year-old lady diagnosed after a 6-month history of bifrontal headache and blurred vision. (a) Left carotid angiogram reveals a giant ophthalmic artery aneurysm. This was clipped through a left pterional approach without attempted decompression. (b) Postoperative angiogram showed occlusion of the internal carotid artery. Patient was immediately brought back to the operating suite and the clip was reapplied after decompressing the aneurysm. (c) Postoperative angiogram ascertains successful clipping.

Table 6 Result of 416 Giant Aneurysms

	Excellent	Good	Poor	Dead
Proximal ligation (34)	24 71%	4 12%	1 3%	5 15%
Simple trapping (29)	18 62%	8 28%	2 7%	1 3%
Direct clipping with or without thrombectomy (208)	128 61.5%	39 19%	24 11.5%	17 8%
Bypass surgery with proximal ligation or clipping or trapping (107)	67 63%	19 18%	11 10%	10 9%
Direct repair with vessel reconstruction (29)	18 62%	6 21%	3 10%	2 7%
Mycotic aneurysm, excision of aneurysm (3)	1	2	—	—
Exploration only, no repair of aneurysm (2)	—	—	—	2
Wrapping (4)	4	—	—	—
Total	260 62.5%	78 19%	41 10%	37 9%
	81.5% (Excellent + Good)			

All grades, with and without subarachnoid hemorrhage.

Illustrative Case 9

This 48-year-old woman presented with a subarachnoid hemorrhage in January 1990. An angiogram at that time demonstrated a 1.0 cm aneurysm of the basilar caput. Clipping of the aneurysm was attempted unsuccessfully at another institution. At that time, the aneurysm was wrapped. The patient subsequently presented one year later to the Mayo Clinic with increasing ataxia and a right hemiparesis. An angiogram demonstrated a partially thrombosed giant aneurysm of the basilar caput (Figure 13a and b). The authors approached this aneurysm through a modified pterional craniotomy, reopening the old bone flap. However there was a tremendous amount of adhesion around the aneurysm with complete obliteration of anatomic landmarks. Accordingly, the perforators off the back wall of the basilar artery could not be clearly identified or dissected free. Therefore, aneurysm clipping was not attempted and the patient was referred for endovascular treatment. During the first GDC coil placement, 95% occlusion of the aneurysm was accomplished (Figure 13c). On follow-up angiogram 3 months later, it appeared that the GDC coils had impacted against the dome and the aneurysm itself had enlarged. Subsequent coils were placed into the aneurysm (Figure 13d and e). A follow-up angiogram several months later again demonstrated impaction of coils with enlargement of the aneurysm. Ten endovascular sessions in all with placement of GDC coils were performed over a 2-year period. The right vertebral artery was also occluded in an attempt to decrease the pulsatile pressure to the aneurysm. The total length of GDC coils placed into the aneurysm dome was 910 cm (Figure 13f and g). Despite these procedures, the patient continued to worsen with progressive ataxia, slurred speech, and right hemiparesis. An MRI scan demonstrated progressive enlargement of the aneurysm with profound compression of the midbrain (Figure 13h). In a lifesaving attempt, the aneurysm was again approached surgically using cardiopulmonary circulatory arrest with profound hypothermia. The cerebral circulation was reduced to 0.5 L/min at a temperature of 15 degrees centigrade for 40 minutes. During this time, the aneurysm dome was opened and a thrombectomy with removal of the GDC coils was performed. Removal of the GDC coils proved to be exceedingly difficult since each coil performed like a gigli saw cutting into the aneurysm wall and several small perforators off the adjacent posterior cerebral artery. After removing the coils and the thrombus, the aneurysm neck was obliterated with a single clip. Despite the use of anticoagulants necessary for the cardiopulmonary bypass, there was no difficulty with hemostasis. Unfortunately, the patient did not awake from surgery and had evidence of severe brainstem injury. The patient subsequently died two weeks later. This case emphasizes several important points. First, difficult aneurysms of the posterior circulation should be treated by experienced neurovascular surgeons. Initially, the aneurysm could have been treated with relatively low morbidity and mortality. Second, wrapping of an aneurysm as the primary treatment is not a viable option considering today's modern neurosurgical and endovascular techniques. Third, GDC coils for giant aneurysms may not be an optimum treatment. Fourth, in retrospect, an alternative treatment to attempted surgical clipping could have been occlusion of the proximal basilar artery.

2. Traumatic, Mycotic, and Neoplastic Aneurysms

These aneurysms are rare in most neurosurgical practices. These aneurysms are often false and lack a true aneurysm wall and, therefore, can rupture easily during the surgical exposure.

Traumatic aneurysms are often seen in the carotid artery at the petrous segment and are associated with a severe closed-head injury and a skull-base fracture. These aneurysms can present with a massive nose bleed a few days after the trauma. They are usually treated with interventional endovascular measures such as balloon occlusion [157]. Rarely, direct surgical repair or bypass surgery is indicated [158]. A peripheral traumatic aneurysm is most commonly seen in the MCA (64%) and ACA (29%) and, again, is associated with severe closed-head injury. Peripheral traumatic aneurysms are exceedingly rare but

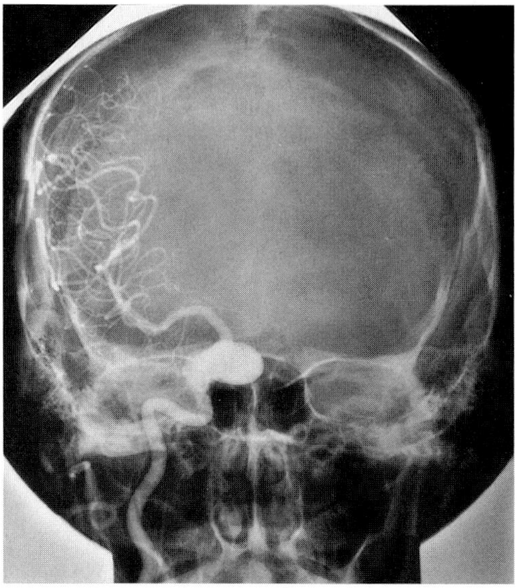

(a)

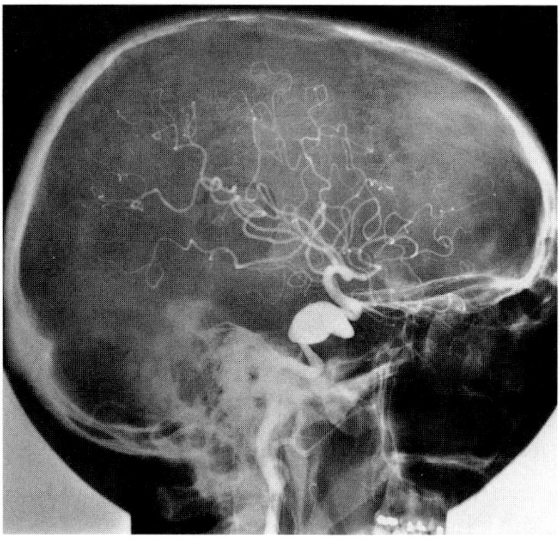

(b)

Figure 12 A 31-year-old man suffering from diplopia. (a)(AP), (b)(Lateral) Preoperative right carotid angiogram showed giant intracavernous aneurysm. There was no definable neck seen on this aneurysm with any angiogram projection. Therefore saphenous vein bypass was recommended. (c)(AP), (d)(Lateral) Postoperative angiogram displays a patent saphenous vein bypass graft from cervical internal carotid to supraclinoidal carotid artery.

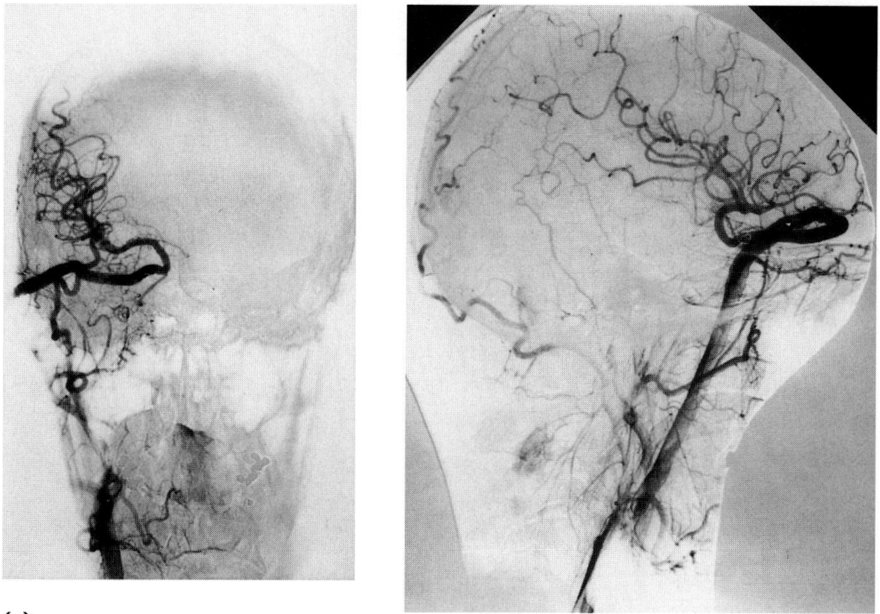

(c)

(d)

Figure 12 Continued

need to be considered when a patient develops a delayed neurological deficit or develops a massive intracranial hemorrhage after trauma. Penetrating trauma is a relatively rare cause of traumatic aneurysms. The mortality for traumatic aneurysms has been reported to be 16% with surgery and 41% if no surgery is performed. Rupture of the aneurysm often occurs approximately 10 days after the initial injury [159].

Mycotic bacterial aneurysms are seen in 4–19% of bacterial endocarditis patients. The most common bacteria cultured are streptococcus or staphylococcus. These aneurysms are typically seen in the peripheral MCA territory (43%) and less frequently in the ACA (16%) and PCA (9%) distributions. Multiple mycotic aneurysms are seen in 18–20% of cases. Proximal arterial involvement is uncommon for bacterial aneurysms. Most patients who develop a mycotic aneurysm are usually septic and moribund. Thus, surgery can have a significant risk from a general medical perspective. There are some reports of regression of mycotic aneurysms with antibiotic therapy alone in a few weeks [160]. If the medical condition is poor or the aneurysm is minimally symptomatic, conservative treatment with serial angiogram followup can be a viable option [161,162]. However, according to Bohmfalk's study, the surgical mortality for these lesions is 26.5% while the mortality for antibiotic therapy alone is 53% [163]. There-

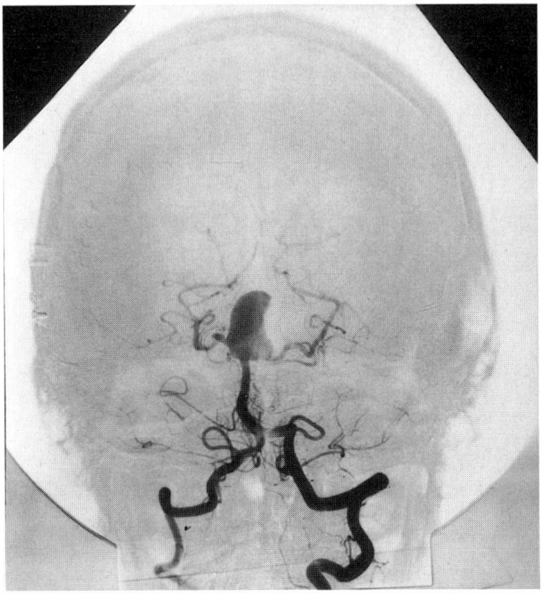

(a)

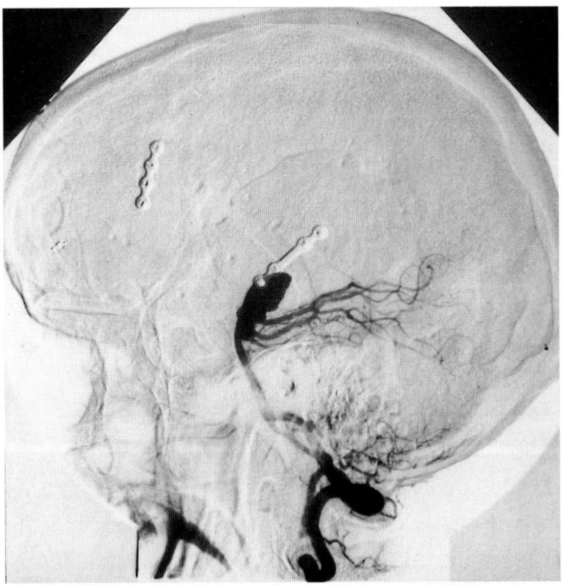

(b)

Figure 13 A 48-year-old lady with history of SAH and previous exploratory surgery. Two previous surgical attempts failed. (a)(AP), (b)(Lateral) Vertebral angiogram deter-

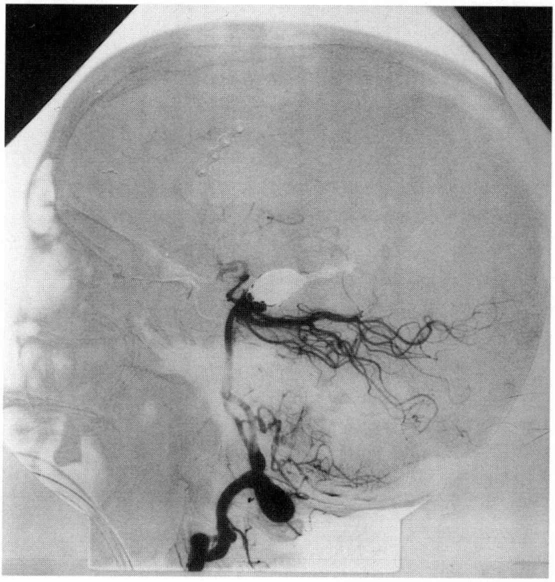

(c)

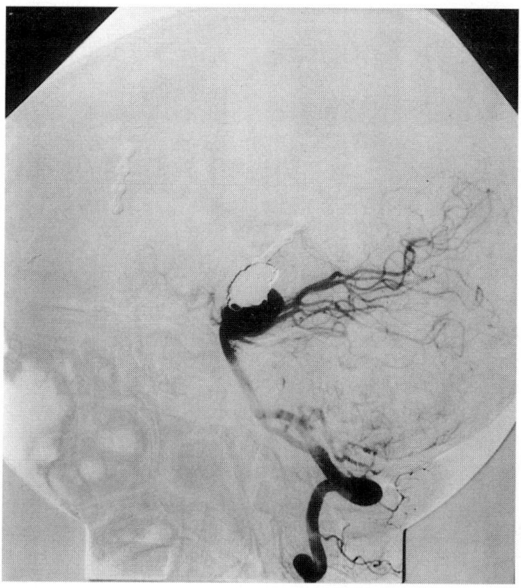

(d)

mined this was wide-base giant basilar-tip aneurysm. (c) After first stage coiling using Guglielmi detachable coil, 95% of aneurysm was occluded. (d) Two months later, coil

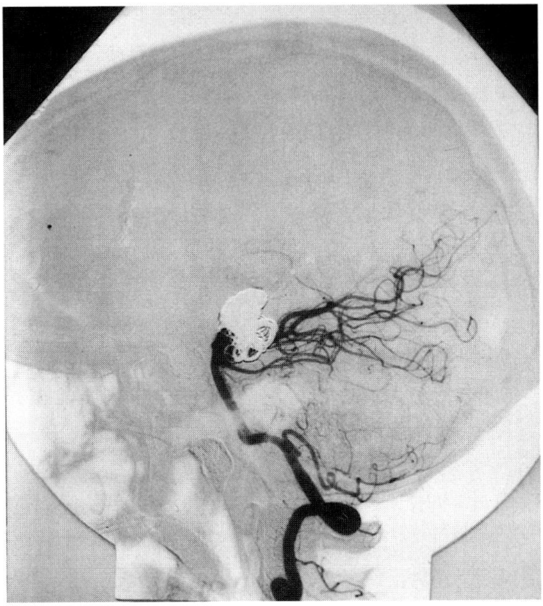

(e)

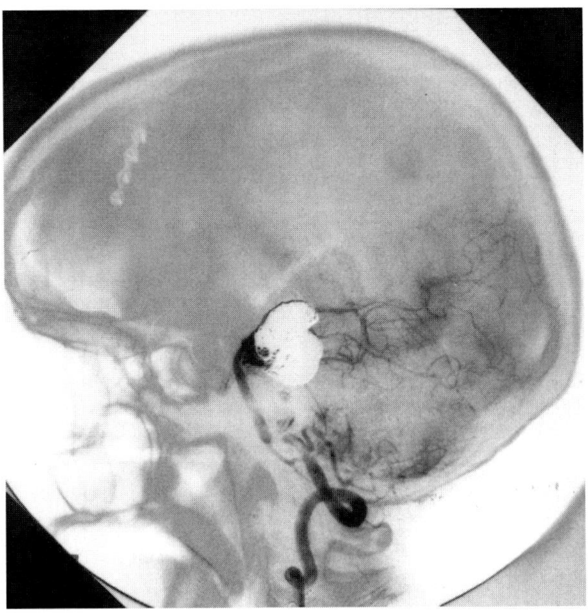

(f)

Figure 13 Continued
was displaced and impacted to the outer dome of aneurysm. Some increase of size of aneurysm was noted. (e) More coil was introduced into the aneurysm. However, more

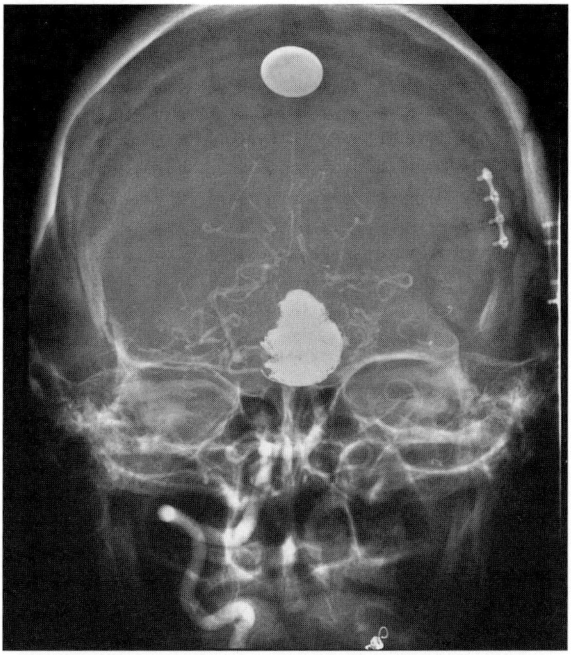

(g)

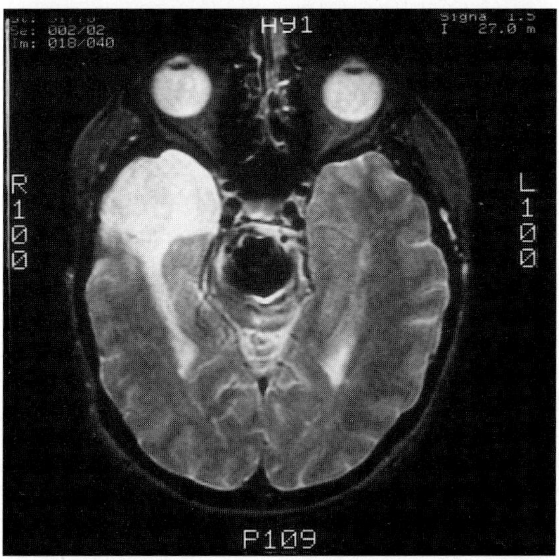

(h)

than 95% occlusion of aneurysm was never achieved. After ten endovascular procedures, patient's aneurysm was two or three times as big as initial size. (f)(AP), (g)(Lateral) Patient was clinically deteriorating and MRI (h) showed significant displacement of midbrain.

fore, if the patient's general medical condition is acceptable, surgery should be considered. Interestingly, fungal aneurysms occur more commonly in proximal major cerebral vessels such as the internal carotid artery. They appear to be more aggressive and can present with a massive SAH. The organisms associated with fungal aneurysms include *Aspergillus* or *Penicillium* and typically occur in patients who are immunocompromised [164].

Neoplastic aneurysms are caused by infiltration of tumor cells across the vessel wall after a neoplastic emboli that occludes the vessel. A cardiac myxoma is the most commonly encountered primary tumor that can cause a neoplastic aneurysm [165]. Some additional cases have been reported with choriocarcinoma and lung cancer. The peripheral MCA territory is the most common site and the mortality from this problem is reported to be 50%.

In traumatic, mycotic, and neoplastic aneurysms there is often no neck that will accept an aneurysm clip. Therefore treatment of these aneurysms usually involves trapping or excision of the diseased vessel segment and aneurysm. Occasionally, it may be technically feasible to reconstruct the artery either through an end-to-end anastomosis or through a distal bypass using the superficial temporal artery. Another unique problem associated with these aneurysms is localization since they often occur in peripheral arteries. We have employed stereotaxis in several cases to localize the mycotic aneurysm easily with minimal morbidity [166].

We have experienced a case of a mycotic aneurysm (Hemophilus influenza) occurring in the distal basilar artery as shown in Illustrative Case 10. Khayata et al. [167] reported a good result in treating mycotic aneurysms with endovascular techniques. This emphasizes that endovascular techniques, which are less invasive, may be better in treating sick, septic patients.

Illustrative Case 10

This patient was a 49-year-old man who presented with chills, fever, and general malaise. The patient was noted to have congestive heart failure and placed in the intensive care unit. His admission blood work was significant for a hemoglobin of 8.0, WBC of 13.1, and an ESR of 78. Seven days later, the patient developed acute cognitive deficits and a CT scan demonstrated a subarachnoid hemorrhage in the prepontine cistern. An angiogram demonstrated either an irregularly shaped or fusiform aneurysm of the basilar caput (Figure 14a). Although all blood cultures were negative, the cardiac ECHO demonstrated aortic valve vegetations consistent with endocarditis. The patient was then transferred to our institution for treatment. Upon review of the angiogram, it was clear that there was an aneurysm of the basilar caput and also one at the origin of the left SCA (Figure 14b). After two weeks of antibiotic therapy, GDC coils were placed into the aneurysm at the origin of the SCA. Coils could not be placed into the basilar caput aneurysm because of it's wide neck. One week later, the basilar caput aneurysm was exposed using a modified pterional craniotomy. The top of the basilar artery including both posterior cerebral and superior cerebellar arteries were covered with yellow friable material. In fact, the GDC coils were visualized and were used as a guide for placement of the aneurysm clip. An immediate postoperative angiogram demonstrated that the aneurysm clip was placed across the basilar artery above the origin of the SCA. The distal basilar artery circulation was supplied by a large left PCA (Fig. 14c). Since the degree of collateral flow and status of the perforators were unknown, the patient was brought immediately back to the operating room, the craniotomy reopened and the clip removed. The basilar tip was then reexplored; the left PCA and some perforating vessels were identified. The aneurysm neck was further identified after removal of the friable yellow grumous material from the basilar caput. The aneurysm clip was then reapplied. A second postoperative angiogram demonstrated no filling of the left PCA during a left vertebral artery injection. However, both PCAs filled from the carotid system (Fig. 14d). The patient awoke in stable neurological condition except for a right third nerve paresis. He subsequently underwent aortic valve replacement and has since returned to his previous employment. A follow-up angiogram six months after surgery demonstrated no change in the clip or GDC coils. This case emphasizes that mycotic aneurysms can be extremely difficult lesions to treat depending on their location. There are often fusiform dilatations of arteries without a definable aneurysm neck for clipping.

3. Dissecting Aneurysms

Dissecting aneurysms in the intracranial circulation are most often seen in the vertebral artery and can present with SAH. Dissection of major arteries in the anterior circulation usually present with symptoms of ischemia. Dissecting aneurysms of the vertebral circulation are often self-limiting and follow-up angiograms typically show reconstitution of the vessel lumen [167]. However, the vertebral artery dissection that presents with SAH can be fatal if not treated. A proximal ligation or balloon occlusion is the usual treatment in these specific cases [168]. Ligation proximal to the PICA origin is preferred to prevent embolic complications or the development of a Wallenberg syndrome [169]. If a segment of the vertebral artery that contains the origin of the PICA needs to be trapped, an occipital artery-PICA anastomosis may be indicated to prevent ischemic complications.

Illustrative Case 11

This 56-year-old woman presented with a gradual increase in headaches and memory loss. The CT and MRI scans demonstrated a 1.5-cm hematoma in the right posterosuperior temporal region (Figure 15a). An angiogram demonstrated an 8-mm diameter aneurysm in the distal MCA involving the posterior temporal branch (Figure 15b). Through a circular

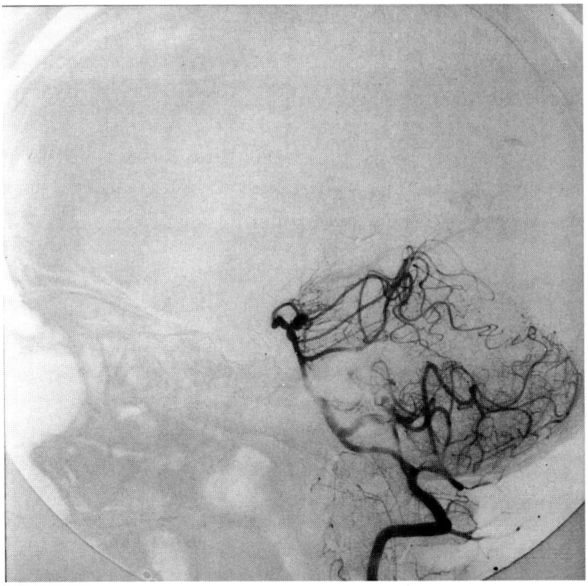

(a)

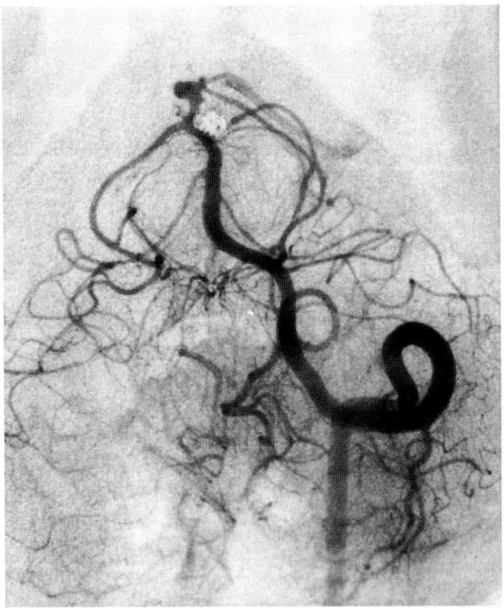

(b)

Figure 14 A 49-year-old man developed subacute bacterial endocarditis and then had a mild subarachnoid hemorrhage. (a) Vertebral angiogram diagnosed a multilobulated aneurysm in the top of the basilar artery. One of the lobules was projecting at the junction of basilar artery and left SCA. GDC coil was placed in basilar SCA aneurysmal lobule (b). Follow-up angiogram revealed increased size of the basilar tip aneurysm. Because of wide base of this aneurysm, endovascular treatment was abandoned. This

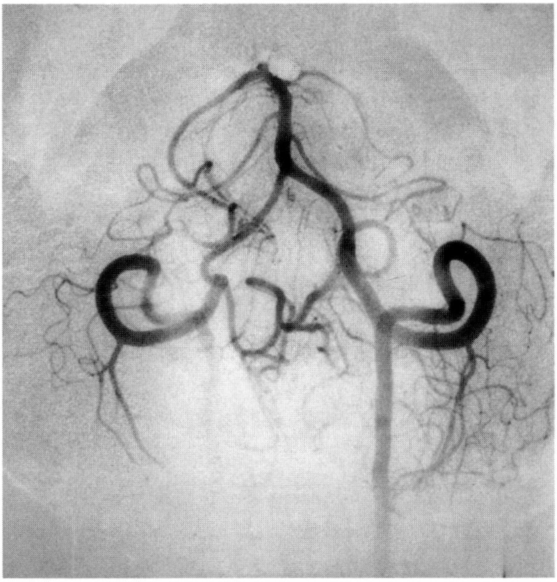

(c)

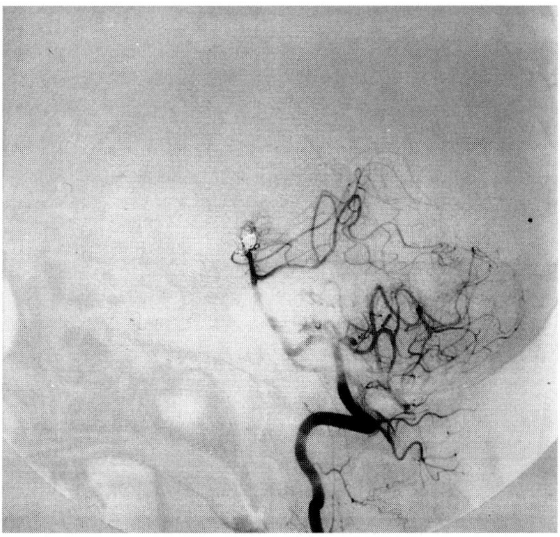

(d)

aneurysm was clipped surgically. Although we are confident that we placed clip across the base of aneurysmal bulge and saved posterior cerebral artery and perforators, post-operative angiogram vertex view (c) indicated clip is across the basilar tip and occluding the posterior cerebral artery. Lateral view (d) showed good visualization of perforators. Bilateral posterior cerebral arteries filled from anterior circulation but aneurysm was not visualized.

craniotomy over the right Chater's point, the distal Sylvian fissure was opened and the aneurysm immediately identified. This aneurysm had no neck and was a fusiform dilatation of the temporal branch. Since the distal branch was significant in size, an STA-MCA anastomosis was performed distal to the lesion and the aneurysm was subsequently trapped. A final pathology report demonstrated that this was a dissecting aneurysm. The patient tolerated the procedure well and a postoperative angiogram demonstrated a patent anastomosis (Figure 15c). This case demonstrates the continued usefulness of an STA-MCA bypass graft. Although it has been discarded as a primary treatment for ischemia, it is still a useful surgical option to preserve blood flow to regions of marginal or branch ischemia. In any neurosurgical procedure in which there is a risk of vascular injury, the STA should be preserved during the initial skin incision and craniotomy.

4. Fusiform Aneurysms

Fusiform aneurysms present with SAH, transient ischemic attacks (TIAs), or mass effect as illustrated in the following case [170]. If SAH or mass effect is the initial presenting symptom, treatment by a proximal ligation or trapping is usual. A balloon occlusion test and other clinical findings will determine if a bypass is needed. In rare situations, some portions of the aneurysm may have a saccular shape that will accept an aneurysm clip. In some cases, the fusiform aneurysm involves important perforators, and occlusion of these vessels carries a significant risk. In such situations, wrapping may be the only alternative. Perhaps the most difficult aneurysms to treat are the giant fusiform basilar trunk aneurysms. We have attempted to treat these with a combination of proximal ligation and distal bypass surgery. In general, our results thus far have been poor.

Illustrative Case 12

This 23-year-old man developed acute onset of headache and drowsiness after sexual intercourse. He was a Grade-2 SAH on admission. An angiogram showed a giant fusiform left M_1 aneurysm. Two days later, an exploration was performed at a local hospital and the aneurysm was felt to be unclippable. The aneurysm was wrapped with muscle and synthetic fibers and then reinforced with acrylic. The patient awoke with a right hemiparesis and aphasia. A second angiogram 10 days after surgery showed enlargement of the aneurysm; the patient was then referred to the Mayo Clinic (Figure 16a and b). Four weeks after the first surgery, a reoperation was performed. Since the aneurysm was wrapped with fibers, muscle, and acrylic, the exposure was extremely difficult. Since the previous surgery had utilized a transsylvian approach, this pathway was completely obliterated with the wrapping material. Therefore, an anterior temporal lobectomy was performed to facilitate exposure of the proximal internal carotid and MCA-M_1 from a different angle. However, because of the acrylic and other wrapping materials, exposure of the aneurysm, proximal and distal vessels, and perforators was challenging and required drilling off the acrylic over the aneurysm. The aneurysm involved the M_1 5 mm from its origin up to the MCA trifurcation. After placing a saphenous vein bypass from the cervical external carotid artery to the proximal M_2 segment, trapping clips were placed across the M_1 just proximal and distal to the aneurysm (Figure 16c). The patient awoke with a mild worsening of the preexisting right hemiparesis but improved significantly with physical therapy.

5. Aneurysm Associated with Arteriovenous Malformations

The association of a cerebral aneurysm with an intracranial arteriovenous malformation (AVM) is well documented. Seven percent of AVMs are associated with intracranial aneurysms [171]. Although some aneurysms can disappear or diminish in size after resection of the AVM, if the aneurysm is accessible during surgery for the AVM, it should be clipped. It is important to note that if the patient presents with SAH, the aneurysm and not the AVM may be the responsible lesion for the hemorrhage.

6. Aneurysm Associated with Moyamoya Disease

Aneurysms associated with moyamoya disease are one of the major causes of hemorrhage in this disease. Approximately 14% of adult cases of moyamoya disease have an intracerebral aneurysm. Alternatively, it is rare for a pediatric moyamoya patient to harbor a cerebral aneurysm. The two types of aneurysms seen in this disease include a microaneurysm, which is thought to be dilatation of a moyamoya vessel (61%), or a saccular aneurysm of the circle of Willis (39%), which is most commonly seen in the posterior circulation [34]. Surgery is indicated if the aneurysm ruptures. Interestingly, after revascularization procedures for moyamoya disease, the microaneurysms appear to regress on subsequent angiography [35].

7. Aneurysms in Pediatric Patients

Aneurysms seen in the young patient have unique features [172]. They are most often giant (27–54%). Although the anterior communicating artery is the most common site in 42%, ICA bifurcation aneurysms are disproportionally frequent in 33% of patients [173]. In our experience [174], 46% of cases had posterior circulation aneurysms. The peak incidence is at less than 2 years of age with a male predominance. The presence of juvenile aneurysms may point to a possible congenital, as opposed to acquired, etiology for some intracranial aneurysms.

8. Aneurysms Associated with Pregnancy

This is an uncommon but difficult clinical situation. Pregnancy does carry some risk for rupture of an intracranial aneurysm because of the endocrine and hemodynamic changes that occur. Over half of aneurysms that rupture in women under the age of 40 are related to pregnancy [175]. The ruptures occur in 1% of patients in the first trimester, 15% in the second trimester, 35% in the third trimester, 13% during labor, and 11% on the first postpartum day [176]. The prognosis in the pregnant woman suffering from SAH is comparable to a routine SAH. If the patient presents with SAH, the aneurysm should be repaired with carefully monitored anesthesia to protect the fetus. In the future, endovascular treatment may be useful in this specific clinical circumstance. If an unruptured aneurysm is diagnosed during pregnancy, surgery can be deferred until the pregnancy is over or, alternatively, after completion of the first trimester.

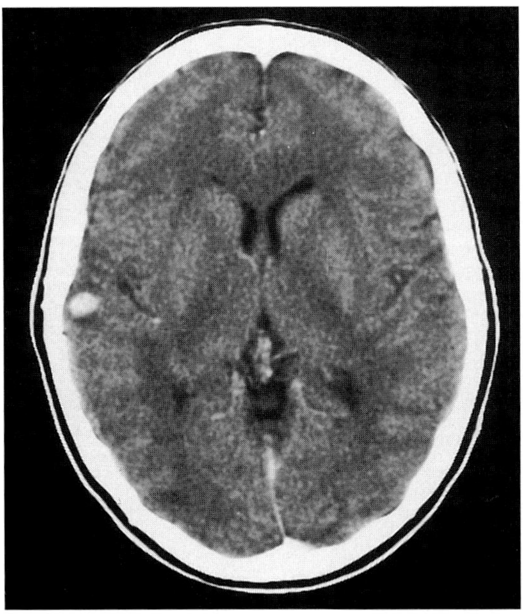

(a)

Figure 15 A 56-year-old lady sought medical attention with gradual memory loss and headache. CT scan indicated a high intensity mass in right posterior temporal area (a). (b) Right carotid angiogram determined this was a distal MCA angular branch aneurysm. Aneurysmal resection and STA-MCA anastomosis to the distal MCA branch was performed. Postoperative angiogram (c) ascertains good patency of the anastomosis.

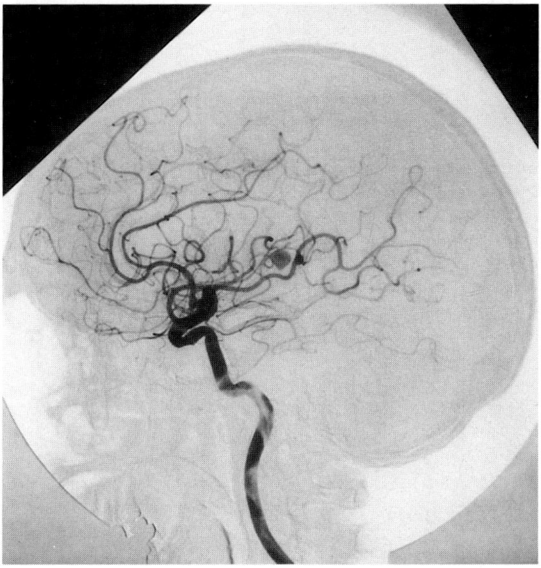

(b)

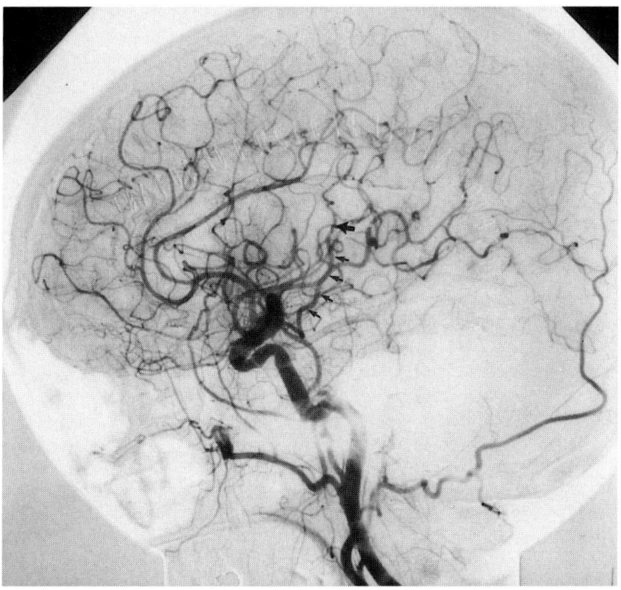

(c)

Figure 15 Continued

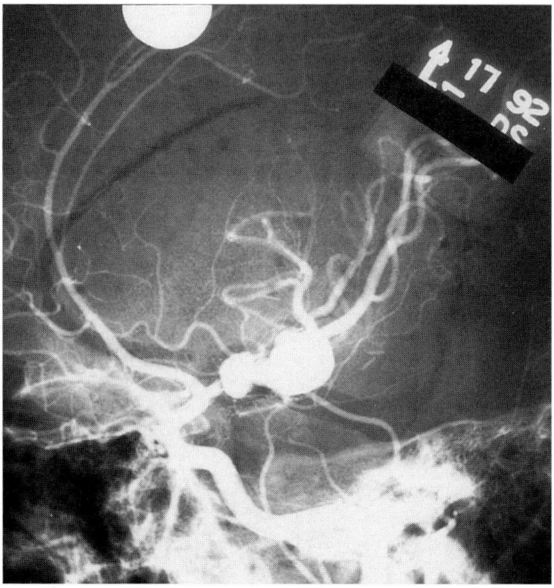

(a)

Figure 16 A 23-year-old man presented after subarachnoid hemorrhage. At a local hospital this aneurysm was explored then wrapped with fabric and acrylic material. a(Oblique), b(Vertex view) Preoperative left carotid angiogram disclosed a fusiform aneurysm involving M_1–M_2. This aneurysm was explored transsuperior temporal lobe approach and found unclippable. Hence this aneurysm was trapped after SVG bypass from external carotid artery to M_2 branch. (c) Postoperative angiogram demonstrates successful bypass.

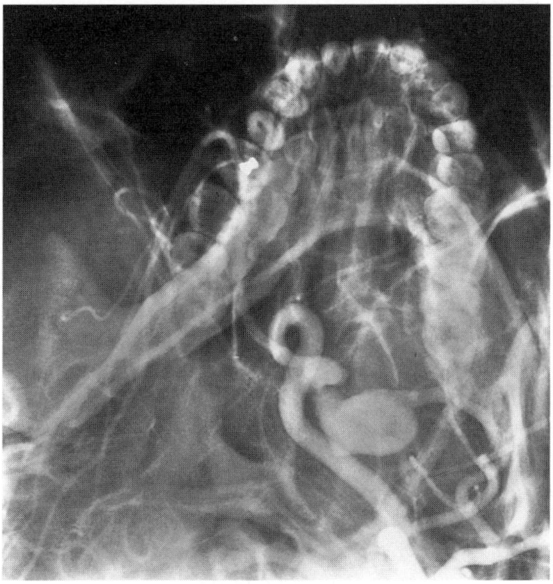

(b)

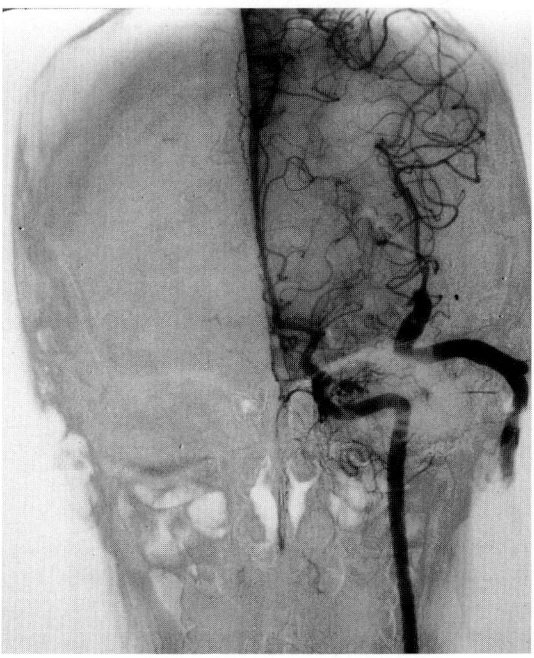

(c)

9. Aneurysms in Multiple Locations

Intracranial aneurysms can be multiple in up to 20% of patients [12,65]. If the patient presents with SAH, occasionally the surgeon may have a dilemma as to which aneurysm was the source of the SAH. Some indications of the responsible aneurysm include irregular shape with a secondary lobule, vasospasm of adjacent arteries, and proximity to the most dense part of the subarachnoid clot [177]. Often the patient's position and craniotomy can be tailored to facilitate clipping of multiple aneurysms under the same anesthetic [66].

X. PERIOPERATIVE MANAGEMENT OF PATIENTS WITH CEREBRAL ANEURYSMS WHO PRESENT WITH A SUBARACHNOID HEMORRHAGE

Several issues merit reemphasis regarding the management of an acute SAH. These issues have been briefly discussed already in other sections of this chapter and elsewhere in this book.

A. Prevention of Rerupture

After the initial medical and neurological stabilization of the patient, the first issue in the early phase of management is prevention of rerupture. As discussed earlier, the greatest risk of rerupture is within the first 24 hours after the initial rupture. The patient should be kept in a quiet room and the blood pressure should be maintained no greater than 140 mm Hg. Poor-grade patients have probable increased intracranial pressure. In these patients, the blood pressure will most likely be high, but should be kept less than 150 mm Hg systolic. This will help ensure adequate perfusion pressure. If the patient is agitated, sedation with mild analgesics or narcotics may be considered. However, it is important not to oversedate so a full neurological assessment can be performed on a regular basis.

B. Prevention and Management of Delayed Arterial Vasospasm and Delayed Ischemic Neurological Deficits (Table 7)

This issue is discussed more extensively in other chapters in this book. Prevention of vasospasm would be the ideal treatment [59–61]. There is some evidence that indicates that clot removal, especially that achieved through the intrathecal administration of tPA, may significantly decrease the risk of delayed arterial spasm [178–183]. The calcium antagonist, nimodipine, has been re-

Table 7 Management of Delayed Arterial Vasospasm

1. Early detection of clinical signs of vasospasm
2. Maintain normal physiological status such as euvolemia, normothermia, normal natremia and normal oxygenation.
3. Nimodipine 60mg po/iv q4 hours or other calcium antagonist
4. Surgical clot removal: tPA application/cisternal drainage/brain shaker, etc.
5. Hypervolemia using packed red blood cells, colloid, albumin solution, fludocortisone 2mg/day or desoxycortisone 20mg/day. Pitressin may be indicated to keep urine output low
   Support CVP 10mmHg, PAWP 19–20 mmHg
6. Induced hypertension with dopamine, dobutamine
7. Balloon angioplasty
8. Topical or intraarterial papaverine injection

ported to decrease significantly the morbidity and mortality in patients of all grades who suffer SAH [184,185]. Therefore nimodipine at a dose of 60 mg po q4 hours should be routinely administered. Although high-dose steroids have been suggested by some to be of benefit, this is not universally accepted and remains controversial [186]. Optimum general care including maintenance of a euvolemic, eunatremic condition may retard the development of symptomatic vasospasm.

If vasospasm becomes symptomatic, an early response is critical. Clinically symptomatic changes need to be closely monitored in the intensive care unit. Volume expansion is indicated and is achieved by the infusion of colloid and occasionally blood [58,72,73]. If clinically significant vasospasm does not respond to these conventional treatments, a cerebral angiogram should be performed for consideration of balloon angioplasty. Higashida [102] reported that this technique significantly improved neurological symptoms in 70% of patients suffering from vasospasm. Recently intraarterial injection of papaverine has been reported to be beneficial [187]. Transcranial doppler is a useful noninvasive technique for monitoring the success of treatment, including volume expansion, in reversing vasospasm [74].

C. Management of Acute Hydrocephalus

As mentioned earlier, acute hydrocephalus can be the cause of progressive neurological deterioration. A poor-grade patient has a greater tendency to develop hydrocephalus because of the increased amount of blood in the basal cisterns. Drainage of CSF through a ventricular catheter is indicated if the hydrocephalus is causing neurological impairment or deterioration. In fact, a poor-grade patient can improve significantly upon placement of a ventricular drain on an emergent basis. Milhorat [188] reported that two-thirds of their patients had significant improvement after placement of a ventricular drain after SAH. However, since acute decompression can be associated with rerupture of an aneurysm, the amount of CSF removed should be carefully controlled [189]. Intermittent ventricular drainage when the intracranial pressure (ICP) increases is preferred as opposed to continuous drainage, which tends to have a greater risk of accidental excessive drainage.

D. Cardiopulmonary Management

If the patient develops neurogenic pulmonary edema or cardiomyopathy after SAH, aggressive respiratory care and cardiopulmonary monitoring are required.

E. Electrolyte and Fluid Management

Maintaining the SAH patient in an euvolemic state is important in preventing the development of symptomatic vasospasm. In Suzuki's series of 1000 cases [190], electrolyte abnormalities developed in 4% of patients. Usually this is hyponatremia that can be severe enough to cause neurological deterioration. In some circumstances, the patient may develop SIADH or cerebral salt wasting [191]. These diagnoses must be made carefully, since in most circumstances hyponatremia is due to fluid mismanagement. The distinction is important since if the patient has the misdiagnosis of SIADH, fluid restriction may lead to the development of symptomatic vasospasm. Therefore routine measurements of urine sodium, serum sodium concentrations and osmolality, and daily body

Table 8 Management of Hyponatremia

1. Check urine sodium, osmolality; if high (Na > 18 mEq/L, Osm 1.5–2.5 times of serum) consider SIADH.
2. Check body weight, fluid balance of last few days; if body weight considerably less than previous weight, consider cerebral salt wasting; fluid balance negative, consider salt wasting and if positive, consider SIADH.
3. Check CVP, PAWP; if low, consider cerebral salt wasting, if high consider SIADH
4. As necessary, change intravenous fluids to normal saline or D5 + 0.9 saline.
5. If SIADH considered, fluid limit < 1000/day, demecrocycline (150–300 mg po q6hr), furosemide (40 mg qD).
6. If cerebral salt wasting considered, colloid infusion, packed red blood cell transfusion, 0.9 saline infusion.
7. If Na < 120, 3% saline infusion may be indicated (25–50 mL/hr).
8. Never over correct hyponatremia to eu- or hyper-natremia. Do not correct more than 25m Eq/L within 24 hours, or 1.3 mEq/L within 1 hour [192].

weights can be useful in sorting out the appropriate diagnosis (Table 8). In the majority of patients, over hydration with a low osmolality solution is the cause of hyponatremia and can be corrected by the appropriate fluid replacement. For SIADH, water restriction to 1000 mL/day is the standard treatment. In some cases, it is necessary to administer 3% sodium solutions or demecrocycline (150–300 mg po QID). In cerebral salt-wasting syndrome, colloid infusion is indicated in addition to sodium and fluid replacement. To correct hyponatremia, the sodium level should not be elevated rapidly (< 25 mEq/L within 24 hours or 1.3 mEq/L per hour), since it may induce demyelination or central pontine myelolysis [192]. Sodium levels should be normalized slowly to a slightly hyponatremic state over 48 hours.

F. Seizure Precaution and Management

Seizures are reported to occur in 1–7% of patients with subarachnoid hemorrhage with or without surgery [193]. The use of prophylactic anticonvulsants is controversial. At our institution, cases in which there is significant temporal lobe retraction are more likely to receive perioperative anticonvulsants.

XI. MAYO CLINIC EXPERIENCE

This patient group consisted of 1947 patients who underwent surgery at the Mayo Clinic from 1969–1990. The mean age was 51.4 years (range 3 months to 88 years) with a male/female ratio of 2 to 3. This group's demographics are similar to other published data; although, because of referral patterns, there were more better-clinical-grade patients, posterior circulation aneurysms (17% compared to the usual 5–10%), and giant aneurysms (21% compared to the usual 5%). Most patients were considered modified Botterell Grade 0 (39%) or Grade 1 (32%) and only 3% who were Botterell Grade 4. The aneurysms were saccular in 59%, globular in 20%, and giant in 21%.

A. Outcome

The outcomes are scaled by Sundt's classification, which is similar to the Glasgow outcome scale (GOS), as follows.

Excellent	Normal employment with normal neurologic exam (GOS 5)
Good	Neurologic deficit, but normal mentation and employment (GOS 4)
Poor	Anything less than full activity (GOS 2–3)
Death	Mortality within 6 months of SAH (GOS 1)

Table 9 Age and Surgical Outcome

Result	Age by decade								Total
	10s	20s	30s	40s	50s	60s	70s	80s	
Excellent	37	68	208	358	420	289	57	8	1445 (74%)
Good	2	8	24	52	62	54	28	1	231 (12%)
Poor	1	7	15	15	46	57	26	4	171 (9%)
Death	1	2	8	18	25	30	12	5	101 (5%)
Total	41	85	255	443	553	430	123	18	

Overall 1445 patients (74%) had an excellent outcome, 231 (12%) had a good outcome, 171 (9%) had a poor outcome, and 101 (5%) died. There were certain trends related with outcome. Younger patients had a better outcome while in the older age group between the 6–8th decade good and poor outcomes increased with reduced excellent outcomes. The mortality did not increase significantly until the 9th decade (Table 9).

There was a direct relation between admit clinical grade and outcome (Table 5). Patients with a good grade on admission had a superior outcome. Over 80% who were Grade 0 (unruptured aneurysm) or Grade 1 had an excellent outcome. Grade 4 had the highest incidence of poor and death outcomes.

Patients with aneurysms in the anterior circulation had a better outcome than patients with posterior circulation lesions (Table 10). Most patients with anterior circulation aneurysms had an excellent outcome (75%), compared to 65% of cases with posterior circulation aneurysms. Basilar caput aneurysms had the highest incidence of poor outcome (with poor and death totaling 30%).

In examining the aneurysm size in relationship to outcome, saccular and globular aneurysms had similar outcomes, while giant aneurysms had a higher death rate (10%, Table 11a). However, an excellent outcome was achieved in 293 patients (69%) with giant aneurysms and in 75% of those who did not have SAH (Table 11b).

Table 10 Anterior Circulation Versus Posterior Circulation

Surgical result	Circulation	
	Anterior	Posterior
Excellent	76%	65%
Good	10%	18%
Poor and death	14%	17%

Table 11a Aneurysmal Size and Surgical Outcome (All grade)

	Size of aneurysm			
Result	Saccular	Globular	Giant	Unknown
Excellent	827 (71%)	213 (75%)	293 (69%)	67 (82%)
Good	130 (11%)	35 (12%)	60 (14%)	6 (7%)
Poor	150 (13%)	30 (9.5%)	28 (7%)	8 (10%)
Death	51 (4%)	7 (2.5%)	41 (10%)	1 (1%)
Total	1158	285	422	82

Table 11b Aneurysm Size and Surgical Outcome (Grade 0/Nonruptured Aneurysm)

	Size of aneurysm		
Result	Saccular	Globular	Giant
Excellent	89%	88%	75%
Good	7%	8%	12%
Poor	2.5%	2%	6%
Death	1.5%	2%	7%

The timing of surgery after SAH and outcome were assessed for cases who underwent surgery (total of 1196 cases, Table 4). Early surgery (day 0–3) was performed in 21% and delayed surgery after the first week was done in 59% of patients. Although previous reports [78,79] have indicated that surgery during the vasospasm period (day 4–11) has a poorer prognosis, our results did not show any difference except for those in Grade 1 with surgery performed between day 4–7. The best outcome in Grade-4 patients was achieved with early surgery (day 0–3).

ACKNOWLEDGMENT

Cases and results are based on experience of patients who underwent surgery by Drs. Thoralf M. Sundt, Jr., David G. Piepgras, and Fredric B. Meyer. The authors acknowledge expert assistance from Ms. Mary Soper in the preparation of this manuscript.

REFERENCES

1. Al-Rodhan NRF, Fox JL. Al–Zahrawi and Arabian neurosurgery 936–1013 AD. *Surg Neurol* 1986; 26: 92–95.
2. de Moulin D. Aneurysms in antiquity. *Arch Chir Neerl* 1961; 13: 49–63.
3. Sundt TM Jr. Surgical Techniques for Saccular and Giant Intracranial Aneurysms. Baltimore: Williams and Wilkins, 1990.
4. Schorstein J. Carotid ligation in saccular intracranial aneurysms. *Br J Surg* 1940; 28: 50–70.
5. Dandy WE. Intracranial aneurysm of internal carotid artery, cured by operation. *Ann Surg* 1938; 107: 654–659.
6. Pool JL, Colton RP. The dissecting microscope for intracranial vascular surgery. *J Neurosurg* 1966; 25: 315–318.
7. Yasargil MG. Microsurgery Applied to Neurosurgery. Stuttgart: George Thieme Verlag, 1969: 119–143.
8. Atkinson JLD, Sundt TM Jr, Houser OW, Whisnant JP. Angiographic frequency of anterior circulation intracranial aneurysms. *J Neurosurg* 1989; 70: 551–555.
9. McCormick WF, Nofzinger JD. Saccular intracranial aneurysm: an autopsy study. *J Neurosurg* 1965; 23: 155–159.
10. Pakarinen S. Incidence, aetiology, and prognosis of primary subarachnoid haemorrhage: a study based on 589 cases diagnosed in a defined urban population during a defined period. *Acta Neurol Scand* 1967; 43(Suppl 29): 1–128.
11. Sekhar LN, Heros RC. Origin, growth, and rupture of saccular aneurysms: a review. *Neurosurgery* 1981; 8: 248–260.
12. Stehbens WE. Intracranial arterial aneurysms. In: Pathology of the Cerebral Blood Vessels. Saint Louis: CV Mosby, 1972: 351–470.
13. Phillips LH II, Whisnant JP, O'Fallon WM, Sundt TM Jr. The unchanging pattern of subarachnoid hemorrhage in a community. *Neurology* 1980; 30: 1034–1040.
14. Jane JA, Kassell NF, Torner JC, Winn HR. The natural history of aneurysms and arteriovenous malformations. *J Neurosurg* 1985; 62: 321–323.
15. Juvela S, Porras M, Heiskanen O. Natural history of unruptured intracranial aneurysms: a long–term follow–up study. *J Neurosurg* 1993; 79: 174–182.
16. Freytag E. Fatal rupture of intracranial aneurysms. *Arch Path* 1966; 81: 418–424.
17. Kiyohara Y, Ueda K, Hasuo Y, et al. Incidence and prognosis of subarachnoid hemorrhage in a Japanese rural community. *Stroke* 1989; 20: 1150–1155.
18. Sahs AL, Nibbelink DW, Torner JC. Aneurysmal Subarachnoid Hemorrhage: Report of the Cooperative Study. Baltimore: Urban and Schwarzenberg, 1981.
19. Drake CG. Progress in cerebrovascular disease. Management of cerebral aneurysms. *Stroke* 1981; 12: 273–283.
20. Ljunggren B, Sonesson B, Saveland H, Brandt L. Cognitive impairment and adjustment in patients without neurological deficits after aneurysmal SAH and early operation. *J Neurosurg* 1985; 62: 673–679.
21. Storey PB. Psychiatric sequelae of subarachnoid hemorrhage. *Br Med J* 1967; 3: 261–266.
22. Sahs AL. Observation on the pathology of saccular aneurysms. In: Intracranial An-

eurysms and Subarachnoid Hemorrhage: A Cooperative Study. Philadelphia: JB Lippincott, 1969: 22–36.

23. Dyste GN, Beck DW. De novo aneurysm formation following carotid ligation: case report and review of the literature. *Neurosurgery* 1989; 24: 88–92.
24. Handa H, Hashimoto N, Nagata I, Hazama F. Saccular cerebral aneurysms in rats: a newly developed animal model of the disease. *Stroke* 1983; 14: 857–886.
25. Hashimoto N, Handa H, Hazama F. Experimentally induced cerebral aneurysms in rats. *Surg Neurol* 1978; 10: 3–8.
26. Rinne JK, Hernesniemi JA. De Novo aneurysms: special multiple intracranial aneurysms. *Neurosurgery* 1993; 33: 981–985.
27. Schievink WI, Piepgras DG, Wirth FP. Rupture of previously documented small asymptomatic saccular intracranial aneurysms. *J Neurosurg* 1992; 76: 1019–1024.
28. Stehbens WE. Aneurysms and anatomical variations of cerebral arteries. *Arch Pathol* 1963; 75: 45–64.
29. Kak VK, Gleadhill CA, Baily IC. The familial incidence of intracranial aneurysms. *J Neurol Neurosurg Psychiat* 1970; 33: 29–33.
30. Lozano AM, LeBlanc R. Familial intracranial aneurysms. *J Neurosurg* 1987; 66: 522–528.
31. Levey AS, Pauker SG, Kassirer JP. Occult intracranial aneurysms in polycystic kidney disease: When is the cerebral arteriography indicated? *N Engl J Med* 1983; 308: 986–994.
32. Neil-Dwyer G, Bartlett JR, Nicholls AC, Narcisi P, Pope FM. Collagen deficiency and ruptured cerebral aneurysms. *J Neurosurg* 1983; 59: 16–20.
33. Crawford T. Some observations on the pathogenesis and natural history of intracranial aneurysms. *J Neurol Neurosurg Psychiat* 1959; 22: 259–266.
34. Kodama N, Suzuki J. Moyamoya disease associated with aneurysm. *J Neurosurg* 1978; 48: 565–569.
35. Waga S, Tochio H. Intracranial aneurysm associated with moyamoya disease in childhood. *Surg Neurol* 1985; 23: 237–243.
36. Kunishio K, Yamamoto Y, Sunami N, Asari S. Agenesis of the left internal carotid artery, common carotid artery, and main trunk of the external carotid artery associated with multiple cerebral aneurysms. *Surg Neurol* 1987; 27: 177–181.
37. Weir B. Aneurysms Affecting the Nervous System. Baltimore: Williams & Wilkins, 1987.
38. Benoit BG, Wortzman G. Traumatic cerebral aneurysms. Clinical features and natural history. *J Neurol Neurosurg Psychiat* 1973; 36: 127–138.
39. Lindsey KW, Bone I, Callander R. Neurology and Neurosurgery Illustrated, Ed 2. New York: Churchill Livingstone, 1991.
40. LeBlanc R. The minor leak preceding subarachnoid hemorrhage. *J Neurosurg* 1987; 66: 35–39.
41. Okawara S-H. Warning signs prior to rupture of an intracranial aneurysm. *J Neurosurg* 1973; 38: 575–580.
42. Drake CG. Report of World Federation of Neurological Surgeons Committee on a Universal Subarachnoid Hemorrhage Grading Scale. *J Neurosurg* 1988; 68: 985–986.

43. Hunt WE, Hess RM. Surgical risk as related to time of intervention in the repair of intracranial aneurysms. *J Neurosurg* 1968; 28: 14–20.
44. Botterell EH, Lougheed WM, Scott JW, Vandewater SL. Hypothermia, and interruption of carotid, or carotid and vertebral circulation, in the surgical management of intracranial aneurysms. *J Neurosurg* 1956; 13: 1–42.
45. Whisnant JP, Sacco SE, O'Fallon WM, Fode NC, Sundt TM Jr. Referral bias in aneurysmal subarachnoid hemorrhage. *J Neurosurg* 1993; 78: 726–732.
46. Fisher CM, Kistler JP, Davis JM. Relation of cerebral vasospasm to subarachnoid hemorrhage visualized by computerized tomographic scanning. *Neurosurgery* 1980; 6: 1–9.
47. Todo T, Usui M, Takakura K. Treatment of severe intraventricular hemorrhage by intraventricular infusion of urokinase. *J Neurosurg* 1991; 74: 81–86.
48. Kassell NF, Torner JC. Aneurysmal rebleeding: a preliminary report from the cooperative aneurysm study. *Neurosurgery* 1983; 13: 479–481.
49. Nishioka H, Torner JC, Graf CJ, Kassell NF, Sahs AL, Goettler LC. Cooperative study of intracranial aneurysms and subarachnoid hemorrhage: a long–term prognostic study. II: Ruptured intracranial aneurysms managed conservatively. *Arch Neurol* 1984; 41: 1142–1146.
50. Graff-Radford NR, Torner J, Adams HP Jr, Kassell NF. Factors associated with hydrocephalus after subarachnoid hemorrhage. *Arch Neurol* 1989; 46: 744–752.
51. van Gijn J, Hijdra A, Wijdicks EFM, Vermeulen M, van Crevel H. Acute hydrocephalus after aneurysmal subarachnoid hemorrhage. *J Neurosurg* 1985; 63: 355–362.
52. Vassilouthis J, Richardson AE. Ventricular dilatation and communicating hydrocephalus following spontaneous subarachnoid hemorrhage. *J Neurosurg* 1979; 51: 341–351.
53. Vassilouthis J. The syndrome of normal–pressure hydrocephalus. *J Neurosurg* 1984; 61: 501–509.
54. Hayashi M, Kobayashi H, Munemoto S, et al. An analysis of time course of intracranial pressure in patients with communicating hydrocephalus following subarachnoid hemorrhage due to ruptured intracranial aneurysms. *Brain Nerve* 1982; 34: 653–660.
55. Black PM, Ojemann RG, Tzouras A. CSF shunts for dementia, incontinence, and gait disturbance. *Clin Neurosurg* 1985; 32: 632–651.
56. Ecker A, Riemenschneider P. Arteriographic demonstration of spasm of the intracranial arteries: with special reference to saccular arterial aneurisms. *J Neurosurg* 1951; 8: 660–667.
57. Weir B, Grace M, Hansen J, Rothberg C. Time course of vasospasm in man. *J Neurosurg* 1978; 48: 173–178.
58. Kassell NF, Sasaki T, Colohan ART, Nazar G. Cerebral vasospasm following aneurysmal subarachnoid hemorrhage: progress reviews. *Stroke* 1985; 16: 562–572.
59. Wilkins RH. Attempted prevention or treatment of intracranial arterial spasm: a survey. *Neurosurgery* 1980; 6: 198–210.
60. Wilkins RH (ed). Cerebral arterial spasm. Proceedings of the Second International Workshop. Baltimore: Williams and Wilkins, 1980.

61. Wilkins RH. Attempts at prevention or treatment of intracranial arterial spasm: an update. *Neurosurgery* 1986; 18: 808–825.
62. Fisher CM, Roberson GH, Ojemann RG. Cerebral vasospasm with ruptured saccular aneurysm—the clinical manifestations. *Neurosurgery* 1977; 1: 245–248.
63. Sakaki T, Kinugawa K, Tanigake T, Miyamoto S, Kyoi K, Utsumi S. Embolism from intracranial aneurysms. *J Neurosurg* 1980; 53: 300–304.
64. Fisher M, Davidson RI, Marcus EM. Transient focal cerebral ischemia as a presenting manifestation of unruptured cerebral aneurysms. *Ann Neurol* 1980; 8: 367–372.
65. Ostergaard JR, Hog E. Incidence of multiple intracranial aneurysms. Influence of arterial hypertension and gender. *J Neurosurg* 1985; 63: 49–55.
66. Yasargil MG (ed). Microneurosurgery, Vol II, Clinical Considerations, Surgery of the Intracranial Aneurysms and Results. Stuttgart: George Thieme Verlag, 1987.
67. Friedamn AH, Drake CG. Subarachnoid hemorrhage from intracranial dissecting aneurysm. *J Neurosurg* 1984; 60: 325–334.
68. Crompton MR. Hypothalamic lesions following the rupture of cerebral berry aneurysms. *Brain* 1963; 86: 301–314.
69. Marion DW, Segal R, Thompson ME. Subarachnoid hemorrhage and the heart. *Neurosurgery* 1986; 18: 101–106.
70. Weir BK. Pulmonary edema following fatal aneurysm rupture. *J Neurosurg* 1978; 49: 502–507.
71. Garfinkle AM, Danys IR, Nicolle DA, Colohan ART, Brem S. Terson's syndrome: a reversible cause of blindness following subarachnoid hemorrhage. *J Neurosurg* 1992; 76: 766–771.
72. Kassell NF, Peerless SJ, Durward QJ, Beck DW, Drake CG, Adams HP. Treatment of ischemic deficits from vasospasm with intravascular volume expansion and induced arterial hypertension. *Neurosurgery* 1982; 11: 337–343.
73. Kassell NF, Drake CG. Timing of aneurysm surgery. *Neurosurgery* 1982; 10: 514–519.
74. Aaslid R, Huber P, Nornes H. Evaluation of cerebrovascular spasm with transcranial Doppler ultrasound. *J Neurosurg* 1984; 60: 37–41.
75. Olsen WL, Brant-Zawadzki M, Hodes J, Norman D, Newton TH. Giant intracranial aneurysms: MR imaging. *Radiology* 1987; 163: 431–435.
76. Wiebers DO, Whisnant JP, O'Fallon WM. The natural history of unruptured intracranial aneurysms. *N Engl J Med* 1981; 304: 696–698.
77. Wiebers DO, Whisnant JP, Sundt TM Jr, O'Fallon WM. The significance of unruptured intracranial saccular aneurysms. *J Neurosurg* 1987; 66: 23–29.
78. Kassell NF, Torner JC, Haley EC Jr, Jane JA, Adams HP, Kongable GL, and participants. The international cooperative study on the timing of aneurysm surgery. Part 1: Overall management result. *J Neurosurg* 1990; 73: 18–36.
79. Kassell NF, Torner JC, Jane JA, Haley EC Jr, Adams HP, and participants. The international cooperative study on the timing of aneurysm surgery. Part 2: Surgical results. *J Neurosurg* 1990; 73: 37–47.
80. Saveland H, Hillman J, Brandt L, Edner G, Jakobsson K-E, Algers G. Overall outcome in aneurysmal subarachnoid hemorrhage. A prospective study from neurosurgical units in Sweden during a 1–year period. *J Neurosurg* 1992; 76: 729–734.

81. Miyaoka M, Sato K, Ishii S. A clinical study of the relationship of timing to outcome of surgery for ruptured cerebral aneurysms. A retrospective analysis of 1622 cases. *J Neurosurg* 1993; 79: 373–378.
82. Wilson CB, Spetzler RF. Operative approaches to aneurysms. *Clin Neurosurg* 1978; 26: 232–247.
83. Nichols DA. Endovascular treatment of the acutely ruptured intracranial aneurysm. *J Neurosurg* 1993; 79: 1–2.
84. Romodanov AP, Shcheglov VI. Intravascular occlusion of saccular aneurysms of the cerebral arteries by means of a detachable balloon catheter. In: Krayenbuhl H, (ed). Advances and Technical Standards in Neurosurgery. New York: Springer–Verlag, 1982: 25–49.
85. Serbinenko FA. Balloon catheterization and occlusion of major cerebral vessels. *J Neurosurg* 1974; 41: 125–145.
86. Higashida RT, Halbach VV, Dowd CF, Barnwell SL, Hieshima GB. Intracranial aneurysms: interventional neurovascular treatment with detachable balloons—results in 215 cases. *Radiology* 1991; 178: 663–670.
87. Guglielmi G, Vinuela F, Sepetka I, Macellari V. Electrothrombosis of saccular aneurysms via endovascular approach. Part 1: Electrochemical basis, technique, and experimental results. *J Neurosurg* 1991; 75: 1–7.
88. Guglielmi G, Vinuela F, Dion J, Duckwiler G. Electrothrombosis of saccular aneurysms via endovascular approach. Part 2: Preliminary clinical experience. *J Neurosurg* 1991; 75: 8–14.
89. Halbach VV, Higashida RT, Dowd CF, Barnwell SL, Hieshima GB. Management of vascular perforations that occur during neurointerventional procedures. *AJNR* 1991; 12: 319–327.
90. Higashida RT, Halback VV, Dormandy B, Bell JD, Hieshima GB. Endovascular treatment of intracranial aneurysms with a new silicone microballoon device: technical considerations and indications for therapy. *Radiology* 1990; 174: 687–691.
91. Hodes JE, Fox AJ, Pelz DM, Peerless SJ. Rupture of aneurysms following balloon embolization. *J Neurosurg* 1990; 72: 567–571.
92. Kwan ESK, Heilman CB, Shucart WA, Klucznik RP. Enlargement of basilar artery aneurysms following balloon occlusion—"water–hammer effect". *J Neurosurg* 1991; 75: 963–968.
93. Guglielmi G, Vinuela F, Duckwiller G, et al. Endovascular treatment of posterior circulation aneurysms by electrothrombosis using electrically detachable coils. *J Neurosurg* 1992; 77: 515–524.
94. Casasco AE, Aymard A, Gobin YP, et al. Selective endovascular treatment of 71 intracranial aneurysms with platinum coils. *J Neurosurg* 1993; 79: 3–10.
95. Swann KW, Heros RC, Debrun G, Nelson C. Inadvertent middle cerebral artery embolism by a detachable balloon: management by embolectomy. Case report. *J Neurosurg* 1986; 64: 309–312.
96. Guglielmi G, Vinuela F, Dion J, Duckwiler G. Response to: endovascular treatment of aneurysms with coils by Hilal SK, Solomon RA. *J Neurosurg* 1992; 76: 338–339.

97. Heilman CB, Kwan ESK, Wu JK. Aneurysm recurrence following endovascular balloon occlusion. *J Neurosurg* 1992; 77: 260–264.
98. Hilal SK, Solomon RA. Endovascular treatment of aneurysms with coils. *J Neurosurg* 1992; 76: 337–338.
99. Fox AJ, Vinuela F, Pelz DM, et al. Use of detachable balloons for proximal artery occlusion in the treatment of unclippable cerebral aneurysms. *J Neurosurg* 1987; 66: 40–46.
100. Mathews D, Walker BS, Purdy PD, et al. Brain blood flow SPECT in temporary balloon occlusion of carotid and intracerebral arteries. *J Nucl Med* 1993; 34: 1239–1243.
101. Zubkov YN, Nikiforov BM, Shustin VA. Balloon catheter technique for dilatation of constricted cerebral arteries after aneurysmal SAH. *Acta Neurochir* 1984; 70: 65–79.
102. Higashida RT, Halbach VV, Cahan LD, et al. Transluminal angioplasty for treatment of intracranial arterial vasospasm. *J Neurosurg* 1989; 71: 648–653.
103. Linskey ME, Horton JA, Rao GR, Yonas H. Fatal rupture of the intracranial carotid artery during transluminal angioplasty for vasospasm induced by subarachnoid hemorrhage. Case report. *J Neurosurg* 1991; 74: 985–990.
104. Swearingen B, Heros RC. Common carotid occlusion for unclippable carotid aneurysms: an old but still effective operation. *Neurosurgery* 1987; 21: 288–295.
105. Tindall GT, Goree JA, Lee JF, Odom GL. Effect of common carotid ligation on size of internal carotid aneurysms and distal intracarotid and retinal artery pressure. *J Neurosurg* 1966; 25: 503–511.
106. Steinberg GK, Drake CG, Peerless SJ. Deliberate basilar or vertebral artery occlusion in the treatment of intracranial aneurysms. Immediate results and long–term outcome in 201 patients. *J Neurosurg* 1993; 79: 161–173.
107. Drake CG. Ligation of the vertebral (unilateral or bilateral) or basilar artery in the treatment of large intracranial aneurysms. *J Neurosurg* 1975; 43: 255–274.
108. Drake CG. The treatment of aneurysms of the posterior circulation. *Clin Neurosurg* 1979; 26: 96–144.
109. Hashi K, Nin K. Complications following carotid ligation combined with EC–IC bypass. *Neurosurgeon* 1984; 4: 359–366.
110. Roski RA, Spetzler RF, Nulsen FE. Late complications of carotid ligation in the treatment of intracranial aneurysms. *J Neurosurg* 1981; 54: 583–587.
111. Higashida RT, Halbach VV, Dowd C, et al. Endovascular detachable balloon embolization therapy of cavernous carotid artery aneurysms: results in 87 cases. *J Neurosurg* 1990; 72: 857–863.
112. Osguthorpe JD, Hungerford GD. Transarterial carotid occlusion. *Arch Otolaryngol* 1984; 110: 694–696.
113. Heros RC. Thromboembolic complications after combined internal carotid ligation and extra–to–intracranial bypass. *Surg Neurol* 1984; 21: 75–79.
114. Drake CG. Giant intracranial aneurysms: experience with surgical treatment in 174 patients. *Clin Neurosurg* 1979; 26: 12–95.
115. Diaz FG, Ausman JI, Pearce JE. Ischemic complications after combined internal carotid artery occlusion and extracranial–intracranial anastomosis. *Neurosurgery* 1982; 10: 563–570.

116. Sundt TM Jr, Piepgras DG, Marsh RW, Fode NC. Saphenous vein bypass graft for giant aneurysms and intracranial occlusive disease. *J Neurosurg* 1986; 65: 439–450.
117. Fukushima T, Day J, Tung H. Intracavernous carotid artery aneurysms. In: Apuzzo MLJ, (ed). Brain Surgery. Complication Avoidance and Management, Vol. 1. New York: Churchill Livingstone, 1993: 925–944.
118. Michenfelder JD. Cerebral preservation for intraoperative focal ischemia. *Clin Neurosurg* 1985; 32: 105–113.
119. Goldman MS, Anderson RE, Meyer FB. Effects of intermittent reperfusion during temporal focal ischemia. *J Neurosurg* 1992; 77: 911–916.
120. Meyer FB, Muzzi DA. Cerebral protection during aneurysm surgery with isoflurane anesthesia. *J Neurosurg* 1992; 76: 541–543.
121. Ausman JI, McCormick PW, Stewart M, et al. Cerebral oxygen metabolism during hypothermic circulatory arrest in humans. *J Neurosurg* 1993; 79: 810–815.
122. Spetzler RF, Hadley MN, Rigamonti D, et al. Aneurysms of the basilar artery treated with circulatory arrest, hypothermia, and barbiturate cerebral protection. *J Neurosurg* 1988; 68: 868–879.
123. Sugita K. Microneurosurgery Atlas. Berlin: Springer–Verlag, 1985.
124. Yasargil MG (ed). Microneurosurgery, Vol I, Microsurgical Anatomy of the Basal Cisterns and Vessels of the Brain, Diagnostic Studies, General Operative Techniques and Pathological Considerations of the Intracranial Aneurysms. Stuttgart: George Thieme Verlag, 1984.
125. Rhoton AL Jr, Saeki N, Perlmutter D, Zeal A. Microsurgical anatomy of common aneurysm sites. *Clin Neurosurg* 1979; 26: 248–306.
126. Gibo H, Carver CC, Rhoton AL Jr, Lenkey C, Mitchell RJ. Microsurgical anatomy of the middle cerebral artery. *J Neurosurg* 1981; 54: 151–169.
127. Gibo H, Lenkey C, Rhoton AL Jr. Microsurgical anatomy of the supraclinoid portion of the internal carotid artery. *J Neurosurg* 1981; 55: 560–574.
128. Harris FS, Rhoton AL Jr. Anatomy of the cavernous sinus. A microsurgical study. *J Neurosurg* 1976; 45: 169–180.
129. Perlmutter D, Rhoton AL Jr. Microsurgical anatomy of the anterior cerebral–anterior communicating–recurrent artery complex. *J Neurosurg* 1976; 45: 259–272.
130. Saeki N, Rhoton AL Jr. Microsurgical anatomy of the upper basilar artery and the posterior circle of Willis. *J Neurosurg* 1977; 46: 563–578.
131. Zeal AA, Rhoton AL Jr. Microsurgical anatomy of the posterior cerebral artery. *J Neurosurg* 1978; 48: 534–559.
132. Hongo K, Kobayashi S, Yokoh A, Sugita K. Monitoring retraction pressure on the brain. An experimental and clinical study. *J Neurosurg* 1987; 66: 270–275.
133. Parkinson D. A surgical approach to the cavernous portion of the carotid artery. Anatomical studies and case report. *J Neurosurg* 1965; 23: 474–483.
134. Parkinson D. Carotid cavernous fistula: direct repair with preservation of the carotid artery. Technical note. *J Neurosurg* 1973; 38: 99–106.
135. Dolenc V. Direct microsurgical repair of intracavernous vascular lesions. *J Neurosurg* 1983; 58: 824–831.

136. Dolenc VV. A combined epi– and subdural direct approach to carotid–ophthalmic artery aneurysms. *J Neurosurg* 1985; 62: 667–672.
137. Sekhar LN, Sen CN, Jho HD, Janecka IP. Surgical treatment of intracavernous neoplasms: a four–year experience. *Neurosurgery* 1989; 24: 18–30.
138. Al-Rodhan NRF, Piepgras DG, Sundt TM Jr. Transitional cavernous aneurysms of the internal carotid artery. *Neurosurgery* 1993; 33: 993–998.
139. Linskey ME, Sekhar LN, Hirsch WL Jr, Yonas H, Horton JA. Aneurysms of the intracavernous carotid artery: natural history and indications for treatment. *Neurosurgery* 1990; 26: 933–938.
140. Heros RC, Ojemann RG, Crowell RM. Superior temporal gyrus approach to middle cerebral artery aneurysms: technique and results. *Neurosurgery* 1982; 10: 308–313.
141. Piepgras DG. Posterior cerebral and superior cerebellar artery aneurysms. In: Apuzzo MLJ, (ed). Brain Surgery. Complication Avoidance and Management, Vol. 1. New York: Churchill Livingstone, 1993: 1083–1100.
142. Peerless SJ, Drake CG. Posterior circulation aneurysms. In: Wilkins RH, Rengachary SS, (eds). Neurosurgery, Vol. 2. New York: McGraw-Hill, 1985: 1422–1437.
143. Sugita K, Kobayashi S, Shintani A, Mutsuga N. Microneurosurgery for aneurysms of the basilar artery. *J Neurosurg* 1979; 51: 615–620.
144. Fujitsu K, Kuwabara T. Zygomatic approach for lesions in the interpeduncular cistern. *J Neurosurg* 1985; 62: 340–343.
145. Sugita K, Kobayashi S, Takemae T, Tada T, Tanaka Y. Aneurysms of the basilar artery trunk. *J Neurosurg* 1987; 66: 500–505.
146. Kawase T, Toya S, Shiobara R, Mine T. Transpetrosal approach for aneurysms of the lower basilar artery. *J Neurosurg* 1985; 3: 857–861.
147. Saito I, Takahashi H, Joshita H, Usui M, Sasaki T, Sano K. Clipping of vertebro–basilar aneurysms by the transoral transclival approach. *Neurol Med Chir (Tokyo)* 1980; 20: 753–758.
148. Kasdon DL, Stein BM. Combined supratentorial and infratentorial exposure for low–lying basilar aneurysms. *Neurosurgery* 1979; 4: 422–426.
149. Spetzler RF, Daspit CP, Pappas CTE. The combined supra– and infratentorial approach for lesions of the petrous and clival regions: experience with 46 cases. *J Neurosurg* 1992; 76: 588–599.
150. Heros RC. Lateral suboccipital approach for vertebral and vertebrobasilar artery lesions. *J Neurosurg* 1986; 64: 559–562.
151. Higashida RT, Halbach VV, Cahan LD, Hieshima GB, Konishi Y. Detachable balloon embolization therapy of posterior circulation intracranial aneurysms. *J Neurosurg* 1989; 71: 512–519.
152. Pia HW, Zierski J. Giant cerebral aneurysms. *Neurosurg Rev* 1982; 5: 117–148.
153. Sundt TM Jr, Piepgras DG. Surgical approach to giant intracranial aneurysms. Operative experience with 80 cases. *J Neurosurg* 1979; 51: 731–742.
154. Tamaki N, Kim S, Ehara K, et al. Giant carotid–ophthalmic artery aneurysms: direct clipping utilizing the "trapping–evacuation" technique. *J Neurosurg* 1991; 74: 567–572.

155. Debrun G, Fox A, Drake CG, Peerless S, Girvin J, Ferguson G. Giant unclippable aneurysms: treatment with detachable balloons. *AJNR* 1981; 2: 167–173.
156. Taki W, Nishi S, Yamashita K, et al. Selection and combination of various endovascular techniques in the treatment of giant aneurysms. *J Neurosurg* 1992; 77: 37–42.
157. Simpson RK Jr, Harper RL, Bryan RN. Emergency balloon occlusion for massive epistaxis due to traumatic carotid–cavernous aneurysm. Case report. *J Neurosurg* 1988; 68: 142–144.
158. Fleisher AS, Patton JM, Tindall GT. Cerebral aneurysms of traumatic origin. *Surg Neurol* 1975; 4: 233–239.
159. Giannotta SL, Weiss MH. Pitfalls in the diagnosis of head injury. *Clin Neurosurg* 1982; 29: 288–299.
160. Morawetz RB, Karp RB. Evolution and resolution of intracranial bacterial (mycotic) aneurysms. *Neurosurgery* 1984; 15: 43–49.
161. Clare CE, Barrow DL. Infectious intracranial aneurysms. *Neurosurg Clin North Am* 1992; 3: 551–566.
162. Ojemann RG. Infectious intracranial aneurysms. In: Fein JM, Flamm ES, (eds). Cerebrovascular Surgery, Vol. III. New York: Springer-Verlag, 1985:1047–1060.
163. Bohmfalk GL, Story JL, Wissinger JP, Brown WE Jr. Bacterial intracranial aneurysm. *J Neurosurg* 1978; 48: 369–382.
164. Ahuja GK, Jain N, Vijayaraghavan M, Roy S. Cerebral mycotic aneurysm of fungal origin. Case report. *J Neurosurg* 1978; 49: 107–110.
165. Roeltgen DP, Weimer GR, Patterson LF. Delayed neurologic complications of left atrial myxoma. *Neurology (Ny)* 1981; 31: 8–13.
166. Steinberg GK, Guppy KH, Adler JR, Silverberg GD. Stereotactic, angiography–guided clipping of a distal, mycotic intracranial aneurysm using the Cosman–Roberts–Wells system: technical note. *Neurosurgery* 1992; 30: 408–411.
167. Khayata MH, Aymard A, Casasco A, Herbreteau D, Woimant F, Merland JJ. Selective endovascular techniques in the treatment of cerebral mycotic aneurysms. *J Neurosurg* 1993; 78: 661–665.
168. Halbach VV, Higashida RT, Dowd CF, et al. Endovascular treatment of vertebral artery dissections and pseudoaneurysms. *J Neurosurg* 1993; 79: 183–191.
169. Yamaura A, Watanabe Y, Saeki N. Dissecting aneurysms of the intracranial vertebral artery. *J Neurosurg* 1990; 72: 183–188.
170. Shokunbi MT, Vinters HV, Kaufmann JCE. Fusiform intracranial aneurysms. Clinicopathologic features. *Surg Neurol* 1988; 29: 263–270.
171. Crawford PM, West CR, Chadwick DW, Shaw MDM. Arteriovenous malformations of the brain: Natural history in unoperated patients. *J Neurol Neurosurg Psychiat* 1986; 49: 1–10.
172. Ferrante L, Fortuna A, Celli P, Santoro A, Fraioli B. Intracranial arterial aneurysms in early childhood. *Surg Neurol* 1988; 29: 39–56.
173. Matson DD. Intracranial arterial aneurysms in childhood. *J Neurosurg* 1965; 23: 578–583.
174. Meyer FB, Sundt TM Jr, Fode NC, Morgan MK, Forbes GS, Mellinger JF. Cerebral aneurysms in childhood and adolescence. *J Neurosurg* 1989; 70: 420–425.

175. Barrett JM, Van Hooydonk JE, Boehm FH. Pregnancy–related rupture of arterial aneurysms. *Obstet Gynecol Surv* 1982; 37: 557–566.
176. Pedowitz P, Perell A. Aneurysms complicated by pregnancy. Part II. Aneurysms of the cerebral vessels. *Am J Obs & Gynec* 1957; 73: 736–749.
177. Nehls DG, Flom RA, Carter LP, Spetzler RF. Multiple intracranial aneurysms: determining the site of rupture. *J Neurosurg* 1985; 63: 342–348.
178. Findlay JM, Weir BKA, Steinke D, Tanabe T, Gordon P, Grace M. Effect of intrathecal thrombolytic therapy on subarachnoid clot and chronic vasospasm in a primate model of SAH. *J Neurosurg* 1988; 69: 723–735.
179. Findlay JM, Weir BKA, Kassell NF, Disney LB, Grace MGA. Intracisternal recombinant tissue plasminogen activator after aneurysmal subarachnoid hemorrhage. *J Neurosurg* 1991; 75: 181–188.
180. Mizoi K, Yoshimoto T, Takahashi A, Fujiwara S, Koshu K, Sugawara T. Prospective study on the prevention of cerebral vasospasm by intrathecal fibrinolytic therapy with tissue–type plasminogen activator. *J Neurosurg* 1993; 78: 430–437.
181. Saito I, Ueda Y, Sano K. Significance of vasospasm in the treatment of ruptured intracranial aneurysms. *J Neurosurg* 1977; 47: 412–429.
182. Taneda M. Effect of early operation for ruptured aneurysms on prevention of delayed ischemic symptoms. *J Neurosurg* 1982; 57: 622–628.
183. Zabramski JM, Spetzler RF, Lee KS, et al. Phase I trial of tissue plasminogen activator for the prevention of vasospasm in patients with aneurysmal subarachnoid hemorrhage. *J Neurosurg* 1991; 75: 189–196.
184. Allen GS, Ahn HS, Preziosi TJ, et al. Cerebral arterial spasm—a controlled trial of nimodipine in patients with subarachnoid hemorrhage. *N Engl J Med* 1983; 308: 619–624.
185. Petruk KC, West M, Mohr G, et al. Nimodipine treatment in poor–grade aneurysm patients. Results of a multicenter double–blind placebo–controlled trial. *J Neurosurg* 1988; 68: 505–517.
186. Chyatte D, Fode NC, Nichols DA, Sundt TM Jr. A preliminary report: effects of high dose methylprednisolone on delayed cerebral ischemia in patients at high risk for vasospasm after aneurysmal subarachnoid hemorrhage. *Neurosurgery* 1987; 21: 157–160.
187. Kaku Y, Yonekawa Y, Tsukahara T, Kazekawa K. Superselective intra-arterial infusion of papaverine for the treatment of cerebral vasospasm after subarachnoid hemorrhage. *J Neurosurg* 1992; 77: 842–847.
188. Milhorat TH. Acute hydrocephalus after aneurysmal subarachnoid hemorrhage. *Neurosurgery* 1987; 20: 15–20.
189. Pare L, Delfino R, Leblanc R. The relationship of ventricular drainage to aneurysmal rebleeding. *J Neurosurg* 1992; 76: 422–427.
190. Takaku A, Shindo K, Tanaka S, Mori T, Suzuki J. Fluid and electrolyte disturbances in patients with intracranial aneurysms. *Surg Neurol* 1979; 11: 349–356.
191. Maroon JC, Nelson PB. Hypovolemia in patients with subarachnoid hemorrhage: therapeutic implications. *Neurosurgery* 1979; 4: 223–226.
192. Ayus JC, Krothapalli RK, Arieff AI. Treatment of symptomatic hyponatremia and

its relation to brain damage. A prospective study. *N Engl J Med* 1987; 317: 1190–1195.

193. Sbeih I, Tamas LB, O'Laroire SA. Epilepsy after operation for aneurysms. *Neurosurgery* 1986; 19: 784–788.

15

Surgical Management of Arteriovenous Malformations of the Brain, Spine, and Dura

Michael K. Morgan
University of Sydney, Sydney, New South Wales, Australia

David G Piepgras and Thoralf M. Sundt†
Mayo Clinic, Rochester, Minnesota

I. INTRODUCTION

Surgical treatment of arteriovenous malformation of the brain had been attempted on at least 9 occasions prior to 1900 [1]. The first report in the literature was that of Giordano in 1890 and on three occasions complete extirpation was claimed to have been achieved prior to the turn of the century [2–5]. In these early cases the patients were reported to have fared well, at least in the immediate postoperative period. In fact, there was no report of a death following surgery until 1902 [6]. The indications for surgery in these early cases was for the management of an unknown but presumably sinnister intracranial space-occupying lesion and diagnosis was not possible prior to exposure.

Before the introduction of cerebral angiography, resection of an arteriovenous malformation was unrewarding despite early optimistic reports. Both Dandy and Cushing had accumulated enough cases by 1928 that they reported their surgical experience. In contrast to a review of case reports to that time (suggesting the majority of patients could be cured with little morbidity or mortality) [1], a series each from Cushing and Dandy suggests that this view was incorrect [7,8]. Dandy concluded from his experience that "the radical attempt at cure is attended by such supreme difficulties and is so exceedingly

†Deceased.

dangerous as to be contraindicated except in certain selected cases" [8]. Cushing and Bailey concluded from their experience that to "extirpate one of these aneurysmal angiomas in its active state would be unthinkable" [7]. With the introduction of angiography the surgeon became armed with information that allowed for the planning of treatment [9].

Olivecrona and Riives were the first to publish a numerically reasonable series supporting surgical resection for selected cases [10]. It was apparent to these authors the "uselessness of partial occlusion of the arterial supply" and that they "were unable to find any proof that Roentgen treatment . . . in any way alters the spontaneous course of the illness" [10]. Furthermore, in their experience, carotid ligation (as recommended by Dandy) was "more dangerous than excision of the malformation" [10] Their decision was "that the choice lies between removing the lesion and leaving it alone." They had excised 43 arteriovenous malformations with 4 deaths (one of which was due to meningitis at a time when antibiotics were not freely available) and one third of survivors were "practically well." Shortly after this report Norlen added 10 operative cases and established postoperative angiography as the investigation of choice in objectively assessing the completeness of removal [11]. At this time the enthusiasm for radical excision was in the ascendency. The advisability of radical excision of cerebral arteriovenous malformations was based on the belief that "in the end, probably most, if not all, patients die of hemorrhage or are completely incapacitated" [10]. However, little was really known of the natural history at this time because of the limited experience with cerebral angiography prior to the Second World War. Potter attempted the first assessment of the natural history with the likely benefits of radical excision [12]. In assessing 12 patients that died with arteriovenous malformations he found that 3 died from unrelated causes and in his opinion, in only one case would "radical operative treatment likely . . . have been possible without risking a severe disablement." From the 58 patients studied the conclusion reached was that "these malformations do not necessarily cause early death or disability." For several decades after Potter's paper, before the development of a computerized axial tomographic scanning, the natural history remained elusive because of difficulties in identifying a population of patients prior to arteriovenous malformation (AVM) rupture. Thus conflicting opinion regarding the advisability of surgery continued [13–16].

Since 1980 the natural history has more clearly been defined. The results of studies by Brown et al., Graf et al., Ondra et al., Crawford et al., Fults and Kelly, and Itoyama et al. have all contributed to this knowledge [17–22]. These authors allow us to conclude that there is an annual risk of hemorrhage of 2 to 4% per year with an annual mortality of 1% per year. For the first year after a hemorrhage the risk of further hemorrhage is 6 to 14%.

II. INDICATIONS FOR SURGICAL RESECTION OF AN ARTERIOVENOUS MALFORMATION OF THE BRAIN

Surgical management of arteriovenous malformation of the brain has been considered for the control of hemorrhage, seizures, nonhemorrhagic neurological deficits, headache, cerebrospinal fluid circulation disorder, and cardiac failure. While certain of these complications have been accepted as reasonable indications for surgery in certain circumstances, others are considered less advisable indications. We will discuss each of these arteriovenous malformation complications in turn.

A. Intracerebral and Subarachnoid Hemorrhage

Cerebral arteriovenous malformation have been known to be a cause for intraparenchymal hemorrhage since 1854 [23]. Of series reported from the past decade, intraparenchymal hemorrhage constitutes 51 to 72% of the modes of presentation [24–32]. For patients with cerebral arteriovenous malformations, the risk for clinically significant first hemorrhage is 2 to 4% per year [17,20–22] and the risk for recurrent hemorrhage is initially 6 to 14% per year declining to a prehemorrhage rate after 5 years [19–21]. Mortality for hemorrhage may approach 30% [17,19,33] and nearly a quarter of survivors from hemorrhage have permanent morbidity [17,33]. Site, size, shunt resistance, presence of seizures, hypertension, age and sex have been shown not to influence the occurrence of hemorrhage [17,20]. However, an increasing venous resistance as caused by venous drainage occlusion [34,35] and the presence of associated arterial aneurysms [17] have both been implicated as factors increasing the propensity for hemorrhage. The risk of hemorrhage in patients with unruptured arteriovenous malformation with an associated arterial aneurysm is 7% per year [36]. The management of intracerebral hemorrhage from an arteriovenous malformation is little different from the management of intraparen-chymal hemorrhage from other causes. It is essential that maximal brain preservation be achieved by optimizing the patients brain perfusion and oxygenation. This may of course necessitate rapid airway control with intubation and ventilation. Measures to control intracranial pressure may need to be introduced and surgical evacuation of the hematoma considered. In deciding whether an intracerebral hematoma should be evacuated, multiple factors need to be considered including the clinical condition of the patient (such as severity and temporal profile of neurological deficit), the site and extent of the hemorrhage, and the anticipated quality of survival [37–41]. It must be borne in mind that very early evacuation may offer a benefit to the local microcirculation that is lost with time [42–44]. We generally recommend surgery if the patient's level of consciousness is deteriorating or focal neurological deficits are increasing. If a neurological deficit is present and most brainstem reflexes are preserved, in the presence of a large lobar or subcortical hematoma we recommend surgical evacuation. In the presence of a large intraventricular hemorrhage causing obtundation, ventricular drainage may prove to be useful [45–48,39]. In the presence of a cerebellar hematoma where there is evidence of brainstem compression, hydrocephalus, or diameter greater than 3 cm, surgical evacuation should be considered [49–55,38]. Although evacuation of brainstem hematomas can be performed with good results [56–59] the role for surgery should be reserved as its general benefit has not been established.

When surgically evacuating the hematoma, resection of the arteriovenous malformation should not be performed at the same procedure unless it has been clearly defined prior to surgery by angiography, is small, and can easily be removed through the hematoma cavity. If these conditions cannot be met then consideration should be given to meeting the arteriovenous malformation at an alternative elective procedure. When evacuating the hematoma, the site and size of the craniotomy should take into account the exposure required for the removal of the arteriovenous malformation. When approaching the arteriovenous malformation, a thin layer of clot should be left undisturbed in order to minimize the risk of intraoperative rupture of the underlying pathology.

The major reason for the elective removal of an arteriovenous malformation is to provide prophylaxis against future hemorrhage. Therefore, a correct assessment of the natural history for a particular patient as well as the individual risks of surgery must be formulated. If a recent hemorrhage has occurred or there is an associated intracranial aneurysm (irrespective of size or site) [36,19,20], especially in a young patient, a great deal of consideration must be given to surgical resection because the risk of hemorrhage from these lesions may be more than 6% per year. On the other hand, in older patients with an asymptomatic lesion without associated arterial aneurysms, only the most favourable surgical lesion (small, easily accessible, and in a noneloquent location) may benefit from surgery as the risk from hemorrhage from these lesions may be less than 2% per year [36]. The calculations of surgical risks will be discussed below. However, the number of variables and their relative importance contributing to the risk of surgery defy their simplification into mathematical formulae. Therefore, the art in decision-making regarding the advisability of surgery in the prophylaxis against hemorrhage remains with the individual neurosurgeon who can only be aided by general guidelines.

B. Seizures

Since 1871, seizures have been known to be associated with arteriovenous malformation of the brain [60]. They are the second most-common modality of presentation. Of large series from the last decade, 15 to 38% of all arteriovenous malformation presentations were by a seizure disorder [24–32,61]. Seizures caused by arteriovenous malformation have a wide spectrum of frequency, severity, and focality. In considering the benefits of resection of arteriovenous malformation for epilepsy control, both Yasargil's and the Mayo Clinic's experience suggest that a clear benefit can be obtained [32,62,280]. Piepgras et al. reported that 83% of patients with preoperative seizures were rendered seizure free by surgery and nearly half of these patients were able to discontinue their anticonvulsant therapy [63]. Therefore, seizures may be an indication for surgery in patients in whom epilepsy reduces their quality of life and who prove refractory to medical control (independently to the benefits from hemorrhage prophylaxis). However, when considering surgery for seizure control the workup and resection should be approached with the rigor that seizure disorders from non-arteriovenous malformation etiologies are subjected.

C. Neurological Deficits Unrelated to Hemorrhage

Because arteriovenous malformations may produce focal arterial hypotension and venous hypertension, neurological deficits may arise in the absence of hemorrhage. In these cases the progress of the deficit is often gradual, inexorable, and associated with large cerebral arteriovenous malformations located in or adjacent to eloquent regions [64]. Elvidge was the first to report that there may be comparitively poor visualization by angiography of arteries surrounding arteriovenous malformation [65]. In the first large series of patients with cerebral arteriovenous malformation studied by angiography it was theorized that "anoxemia of the brain due to shunting of the blood" was responsible for progressive neurological deficits, cognitive impairment, and cerebral atrophy" [10]. Shortly thereafter, it was noted that upon resection there was an improvement in angiographic visualization of vessels surrounding the arteriovenous malformation [11]. This phenomenon of a preferential diversion of blood flow to the lower resistance arteriovenous malformation has been termed "steal" [66]. Recently it has been estimated that 1.5% of patients per year with arteriovenous malformation undergo a functional decline [17]. When this is not caused by hemorrhage it can often be accounted for by "steal." Cerebral blood flow studies have demonstrated that an arteriovenous malformation reversibly impairs perfusion of the brain [67–76] and in extreme cases, results in permanent loss of tissue [77,78]. While the relative contributions of regional arterial hypotension and venous hypertension may vary from case to case [67,79–83] the common finding in patients so affected is that there is a high shunt flow and either the arterial feeders or venous drainage (or both) are in the vicinity of eloquent brain.

While patients with nonhemorrhagic neurological deficits may be the group of patients most continuously affected by the arteriovenous malformation, they are often difficult to treat because of the risks of surgery (see below) as both the size and eloquent location may preclude surgical extirpation. In such cases consideration should be given to interventional neuroradiological procedures to provide temporary relief of symptoms [84–86] and focussed irradiation on feeding vessels to reduce the flow [87]. While these procedures may not reduce the risk of hemorrhage in large arteriovenous malformations they may still reduce flow sufficiently to alleviate symptoms.

D. Headache

Even in the absence of hemorrhage, headache has been linked with cerebral arteriovenous malformations. In a detailed description of 12 cases, Mackenzie suggested that arteriovenous malformations may be responsible for headache [88]. Furthermore, reported cases of headache in association with raised intracranial pressure caused by venous hypertension and cerebrospinal fluid circulatory disturbances are reported [67,79,82,83]. However, in the absence of raised intracranial pressure, patients with cerebral arteriovenous malformation have no higher incidence of headaches than the normal population [89,90] and therefore, in the absence of papilloedema, a recommendation for surgery to treat headache is not currently advisable. The authors have seen cases of migraine ipsilateral to the arteriovenous malformation that have not changed in nature after arteriovenous malformation resection for hemorrhage prophylaxis.

E. Cerebrospinal Fluid Circulation Disorder

Cerebrospinal fluid (CSF) circulatory disturbance can be caused by an arteriovenous malformation, by hemorrhage (with the subsequent development of communicating hydrocephalus), mechanical obstruction to CSF flow of a draining vein (e.g., a varix of the vein of Galen), or by venous hypertension reducing CSF absorption [29,91]. The incidence of CSF circulation disturbance as a primary mode of presentation was less than 5% of the cases in several large series [29,30,32]. However, it may be expected to be a frequent accompaniment of very large arteriovenous malformations or those in which subarachnoid hemorrhage has occurred. The choice between ablating the primary pathology (e.g., resecting the arteriovenous malformation) and providing a CSF diversion pathway in the management of CSF circulation disorders will depend on the nature and magnitude of the CSF disturbance, the surgical risks of AVM resection, and other indications for considering surgical resection.

F. Cardiac Failure

Cardiac failure is a rare cause for presentation and in its most life-threatening form is almost totally confined to children in the first three months of life.

Wallace et al. demonstrated in 1965 that arteriovenous malformations of large size can lower total peripheral resistance, increase total blood volume, and increase cardiac output [92]. The almost exclusive confinement to young children of cardiac failure caused by arteriovenous shunting is likely due to the magnitude of the shunt in proportion to their normal cardiac output [93–105].

The indication for intervention at such a young age is failure of medical management of the cardiac failure with impending death. However, surgical intervention carries with it a 90% operative mortality for the most typical arteriovenous fistulae causing cardiac failure in this age group up (i.e., vein of Galen malformations) [96,98,100,101,103,104]. Therefore, surgery should only be considered if the arteriovenous fistula is simple and interventional neuroradiological approaches cannot even offer temporary relief [32,98,106–108]. It may well be that even temporary reduction in the arteriovenous flow may be enough to allow the patient to grow sufficiently so that fistula flow no longer compromises cardiovascular function. Therefore, in time, surgical intervention can be dictated by other considerations.

III. PERIOPERATIVE MANAGEMENT

In addition to the perioperative management normally afforded a patient undergoing cranial surgery, special consideration needs to be given to preoperative evaluation (i.e., angiography, computerized tomography (CT) and magnetic resonance imaging (MRI) scanning, and physiological studies) and preoperative preparation (i.e., embolization).

A. Preoperative Evaluation

1. Angiography

High-quality angiography with the availability of superselective catheterization, stereoscopic imaging, and selective amytal testing remains the cornerstone for the evaluation and planning of surgical resection. The arterial feeders can be identified and their location at surgery anticipated. In addition, angiography identifies the area of supply to the normal parenchyma of these feeding vessels. Function of these regions of brain can then be deduced by anatomical location and, in some cases, amytal testing. Furthermore, arterial aneurysms can be identified that would aid in evaluating the likely natural history of the lesion [36]. Another aspect to note is the diameter, length, and tortuosity of the feeding arteries. Operative complications of normal perfusion pressure breakthrough might be anticipated in the presence of large diameter, long, straight arterial feeders whose connections with the nidus are greater than 300 micrometers (see below) [89,109–112]. Finally, evaluation of the possibility of preoperative embolisation largely hinges on the anatomy of the feeding arteries (e.g., size and tortuosity). The location, size, and compactness of the arteriovenous malformation nidus can all be assessed by angiography. The most important information regarding the prediction of surgical complication is the size and location [26,27,30,32,62,64,113–117]. Evaluation of the venous drainage is imperative in order to plan the surgical resection in such a way as to preserve major venous drainage until the majority of arterial input has been curtailed. Furthermore, if the size of the venous draining system is large and involves eloquent brain it may be anticipated that postoperative venous thrombosis could lead to significant complications [118].

2. CT and MRI Scanning

Most patients present with CT scans that contribute to the diagnosis of arteriovenous malformation and hemorrhage. However, MRI scans are of particular use because they demonstrate more clearly the relationship of the nidus to the surrounding brain and are more frequently diagnostic. The MRI technique is very useful in the preoperative planning especially in calculating AVM size and relationship to the ventricles, sulci, and the surface presentation. In patients in whom surgery is unlikely to be considered, if the CT-scan lesion proves to be an AVM (e.g., asymptomatic elderly patient in eloquent brain) the risks of angiography may be avoided with a diagnostic MRI. The MRI technique is also useful in diagnosing hemorrhage and defining the hematoma–AVM boundary. This is often more difficult with a CT scan.

Another utility of these radiological investigations is the coupling to stereotactic localization for either stereotactic guided craniotomy (either for lesion resection or feeding vessel localization) [119–126] or for functional positron emission tomography (PET) scanning [127]. This latter embryonal application enables the identification of the function of adjacent brain.

3. Other Preoperative Investigations

Other preoperative investigations that have been utilized include transcranial doppler, cerebral blood flow determination by xenon-133 methodology, SPECT scanning, and PET scanning [67–76,128–134]. These investigations provide physiological data that may contribute to our further understanding of the hemodynamics of these lesions and the way in which they affect the surrounding brain. However, as the most important factors that determine complications from surgery are size and location, these physiological studies seldom add to the information gained from angiography and MRI scanning in evaluation of surgical resectability. The first direct attempt at physiological studies of cerebral arteriovenous malformation was reported in 1948 by Shenkin, Spitz, Grant, and

Kelty [137]. They calculated the average cerebral blood flow in 2 patients with arteriovenous malformations to be approximately 3 times normal. This methodology was not adopted into clinical practice. However, with the recent evolution of studies of cerebral blood flow and metabolism, renewed interest has developed in studying the effects of an arteriovenous malformation upon the brain. It could well be that the more sophisticated physiological studies will contribute significantly to our understanding and management of these lesions in the future.

B. Preoperative Preparation

The usual preoperative preparation for a craniotomy needs to be made including appropriate blood cross-match and anticonvulsant loading (for supratentorial lesions). As the incidence of postoperative seizures in patients not previously experiencing seizures is 20% [32,62], we do not believe there is a place for withholding anticonvulsants in supratentorial lesions. A major consideration before surgery is whether or not to attempt preoperative embolization.

1. Preoperative Embolization

The technique of preoperative embolization has evolved rapidly over the past two decades. Since Serbinenko introduced intraarterial navigation into cortical arterial branches in 1979 [139] much progress has been made with the development of microcatheters and embolization [64,73,84,85,140–150]. Vinuela et al., evaluating 101 cases of embolization followed by surgery, concluded that a benefit to surgical resection generally occurred if more than 75% of the arteriovenous malformation had been obliterated by embolization (achieved in 31% of patients) and that it may help if more than 50% of the arteriovenous malformation had been obliterated (achieved in 80% of patients) but was unlikely to be of appreciable benefit if less than 50% occlusion was achieved [150]. They performed their last 300 catheterizations without technical complications. Offsetting somewhat the benefit of preoperative embolization are the neurological deficits that may result, the risk of hemorrhage following embolization, and the possibility of increasing the surgical difficulties. In the large series from Vinuela et al. 6% of patients developed severe neurological deficits from occlusion of parenchymal vessels. Furthermore, 2% of patients suffered serious intracerebral hemorrhage (4 and 5 days post embolization; one fatality) thought to be on the basis of progressive thrombosis of draining veins not associated with concomitant thrombosis of the arteriovenous malformation [150]. This point has been previously raised in the analysis of staged obliteration of arteriovenous malformations [151]. Finally, concern has been expressed that incomplete obliteration may result in enlargement of previously small, deeply placed feeding vessels whose walls become more attenuated and more difficult to secure at surgery [118,145,146]. Fourteen experts had their opinion sought on this issue and their opinions were divided, although eight felt that embolization ran the risk of enlarging deep collaterals [150]. In conclusion, the role of preoperative embolization is yet to be fully defined; however, if it has a role, it is likely to be for those that have a large arteriovenous malformation and in whom it is anticipated that extensive obliteration will occur.

IV. OPERATIVE METHODS

The surgical methods utilized in the management of arteriovenous malformation of the brain are clearly critical in minimizing complications. Not only is careful planning of the surgical strategy necessary but also consideration needs to be given to operative equipment.

A. Operative Equipment

Intraoperative complications may be reduced with appropriate surgical strategies and the use of optimal operating equipment. Equipment of particular importance for surgery of arteriovenous malformations includes the operating microscope, bipolar coagulation forceps, graduated suction, and microclips. The operating microscope provides the illumination and magnification necessary to accurately disect sulci (so frequently necessary in surgery for arteriovenous malformation) and to identify feeding and draining vessels, particularly in the depths of the wound. With the mobility provided by modern microscope stands there is no longer the restriction that hampered older microscope designs. Bipolar forceps must be well cleaned in order to effect coagulation with a low risk for vessel rupture. Irrigation as well as minimal vessel retraction while coagulating also reduce the chance of vessel rupture. Graduated suction units allow for controlled suction that reduces the risk of arteriovenous malformation damage. Microclips offer the ability to temporarily clip vessels as an aid in their coagulation and permanently occlude vessels where appropriate [62,152]. The small feeding vessels with attenuated walls deep in the bed frequently rupture with coagulation. Application of microclips to these vessels before coagulation improves the control of these vessels.

B. Surgical Strategies

Surgical strategies employed for specific lesions must be individually assessed as it is difficult to provide rules for all contingencies and manifestations. However, general guidelines are useful and these will be discussed in terms of prevention of hemorrhage, strategy of resection, and approach to each of the components of the arteriovenous malformation and their location.

1. Prevention of Hemorrhage

Surgical strategies that reduce the risk of intraoperative hemorrhage include a well-placed large craniotomy flap, avoidance of premature venous occlusion, and immaculate hemostasis of the surgical bed. A well-placed large craniotomy flap allows for an increase in control by maximizing the potential approaches, optimizing the angles of the line of sight, and the facilitation of retraction. Preservation of the major draining vein is imperative until all the feeding arteries have been obliterated. Premature occlusion of this vein may lead to rupture of the arteriovenous malformation or to an increase in turgor, which detracts from the ability to retract the arteriovenous malformation nidus. Finally, immaculate hemostasis is required. All small bleeding points should be secured by bipolar coagulation. If hypotension is present, this should be corrected. However, marked elevation in blood pressure may lead to normal perfusion pressure breakthrough and should be limited in time and extent.

2. General Strategy of Resection

The strategy of resection may be classified into one of three approaches: coagulation, marginal resection, and zone resection. Direct coagulation of the nidus is possible under two circumstances: firstly, if the nidus is no greater than 1 cm in diameter and, secondly, if most of the arterial input has been arrested and the nidus becomes relatively slack. Then bipolar coagulation of the lesion margin may allow it to retract away from normal brain, reducing the amount of retraction necessary. Marginal resection is necessary in dealing with most arteriovenous malformations. This technique involves a dissection of the nidus wall from the surrounding parenchyma. With the use of bipolar forceps and suction as the predominant instruments, a very thin layer of brain can be removed from around the lesion, establishing a plane of dissection. This can be extended circumferentially in such a way as to maintain a fairly even depth of dissection. The input feeding vessels can be dealt with in the manner described above.

The final strategy is that of zone resection. In this technique a region is chosen at a distance from the nidus in "silent" brain that allows a safe dissection without abutting the nidus. In this approach feeding vessels will be encountered but they are likely to be less numerous than would be found with marginal resection. It is always important to preserve arterial supply to normal brain. It may be more difficult to anticipate the destination of arteries by the zone resection technique and if there is doubt the vessel should be followed to the lesion.

For each individual arteriovenous malformation it should be planned in advance which resection strategy will be employed and, if more than one strategy is required (as is frequently the case), along which margins the various techniques should be utilized. Hinging on this decision is the necessity to gain access not only to the nidus, but also to the feeding arteries and draining veins. In many cases, especially with marginal resection, it will also be advantageous to have access to the more proximal origin of the feeding arteries (e.g., Sylvian fissure opening for access to the middle cerebral artery for opercular lesions). Access to these various components of arteriovenous malformations (i.e., nidus, feeding arteries, and draining veins) is by one of four major routes and these must be considered for each component. These routes are either via a surface (e.g., convexity, interhemispheric, and basal), sulci (or fissure), hematoma cavity, or silent brain. After analyzing all these general strategies a plan of action can be formulated.

3. Regional Strategies

With the above guidelines a general approach to different regions can be formulated.

a. *Supratentorial AVMs*

Anterior frontal arteriovenous malformations can often be resected entirely with a zone approach. Mid-frontal lesions (excluding the dominant opercular site and the dominant supplementary motor area) can generally be resected on their anterior extent by a zone resection before the posterior limits via a marginal approach. In the dominant supplementary motor area, dominant frontal operculum, sensory-motor cortex, parietal cortex, insular cortex, and dominant superior temporal gyrus a marginal approach is utilized. For other temporal locations a zone resection is generally performed. For occipital lesions with preserved vision and nidus diameter no greater than 4 cm, a marginal approach is recommended.

If feeding arteries arise from nonterminal branches of the internal carotid artery, the approach should allow for a wide Sylvian dissection as should opercular lesions. This is sometimes difficult where the predominant venous drainage is via the superficial middle cerebral vein. For temporal lobe lesions fed from P_1 and P_2 branches of the posterior cerebral artery, an infratemporal approach may prove desirable and this may also be aided by Sylvian fissure dissections for P_1 feeding vessels. For lesions with an anterior cerebral or more distal posterior cerebral artery involvement, the midline must be accessible and the interhemisphere fissure opened. Lesions in and about the transverse fissure may best be approached via the midline posteriorly in the interhemispheric fissure. Where draining veins to the superior sagittal sinus make an ipsilateral approach to the interhemispheric fissure difficult, we have found a contralateral approach desirable. In this technique a window in the falx is cut to gain access to feeding arteries. Ventricular lesions should be approached through the most direct noneloquent route.

b. *Infratentorial AVMs*

Cerebellar hemisphere lesions can be resected via a zone approach with the exception of lesions in proximity to the deep nuclei, which require a marginal dissection. Often very little deficit arises with this approach even when a very large lesion is resected. Cerebellar vermian lesions require a marginal resection as the fourth ventricle is approached. Brainstem lesions are particularly treacherous and require a marginal approach in all locations. Tectal lesions can be approached in the same manner as a pineal region tumor (infratentorial-supracerebellar, suboccipital-transtentorial, or interhemispheric-splenial approaches), lateral brainstem lesions via a cerebello-pontine angle approach (supplemented by adding a subtemporal-transtentorial exposure when necessary), and fourth ventricular lesions and dorsal closed medullary lesions can be approached through a midline vermian split exposure.

c. *Deep AVMs*

When exposing deep and small lesions, stereotactic guidance may well be of assistance. With this technique it may be possible to identify any or all components of the arteriovenous malformation [119–127].

V. COMPLICATIONS OF ARTERIOVENOUS MALFORMATION RESECTION

A review of results from surgical series on arteriovenous malformations of the brain from 1948 until 1991 demonstrates considerable variation in morbidity and mortality, and series mortality ranges from 00 to 12.5% [13,24–25,27,30–32,62,64,113,115,153–159]. Series morbidity ranges from 3 to 30% [25–27,30,31,64,154,157–159] (Table 1). While the average series reported since 1980 appears to have fewer bad results when compared with those before 1980, there were series prior to 1980 with less than a 5% mortality [13,154,158] and less than 7% combined morbidity and mortality [154,158]. Conversely, there are large series reported since 1980 from highly regarded centers with series mortality of greater than 10% [24,27]. Therefore, the improvements in surgery that have occurred have not been reflected in a uniform reduction in morbidity and mortality. This can be explained in part by the method of reporting and in part on the increasing complexity of cases now considered surgically operable. An example of the former influence can be seen in the excellent series from Davis and Symon who reported a 1.5% mortality [25]. However, if the patients

Table I Literature Review of Morbidity and Mortality Rates for AVM Resection

Series	Number	Mortality (%)	Morbidity (%)
Paterson and McKissock, 1956 [160]	36	8	—
Perret and Nishioka, 1966 [157]	119	12	—
Forster et al., 1972 [13]	95	4	—
Drake, 1979 [153]	140	11	—
Pertuiset et al., 1979 [31]	162	11	—
Pellettieri, 1979 [113]	112	8	16
Nornes et al., 1979 [154]	63	1.6	3
Wilson et al., 1979 [159]	65	6	28
Parkinson and Bacher, 1980 [156]	90	4	—
Suzuki et al., 1982 [158]	147	3	3
Albert, 1982 [24]	124	12	—
Luessenhop and Rosa, 1984 [64]	90	2	11
Jomin et al., 1985 [27]	119	12.5	30
Davis and Symon, 1985 [25]	69	1.5	8.7
Yasargil et al., 1988 [32]	414	2	—
Steinmeier et al., 1989 [115]	48	0	10
Sundt et al., 1990 [152]	279	2.5	—
Heros et al., 1990 [26]	153	0.6	7.8
Morgan et al., 1992 [30]	112	3.6	18

with a poor neurological condition on admission and who died postoperatively were included, there would have been a 10% mortality. A reflection of the lower threshold for operability with the passage of time can be seen when comparing the earlier series of Paterson and McKissock in 1957 where 37% of patients with arteriovenous malformations underwent surgery [160] to series in the 1970s where 56 to 64% of cases underwent surgery [13,161,169], finally to Yasargil's series of 500 patients of whom 83% underwent surgery [1].

Complications of surgery can be postoperative or intraoperative hemorrhage, normal perfusion pressure hyperfusion breakthrough, obstructive venous hypertension, new neurological deficits, new seizure development, extracerebral hematomas, complications of blood-product replacement, infections, and deep venous thrombosis. Several attempts at complication forecasting have been made and these will be discussed after reviewing the complications.

A. Intraoperative and Postoperative Hemorrhage

Causes for morbidity and mortality as a result of surgery for arteriovenous malformations of the brain are as diverse as the reported series incidence of complications. However, the complication most feared is that of hemorrhage. In the series of supratentorial arteriovenous malformations from the Mayo Clinic, there was a 7% incidence of reoperation for postoperative hemorrhage. Of these 16 patients, the cause was thought to be incomplete resection in 12, normal perfusion pressure breakthrough or venous obstruction in 3, and an epidural hematoma in 1 [62]. In a recent series by Morgan et al. [30] there were 24 operative complications of which 10 were caused by hemorrhage (9% of all operated cases). The cause for hemorrhage in this series was thought to be intraoperative arteriovenous malformation rupture in 4 cases (3 deaths), normal perfusion pressure breakthrough in 3 cases (1 death), epidural hematoma in 2 cases, and an intracerebral hemorrhage after commencing heparin to manage pulmonary emboli in 1 case. Hemorrhage accounted for all deaths in the series. Seven percent of Yasargil's series required reexploration for hemorrhage [32]. The 6 deaths in this group were all from the group of 12 patients with residual arteriovenous malformation. Hemorrhage of unknown etiology (oozing from resection bed) accounted for 11 cases and epidural or subdural hematomas in 3 cases. From these recent series, it is clear that a significant proportion of morbidity and mortality is related to hemorrhage, of which hemorrhage from the arteriovenous malformation (intraoperatively or from residual lesions postoperatively) is the most common. Hemorrhage caused by venous thrombosis or normal perfusion pressure breakthrough will be discussed below. Factors of predictive value for the occurrence of hemorrhage include arteriovenous malformation size [30,116]. In an analysis of variables predicting occurrence of complications, size had been found to be the most important factor [30,64,115,116,160]. This must, in part, be related to the risk of intraoperative rupture of the arteriovenous malformation and the risk of leaving undetected residual arteriovenous malformation. In our experience arteriovenous malformations of less than 4 cm rarely present problems with hemorrhage [30].

Another factor that may be of importance in the risk of intraoperative rupture is distance from the convexity surface [114,116,161]. While there is no statistical evidence supporting the increased risks of deeply placed lesions, logic would dictate that for an equivalent size, the risk from deeply placed lesions in terms of hemorrhage would be greater than superficial convexity lesions. This attitude is clearly supported in the literature by those that have incorporated a measure of depth in their grading system [114,116,161].

Factors that predict postoperative venous occlusion must be related to the size of the draining vein, the distribution of tributaries to this vein, and the flow through the arteriovenous malformation into this vein. A study to evaluate these factors has not been done because it is difficult to distinguish the difference between normal perfusion pressure breakthrough and hemorrhage or edema from venous thrombosis [62,118]. However, applying the basic principles understood to contribute to the occurrence of venous thrombosis, it would be anticipated that the slower the flow in the vessel the more likely it is that thrombosis will ensue.

Several measures can be taken to minimize the risk of intra- and postoperative hemorrhage from arteriovenous malformation resection. These can be divided into preoperative measures (embolization), intraoperative measures (large flap, single stage, utilization of microscope, microclips, good bipolar technique, graduated suction, preservation of vein until late in dissection, effective hemostasis), and postoperative measures (early angiography). Preoperative and intraoperative measures aimed at reducing hemorrhage from residual arteriovenous malformation occurs in most large series. Even the most experienced neurosurgeon can, on occasions, be surprised to find residual arteriovenous malformations. Sundt et al. reported there was a 5% postoperative hemorrhage rate from residual arteriovenous malformation [67]. Yasargil's rate of reoperation from hemorrhage from retained residual arteriovenous malformation was 3% [32]. However, for some time now this complication has been avoided at the Mayo Clinic by performing immediate or early postoperative cerebral angiography and immediate reoperation for residual arteriovenous malformation. This is now the recommended practice even with meticulous surgery.

B. Normal Perfusion Pressure Breakthrough

Few subjects are more controversial in neurosurgery than "normal pressure hyperperfusion breakthrough" or normal perfusion pressure breakthrough. The redistribution of blood flow following the obliteration of a cerebral arteriovenous malformation has been cited as a cause for hemorrhage and edema complications. Spetzler et al. named this disorder normal perfusion pressure breakthrough based on clinical observations of complications (3 patients, of whom 2 died of brain swelling and one developed hemiplegia) and an animal model [163]. Their hypothesis was that the arteriovenous shunt creates hypoperfusion of the cerebral parenchyma (without infarction) that impairs cerebral autoregulation. Autoregulation is thought to remain impaired after the restoration of normal perfusion pressure on shunt ablation resulting in hyperemia and possibly disruption of the capillary bed with its obvious sequalae.

Gowers was the first to predict this possibility, in general terms, in 1888 with his description of "congestive apoplexy" as the most severe complication of cerebral congestion (or hyperemia) [164]. He defined "partial active congestion" as that occurring "when an artery is obstructed, and the adjacent branches of the main vessel receives too much blood." As the first successful removal of a cerebral arteriovenous malformation was not published until after this description, the "partial active congestion" hypothesis is unlikely to have arisen in relation to such surgery. Nonetheless, it fits well the characteristics of the normal perfusion pressure breakthrough syndrome. Many cases have been reported that are thought to represent this complication [30,31,62,72,73,111,153,159,

161,165–173]. There are several reported series in which this complication constitutes the major cause of morbidity and mortality unrelated to technical error or poor preoperative neurological condition [30,31,100,136,159,161,166,171]. The highest reported incidence is that of Batjer et al. who reported "hyperemic complications" (defined as "unexpected or abnormal degrees of intraoperative brain swelling or hemorrhage unrelated to technical error or concealed ventricular hemorrhage . . . and CT evidence of edema associated with neurological deficit not related to inadvertent proximal vascular occlusion or intraoperative brain retraction as well as hemorrhage after angiographically proven complete AVM resection") in 13 of 62 patients (21%) [129]. Of these patients with hyperemic complications, 7 either died or were not capable of independence. Spetzler et al. [73] and Andrews et al. [176] have thought this complication to be sufficiently frequent in larger arteriovenous malformations that they advocate routinely a staged ablation for these larger lesions in order to minimize the risk of its occurrence (however, the merits of this strategy have been questioned [118,151,156]). The vast majority of reported cases of normal perfusio pressure breakthrough occur in large-flow arteriovenous malformations or fistulae.

Despite the reported cases of normal perfusion pressure breakthrough, doubt does exist with regard to the mechanism of edema and hemorrhage. Sundt reported difficulty in differentiating complications of normal perfusion pressure breakthrough from delayed venous thrombosis [118]. There are several large reported series where the complication of normal perfusion pressure breakthrough has not been reported [1,177,178].

Examining the clinical evidence upon which the diagnosis of normal perfusion pressure has been deduced, there are two frequently quoted sources of information. These are firstly the pressure changes within parenchymal feeding arteries and secondly the cerebral blood-flow changes observed consequent to arteriovenous shunt ablation. Nornes and Grip suggested that the degree to which there is an increase in pressure within feeding arteries is proportional to the risk for the development of normal perfusion pressure breakthrough [111]. They identified three patients developing brain swelling following arteriovenous malformation resection in which the feeding-artery pressure increased from 40 to 80 mm Hg, 50 to 75 mm Hg, and 57 to 85 mm Hg. Barrow measured changes in pressure from 35 to 75 mm Hg following excision of an arteriovenous malformation in a patient he identified as developing normal perfusion pressure breakthrough [79]. However, many cases in which no complications ensued also experienced similar changes in pressure of the feeding arteries following arteriovenous malformation resection [67,69,73,87]. This is not surprising as the maximum pressure that can be achieved in these conducting vessels is the systemic arterial pressure and for this to be responsible for hemorrhage and edema, the regional cerebral microcirculation must be pathologically deficient in protecting the capillary bed. Changes in feeding artery pressure alone are insufficient evidence in support of the existence of normal perfusion pressure breakthrough. The second category of clinical evidence cited as supporting the existence of normal perfusion pressure breakthrough is from cerebral blood-flow data. Young et al. (utilizing ^{133}Xe) [276] and Barnett et al. (utilizing thermister Peltier stack arrays) [67] reported 2 cases each in which an increase in cerebral blood flow was seen to occur in patients said to develop clinical evidence of normal perfusion pressure breakthrough. However, the postexcision cerebral blood-flow results in Barnett's series were below normal in one case and only slightly elevated in the other. In Young's series one of the cases allegedly developing normal perfusion pressure breakthrough had normal postexcision cerebral blood flow. In addition, cerebral blood-flow recordings from several patients not developing clinical evidence of normal perfusion pressure breakthrough have been found to show a more dramatic increase in cerebral blood flow upon arteriovenous malformation ablation than the above cases of normal perfusion pressure breakthrough [67,72,73]. Experimental evidence for hyperemia following the ablation of arteriovenous shunt does exist [163,179–181]. However, this is not associated with loss of CO_2 reactivity [180] or blood-brain-barrier disruption (unless hypertension is induced) [179,180,182].

Therefore, there is no firm evidence, as yet, that the microcirculation in patients with arteriovenous malformation is not capable of coping with changes in cerebral blood flow occurring with shunt ablation. Furthermore, there is insufficient evidence to support the basis for this phenomenon, i.e., that autoregulation is impaired by chronic noninfarctional hypoperfusion. However, despite these deficits in knowledge we are inclined to believe that the complication of normal perfusion pressure breakthrough does occur in a few selected cases of large flow arteriovenous malformations (Figure 1).

With such controversy as to the nature of normal perfusion pressure breakthrough it is difficult to recommend treatment for this complication. It is difficult to believe on theoretical grounds that a staged ablation reduces the risk of this complication because the nature of ablation is to reduce a percentage of feeding vessels totally rather than reduce all feeding vessels by a percentage. This means, for staged procedures, while the resistance is increased in some areas of the arteriovenous malformation it will be reduced in others (by reducing outflow venous pressure). For these areas of reduced resistance the risk for normal perfusion pressure may even be increased [151]. Experimentally it has been demonstrated that hypertension after ablation of the arteriovenous shunt may lead to blood-brain-barrier disruption [179,182] and clinically this has been found to be the case following carotid endarterectomy in the presence of a high-grade hemodynamically significant stenosis (another example of a sudden reversal of chronic noninfarctional hypoperfusion) [183–187]. Therefore, it is our general practice to aggressively avoid any increase in systemic arterial pressure above 120 mm Hg systolic. Furthermore, as CO_2 reactively could well be retained in these patients [77] strict control of arterial $PaCO_2$ is also instituted to prevent hypercapnea. If profound swelling occurs that necessitates drastic action then the use of early barbiturate coma, hypotension, hyperventilation, and intracranial pressure monitoring may be of assistance. The use of mannitol may exacerbate the problem by crossing the disrupted blood-brain-barrier as well as further increasing cerebral blood flow.

C. Obstructive Venous Hypertension

Of the 273 cases from the Mayo Clinic of arteriovenous malformation resections, there were 14 patients in whom obstruction of the venous drainage represents a possible or probable cause of death or postoperative deterioration [62,118,188]. The mechanism for this complication is related to stasis of blood in the redundant drainage system of the arteriovenous malformation with subsequent propagation of thrombus (Figure 2). The risk for the development of this complication would presumably be highest in high-flow arteriovenous malformations with large varicose draining veins that widely communicate with critical venous systems, e.g., vein of Galen. In addition, abnormalities of the venous system that may exist with arteriovenous malformation [34,35,189,190] may further increase this risk of postoperative thrombosis. It would seem reasonable to minimize the risk of this complication by ligating the venous outflow immediately proximal to the first normal venous tributary and to avoid dehydration in the perioperative period.

D. New Neurological Deficits

The two major causes for neurological deficits resulting from arteriovenous malformation resection (excluding the above 3 categories of complications) are dissection of nonsilent brain and occlusion of arteries with a parenchymal distribution. These complications account for a variable percentage of most large series. In a series from Sydney the incidence of such deficits was 8% [30]. In order to avoid sacrificing an artery of functional importance it is imperative to make a thorough study of a high-quality superselective angiogram. At the time of surgery it is important to trace all arteries to the nidus to ensure that they do not continue to supply the brain. In resecting arteriovenous malformations it must be borne in mind that adjacent brain may be damaged irrespective of the proximity the dissection takes to the nidus. Therefore, arteriovenous malformation in the region of eloquent brain is more likely to result in postoperative deficits than resection from silent brain [26,27,62,64,113,114,117]. With MRI scanning the 3-dimensional perspective of these lesions is readily apparent. This enables a careful analysis of the proximity of critical areas. It may well be that patients

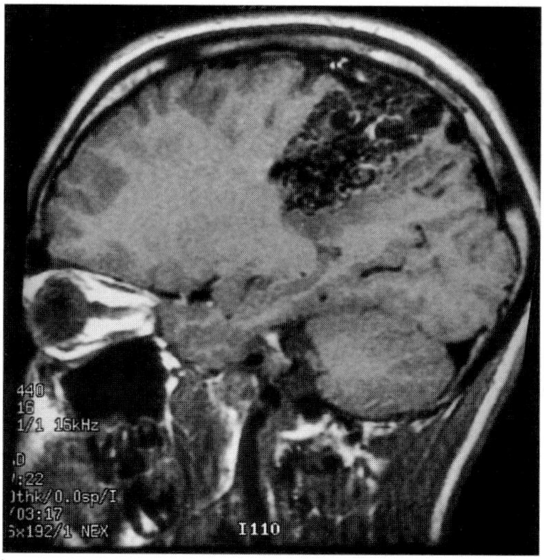

(a)

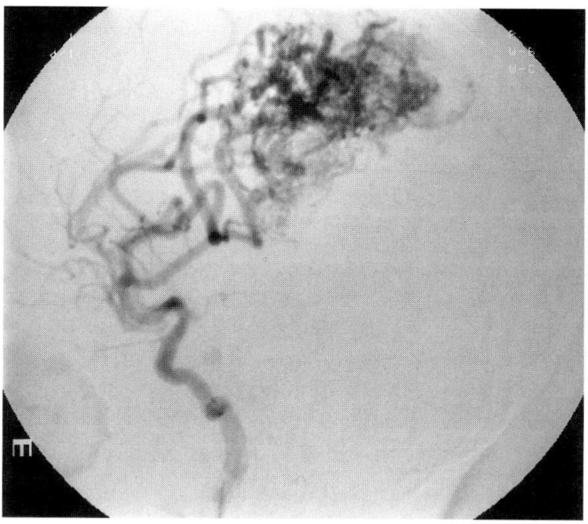

(b)

Figure 1 This 20-year-old male presented with a small intracerebral hemorrhage resulting in no permanent neurological deficit. MRI (a) and cerebral angiography (b and c) demonstrated this to be a 6-cm right parietal convexity arteriovenous malformation fed by anterior, middle, and posterior cerebral arteries. Surgical resection of the lesion was performed without intraoperative complications and immediately following surgery, angiography confirmed nonfilling of the lesion (d and e).

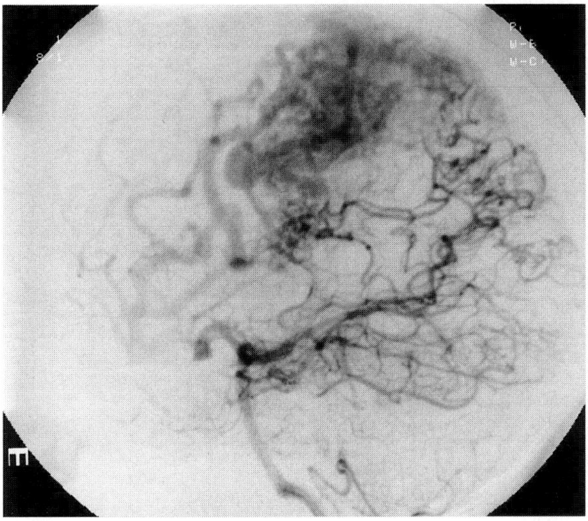

(c)

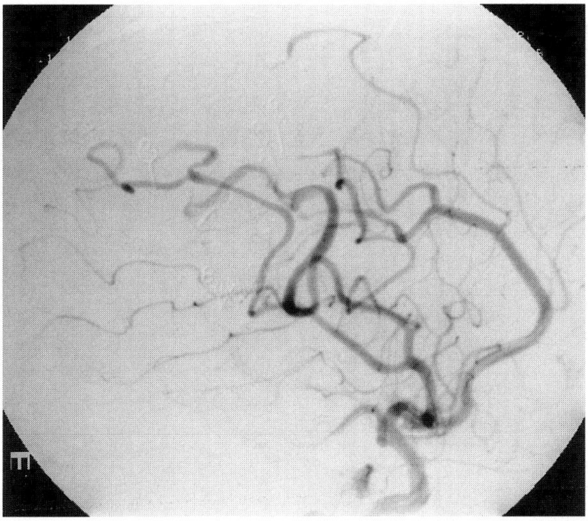

(d)

In the early postoperative period this patient had a left-arm paresis that was recovering to be antigravity on the morning of the sixth postoperative day. CT scan in this interval (f) was unremarkable. Because of the concern for the potential of postresection brain swelling he was maintained at a systolic blood pressure below 110 mm Hg in this post-operative interval. However, his blood pressure significantly increased on the sixth day and he sustained a catastrophic intracerebral and intraventricular hemorrhage at this

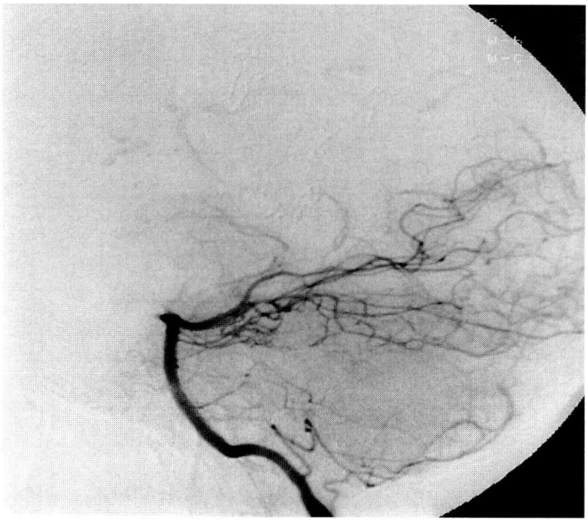

(e)

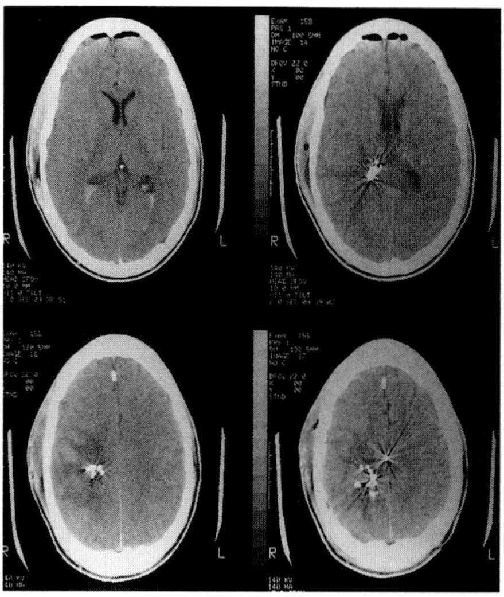

(f)

Figure 1 Continued

time (g). The source of the hemorrhage was presumed to be related to the blood pressure change and is likely to represent a ruptured feeding artery or hemorrhage from the parenchymal capillary bed. Therefore, this may represent a case of normal perfusion pressure breakthrough and underscores the importance of good postoperative blood pressure control.

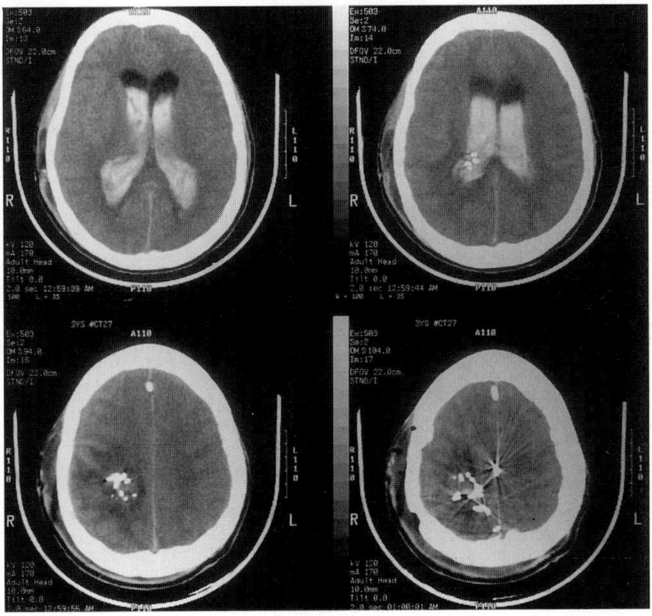

(g)

Figure 1 Continued

will accept certain neurological deficits (e.g., visual field defect) in exchange for prophylaxis against future hemorrhage. However, it must be remembered that the expected location for cerebral function may be incorrect in patients with arteriovenous malformations. For this reason, some surgeons perform the surgery using local anaesthesia and proceed with cortical mapping prior to arteriovenous malformation resection [191,192]. An alternate approach being developed is the use of activated PET scanning linked to anatomical radiological modalities through stereotactic methodology [127]. In this way images of suspected critical areas (e.g. language) can be superimposed on MRI images. Progress in the development of aids that help avoid damaging critical areas at the time of surgery is proceeding constructively.

E. Other Causes of Morbidity and Mortality

In addition to the above problems that arise from arteriovenous malformation resection, other complications must be anticipated. In a recent series from Sydney in which complications of surgery were rigorously defined (including worsening of neurological status, reoperation, infection, new seizures, and prolonged admission) there was an 8% incidence of complications excluding the above 4 categories [30]. These complications can be explained in terms of complications

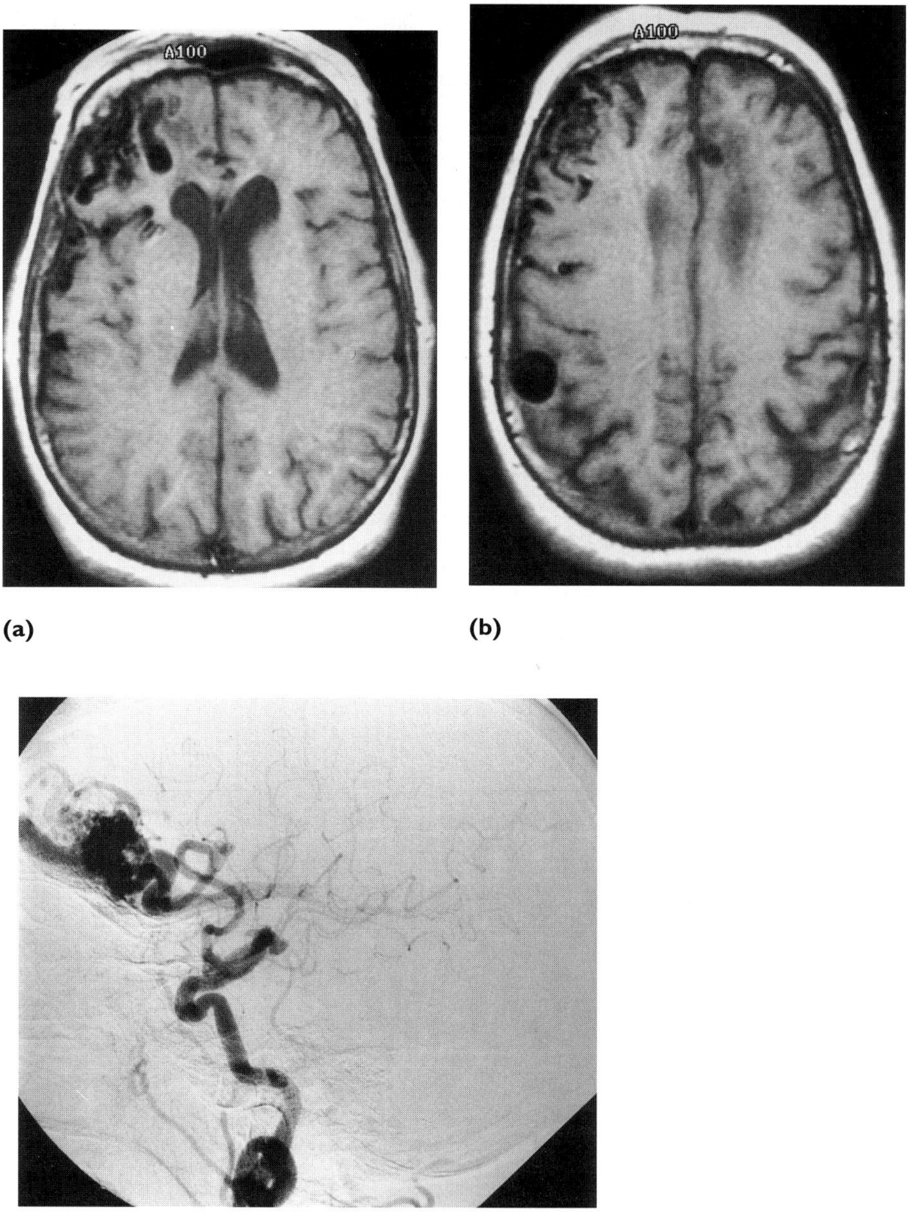

(a) (b)

(c)

Figure 2 The case of this 62-year-old female illustrates the potential problems of propagated venous thrombosis following surgical resection. Her right frontal arteriovenous malformation (a and b) was discovered after investigation for seizures. The large superficial parietal globular flow void identified on MRI (b) was confirmed to be

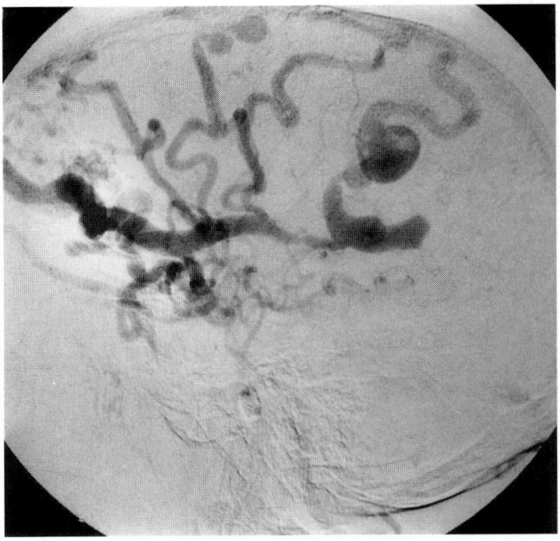

(d)

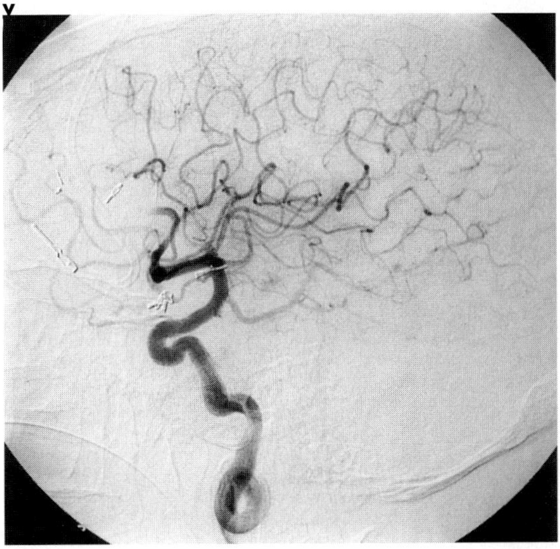

(e)

a venous varix in the arteriovenous malformation drainage system (c and d). Following complete surgical excision of the arteriovenous malformation without intraoperative complications the patient developed a delayed onset of left hemiparesis. Cerebral angiography confirmed complete ablation (e and f) with nonfilling of the venous system containing the varix (compare d with f). A noncontrast CT scan demonstrated the hyperdensity within the thrombosed superficial venous drainage (g).

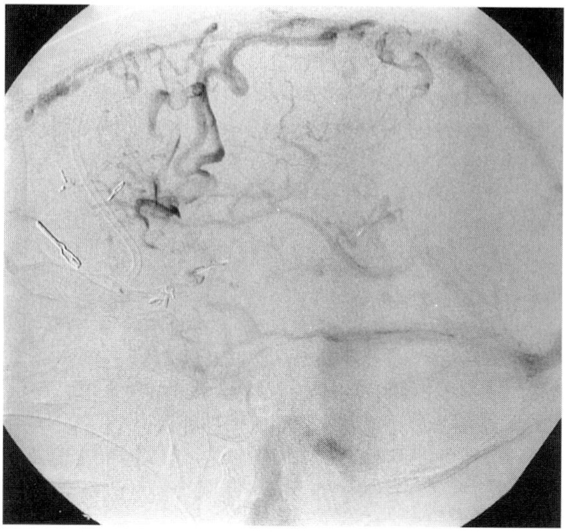

(f)

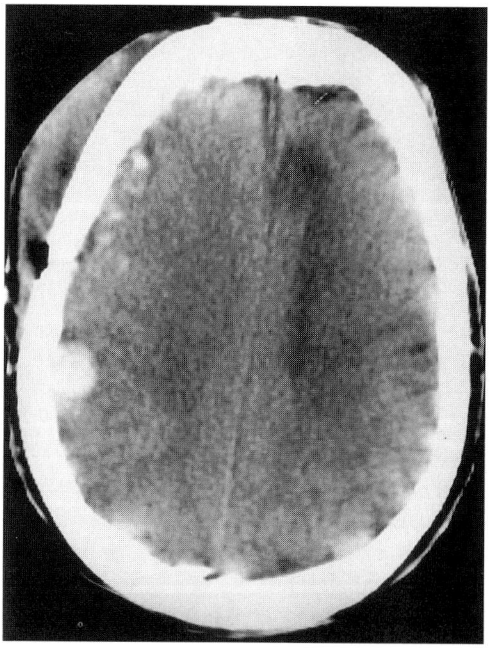

(g)

Figure 2 Continued

to be anticipated with resection of any vascular cerebral lesion. Included are new seizure development, vasospasm (Figure 3), complications of embolization (Figure 4), extradural hematoma, complications of blood product replacement, infection, and deep venous thrombosis or pulmonary embolus.

A review of supratentorial resection from the Mayo Clinic revealed that 6% of patients that had no history of seizures prior to surgery developed new ongoing seizures [62,63]. However, 83% of patients that had seizures preoperatively had no seizures in followup. This experience is similar to that of Yasargil [32].

F. Complication Forecasting Schemes

In an effort to incorporate those factors thought to increase the risk of surgery into a formula, several authors have produced grading systems to assess "operability" [64,114–116,161,193,194]. Factors that have been cited to influence the risk of surgical complications include arteriovenous malformation size [26,27,30,32,62,64,164,113,114,116,117,194], location in eloquent cortex [26,62,113–115,117], angiographic evidence of steal [129], and deep venous drainage [26,114,115,117]. Of these factors, proximity to eloquent cortex and size are the most important factors [30,115,116,194]. It is important to keep in mind when evaluating grading systems that not all variables are independent of each other and therefore to incorporate two related variables biases the equation. An example of this would be if an arteriovenous malformation of 7 cm or greater is considered. It is highly likely that such a lesion would be adjacent to eloquent cortex, demonstrate angiographic evidence of steal, have a large number of feeding arteries, derive some supply from deep perforating vessels, and possess deep venous drainage. It may well be that only size and location are the variables that contribute to the risk of surgery and that in statistical analysis the other variables contribute little to the predictive power of forecasting equations. Despite the interdependence of these variables they have been incorporated into grading systems in a manner suggesting their independence.

Luessenhop and Gennarelli introduced the first grading system based on size in 1977 [64]. Subsequent grading systems incorporated more variables and became more complex. Spetzler and Martin proposed a grading system based on size, pattern of venous drainage, and location in proximity to eloquent cortex [114]. They found that the results of surgery tended to correlate with the grade but they did not statistically analyse the individual factors and their relative importance. Shi and Chen proposed a more complex scheme grading size, location and depth, arterial supply and venous drainage [161]. This resulted in a 7-tier system that again tended to correlate with surgical risks but failed to analyse the individual factors that contributed to this outcome.

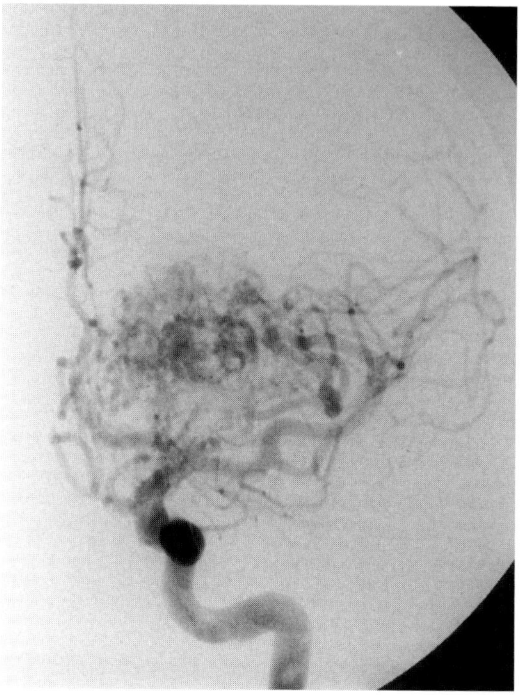

(a)

Figure 3 Another cause for postoperative neurological deterioration is vasospasm. This 48-year-old female with a left frontal basal arteriovenous malformation (a) underwent resection involving an extensive dissection from within the Sylvian fissure. She was neurologically normal following the surgery but on day 10 developed dysphasia and underwent another angiogram that demonstrated the presence of left middle cerebral artery vasospasm (b). She responded to the intraarterial administration of papaverine both angiographically (c) and clinically with complete resolution of her dysphasia.

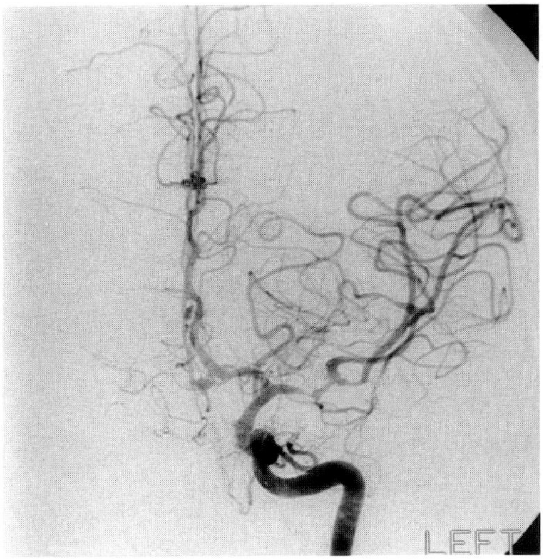

(b)

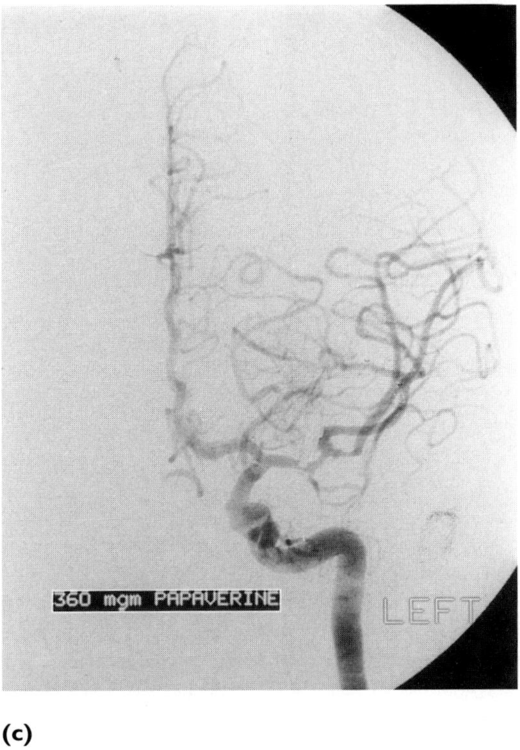

(c)

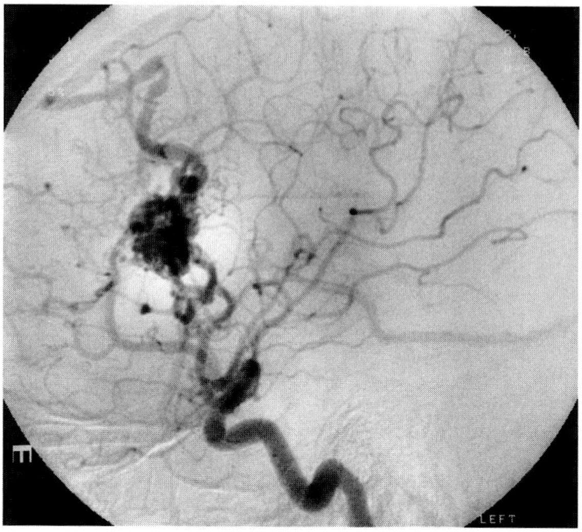

(a)

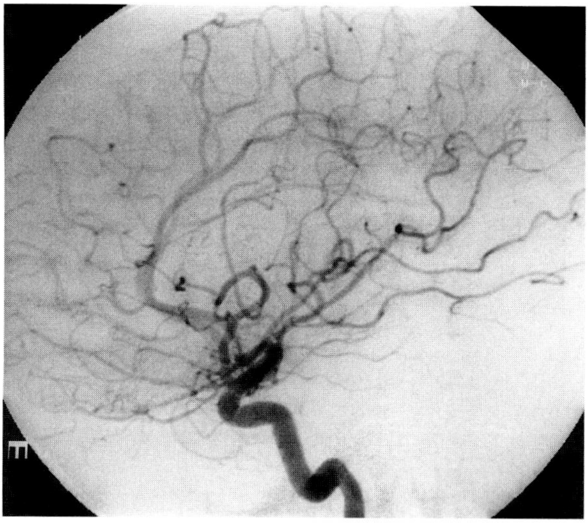

(b)

Figure 4 The risks of preoperative angiography includes that of postembolization rupture. In this case of a left frontal arteriovenous malformation (a) there was an excellent angiographic result with nonvisualisation of either nidus or early draining vein (b). However, 10 hours following the embolization procedure, while straining, the patient developed a rapidly progressive aphasia and right hemiparesis from an intracerebral hemorrhage (c). This was urgently evacuated and the arteriovenous malformation resected (d).

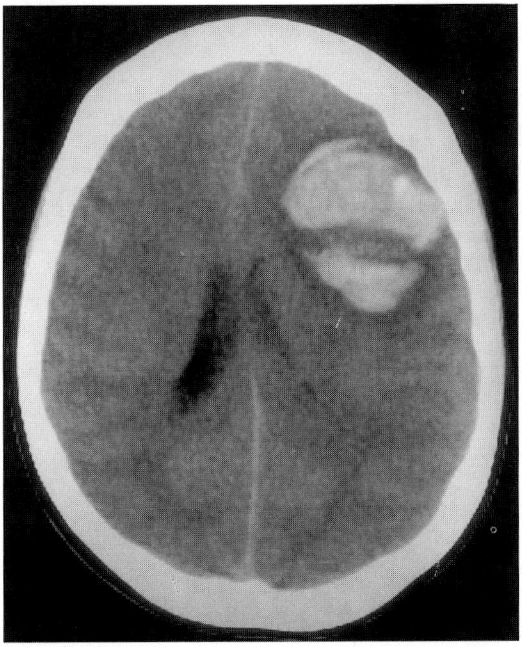

(c)

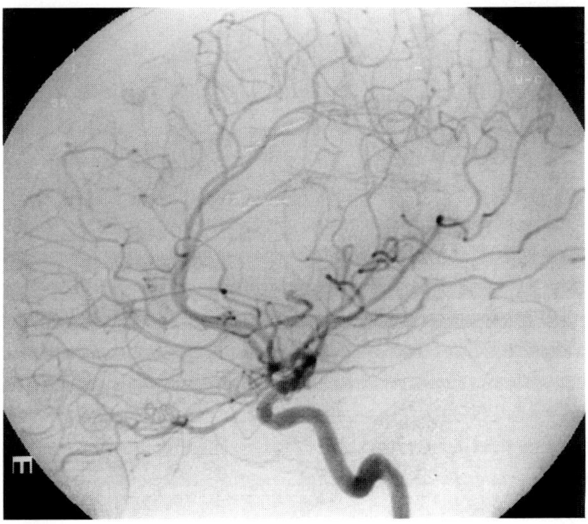

(d)

A comparison of these three systems (in addition to that of Pellettieri et al., which does not assess complications but outcome [113] applied to a different series of patients suggested that Spetzler and Martin's system correlated best with postoperative neurological deterioration. More recently, Pertuiset et al. introduced a very complex grading system including variables of "sectorization," "determination," calibre and straightening of feeding vessels, volume, vascular autoregulation, circulatory velocity of red blood cells in neck arteries, and "cellular steal" [193]. In each category the patient was graded 0 to 5 unless the variable suggested inoperability and then it was assigned 10. They found that the results of 67 cases with 8 deaths correlated with the scoring system. However, this proves to be a cumbersome grading system with only 27 of 66 patients undergoing all the investigations required for assessment. Furthermore, as the aim was to establish "operability" and ability to identify inoperability is necessary to grade some of the variables, this system is not particularly helpful. We believe that while there are grading systems that appear to correlate with outcome, they should not replace the experienced neurosurgeon's assessment of operability. It is of interest that one of the first authors of the original grading system, Luessenhopp, recently stated that "I do not think that determination of operative mortality and morbidity in a large number of cases according to a simplified grading system is particularly useful" [194]. He further commented that in his experience there were only two factors of importance and these are how big the malformation is and where it is, and that patterns of venous drainage were frequently not a feature bearing on surgical difficulty. Therefore when utilizing a grading system it must be remembered that some factors that have been included may not have any bearing on complications and other factors that may be of great importance may not have been taken into consideration.

VI. NONSURGICAL ALTERNATIVES

Radiation therapy has regained popularity as an alternative to surgery for arteriovenous malformations of the brain with the development of sharp, accurate focusing of energy. While results with conventional radiation have been variable, an overall good result by this technique can be expected in 40% of cases [87]. Considerable progress has been made in treating arteriovenous malformations with the development of Gamma Knife radiosurgery, stereotactic linear accelerator radiosurgery, and Bragg peak therapy. The results with both Gamma Knife and stereotactic linear accelerator radiosurgery appear to be similar although the Gamma Knife technique has a longer history. Lecksell pioneered this technique over 4 decades ago and has gained considerable experience with the management of arteriovenous malformations [195]. It can be expected that with

Gamma Knife radiosurgery, treatment is most effective for lesions less than 3 cm in diameter (85% obliteration expected by 2 years), no change in the natural history of the lesion is likely before complete obliteration occurs, and 3% of patients will develop radiation necrosis within 12 months of treatment [87]. Results utilizing stereotactic linear accelerator technology appear to be similar at this early stage of result collation. Lesions greater than 2.5 cm in diameter have an obliteration rate comparable to conventional radiotherapy (i.e., 40% obliteration). Smaller lesions respond with a similar obliteration rate to Gamma Knife radiosurgery with a 10% development of radiation necrosis within 2 years of commencing treatment [196]. Again, no protection appears to be offered until obliteration has occurred.

The use of Bragg peak therapy has likewise proven to be effective in lesions up to 70 cm^3 (80% obliteration rate by 2 years following treatment) with a better response from smaller lesions [87]. Serious permanent neurological complications at 2 years are 2 to 4% by this technique. However, when considering all cases treated, there appears to be no change from the natural history of the primary disease state for 8 years [197].

It may well be that all three forms of therapy offer similar results in terms of size of lesion that responds best, latency period before protection, and incidence of radiation necrosis. Hopefully, these forms of treatment will, with further development, may be able to treat a wider spectrum of lesions effectively and safely. It must also be considered that the lesions treated in these series are often those deemed unsuitable for surgical resection and therefore these results must be considered in this light.

When approaching the decision-making process that determines whether focussed irradiation or surgical resection is utilized in managing an individual lesion it is possible to design an algorithm (Figure 7) based on the following 5 generalizations (note, some of these figures are approximations based on a number of studies with disparate results). 1. Arteriovenous malformations of size greater than 3 cm in diameter are not likely to be obliterated by focussed irradiation [87]. 2. On average, there is a latency of 2 years between treatment and protection by focussed irradiation [87]. 3. Radiation necrosis follows focussed irradiation treatment in 10% of cases and this will be symptomatic only in eloquent brain [87]. 4. The risk of hemorrhage from an arteriovenous malformation is 4% for the 2 years after diagnosis in the absence of presentation by hemorrhage or angiographically demonstrated arterial aneurysms. If presentation by hemorrhage occurs or there is an associated aneurysm found at angiography, the risk of hemorrhage over 2 years is 14% [13,16–22,198–203] 5. The risk of death from hemorrhage is 29% and the risk of permanent neurological deficit is 17% [17].

With increasing knowledge, further development, and refinement of irradiation this algorithm will require modification.

VII. SPECIAL SURGICAL CONSIDERATIONS

A. Arteriovenous Malformations and Pregnancy

When considering the implications of pregnancy in patients with arteriovenous malformations of the brain, both the patient and the fetus need to be considered. It has long been held that pregnancy increases the risk of rupture of arteriovenous malformations of the brain [204]. This has resulted in the advise that pregnancy should be avoided. In addition, there is a philosophy that surgical excision should be considered as soon as possible after presentation of a pregnant patient with an arteriovenous malformation rupture because of reports that the risk of recurrent hemorrhage is increased by pregnancy [204–206]. However, more recently these positions have been challenged. In a retrospective study of patients known to have an arteriovenous malformation, 540 pregnancies were reviewed [207]. It was found that 17 pregnancies were associated with hemorrhage. It was estimated that the risk of first hemorrhage during the 40 weeks of pregnancy and the subsequent 12 weeks postpartum to be 3.5%. This figure was found to be no higher than that expected for age-matched nonpregnant women. In this study 375 live births occurred by vaginal delivery and 63 by Caesarean section without hemorrhage. The conclusion from this study is that pregnancy does not increase the risk of hemorrhage. In another recent study reviewing all case reports and series of subarachnoid hemorrhage in pregnancy, the ratio of arteriovenous malformation to aneurysm hemorrhage was approximately 1 to 3 [208]. Of particular importance is that 74% of patients with arteriovenous malformation hemorrhage had a prior pregnancy free of hemorrhage. Therefore, the lack of previous trouble is no assurance that hemorrhage should not occur during subsequent pregnancies. It was also revealed that maternal mortality from hemorrhage was 28%, a figure similar to that found by the Mayo Clinic for all first hemorrhage patients [17]. This study also confirmed that very few patients sustain a hemorrhage during labor.

Therefore, it is likely that avoidance of pregnancy will not reduce the risk of hemorrhage from an arteriovenous malformation of the brain. However, it must be considered that certain aspects of management may have an adverse effect upon the fetus including anticonvulsants, steroids, surgery, diuretics, and the effects of maternal hemorrhage or seizures. While it is well known that anticonvulsants may predispose to the development of fetal anomalies it is also known that avoidance of anticonvulsants with the subsequent risk of seizure and possible fetal hypoxia may adversely effect the fetus [94,209–213].

In the management of hemorrhage (or in the course of surgery) fetal dehydration may occur from the administration of mannitol or other diuretics [214], high doses of glucocorticoids may cause neonatal hypoadrenalism, and induced hypotension may produce uterine hypoperfusion [215–217]. In addition, it is known that if a hemorrhage occurs, there is an increased risk to the fetus. Of 14 pregnancies complicated by arteriovenous malformation rupture reported in one series, 3 resulted in abortion and 11 in healthy full-term infants [207]. Therefore, the advisability of avoiding pregnancy should be based on consideration of the fetus rather than the risk to the mother. However, if an arteriovenous malformation is diagnosed during the course of pregnancy this should be managed in a similar way to management of a nongravid patient with appropriate precautions taken for the fetus (e.g., shielding during angiography).

B. Associated Arterial Aneurysms

The prevalence of patients with cerebral arterial aneurysms found to occur in association with intracranial arteriovenous malformations ranges from 2.7 to 17.6% [1,29,36,157,160,218–220]. The two largest series, each of over 400 patients, reported an aneurysm prevalence of 7 and 10% each [1,157]. A recent study from the Mayo Clinic specifically studied unruptured arteriovenous malformations of the brain in association with intracranial arterial aneurysms diagnosed between 1974 and 1985 (therefore, reviewing angiograms of more recent vintage than many of the other studies) [36]. It was found that nearly 18% of 91 patients with arteriovenous malformations had aneurysms. This compares with a prevalence of asymptomatic aneurysms unassociated with arteriovenous malformations of 1% [221]. Clearly, the prevalence rate of aneurysms among patients with arteriovenous malformations is considerably higher than would be predicted by chance.

The location of many arterial aneurysms in patients with arteriovenous malformations has long been known to be atypical with a predilection for a location on the arterial feeding network of the arteriovenous malformation [1,157,219–241]. Recently it has been shown that aneurysms have a tendency to be located more proximally in the arterial feeding network of large arteriovenous malformations and closer to the nidus in smaller lesions [36].

While it has been argued that a maldevelopment of the arterial system may occur to account for both the arteriovenous malformation and the aneurysm [1,222,224] it is more likely that the abnormalities of flow and pressure (caused by the presence of the low-resistence arteriovenous malformation) interplay in such a way as to result in the production of the aneurysm [161,229,239,242]. It must be considered that the falloff in transmural pressure within the feeding artery system will be greatest in those lesions with a higher flow. As pressure plays a role in aneurysm formation, it can be appreciated that the higher flow lesions are likely to demonstrate a propensity for more proximal aneurysm formation than low-flow lesions; a distribution found to be the case in a clinical series [36]. Thus, the mechanism for aneurysm formation in association with arteriovenous malformations is similar to that arising in the absence of this association [189,243,244]. When both arteriovenous malformation and aneurysm are present it has been suggested that the most likely source of hemorrhage is the arteriovenous malformation [157,220,229,238]. However, the management mortality for aneurysmal hemorrhage is greater than that for arteriovenous malformation hemorrhage and therefore there is a tendency for retrospective surgical studies to underestimate the incidence of aneurysmal rupture. In a recent prospective study from the Mayo Clinic of combined, initially unruptured lesions, the source of hemorrhage could only be confidently identified in two out of six cases and for these 2 cases the source of hemorrhage was one each from the aneurysm and the arteriovenous malformation [36].

The management of arteriovenous malformation and aneurysm in one patient is dependent on several factors. If the aneurysm has ruptured this should be dealt with in a similar way to any ruptured cerebral aneurysm providing it is accessible without compromising arteriovenous malformation drainage. If it is likely that a direct surgical approach to the aneurysm is too difficult then an endovascular approach may be possible. On the other hand, if the aneurysm has not ruptured then surgical considerations are focused on the etiology of the aneurysm, (i.e., the arteriovenous malformation) and the risk–benefit ratio of its repair, bearing in mind the 7% annual risk of hemorrhage when both lesions are present [36]. The decision of whether or not to repair the aneurysm depends on two conflicting results of arteriovenous malformation resection. As the aneurysm is likely to be produced by the high flow within its parent artery supplying the arteriovenous malformation it can be expected that the force of propagation can be reduced by resection of the arteriovenous malformation alone. Indeed, this has been shown to be the case in clinical practice [239] (Figure 5). However, because of the rapid increase in pressure within the feeding artery network attended on arteriovenous shunt ablation, there is a risk of aneurysm rupture at the time of arteriovenous malformation repair. This too, has been reported [153]. Therefore, it seems reasonable that if arteriovenous malformation obliteration is contemplated, accessible associated aneurysms should be repaired before shunt obliteration has occurred. Again, this might be more appropriately performed via an endovascular technique [245]. As there is a 7% risk per year of hemorrhage when both aneurysms and arteriovenous malformation are present, and the risk is likely increased if either lesion has previously ruptured, a great deal of consideration needs to be given to ablating these lesions.

VIII. SURGICAL MANAGEMENT OF DURAL ARTERIOVENOUS MALFORMATIONS OF THE SPINE AND CRANIUM: INTRODUCTION

Abnormal arteriovenous shunts may be located predominantly or exclusively within the intracranial or spinal dura. The earliest reported intracranial case was likely that of Sachs in 1931 [246]. However, the first diagnosis of a spinal dural arteriovenous malformation did not occur until the development of selective spinal angiography in the 1960s [247]. The debate with regard to the true location of the point of transition from artery to vein has only recently been resolved [248–251] despite the fact that the first successful operation for a spinal dural AVM likely occurred in 1914 [246]. Characteristic of all these lesions is venous drainage either into a dural venous sinus or into a vein within the subarachnoid space (connecting the fistula with veins of the central nervous system).

Early attempts at cure of intracranial dural arteriovenous malformations were directed at proximal arterial ligation [253] with the occasional addition of venous occlusion [254]. Although, reports of symptomatic improvement suggested these remote forms of surgery to be of benefit, the postoperative angiography seldom confirmed cure [81] and it became apparent that the best form of cure was total excision of the nidus when possible [81,255–257].

IX. INDICATIONS FOR TREATMENT

A. Pulsatile Tinnitus

This is the most common symptom of transverse and sigmoid dural sinus arteriovenous malformations [258]. While a conservative course is reasonable for the majority of these lesions, this symptom, on occasion, can be so disabling or be associated with other more alarming signs (e.g., impaired vision or papilledema) that intervention is warranted [258]. However, the incapacity of the patient may be ameliorated by measures short of complete ablation (e.g., partial obliteration by embolization) and more aggressive attempts at cure may not be warranted.

B. Venous Sinus Hypertension

Venous sinus hypertension is the most frequent reason for intervention. The reason for the venous sinus hypertension is often a combination of partial sinus thrombosis, partial sinus outflow thrombosis, and arterial inflow into the venous sinus. Dural arteriovenous fistulae that drain into the cavernous sinus may cause symptomatic hypertension of this structure resulting in exophthalmos, extraocular muscle palsy, and impaired vision. When symptomatic venous sinus hypertension results from fistulae involvement of the superior sagittal, transverse, or sigmoid sinus, a CSF malabsorption syndrome may occur. This takes the form of pseudotumor cerebri with headache, visual impairment, and papilledema. While some dural arteriovenous malformations appear to spontaneously resolve [259–262] this is seen in no more than 10% of cases [263]. Unrelenting symptomatic venous hypertension is an indication for intervention aimed at

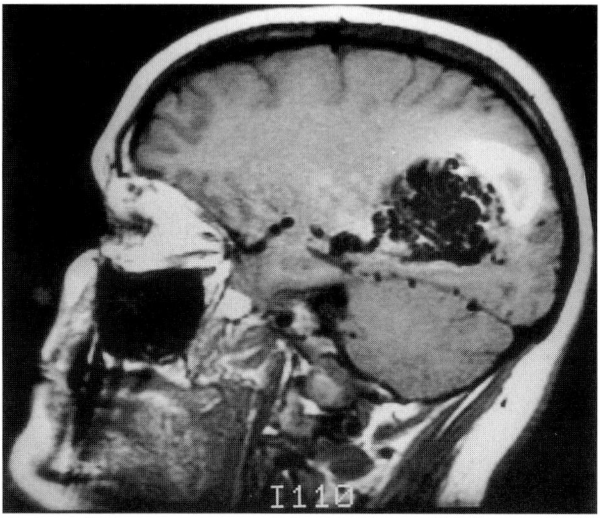

(a)

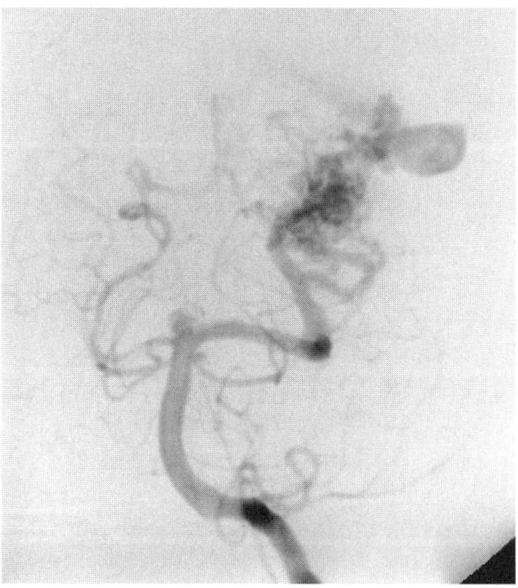

(b)

Figure 5 Management of aneurysms associated with arteriovenous malformations requires the consideration that removal of the high flow of an arteriovenous malformation may reverse the forces propagating aneurysm formation with subsequent involution of the aneurysm. This is seen with this patient with a left trigonal arteriovenous malforma-

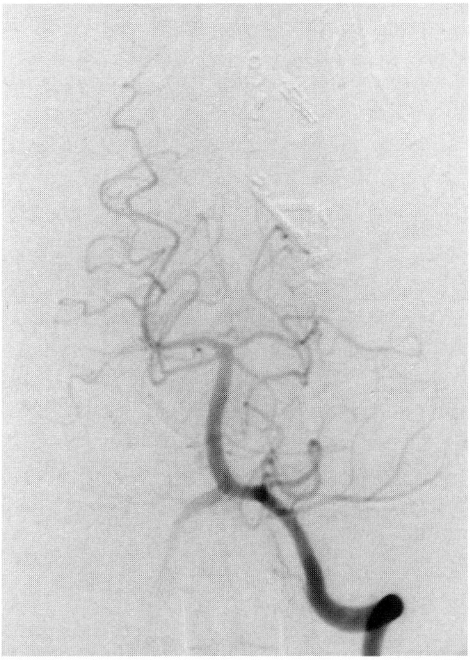

(c)

tion (a and b), which became angiographically occult within 12 months (c). However, there is some danger that the acute rise in feeding artery pressure on arteriovenous malformation ablation may rupture the unsecured aneurysm and to minimize this risk, blood pressure must be kept low. If aneurysm surgery is straightforward, this may be considered to be performed prior to, or at the time of, arteriovenous malformation resection.

significantly reducing or obliterating the nidus and whenever vision is threatened intervention should be considered.

C. Venous Compression Syndromes

Trigeminal neuralgia and hemifacial spasm have been ascribed to compression from the draining veins of dural arteriovenous malformations [80,264]. As with other compressive causes for these syndromes, they respond well to microvascular decompression and, for this pathology, ligation of the offending vein or direct obliteration of the arteriovenous malformation will successfully address the clinical problem. The indications for intervention are identical for the indications of managing these syndromes arising from other etiologies.

D. Parenchymal Venous Hypertensive Syndromes

When venous drainage from the dural arteriovenous malformation involves the normal venous anatomy of the central nervous system secondarily, parenchymal venous hypertensive syndromes may arise. The central nervous system involved may be adjacent or remote. The most common of these syndromes is the caudal cord venous hypertensive syndrome of a progressive painful mixed upper and lower motor neuron weakness of the legs. This syndrome, resulting from venous hypertension within the coronal venous plexus of the caudal spinal cord, usually arises from a spinal dural arteriovenous malformation but may arise from intracranial dural arteriovenous malformations with the appropriate venous drainage [248,250,251,265–268]. Focal neurological deficits and seizures are the clinical manifestations of cerebral venous hypertension and the particular clinical manifestations of cerebral venous hypertension and the particular clinical manifestation obviously relates to the location of the involved veins. Again, the site of the arteriovenous fistula may be remote from brain involved in cerebral systoms, but more commonly adjacent dural arteriovenous malformations are implicated. [80,256,269]. Treating these disorders successfully involves disconnecting the parenchymal venous system from the draining vein of the arteriovenous malformation. While this can be achieved by obliterating the nidus, it can also be successfully and more simply treated by dividing the draining vein or veins. The main risk with the later procedure is that the development of collateral venous drainage may lead to future problems. However, for the most part, this form of treatment appears to be successful in ameliorating the clinical syndromes of parenchymal venous hypertension [248,269–271].

E. Intracranial Hemorrhage

Leptomeningeal venous drainage, aneurysmal venous dilatation within the subarachnoid space, and Galenic drainage from intracranial dural arteriovenous malformations are associated with a risk of intracranial hemorrhage [266]. The site of hemorrhage is from the leptomeningeal venous connections rather than the nidus [80,272–276]. While this sinister venous drainage is most commonly seen with dural arteriovenous malformations located at the tentorial–incisural, Sylvian–middle fossa, and orbito–anterior falcine locations, there is no intracranial location of these malformations that has not been associated with such venous drainage [272]. As with parenchymal venous hypertensive syndromes, effective management can be achieved by disconnecting the arteriovenous malformation from the normal parenchymal venous circulation. This can be accomplished by either obliteration of the nidus or ligation of the draining vein. In the majority of patients with this pattern of drainage, treatment should be considered irrespective of the clinical presentation (Figure 6).

X. PREOPERATIVE MANAGEMENT

A. Myelography

Dural arteriovenous malformations may be suspected to be present on myelography with the appearance of a serpiginous filling defect on the dorsum of the caudal spinal cord or cauda equina. False positive myelography can occur because of thrombosis of the dural malformation or (when only the cauda equina is involved) because of redundant nerve roots associated with lumbar spinal stenosis.

B. CT and MRI Scanning

Computerized tomography scans may demonstrate a prominent draining vein (e.g., superior ophthalmic vein in the case of a cavernous sinus dural arteriovenous malformation) and MRI scan may also demonstrate prominent flow voids consistent with arteriovenous malformation venous drainage. A T2 weighted MRI scan may also demonstrate hyperintensity as a consequence of parenchymal venous hypertension. Both these investigations may therefore be useful, particularly in the screening phase, although neither is ensured to detect dural arteriovenous malformations.

C. Angiography

The decision regarding the most appropriate method of management—including conservative, transvascular approaches, focussed irradiation, or surgery—depend not only on clinical factors but also on angiographic assessment. All cranial dural arteriovenous malformations have been associated with venous drainage that may be sinister (i.e., leptomeningeal). Furthermore, even caudal cord venous hypertension syndromes have resulted from cranial dural arteriovenous malformations demonstrating that the clinical manifestations of these types of arteriovenous malformations may well be remote to the actual fistulae. Therefore, angiography is necessary to best manage dural arteriovenous malformations and should be performed in all patients that would be considered a low risk for this procedure. Complete spinal (including sacral vessels) and cranial angiography may be required to pursue the occasional elusive arteriovenous malformation.

D. Preoperative Embolization

Preoperative embolization plays an important role in reducing bleeding from those arteriovenous malformations where control of the feeding arteries may be difficult and risk of hemorrhage during exposure is high. This is particularly

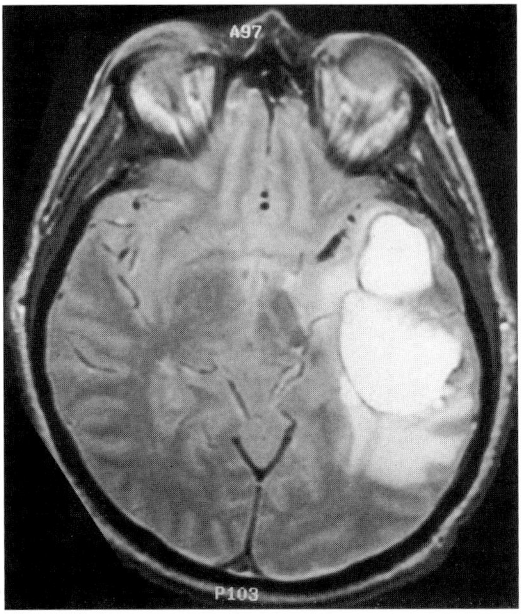

(a)

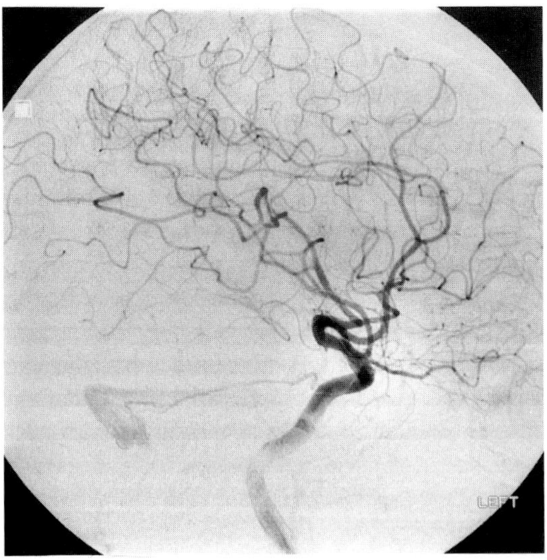

(b)

Figure 6 Significant intracerebral hemorrhage can arise in the distribution of parenchymal venous drainage from dural arteriovenous malformations (a). This 60-year-old male had a pure dural arteriovenous malformation fed by the left internal and

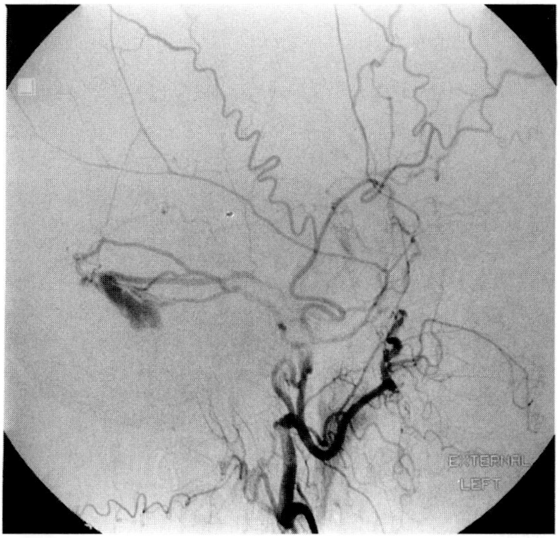

(c)

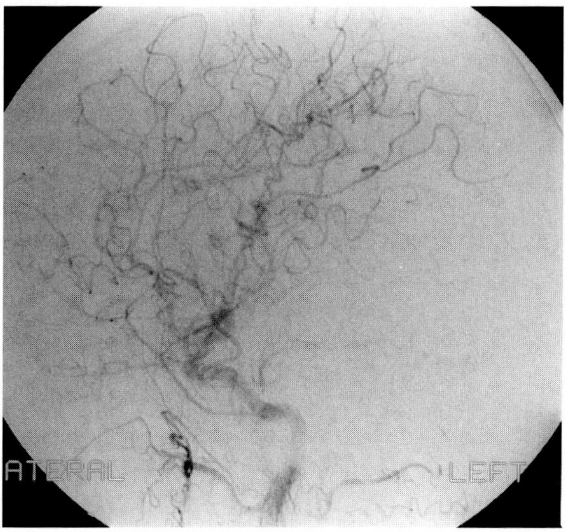

(d)

external carotid meningeal arteries associated with impaired sigmoid sinus drainage (b and c). In this case the propensity for repeat hemorrhage caused by venous hypertension could be easily eliminated by resecting the dural arterial connections to the sigmoid sinus and packing the sinus (d).

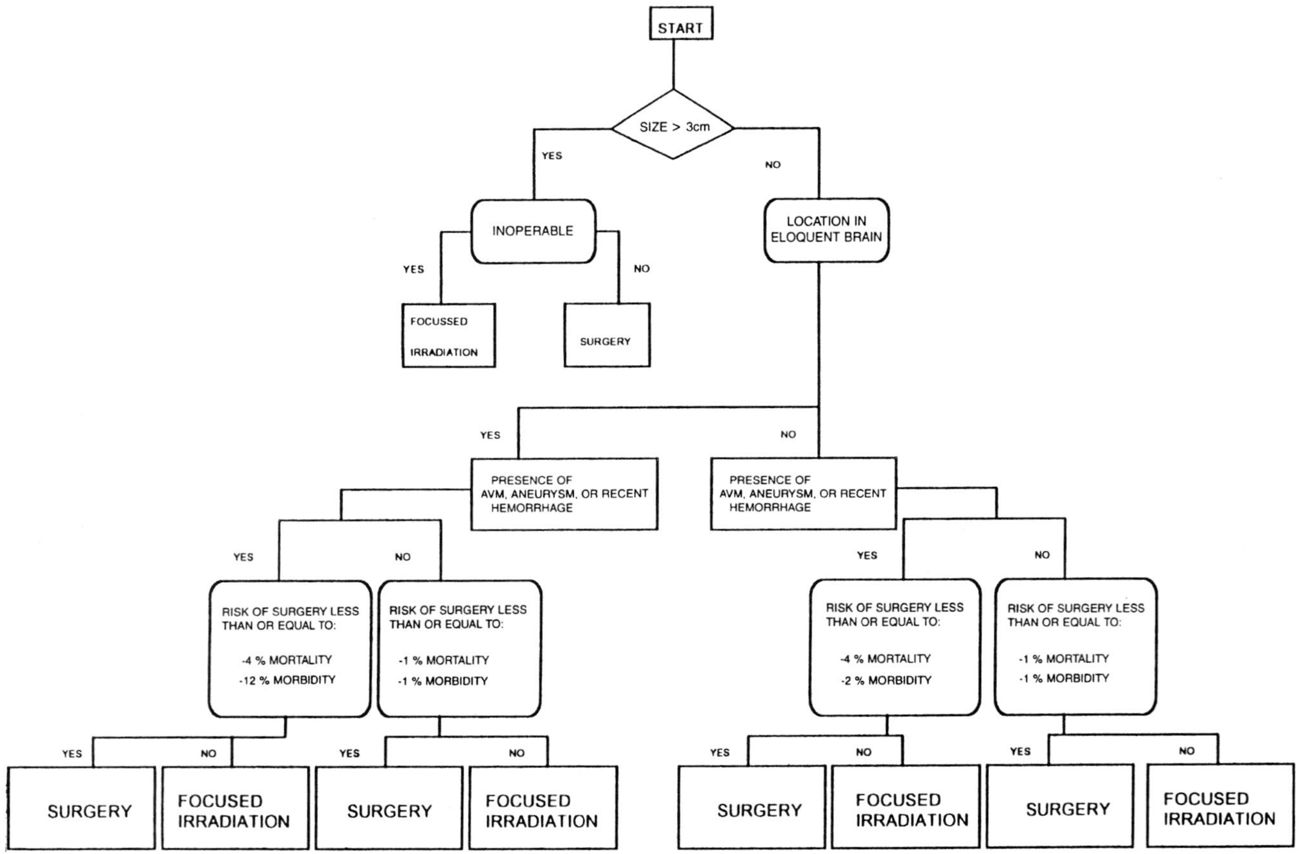

Figure 7 This is an example of a paradigm that may be used in aiding the decision-making process with regard to management of AVM by surgery versus focussed irradiation. See text for the statistics used to derive the morbidity, mortality risk for each group.

true for arteriovenous malformations of the transverse and sigmoid sinus [258].

XI. SURGICAL STRATEGIES

A. Interruption of Venous Drainage Within the Subarachnoid Space

When the surgical aim is to prevent intracranial hemorrhage or to reverse a parenchymal venous hypertensive syndrome (of the brain or spinal cord) an adequate strategy may be to do no more than ligation of the offending draining vein. Once this has been achieved the arteriovenous malformation will have been rendered relatively benign and complete ablation of the arteriovenous malformation should follow only when it is considered sufficiently easy that no significant extra morbidity will be incurred by this surgery.

B. Obliteration of the Arteriovenous Malformation

When the surgical aim is to prevent venous sinus hypertension it is necessary to obliterate the involved segment of dural venous sinus.

C. Regional Strategies

Observation without invasive interventional therapy is indicated for lesions without sinister venous drainage and lesions with benign symptomatology. For lesions of the tentorial–incisura, Sylvian region, and anterior cranial fossa, surgical strategies need to be individualized according to the above principles. Frequently the main aim of surgery at these locations is the disconnection of the AVM in the dura from the leptomeningeal venous circulation. We have found the indications for direct surgery on superior sagittal sinus lesions to be sufficiently unusual to cause resection of the involved sinus and dura to be rare. The three regions that are approached with a standard technique and that sometimes involve more than venous disconnection (although in certain circumstances this may be all that is required) are lesions of the transverse–sigmoid sinus, cavernous sinus, and the spine. However before patients with these lesions (with the exception of spinal dural AVMs) are considered for surgery they must have been evaluated by the interventional neuroradiologist for possible endovascular obliteration. Therapy by this technique is highly successful now that a combination of arterial and venous approaches to the pathology are employed. Seventy-nine cases of cranial dural arteriovenous malformations were surgically treated at the Mayo Clinic between 1974 and 1992 with 3 deaths (2 secondary to intraoperative hemorrhage prior to the use of preoperative hemorrhage) and an excellent outcome achieved in 66 cases [258].

1. Transverse–Sigmoid

This is the lesion most commonly considered for surgical therapy. Of the 79 surgically treated cranial dural arteriovenous malformations between 1974 and 1992 at the Mayo Clinic, 61 were in this transverse–sigmoid. The craniotomy flap must extend to expose both sides of the transverse and sigmoid sinus for the entire length of the involved dura. To facilitate this and to reduce the volume of hemorrhage we recommend preoperative embolization and the use of a high-speed drill with a diamond bit in turning the flap. The sinus ligation is effected by incising along the infratentorial and supratentorial dura parallel to the sinus followed by medial ligation. Subsequent gentle lateral retraction of the involved sinus allows the tentorial attachment to be progressively divided to the transverse–sigmoid junction. At this point it is necessary to drill further the petrous bone to gain anterior exposure of the proximal sigmoid sinus controlling bleeding with bone wax. The sigmoid sinus can now be firmly packed with surgicel. Even large veins connected with the sinus may be sacrificed when retrograde flow is observed (evident by their arterialized color). Closure of the dura is accomplished with a graft (e.g., fascia lata) [258].

2. Cavernous

For the most part, the cavernous sinus lesion is becoming a lesion rarely treated by surgery. If it is not possible to endovascularly catheterize draining veins because of technical difficulties or because of the dangers of exacerbating drainage into pial vessels, a direct approach to the cavernous sinus with the aim of packing may be indicated in some cases. The surgical approach described by Vinko Dolenc gives an excellent exposure of the sinus [277]. Before opening the sinus the arterial inflow to the sinus should be arrested with temporary clamps on the ipsilateral external and internal carotid artery in the neck and temporary clips placed on the ophthalmic and adjacent internal carotid artery intracranially. This reduces the tension within the sinus sufficiently to enable packing with surgicel upon opening. It is usually necessary to open the sinus in several locations to ensure adequate ablation. While the arterial input is temporarily arrested EEG monitoring will indicate the safety of this maneuver and will also help identify unacceptable internal carotid artery narrowing after the temporary clips and clamps are removed. Following release of the temporary arterial arrest into the sinus, intraoperative angiography should be performed to assess the state of the internal carotid artery as some of the packing may have to be removed. If this is not possible to reverse, consideration must be given to an interposition saphenous vein bypass graft between the cervical carotid and the intracranial internal carotid arteries with trapping of the sinus segment. Because of the magnitude of such surgery and the usually benign nature of the disease, the indications for such a procedure are very limited.

3. Spinal

The nidus may be easily approached by a limited laminectomy with a lateral enough exposure to gain access to the involved nerve root axilla. Following the laminectomy the dura is opened reflected laterally on the origin of the vein connecting the arteriovenous malformation with the coronal venous plexus. This vein is then ligated and divided followed by ablation of the arteriovenous malformation nidus either by excising the involved dura or more simply by bipolar coagulation with one blade of the forceps placed extradurally and one placed intradurally.

When the nidus is not readily accessed the laminectomy exposure should be such that the draining vein will be easily identified for ligation and division. The nidus may be left undisturbed with a reasonable expectation of surgical success [250,251,266]. Surgical management of this disorder is simple, effective, and carries a low morbidity [279]. We consider this the first line in treatment for lesions in this location in contrast to dural arteriovenous malformations in other locations where an endovascular technique is the usual preferred mode of treatment.

XII. SURGICAL MANAGEMENT OF ARTERIOVENOUS MALFORMATIONS OF THE SPINAL CORD: INTRODUCTION

In many institutions parenchymal arteriovenous malformations of the spinal cord are less common lesions than spinal dural arteriovenous malformations [251,278] although this experience is not uniformly reported [279,281]. Spinal dural arteriovenous malformations have been discussed in the previous section but the difference between parenchymal and dural arteriovenous malformations deserves highlighting. Like arteriovenous malformations of the brain, the most common mode of presentation of spinal parenchymal arteriovenous malformations is hemorrhage with a similar age and sex distribution. Whereas the spinal dural arteriovenous malformations present a venous hypertensive syndrome and occur in males (85%) older on average than their parenchymal counterpart, spinal parenchymal arteriovenous malformation may even be clinically apparent at birth [280–282]. The parenchymal arteriovenous malformations can be classified into medullary arteriovenous malformations and arteriovenous fistulae. The medullary lesions can be subclassified into glomus lesions, which are tightly packed lesions confined to the cord, and juvenile lesions, which involve cord, canal, and adjacent structures. The direct arteriovenous fistulae may be intramedullary or paramedullary. As with arteriovenous malformations of the brain, associated arterial and venous aneurysms are common.

XIII. INDICATIONS FOR TREATMENT

In comparison with the counterpart lesion of the brain, spinal parenchymal arteriovenous malformations do not carry the same risk of death. Even after excluding 20% of cases from surgery (presumably in part based on perceived operability) Rosenblum et al. found that surgery resulted in a 2% mortality and a neurological deterioration in 14% with residual arteriovenous malformation being present in 41% of cases [280]. Yasargil et al. had a mortality of 5% and a clinical deterioration in 20% of patients with 27% of patients undergoing surgery having an incomplete resection [281]. Clearly, even in the best hands, surgery for spinal parenchymal arteriovenous malformations is difficult. Factors that are likely to increase the risk of ablation by surgery include anterior location, a diffuse lesion, extension over more than 2 vertebral segments, arterial supply including sulcocommisural branches of the anterior spinal artery, venous drainage predominantly dorsal, and a cervical location (the latter factor on the basis of the greater neurological deficit expected if a complication were to ensue) [281]. As with arteriovenous malformations of the brain, the presence of an arterial aneurysm likely indicates an increased propensity for hemorrhage [280] although hemorrhage is certainly seen in the absence of aneurysm. As the true natural history for spinal arteriovenous malformations is unknown it is difficult to be dogmatic with regard to indications for surgery. At present our indications are to consider surgery only for symptomatic lesions without concomitant unfavorable anatomical factors. As more knowledge is gained, the true indications for surgical therapy will hopefully become more accurately defined.

XIV. PREOPERATIVE MANAGEMENT

Good quality selective angiography is essential in the preoperative evaluation of these lesions. In addition, MRI scanning with transverse cuts adds further information in the evaluation of these lesions and the relationship to adjacent hemorrhage. Dexamethasone is commenced and if intraoperative radiological localization is not possible, accurate spinal marking should be obtained by the neuroradiologist at the time of spinal angiography.

XV. SURGICAL STRATEGIES

As with arteriovenous malformations of the brain, a good exposure is imperative. This is facilitated by a laminectomy considerably above the cephalad pole and below the caudal pole of the lesion. In addition, it is necessary to be as wide in the laminectomy as the lateral gutters of the spinal canal. Sectioning of the dentate ligament may further enhance exposure by facilitating mobility of the cord. The dissection must be carried out with the aid of the operating microscope and the dissection must be exclusively on the margin of the lesion. Monitoring cord function intraoperatively with evoked potentials may aid the dissection. Cephalad and caudal extension of the pial incision is frequently required to gain maximal exposure of the arteriovenous malformation. Retraction of the pia can be achieved by suturing to the reflected dura. Further dissection can be facilitated by gently coagulating the lesion by bipolar diathermy which effectively shrinks the lesion.

REFERENCES

1. Yasargil MG. Microneurosurgery Volume III A. New York: Thieme Medical Publishers, 1987.
2. Giordano D. Contributo alla cura delle lesioni traumatiche ed ella trapenazione del cranio. *Gazz med ital* 1890; 41: 5–15.
3. Guldenarm JA, Winkler C. Cerebral verschijnselen na een trauma van den schedal. *Ned T Geneesk* 1891; 4: 217–230.
4. Lucas-Championiere MJ. *Bull Soc Chir (Paris)* 1909; 35: 318–322.
5. Starr MA, McCosh AJ. A contribution to the localization of the muscular sence. *Amer J Med Sci* 1894; 108: 517–520.
6. Von Bergmann E. Zur Kasuistik operativer Hirntumoren. *Arch Klin Chir* 1901/1902; 63: 936–958.
7. Cushing H, Bailey P. *Tumours Arising from the Blood Vessels of the Brain. Angiomatous Malformations and Hemangioblastomas.* Vol III. Springfield IL: Thomas, 1928.
8. Dandy WE. Arteriovenous aneurysm of the brain. *Arch Surg* 1928; 17: 190–243.
9. Moniz E. Angiomes cerebraux. Importance de langiographie cerebrale dans leur diagnostic. *Bull Acad Med (Paris)* 1935; 3: 113.
10. Olivecrona H, Riives J. Arteriovenous aneurysms of the brain. Their diagnosis and treatment. *Arch Neurol Psych* 1948; 59: 567–602.
11. Norlen G. Arteriovenous aneurysms of the brain: report of ten cases of total removal of the lesion. *J Neurosurg* 1949; 6: 475–494.
12. Potter JM. Angiomatous malformations of the brain. Their nature and prognosis. *Ann Royal College Surg Engl* 1955; 16: 227–243.
13. Forster DMC, Steiner L, Hakanson S. Arteriovenous malformations of the brain. A long–term clinical study. *J Neurosurg* 1972; 37: 562–570.

14. Mingino S. Supratentorial arteriovenous malformations of the brain. *Adv Technical Standards Neurosurgery* 1978; 5: 93–123.
15. Morello G, Borghi GP. Cerebral angiomas. A report of 154 personal cases and a comparison between the results of surgical excision and conservative treatment. *Acta Neurochir* 1973; 28: 135–155.
16. Troupp H, Marttila I, Halonen V. Arteriovenous malformations of the brain: prognosis without operation. *Acta Neurochir* 1970; 22: 125–128.
17. Brown RD, Wiebers DO, Forbes G, O'Fallon WM, Piepgras DG, Marsh WR, Maciunas RJ. The natural history of unruptured intracranial arteriovenous malformations. *J Neurosurg* 1988; 68: 352–357.
18. Crawford PM, West CR, Chadwick DW, Schaw MDM. Arteriovenous malformation of the brain. Natural history in unoperated patients. *J Neurol Neurosurg Psychiat* 1986; 49: 1–10.
19. Fults D, Kelly DL Jr. Natural history of arteriovenous malformations of the brain: a clinical study. *Neurosurgery* 1984; 15: 658–662.
20. Graf CJ, Perrett GE, Torner JC. Bleeding from cerebral arteriovenous malformations as part of their natural history. *J Neurosurg* 1983; 58: 331–337.
21. Itoyama Y, Uemura S, Ushio Y, Kuratsu JI, Nonaka N, Wada H, Sano Y, Fukukumura A, Yoshida K, Yano T. Natural course of unoperated intracranial arteriovenous malformations: study of 50 cases. *J Neurosurg* 1989; 71: 805–809.
22. Ondra SL, Troupp H, George ED, Schwab K. The natural history of symptomatic arteriovenous malformations of the brain: a 24–year follow–up assessment. *J Neurosurg* 1990; 73: 387–391.
23. Luschka H. Cavernose blutgeschwulst des gehirns. *Virchows Arch* 1854; 6: 458–470.
24. Albert P. Personal experience in the treatment of 178 cases of arteriovenous malformations of the brain. *Acta Neurochir* 1982; 61: 207–226.
25. Davis CH, Symon L. The management of cerebral arteriovenous malformations. *Acta Neurochir* 1985; 74: 4–11.
26. Heros RC, Korosue K, Diebold PM. Surgical excision of cerebral arteriovenous malformations: late results. *Neurosurgery* 1990; 26: 570–578.
27. Jomin M, Lesain F, Lozes G. Prognosis for arteriovenous malformations of the brain in adults based on 150 cases. *Surg Neurol* 1985; 23: 362–366.
28. Moody RA, Poppen JL. Arteriovenous malformations. *J Neurosurg* 1970; 32: 503–511.
29. Morgan MK, Johnston I. Intracranial arteriovenous malformations: an 11 year experience. *Med J Aust* 1988; 148: 65–68.
30. Morgan MK, Johnston IH, Hallinan JM, Weber NC. Complications of surgery for arteriovenous malformations of the brain. *J Neurosurg* 1993; 78: 176–182.
31. Pertuiset B, Sichez JP, Philippon J, Fohanna D, Horn YE. Mortality and morbidity following the surgical excision of 162 intracranial arteriovenous malformations (1958–1978). *Rev Neurol* 1979; 135: 319–327.
32. Yasargil MG, Curcic M, Kis M, Teddy PJ, Valavanis A. Microneurosurgery Volume III B. New York: Thieme Medical Publishers, 1988.
33. Luessenhop AJ. Natural history of cerebral arteriovenous malformations. In: Wilson CB, Stein BM (eds). Intracranial Arteriovenous Malformations. Baltimore: Williams and Wilkins, 1984: 12–23.

34. Dobbelaere P, Jomin M, Clarrisse J, Laine E. Interet pronostique de letude du drainage verneux de aneurysms arterio–veneux cerebraux. *Neurochirugie* 1979; 25: 178–184.
35. Vinuela F, Nombela L, Roach MR, Fox AJ, Pelz DM. Stenotic and occlusive disease of the venous drainage system of deep brain AVM's. *J Neurosurg* 1985; 63: 180–184.
36. Brown RD, Wiebers DO, Forbes GS. Unruptured intracranial aneurysms and arteriovenous malformations: frequency of intracranial hemorrhageand relationship of lesions. *J Neurosurg* 1990; 73: 859–863.
37. Kanno T, Sano H, Shinomiya T, Katada K, Nagata J, Hoshino M, Mitsuyama F. Role of surgery in hypertensive intracerebral hematoma. *J Neurosurg* 1984; 61: 1091–1099.
38. Luessenhop AJ, Shevlin WA, Ferrero AA, McCullough DC, Barone BM. Surgical management of primary intracerebral hemorrhage. *J Neurosurg* 1967; 27: 419–427.
39. Piepgras DG, Redmond MJ. Surgical management of intracerebral hemorrhage. In: Schmidek HH, Sweet WH (eds). Operative Neurosurgical Techniques. Indications, Methods and Results. Philadelphia: WB Saunders, 1988: 881–888.
40. Volpin L, Cervellini P, Colombo F, Zanusso M, Benedetti A. Spontaneous intracerebral hematomas. A new proposal about the usefulness and limits of surgical treatment. *Neurosurgery* 1984; 15: 663–666.
41. Waga S, Yamamota Y. Hypertensive putaminal hemorrhage: treatment and results. Is surgical treatment superior to conservative one? *Stroke* 1983; 14: 480–485.
42. Kaneko M, Koba T, Yokoyama T. Early surgical treatment for hypertensive intracerebral hemorrhage. *J Neurosurg* 1977; 46: 579–583.
43. Nehls DG, Mendelow AD, Graham DI, Sinar EJ, Teasdale GM. Experimental intracerebral hemorrhage: progression of hemodynamic changes production of a spontaneous mass lesion. *Neurosurgery* 1988; 23: 439–444.
44. Nehls DG, Mendelow AD, Graham DI, Teasdale GM. Experimental intracerebral hemorrhage: early removal of a spontaneous mass lesion improves late outcome. American Association of Neurological Surgeons. Toronto, Ontario, April 24–28, 1988.
45. Kase C, Williams J, Wyatt D, Mohr JP. Lobar intracerebral hematomas: clinical and CT analysis of 22 cases. *Neurology* 1982; 32: 1146–1150.
46. Little JR, Blomquist GA, Ethier R. Intraventricular hemorrhage in adults. *Surg Neurol* 1977; 8: 143–147.
47. Ojemann RG, Heros RC. Spontaneous brain hemorrhage. *Stroke* 1983; 14:468.
48. Pia HW. The surgical treatment of intracerebral and intraventricular hematomas. *Acta Neurochir* 1972; 27: 149–152.
49. Auer LM, Auer T, Sayama I. Indications for surgical treatment of cerebellar hemorrhage and infarction. *Acta Neurochir* 1986; 79: 74–79.
50. Fisher CM, Picard EH, Polak A. Acute hypertensive cerebellar hemorrhage: diagnosis of surgical treatment. *J Nerv Ment Dis* 1965; 140: 38–57.
51. Freeman RE, Onofrio BM, Okazaki H, Dinapoli RP. Spontaneous intracerebellar hemorrhage. Diagnosis and surgical treatment. *Neurology* 1973; 23: 84–90.
52. Heros RC. Cerebellar hemorrhage and infarction. *Stroke* 1982; 13: 106–109.

53. Little JR, Tubman DE, Ethier R. Cerebellar hemorrhage in adults: diagnosis by computerized tomography. *J Neurosurg* 1978; 48: 575–579.
54. McKissock W, Richardson A, Walsh LS. Spontaneous cerebellar haemorrhage: a study of 34 consecutive cases treated surgically. *Brain* 1960; 83: 1–9.
55. Yoshida S, Sasaki M, Oka H, Gotoh O, Yamada R, Sano K. Acute hypertensive cerebellar hemorrhage with signs of lower brainstem compression. *Surg Neurol* 1978; 10: 79–83.
56. Cioffi FA, Tomasello F, D'Avanzo R. Pontine hematomas. *Surg Neurol* 1981; 16: 13–16.
57. Konovaslow AN, Spallone A, Makhmudow UB, Kukhlajeva JA, Ozerova VI. Surgical management of hematomas of the brain stem. *J Neurosurg* 1990; 73: 212–216.
58. Koos WT, Sunder-Plassmann M, Salah S. Successful removal of a large intrapontine hematoma. Case report. *J Neurosurg* 1969; 31: 690–694.
59. Murphy M. Successful evacuation of acute pontine hematoma. *J Neurosurg* 1972; 37: 224–225.
60. Morris H. Venous vascular tumour of cerebrum. *Trans Path Soc London* 1871; 22: 22–24.
61. Leblanc R, Feindel W, Ethier R. Epilepsy from cerebral arteriovenous malformations. *Can J Neurol Sci* 1983; 10: 91–95.
62. Sundt TM Jr, Piepgras DG, Stevens LN. Surgery for supratentorial arteriovenous malformations. *Clin Neurosurgery* 1990; 37: 49–115.
63. Piepgras DG, Sundt TM Jr, Ragoowansi AT, Stevens L. Seizure outcome in patients with surgically treated cerebral arteriovenous malformations. *J Neurosurg* 1993; 78: 5–11.
64. Luessenhop AJ, Rosa L. Cerebral arteriovenous malformations. Indications for and results of surgery and the role of intravascular techniques. *J Neurosurg* 1984; 60: 14–22.
65. Elvidge AR. The cerebral vessels studied by angiography. In: Penfield W (ed). The Circulation of the Brain and Spinal Cord. Baltimore: Williams and Wilkins, 1938: 110–149.
66. Murphy JP. Cerebrovascular Disease. Chicago: Yearbook Medical Publishers, 1954: 408.
67. Barnett GH, Little JR, Ebrahim ZY, Jones SC, Friel HT. Cerebral circulation during arteriovenous malformation operation. *Neurosurgery* 1987; 20:836–842.
68. Hashimoto K, Nishimura T, Kozuka T, Hayashi M. Cerebral hemodynamics in arteriovenous malformations: evaluation by single–photon emission CT. *AJNR* 1987; 8: 193–197.
69. Hassler W, Steinmetz H. Cerebral hemodynamics in angioma patients: an intraoperative study. *J Neurosurg* 1987; 67: 822–831.
70. Menon D, Weir B. Evaluation of cerebral blood flow in arteriovenous malformations by the xenon 133 inhalation method. *Can J Neurol Sci* 1979; 6: 411–416.
71. Okabe T, Meyer JS, Okayasu H, Harper R, Rose J, Grossman RG, Centene R, Tachibana H, Lee YY. Xenon–enhanced CT CBF measurements in cerebral AVM's before and after excision. *J Neurosurg* 1983; 59: 21–31.
72. Rosenblum BR, Bonner RF, Oldfield EH. Intraoperative measurement of cortical

blood flow adjacent to cerebral AVM using laser doppler velocimetry. *J Neurosurg* 1987; 66: 396–399.

73. Spetzler RF, Martin NA, Carter LP, Flom RA, Raudzens PA, Wilkinson E. Surgical management of large AVM's by staged embolization and operative excision. *J Neurosurg* 1987; 67: 17–28.
74. Takeuchi S, Kikuchi H, Karasawa J, Narvo Y, Hashimoto K, Nishimura T, Kozuka T, Hayashi M. Cerebral hemodynamics in arteriovenous malformations: evaluation by single–photon emission CT. *AJNR* 1987; 8: 193–197.
75. Yamada S. Arteriovenous malformations in the functional area: surgical treatment and regional cerebral blood flow. *Neurol Res* 1982; 4: 283–322.
76. Young WL, Prohovnik I, Ornstein E, Sisti MB, Solomon RA, Stein BM, Ostapkovich N. Monitoring of intraoperative cerebral hemodynamics before and after arteriovenous malformation resection. *Anesth Analg* 1988; 67: 1011–1014.
77. Norman MG, Becker LE. Cerebral damage in neonates resulting from arteriovenous malformation of the vein of Galen. *J Neurol Neurosurg Psychiat* 1974; 37: 252–258.
78. Takashima S, Becker LE. Neuropathology of arteriovenous malformation in children. *J Neurol Neurosurg Psychiat* 1980; 43: 380–385.
79. Barrow DL. Unruptured cerebral arteriovenous malformations presenting with intracranial hypertension. *Neurosurgery* 1980; 23: 484–490.
80. Lasjaunias P, Chiu M, Brugge KT, Tolia A, Hurth M, Bernstein M. Neurologic manifestations of intracranial dural arteriovenous malformations. *J Neurosurg* 1986; 64: 724–730.
81. Obrader S, Sato M, Silvela J. Clinical syndromes of arteriovenous malformations of the transverse–sigmoid sinus. *J Neurol Neurosurg Psychiat* 1975; 38: 436–451.
82. Vassilouthis J. Cerebral arteriovenous malformation with intracranial hypertension. *Surg Neurol* 1979; 11: 402–404.
83. Weisberg LA, Pierce JF, Jabbari B. Intracranial hypertension resulting from a cerebrovascular malformation. *South Med J* 1977; 70: 624–626.
84. Fox AJ, Girvin JP, Vinuela F, Drake CG. Rolandic arteriovenous malformations: improvement in limb function by IBC embolization. *AJNR* 1985; 6: 572–582.
85. Kusske JA, Kelly WA. Embolization and reduction of the "steal" syndrome in cerebral arteriovenous malformations. *J Neurosurg* 1974; 40: 313–321.
86. Wolpert SM, Barnett FJ, Prager RJ. Benefits of embolization without surgery for cerebral arteriovenous malformations. *AJR* 1982; 138: 99–102.
87. Ogilvy CS. Radiation therapy for arteriovenous malformation: a review. *Neurosurgery* 1990; 26: 725–735.
88. Mackenzie I. The clinical presentation of cerebral angioma. A review of 50 cases. *Brain* 1953; 76: 184–214.
89. Mohr JP. Neurological manifestations and factors related to therapeutic decisions. In: Wilson CB, Stein BM (eds). Intracranial Arteriovenous Malformations. Baltimore: Williams and Watkins, 1984; 5–6.
90. Ozer MN, Sencer W, Block J. A clinical study of cerebral vascular malformations: the significance of migraine. *J Mt Sinai Hospital NY* 1964; 31: 403–423.
91. Johnston I. The definition of a reduced CSF absorption syndrome: a reappraisal of

benign intracranial hypertension and related conditions. *Med Hypotheses* 1976; 1: 10–14.

92. Wallace JM, Nashold BS Jr, Slewka AP. Hemodynamic effect of cerebral arteriovenous aneurysms. *Circulation* 1965; 31: 696–704.
93. Glatt BS, Rowe RD. Cerebral arteriovenous fistula associated with congestive heart failure in the newborn. *Pediatr* 1960; 26: 596–603.
94. Goldman AS, Yaffe SJ. Fetal trimethadione syndrome. *Teratology* 1978; 17: 103–106.
95. Hernandez A, Schwartz HG, Goldring S. Cerebral arteriovenous fistulas and congenital heart disease. *Case report Pediatr* 1965; 66: 722–728.
96. Hoffman HJ, Chuang S, Hendrick EB, Humpherys RP. Aneurysms of the vein of Galen. Experience of the Hospital for Sick Children, Toronto. *J Neurosurg* 1982; 57: 316–322.
97. Jacques S, Garner JT, Shelden H, Johnson PE Jr, Johnson D. Severe neonatal cardiac insufficiency due to arteriovenous fistula of the vein of Galen. *G Ital Cardiol* 1984; 14: 671–677.
98. Johnston IH, Whittle IR, Besser M, Morgan MK. Vein of Galen malformation: diagnosis and management. *Neurosurgery* 1987; 20: 747–758.
99. Levine OS, Jamieson AG, Nellhaus G, Gold AP. Cardiac complications of cerebral arteriovenous fistula in infancy. *Pediatrics* 1962; 30: 563–575.
100. Long DM, Seljeskok EL, Chou SN, French LA. Giant arteriovenous malformations of infancy and childhood. *J Neurosurg* 1974; 40: 304–312.
101. Marasini M, Ribaldone D, Pannizzon G, Lazzaroni F, Tarcone G, Cantoni LG. Severe neonatal heart failure and arteriovenous fistula of the vein of Galen. *G Ital Cardiol*; 14: 671–677.
102. Mori K, Murata T, Hashimoto N, Handa H. Clinical analysis of arteriovenous malformations in children. *Child's Brain* 1980; 6: 13–25.
103. Salazar J, Eiras J, Mengual J, Felipe J, Caravilla LI, Garcia MD. Aneurysm of the vein of Galen with neonatal cardiac insufficiency. Success of early neurosurgical treatment. *Pediatric* 1987; 42: 167–170.
104. Schwechheimer K, Kuhl G. Arteriovenous angioma of the vein of Galen causing cardiac failure in the neonate. Report on clinical and pathological findings in two cases. *Neuropediatrics* 1983; 14: 184–187.
105. Ventureyra EC, Ivan LP, Naliovi N. Deep seated giant arteriovenous malformations in infancy. *Surg Neurol* 1978; 10: 365–370.
106. Mickle JP, Quisling RG. The transtorcular embolization of vein of Galen aneurysm. *J Neurosurg* 1986; 64: 731–735.
107. Quisling M. Vein of Galen malformation. In: Hoffman HJ, (ed). Neurosurgery, Advances in Paediatric Neurosurgery. State of the Art Reviews. Philadelphia: Hanley and Belfus, 1986: 129–131.
108. So SC. Cerebral arteriovenous malformations in children. *Child's Brain* 1978; 4: 242–250.
109. Luessenhop AJ, Mujica PH. Embolization of segements of the circle of Willis and adjacent branches for management of certain inoperable cerebral arteriovenous malformations. *J Neurosurg* 1981; 54: 573–582.

110. Luessenhop AJ, Presper JH. Surgical embolization of cerebral arteriovenous malformations through internal carotid and vertebral arteries. *J Neurosurg* 1975; 42: 443–451.
111. Nornes H, Grip A. Hemodynamic aspects of cerebral arteriovenous malformations. *J Neurosurg* 1980; 53: 456–464.
112. Russell EJ, Berenstein A. Neurologic applications of interventional radiology. *Neurol Clinics* 1984; 2: 873–902.
113. Pellettieri L. Surgical versus conservative treatment of intracranial arteriovenous malformations. *Acta Neurochir Suppl* 1979; 29: 1–86.
114. Spetzler RF, Martin NA. A proposed grading system for arteriovenous malformations. *J Neurosurg* 1986; 65: 476–483.
115. Steinmeier R, Schramm J, Muller HG, Fahlbusch R. Evaluation of prognostic factors in cerebral arteriovenous malformations. *Neurosurgery* 1989; 24: 193–200.
116. Tamaki N, Ehara K, Lim TK, Kuwamura K, Obora Y, Kanazawa Y, Yamashita H, Matsumoto S. Cerebral arteriovenous malformations: Factors influencing the surgical difficulty and outcome. *Neurosurgery* 1991; 29: 856–863.
117. Zabramski JM, Spetzler RF. Comments. *Neurosurgery* 1988; 22 :509.
118. Sundt TM Jr. Controversies in the surgical management of hemorrhagic cerebrovascular disease. *Clin Neurosurgery* 1990; 37: 12–18.
119. Cahan LD, Rand RW. Stereotactic coagulation of a paraventricular arteriovenous malformation. Case report. *J Neurosurg* 1978; 39: 770–774.
120. Davis DH, Kelly PJ. Stereotactic resection of occult vascular malformations. *J Neurosurg* 1990; 72: 698–702.
121. Kandel EI, Peresedov VV. Stereotaxic clipping of arterial aneurysms and arteriovenous malformations. *J Neurosurg* 1977; 46: 12–23.
122. Kelly PJ. Volumetric stereotactic surgical resection of intra–axial brain lesions. *Mayo Clin Proc* 1988; 63: 1186–1198.
123. Kelly PJ, Alker GJ, Zoll JG. A microstereotactic approach to deep–seated arteriovenous malformations. *Surg Neurol* 1982; 17: 260–262.
124. Riechert T, Mundinger F. Combined stereotaxic operation for treatment of deep–seated angiomas and aneurysms. *J Neurosurg* 1964; 21: 358–363.
125. Siti MB, Solomon RA, Stein BM. Stereotactic craniotomy in the resection of small arteriovenous malformations. *J Neurosurg* 1991; 75: 40–44.
126. Yamada S, Ritland S, Knierim D. Stereotactic localization of deep–seated arteriovenous malformations in the functional area. *Appl Neurophysiol* 1983; 46: 231–235.
127. Leblanc R, Meyer E. Functional PET scanning in the assessment of cerebral arteriovenous malformations. *J Neurosurg* 1990; 73: 615–619.
128. Batjer HH, Devous MD Sr, Meyer YJ, Purdy PD, Samson DS. Cerebrovascular hemodynamics in arteriovenous malformations complicated by normal perfusion breakthrough. *Neurosurgery* 1988; 22: 503–509.
129. Batjer HH, Devous MD Sr, Seibert GB, Purdy PD, Ajmani AK, Delarosa M, Bonte FJ. Intracranial arteriovenous malformation: relationships between clinical and radiographic factors and ipsilateral steal severity. *Neurosurgery* 1988; 23: 322–328.
130. Deutsch G. Blood flow changes in arteriovenous malformation during behavioural activation. *Ann Neurol* 1983; 13: 38–43.

131. Ewing JR, Robertson WM, Brown GG, Welch KMA. ^{133}Xenon inhalation: accuracy in detection of ischemic cerebral regions and angiographic lesions. In: Wood JH (ed). *Cerebral Blood Flow.* New York: McGraw-Hill, 1987: 202–219.
132. Hassler W. Hemodynamic aspects of cerebral angiomas. *Acta Neurochir (wien)* 1986; Suppl 37: 1–136.
133. Homan RW, Devous MD Sr, Stokely EM, Bonte FJ. Quantification of intracerebral steal in patients with arteriovenous malformation. *Arch Neurol* 1986; 43: 779–785.
134. Lindegaard KF, Grolimund P, Aaslid R, Nornes H. Evaluation of cerebral AVM's using transcranial doppler ultrasound. *J Neurosurg* 1986; 65: 335–344.
135. Hassler W, Gilsbach J. Intra– and perioperative aspects of the hemodynamics of supratentorial AVM. *Acta Neurochir (Wien)* 1984; 73: 35–44.
136. Pertuiset B, Ancri D, Clergue F. Preoperative evaluation of hemodynamic factors in cerebral arteriovenous malformations for selection of a radical surgical tactic with special reference to vascular autoregulation disorders. *Neurol Res* 1982; 4: 209–233.
137. Shenkin HA, Spitz EB, Grant FC, Kelty SS. Physiologic studies of arteriovenous anomalies of the brain. *J Neurosurg* 1948; 5: 165–172.
138. Tyler JL, Leblanc R, Meyer E, Dagher Y, Yamamoto YL, Diksic M, Hakin A. Hemodynamic and metabolic effects of cerebral arteriovenous malformations studied by positron emission tomography. *Stroke* 1989; 20: 890–898.
139. Serbinenko FA. Six hundred endovascular neurosurgical procedures in vascular pathology. A ten–year experience. *Acta Neurochir Suppl* 1979; 28: 310–311.
140. Bank WO, Kerber CW, Cromwell LD. Treatment of intracerebral arteriovenous malformations with isobutyl 2–cyanoacrylate. Initial clinical experience. *Radiology* 1981; 139: 609–616.
141. Berenstein AB, Choi IS, Rupersmith MT, Flamm E, Kricheff II, Madrid MM. Complications of endovascular embolization in 202 patients with cerebral arteriovenous malformations. *AJNR* 1989; 10: 876.
142. Berenstein A, Kricheff II. Catheter and material selection for transarterial embolization: technical considerations. Part I. Catheters. *Radiology* 1979; 132: 619–630.
143. Berenstein A, Kricheff II. Catheter and material selection for transarterial embolization: Part II. Materials. *Radiology* 1979; 132:631–639.
144. Debrun G, Vinuela F, Fox AJ, Drake CG. Embolization of cerebral arteriovenous malformations with bucrylate. *J Neurosurg* 1982; 56:615–627.
145. Fournier D, TerBrugge KG, Willinsky R, Lasjaunias P, Montanera W. Endovascular treatment of intracerebral arteriovenous malformations: experience in 49 cases. *J Neurosurg* 1991; 75:228–233.
146. Hilal SK, Khandji AJ, Chi LT, Stein BM, Bello JA, Silver AJ. Synthetic fiber–coated platinum coils successfully used for the endovascular treatment of arteriovenous malformations, aneurysms and direct arteriovenous fistulas of the CNS. *AJNR* 1988; 9:1030.
147. Picard L, Moret J, Lepoire J. Endovascular treatment of intracerebral arteriovenous angiomas. Techniques, indications, and results. *J Neuroradiol* 1984; 11:9–28.

148. Purdy PD, Samson D, Batjer HH, Risser RC. Preoperative embolization of cerebral arteriovenous malformations with polyvinyl alcohol particles: experience in 15 adults. *AJNR* 1990; 11: 501–510.
149. Scialfa G, Scotti G. Superselective injection of polyvinyl alcohol microemboli for the treatment of cerebral arteriovenous malformations. *AJNR* 1985; 957–960.
150. Vinuela F, Dion JE, Duckwiler G, Martin NA, Lylyk P, Fox A, Pelz D, Drake CG, Girvin JJ, Debrun G. Combined endovascular embolization and surgery in the management of cerebral arteriovenous malformations: experience with 101 cases. *J Neurosurg* 1991; 75: 856–864.
151. Morgan MK, Sundt TM Jr. The case against staged operative resection of cerebral arteriovenous malformations. *Neurosurgery* 1989; 25: 429–436.
152. Sundt TM Jr. Operative techniques for arteriovenous malformations of the brain. In: Barrow DL, (ed). Intracranial Vascular Malformations: Neurosurgical Topics. Park Ridge, Ill: American Association of Neurological Surgeons; 1990: 111–124.
153. Drake CG. Considerations for and experience with surgical treatment in 166 cases. *Clin Neurosurg* 1979; 26: 145–206.
154. Nornes H, Ludar T, Wikeby P. Cerebral arteriovenous malformations. Results of microsurgical management. *Acta Neurochir* 1979; 50: 243–257.
155. Olivecrona H, Ladenheim J. Congenital Arteriovenous Aneurysms of the Carotid and Vertebral Arterial Systems. Berlin: Springer-Verlag, 1957.
156. Parkinson D, Bacher G. Arteriovenous malformations: summary of 100 consecutive supratentorial cases. *J Neurosurg* 1980; 53: 285–299.
157. Perret G, Nishioka H. Arteriovenous malformations. An analysis of 545 cases of craniocerebral arteriovenous malformations and fistulae reported to the cooperative study. *J Neurosurg* 1966; 25: 467–490.
158. Suzuki J, Onuma T, Kayama T. Surgical treatment of intracranial arteriovenous malformation. *Neurological Res* 1982; 4: 191–207.
159. Wilson CB, U HS, Dominique J. Microsurgical treatment of intracranial vascular malformations. *J Neurosurg* 1979; 51: 446–454.
160. Paterson JH, McKissock WA. A clinical survey of intracranial angiomas with special reference to their mode of progression and surgical treatment. A report of 110 cases. *Brain* 1956; 79: 233–266.
161. Shi YQ, Chen XC. A proposed scheme for grading intracranial arteriovenous malformations. *J Neurosurg* 1986; 65: 484–489.
162. Luessenhop AJ, Ferraz FM, Rosa L. Estimate of the incidence and importance of circulatory breakthrough in the surgery of cerebral arteriovenous malformations. *Neurol Res* 1982; 4: 177–190.
163. Spetzler RF, Wilson CB, Weinstein P, Mehdorn M, Townsend J, Telles D. Normal perfusion pressure breakthrough theory. *Clin Neurosurg* 1978; 25: 651–672.
164. Gowers WR. A Manual of Disease of the Nervous System. Philadelphia: P. Blakiston, 1888: 764–773.
165. Aoki N, Mizutani H. Arteriovenous malformation in the territory of the occluded middle cerebral artery with massive intraoperative brain swelling. Case report. *Neurosurgery* 1985; 16: 660–662.

166. Batjer HH, Devous MD Sr, Seibert GB, Purdy PD, Bonte FJ. Intracranial arteriovenous malformation: relationship between clinical factors and surgical complications. *Neurosurgery* 1989; 24: 75–79.
167. Batjer HH, Purdy PD, Giller CA, Samson DS: evidence of redistribution of cerebral blood flow during treatment for an intracranial arteriovenous malformation. *Neurosurgery* 1989; 25: 599–605.
168. Bonnal J, Born JD, Hans P. One–stage excision of high–flow arteriovenous malformations. *J Neurosurg* 1985; 62: 128–131.
169. Day AL, Friedman WA, Sypert GW, Mickle P. Successful treatment of the normal perfusion pressure breakthrough syndrome. *Neurosurgery* 1982; 11: 625–630.
170. Doberstein C, Martin NA, Hawkins R, Vinuela F, Thomas K, Zane C, Becker DP. Assessment of cerebral autoregulation in patients with arteriovenous malformations. *J Cerebral blood flow metabolism II* 1991; Suppl 2: S 47.
171. Morgan MK, Johnston IH, Sundt TM Jr. Normal perfusion pressure breakthrough complicating surgery for the vein of Galen malformation: report of three cases. *Neurosurgery* 1989; 24: 406–436.
172. Morgan MK, Sundt TM Jr, Houser OW. Arterio–inferior sagittal sinus fistula: case report. *Neurosurgery* 1989; 25: 971–975.
173. Mullan S, Brown FD, Patronas MJ. Hyperemic and ischemic problems of surgical treatment of arteriovenous malformations. *J Neurosurg* 1979; 51: 757–764.
174. U HS. Microsurgical excision of paraventricular arteriovenous malformations. *Neurosurgery* 1985; 16: 293–303.
175. Yamada K, Hayakawa T, Yashimine T, Nakao K, Ushio Y, Mogami H. Surgery of high–flow arteriovenous malformation. With special reference to normal perfusion pressure breakthrough phenomenon. *No Shinkei Geka* 1986; 14: 741–748.
176. Andrews BT, Wilson CB. Staged treatment of arteriovenous malformations of the brain. *Neurosurgery* 1987; 21: 314–323.
177. Malis LI. Arteriovenous malformations of the brain, in Youmans JR (ed). Neurologic Surgery. Vol 3. Philadelphia: WB Saunders, 1982; 1786–1806.
178. Parkinson D. Staged treatment of arteriovenous malformations. *J Neurosurg* 1988; 68: 658–659.
179. Morgan MK, Johnston I, Besser M, Baines D. Cerebral arteriovenous malformation, steal, and the hypertensive breakthrough threshold. An experimental study in rats. *J Neurosurg* 1987; 66: 563–567.
180. Morgan MK, Anderson RE, Sundt TM Jr. The effects of hyperventilation on cerebral blood flow in the rat with an open and closed carotid–jugular fistula. *Neurosurgery* 1989; 25: 606–612.
181. Morgan MK, Anderson RE, Sundt TM Jr. A model of the pathophysiology of cerebral arteriovenous malformations by a carotid–jugular fistula in the rat. *Brain Research* 1989; 496: 241–250.
182. Sakaki T, Tsujimoto S, Nishitani M, Ishida Y, Morimoto T. Perfusion pressure breakthrough threshold of cerebral autoregulation in the clinically ischemic brain: an experimental study in cats. *J Neurosurg* 1992; 76: 478–485.
183. Bernstein M, Fleming JFR, Deck JHN. Cerebral hyperperfusion after carotid endarterectomy. A cause of cerebral haemorrhage. *Neurosurgery* 1984; 15: 50–56.

184. Piepgras DG, Morgan MK, Sundt TM Jr, Yanagihara T, Mussman LM. Intracerebral hemorrhage after carotid endarterectomy. *J Neurosurg* 1988; 68: 532–536.
185. Schroeder T, Sillesen H, Sorensen O, Engell HC. Cerebral hyperperfusion following carotid endarterectomy. *J Neurosurg* 1987; 66: 824–829.
186. Solomon RA, Loftus CM, Quest DO, Correll JW. Incidence and etiology of intracerebral hemorrhage following carotid endarterectomy. *J Neurosurg* 1986; 64: 29–34.
187. Sundt TM Jr, Sharbrough FW, Piepgras DG, Kearns TP, Messick JM, O'Fallon WM. Correlation of cerebral blood flow and electroencephalographic changes during carotid endarterectomy. With results of surgery hemodynamics of cerebral ischaemia. *Mayo Clin Proc* 1981; 56: 533–543.
188. Al-Rodhan NRF, Sundt TM Jr, Piepgras DG, Nichols DA, Rufenacht D, Stevens LN. Occlusive hyperemia: a theory for the hemodynamic complications following resection of intracerebral arteriovenous malformations. *J Neurosurg* 1993; 78: 167–175.
189. Ferguson GG. Physical factors in the initiation, growth and rupture of human intracranial saccular aneurysms. *J Neurosurg* 1972; 37: 666–677.
190. Miyasaka Y, Yada K, Ohwada T, Kitahara T, Kurata A, Irikura K. An analysis of the venous drainage system as a factor in haemorrhage from arteriovenous malformations. *J Neurosurg* 1992; 76: 239–243.
191. Garretson HD. Intracranial arteriovenous malformations. In: Wilkins RH, Rengachary SS (eds). *Neurosurgery* New York:McGraw-Hill, 1985; 1448–1458.
192. Girvin JP, Fox AJ, Vinuela F, Drake CG. Intraoperative embolization of cerebral arteriovenous malformations in the awake patient. *Clin Neurosurg* 1984; 31: 188–247.
193. Pertuiset B, Ancri D, Kinuta Y, Haisa T, Bordi L, Lin C, Mahdi M, Arthuis F. Classification of supratentorial arteriovenous malformations. A score system for evaluation of operability and surgical strategy based on an analysis of 66 cases. *Acta Neurochir* 1991; 110: 6–16.
194. Luessenhop AJ. AVM grading in assessing surgical risk. *J Neurosurg* 1987; 66: 637.
195. Lecksell L. The stereotactic method of radiosurgery of the brain. *Acta Chir Scand* 1951; 102: 316–319.
196. Colombo F, Benedetti A, Pozza F, Marchetti C, Chierego G. Linear acceleration radiosurgery of cerebral arteriovenous malformations. *Neurosurgery* 1989; 24: 833–840.
197. Kjellberg RN. Proton beam and radio–surgery. Toronto Stroke Workshop. Toronto, Ontario, Sep 14–16, 1988.
198. Guidetti B, Delitala A. Intracranial arteriovenous malformations. Conservative and surgical treatment. *J Neurosurg* 1980; 53: 149–152.
199. Heros RC, Tu TK. Is surgical therapy needed for unruptured arteriovenous malformations? *Neurology* 1987; 137: 279–286.
200. Jane JA, Kassell NF, Torner JC, Winn HR. The natural history of aneurysms and arteriovenous malformations. *J Neurosurg* 1985; 62: 321–323.
201. Locksley MB. Report on the cooperative study of intracranial aneurysms and subarachnoid haemorrhage. Section V, Part I. Natural history of subarachnoid haemorrhage, intracranial aneurysms and arterial malformations. Based on 6368 cases in the cooperative study. *J Neurosurg* 1966; 25: 219–239.

202. Porter AJ, Bull J. Some aspects of the natural history of cerebral arteriovenous malformation. *Brit J Radiol* 1969; 42: 667–675.
203. Svien HJ, McRae JA. Arteriovenous anomalies of the brain: fate of patients not having definite surgery. *J Neurosurg* 1965; 23: 23–28.
204. Robinson JL, Hall CJ, Sedzimir CB. Subarachnoid hemorrhage in pregnancy. *J Neurosurg* 1972; 36: 27–33.
205. Amias AG. Cerebral vascular disease in pregnancy. I. Haemorrhage. *J Obstet Gynecol Br Commonwealth* 1970; 77: 100–120.
206. Robinson JL, Hall CJ, Sedzimir CB. Arteriovenous malformations, aneurysms, and pregnancy. *J Neurosurg* 1974; 41: 63–70.
207. Horton JC, Chambers WA, Lyons SL, Adams RD, Kjellberg RN: Pregnancy and the risk of hemorrhage from cerebral arteriovenous malformations. *Neurosurgery* 1990; 27: 867–872.
208. Dias MS, Sekhar LN. Intracranial haemorrhage from aneurysms and arteriovenous malformations during pregnancy and puerperium. *Neurosurgery* 1990; 27: 855–866.
209. Hanson JW, Smith DW. The fetal hydantoin syndrome. *J Pediatr* 1975; 87: 285–290.
210. Janz D. The teratogenic risk of anti epileptic drugs. *Epilepsia* 1975; 16: 159–169.
211. Montouris GD, Fenichel GM, McLain LW. The pregnant epileptic: a review and recommendations. *Arch Neurol* 1979; 36: 601–603.
212. Segal S, Anyan WR, Cohen SN, Freeman J, Hill RM, Kauffman RE, Pruitt AW, Shinefeld HR, Vickers SM. Anticonvulsants and pregnancy (American Academy of Pediatrics Committee on Drugs). *Pediatrics* 1979; 63: 331–333.
213. Zakai EH, Mellman WJ, Neiderer B, Hanson JW. The fetal trimethadione syndrome. *J Pediatr* 1975; 87: 280–284.
214. Bruns PD, Linder RO, Drose VE, Battaglia F. The placental transfer of water from fetus to mother following intravenous infusion of hypertonic mannitol to the maternal rabbit. *Am J Obstet Gynecol* 1963; 86:160–166.
215. McDowell DG, Keaney NP, Turner JM, Lane JR, Okuda Y. The toxicity of sodium nitroprusside. *Br J Anaesth* 1974; 46: 327–332.
216. Naulty J, Cefalo RC, Lewis PE. Fetal toxicity of nitroprusside in the pregnant ewe. *Am J Obstet Gynaecol* 1981; 139: 708–711.
217. Rosen MA. Cerebrovascular lesions and tumors in the pregnancy patient. In: Newfield P, Cottrell JE, (eds). Handbook of Neuroanesthesia: Clinical and Physiologic Essentials. Boston:Little, Brown, 1983: 227–244.
218. Cronquist S, Troupp H. Intracerebral arteriovenous malformation and arterial aneurysm in the same patients. *Acta Neurol Scand* 1966; 42: 307–316.
219. Okamoto S, Handa H, Hashimoto N. Location of intracranial aneurysms associated with cerebral arteriovenous malformation. Statistical Analysis. *Surg Neurol* 1984; 22: 335–340.
220. Suzuki J, Onuma T. Intracranial aneurysm associated with arteriovenous malformations. *J Neurosurg* 1979; 50: 742–746.
221. Atkinson JLD, Sundt TM Jr, Houser OW, Whisnant JP. Angiographic frequency of anterior circulation intracranial aneurysms. *J Neurosurg* 1989; 70: 551–555.

222. Anderson RM, Blackwood W. The association of arteriovenous angioma and saccular aneurysm of the arteries of the brain. *J Path Bact* 1959; 77: 101–110.
223. Arai H, Sugiyama Y, Kawakami S, Miyazawa N. Multiple intracranial aneurysms and vascular malformations in an infant. Case report. *J Neurosurg* 1972; 37: 357–360.
224. Arieta S, Gray EW. Progressive multiform angiosis. Association of a cerebral angioma, aneurysm and other vascular changes in the brain. *Arch Neurol Psych* 1944; 51: 182–189.
225. Batjer HH, Suss RA, Samson D. Intracranial arteriovenous malformations associated with aneurysms. *Neurosurgery* 1986; 18: 29–35.
226. Boyd-Wilson JS. The association of cerebral angiomas with intracranial aneurysms. *J Neurol Neurosurg Psychiatry* 1959; 22: 218–223.
227. Caram PC. Simultaneous occurrence of intracranial aneurysm and angioma. Case report. *J Neurosurg* 1959; 16: 230–232.
228. Fine R, Paterson A, Steven L, Gaylor JB. Simultaneous occurrence of intracranial aneurysm and arteriovenous malformation. *Brit Med J* 1960; 112: 711–712.
229. Gacs G, Vinuela F, Fox AJ, Drake CG. Peripheral aneurysms of the cerebellar arteries. Review of 16 cases. *J Neurosurg* 1983; 58: 63–68.
230. Garza-Mercade R, Rangel RA, Garza-Vasquez JF. Coexistence of bilateral aneurysms of the internal carotid arteries and an arteriovenous malformation of the left frontal lobe. *Surg Neurol* 1984; 21: 267–271.
231. Gibson RM, Rocha Melo AN. Angiographic finding of an aneurysm and arteriovenous malformation in the posterior cranial fossa in a case of subarachnoid hemorrhage. *J Neurol Neurosurg Psychiat* 1960; 23: 237–238.
232. Hayashi S, Arimoto T, Itakuru T, Fujii T, Nishiguchi T, Komai N. The association of intracranial aneurysm and arteriovenous malformations of the brain. Case report. *J Neurosurg* 1981; 55: 971–975.
233. Higashi K, Hatano M, Yamashita T, Inove S, Matsumura T. Coexistence of posterior inferior cerebellar artery aneurysm and arteriovenous malformation fed by the same artery. *Surg Neurol* 1979; 12: 405–408.
234. Kikuchi K, Kowada M, Yoneya M. Association of arteriovenous malformation and intracranial aneurysm in the posterior fossa. *Surg Neurol* 1984; 22: 499–502.
235. Koulouris S, Rizzoli HV. Coexisting intracranial aneurysm and arteriovenous malformation. Case report. *Neurosurg* 1981; 8: 219–222.
236. Mabuchi S, Kamiyama H, Abe H. Distal aneurysm of the superior cerebellar artery and posterior inferior cerebellar artery feeding an associated arteriovenous malformation. Case report. *Neurosurgery* 1992; 30: 284–287.
237. Miyasaka K, Wolpert SM, Prager RJ. The association of cerebral aneurysm infundibula, and intracranial arteriovenous malformations. *Stroke* 1982; 13: 196–203.
238. Nehls DG, Carter LP. Multiple unusual aneurysms and arteriovenous malformation in a single patient. A case report. Part I. *Neurosurgery* 1985; 17: 97–100.
239. Shenkin HA, Jenkins F, Kim K. Arteriovenous anomaly of the brain associated with cerebral aneurysm. Case report. *J Neurosurg* 1971; 34: 225–228.
240. Voigt K, Beck U, Reinshagen G. A complex cerebral vascular malformation studied

by angiography: multiple aneurysms, angiomas and arterial ectasia. *Neuroradiology* 1973; 5: 117–123.

241. Waga S, Itoh H, Kojima T. Posterior inferior cerebellar artery aneurysm associated with arteriovenous malformation fed by the same artery. *Surg Neurol* 1985; 23: 617–620.
242. Hashimoto N, Handa H, Nagata I, Hazama F. Experimentally induced cerebral aneurysms in rats. Part V. Relation of hemodynamic consequences in the Circle of Willis to formation of aneurysms. *Surg Neurol* 1980; 13: 41–45.
243. Ferguson GG. Turbulence in human intracranial saccular aneurysms. *J Neurosurg* 1970; 33: 485–497.
244. Stehbens WE. Etiology of intracranial berry aneurysms. *J Neurosurg* 1981; 70: 823–831.
245. Guglielmi G, Vinuela F, Dion J, Duckwiler G. Electrothrombosis of saccular aneurysm via endovascular approach. *J Neurosurg* 1991; 75: 8–14.
246. Sachs E. The Diagnosis and Treatment of Brain Tumours. London:Kimpton.
247. Di Chiro G, Doppman JL, Ommaya AK. Selective arteriography of arteriovenous aneurysms of spinal cord. *Radiology* 1967; 88: 1065–1077.
248. Logue V, Aminoff MJ, Kendall BE. Results of surgical treatment for patients with a spinal angioma. *J Neurol Neurosurg Psychiatry* 1974; 37: 1074–1081.
249. Merland, JJ, Riche MC, Chirac J. Intraspinal extrameduulary arteriovenous fistulae draining into the medullary veins. *J Neuroradiol* 1980; 7: 271–320.
250. Oldfield EH, DiChiro G, Quindlen EA, Reith KG, Doppman JL. Successful treatment of a group of spinal cord arteriovenous malformations by interruption of dural fistula. *J Neurosurg* 1983; 59: 1019–1030.
251. Symon L, Kuyama H, Kendall B. Dural arteriovenous malformations of the spine. Clinical features and surgical results in 55 cases. *J Neurosurg* 1984; 60: 238–247.
252. Elsberg CA. Diagnosis and Treatment of Surgical Diseases of the Spinal Cord and its Membranes. Philadelphia: WB Saunders, 1916: 194–204.
253. Travers B. A case of aneurysm of anastomosis in the orbit, by ligation of the common carotid artery. *Med Clin Tr* 1811; 2: 1–16.
254. Fontaine R, Dany A, Briot B. Fistules arterio–veineuses posttraumatiques de la region parieto–occipitale droite du crane et de la dure–mere sous–jacente. Role probable des canaux derivatifs du type Sucquet. *Neurochir* 1957; 3: 30–39.
255. Debrun G, Chartres A. Infra and supratentorial arteriovenous malformations. A general review about 2 cases of spontaneous supratentorial arteriovenous malformation of the dura. *Neuroradiology* 1972; 3: 184–192.
256. Kosnik EJ, Hunt WE, Miller CA. Dural arteriovenous malformations. *J Neurosurg* 1974; 40: 322–326.
257. Laine E, Galibert P, Lopez C, Delahousse J, Delandtsheer JM, Christiaens JL. Anevrysmes arterio–veineux intra–duraux (developpes dans l'epaisseur de la dure-mere) de la fosse posterieure. *Neurochirurgie* 1963; 9: 147–158.
258. Sundt TM Jr, Piepgras DG. The surgical approach to arteriovenous malformations of the lateral and sigmoid dural sinuses. *J Neurosurg* 1983; 59: 32–39.
259. Bitoh S, Sakaki S. Spontaneous cure of dural arteriovenous malformation in the posterior fossa. *Surg Neurol* 1979; 12: 111–114.

260. Hansen JH, Sogaard I. Spontaneous regression of an extra– and intracranial arteriovenous malformation. Case report. *J Neurosurg* 1976; 45: 338–341.
261. Magidson MA, Weinberg PE. Spontaneous closure of a dural arteriovenous malformation. *Surg Neurol* 1976; 6: 107–110.
262. Olutola PS, Eliam M, Molot M, et al. Spontaneous regression of a dural arteriovenous malformation. *Neurosurgery* 1983; 12: 687–690.
263. Debrun GM. Embolization techniques in the treatment of vascular lesions involving the cavernous sinus. In: Dolenc VV (ed). The Cavernous Sinus. A Multidisciplinary Approach to Vascular and Tumorous Lesions New York: Springer, 1987: 173–181.
264. Harders A, Gilsbach J, Hassler W. Dural AV malformation of the lateral and sigmoid sinuses as possible cause of trigeminal neuralgia: a case report. *Acta Neurochir* 1982; 66: 95–102.
265. Gaensler EHL, Jackson DE Jr, Hallbach VV. Arteriovenous fistulas of the cervico—medullary junction as a cause of myelopathy: radiographic findings in two cases. *AJNR* 1990; 11: 518–521.
266. Vinuela F, Fox AJ, Pelz DM, Drake CG. Unusual clinical manifestations of dural arteriovenous malformations. *J Neurosurg* 1986; 64: 554–558.
267. Willinsky R, TerBrugge K, Lasjaunias P, Montanera W. The variable presentation of craniocervical and cervical dural arteriovenous malformations. *Surg Neurol* 1990; 34: 118–123.
268. Wrobel CJ, Oldfield EH, Di Chiro G, Tarlov EC, Baker RA, Doppman JL. Myelopathy due to intracranial dural arteriovenous fistulas draining intrathecally into spinal medullar veins. *J Neurosurg* 1988; 69: 934–939.
269. Hurst RW, Hackney DB, Goldberg HI, Davis RA. Reversible arteriovenous malformation–induced hypertension as a cause of neurological deficits. *Neurosurgery* 1992; 30: 422–425.
270. Martin NA, King WA, Wilson CB, Nutik S, Carter LP, Spetzler RF. Management of dural arteriovenous malformations of the anterior cranial fossa. *J Neurosurg* 1990; 72: 692–697.
271. Morimoto T, Yoshida S, Basugi N. Dural arteriovenous malformation in the cervical spine presenting with subarachnoid hemorrhage: case report. *Neurosurgery* 1992; 31: 118–121.
272. Awad IA, Little JR, Akrawi WP, et al. Intracranial dural arteriovenous malformations: Factors predisposing to an aggressive neurologic course. *J Neurosurg* 1990; 72: 839–850.
273. Enker SH. Progression of a dural arteriovenous malformation resulting in an intracerebral hematoma: a case report. *Angiology* 1979; 30: 198–204.
274. Grady MS, Pobereskin L. Arteriovenous malformations of the dura mater. *Surg Neurol* 1987; 28: 135–140.
275. Grisoli F, Vincentelli F, Fuchs S, et al. Surgical treatment of tentorial arteriovenous malformations draining into the subarachnoid space. *J Neurosurg* 1984; 60: 1059–1066.
276. Malik GM, Pearce JE, Ausman JI, et al. Dural arteriovenous malformations and intracranial hemorrhage. *Neurosurgery* 1984; 15: 332–339.

277. Dolenc VV. *Anatomy and Surgery of the Cavernous Sinus*. New York: Springer, 1989.
278. Logue V. Angiomas of the spinal cord: review of the pathogenesis, clinical features, and results of surgery. *J Neurol Neurosurg Psych* 1979; 42: 1–11.
279. Morgan MK, Marsh WR. Management of spinal dural arteriovenous malformations. *J Neurosurg* 1989; 70: 832–836.
280. Rosenblum B, Oldfield EH, Doppman JL, DiChiro G. Spinal arteriovenous malformations: a comparison of dural arteriovenous fistulas and intradural AVM's in 81 patients. *J Neurosurg* 1987; 67: 795–802.
281. Yasargil MG, Symon L, Teddy PJ. Arteriovenous malformations of the spinal cord. *Advanced Tech Standards Neurosurg* 1984; 11: 61–102.
282. Morgan MK, Chaseling R, Johnston I, De Silva M. Spinal arteriovenous malformation presenting at birth. Case report. *Neurosurgery* 1986; 19: 637–640.
283. Garcia JH, Williams JP, Tanaka J. Spontaneous thrombosis of deep veins: a complication of arteriovenous malformation. *Stroke* 1975; 6: 164–171.
284. Gomez MR, Whiten CF, Nolke A, Bernstein J, Meyer JS. Aneurysmal malformation of the great vein of Galen, causing heart failure in early infancy: report of five cases. *Pediatrics* 1963; 31: 400–411.
285. Solomon RA, Michelsen WJ. Defective cerebrovascular autoregulation in regions proximal to arteriovenous malformation of the brain. A case report and topic review. *Neurosurgery* 1984; 14: 78–82.

16

Stereotactic Radiosurgery for the Treatment of Arteriovenous Malformation

Robert J. Coffey
Mayo Clinic, Rochester, Minnesota

I. INTRODUCTION

Barely a dozen years ago, stereotactic neurosurgery and radiosurgery in particular were practiced at only a few centers scattered throughout the world. More recently interest in stereotactic techniques, including radiosurgery, has led to an exponential growth in the number of neurosurgical centers equipped to perform radiosurgery and to a similar increase in the number of patients being treated for a variety of intracranial disorders [1]. The first few patients with small intracranial arteriovenous malformations (AVMs) were treated by Leksell, Steiner, and colleagues, using Gamma Unit I in Stockholm, Sweden, over 25 years ago [2–4]. By now, the quantity of AVM patients that have been treated using a variety of radiosurgical devices numbers in the tens of thousands. Instrumentation used to perform radiosurgery on AVMs includes the Leksell Cobalt-60 gamma unit, or "Gamma Knife" (both the Model-U and the newer Model-B now available in the United States), various linear-accelerator-based systems (LINAC radiosurgery), and a few charged particle beam units (protons, helium ions) [2,3,5–15]. As of this writing the author believes that radiosurgery is now the most commonly used treatment for AVMs in the industrialized world. Recent advances in neuroimaging and computer technology have increased the speed, safety, and possibly the efficacy of radiosurgery. Current data suggest that earlier notions regarding the size of AVMs that could be treated and the types of patients who should be treated need to be broadened.

To investigate the role of clinical factors such as AVM size and location, and radiation dose on patient outcome, we studied 121 consecutive patients with parenchymal cerebral AVMs treated over a four-year period (1990–1993) using the Leksell Gamma Unit at the Mayo Clinic in Rochester, Minnesota (Figure 1). The results of early followup in this patient cohort were published in 1995. Although our group has treated hundreds more patients since then, the author believes that a more thorough and longer term analysis of this initial patient series is the most informative approach to the topic.

II. PATIENT POPULATION AND CHARACTERISTICS OF AVMS

A. Patient Population

Between January, 1990 and December 1993 we treated 121 consecutive patients believed to have parenchymal cerebral AVMs using the Leksell Gamma Knife and we reported the early results in a series of articles [16,17]. Patients with

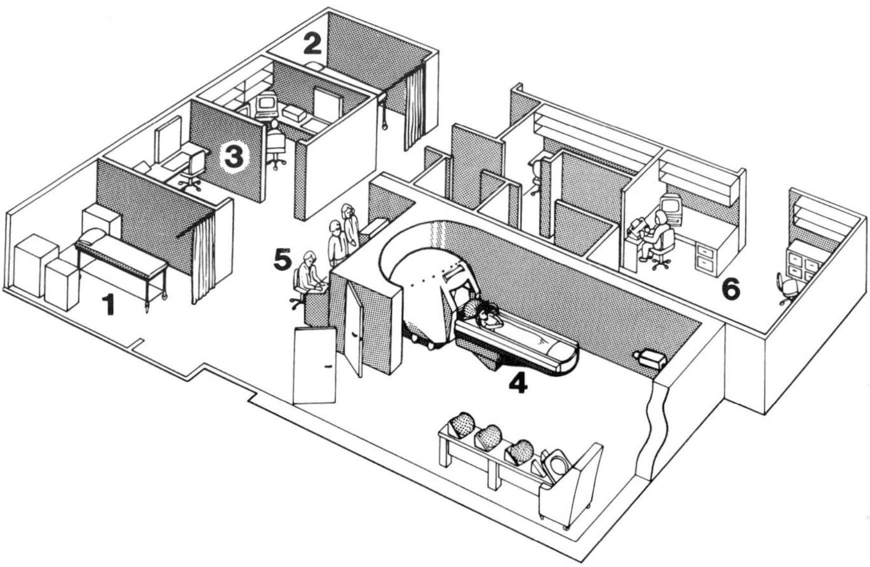

Figure 1 The Gamma Knife facility at the Mayo Clinic, Rochester, MN. 1. Headframe application area, 2. patient holding area, 3. dose planning and radiation physics workstation, 4. gamma unit treatment room, 5. control console and monitors, 6. administrative office and patient records. In 1997 the Model U was replaced with the newer Model B unit.

dural AVMs (dural arteriovenous fistulae) and angiographically occult vascular malformations (including cavernous malformations) were excluded from the analysis. The clinical characteristics of our patient population are summarized in Table 1. Seventy-five percent of the AVMs had a volume of 10 cm^3 or smaller and 25 percent had a volume greater than 10 cm^3. Fifty-three AVMs (44%) had bled at least once before treatment and most patients were ambulatory and able to care for themselves (mean Karnofsky performance rating, 86). Before referral for radiosurgery, 13 patients (11%) had undergone craniotomy either for attempted removal of the AVM (n=8), or removal of an intracerebral hematoma (n=5), or to clip an associated aneurysm (n=2). Thirteen patients underwent embolization to reduce the dimensions of the AVM prior to planned radiosurgical treatment or prior to attempted surgical resection before referral for radiosurgery. Four patients had their AVMs treated elsewhere using proton beam therapy (n=2) or gamma knife radiosurgery (n=2) between two and seven years before treatment at our institution. In one of the latter patients, obliteration of the nidus within the original treatment field had occurred; however, an additional previously obscure nidus compartment became apparent and required further treatment (Figure 2). The AVMs in the other three patients had not changed appreciably since their original pretreatment angiograms elsewhere.

Subsequent followup after our initial report revealed that another five patients had vascular malformations that were more complex than was appreciated initially and that should be excluded from the analysis of this series of ordinary parenchymal AVMs (3 vein of Galen malformations and fistulae and 2 other direct arteriovenous fistulae). Exclusion of these individuals does not alter the overall demographics of the patient population nor the angiographic or clinical results.

B. Features of AVMs Treated Using Radiosurgery

The location of the AVMs is summarized in Table 2. Although 78 malformations occupied a lobar location, most were deep within the hemispheric white matter, predominantly on the left (dominant) side. Thirty-six AVMs involved the basal ganglia, thalamus, brainstem, or cerebellum thus representing high-risk locations for open surgical excision. In fact, 46 AVMs (38%) were judged inoperable by experienced cerebrovascular surgeons because conventional surgery carried an unacceptable risk of death or severe neurologic morbidity.

The sizes of the AVMs in this series, expressed as volume (in cm^3), are listed in Table 3. Fifty patients (41%) had AVMs $\leq$ 4 cm^3, approximately equivalent to an average diameter $\leq$ 2 cm. Forty patients had AVM volumes between 4 and 10 cm^3 (average diameter between 2 and 2.7 cm). The remaining 31 patients (26%) had AVM volumes substantially larger than 10 cm^3 and had an average nidus diameter > 3 cm. Because AVM volumes increase exponentially

Table 1 Clinical Features of 121 Patients with AVMs Treated Using Radiosurgery

AVM Volume	Age (yrs)		Sex		Hemorrhage number	Headache number	Seizures number	Neurological deficit number	Karnofsky rating	
	Mean	Range	M	F					Mean	Range
≤10 cm^3 (n=90)	38	(11–78)	46	44	40 (44%)	53 (59%)	37 (44%)	34 (38%)	86	(40–100)
>10 cm^3 (n=31)	38	(3–60)	15	16	13 (42%)	24 (77%)	22 (71%)	10 (32%)	86	(50–100)
Total series (n=121)	38	(3–78)	61	60	53 (44%)	77 (64%)	59 (49%)	44 (36%)	86	(40–100)

as a factor of the radius cubed (r^3), relatively small increments in nidus dimensions lead to dramatic increments in nidus volume, especially if the lesion is roughly spherical or "solid." For irregular, tubular-shaped, or "c" shaped AVMs within the lateral ventricles or cerebral fissures, a single dimension may be large (> 5–6 cm), but the overall lesion volume may be quite manageable (on the order of 15 cm^3 or smaller). As described below, both MRI and conventional angiography are necessary to determine the dimensions, shape, and volume of the nidus in such cases.

III. OPERATIVE PROCEDURES

A. Headframe Application and Stereotactic Imaging

At first we performed radiosurgical procedures in the inpatient setting. Presently patients are admitted to the hospital early in the morning on the day of treatment. Evaluation by the neurology, neurosurgery, and radiation oncology staff is completed beforehand, as are a general medical examination, and any appropriate subspecialty consultations or diagnostic tests.

Patients with cortical or hemispheric AVMs have supratherapeutic doses of their usual anticonvulsant medication administered the evening before and morning of radiosurgery. Previously unmedicated patients are loaded with oral and/or parenteral phenytoin. Patients who have had frequent seizures also receive intravenous or oral phenobarbitol on the evening before and morning of treatment. Phenobarbital is continued for two days after treatment as additional insurance against early post-treatment seizures. Corticosteroids are *not* administered routinely before radiosurgery unless the patient is already taking such medications. No hair is shaved before or during the procedure. Unless the patient has valvular heart disease, a cardiac prosthesis, or another unusual condition, antibiotics are not administered. Patients on coumadin or other anticoagulant medication are requested to discontinue medication for two days before radiosurgery. However, this precaution is probably unnecessary, as the rare instances of scalp pin site bleeding are controlled easily by a single suture and/or direct pressure at the time of headframe removal.

With the exception of infants and very young children (below 9 years old), the vast majority of patients can undergo stereotactic headframe placement, neuroimaging procedures, and radiosurgery under local anesthesia and parenteral sedation. For more anxious adults, or those with cardiac illness, an anesthesiologist or nurse anesthetist is in attendance. Young children and demented adults may not tolerate the process of headframe application without major sedation, but they can undergo imaging procedures and treatment without difficulty. In such patients, an anesthesiologist administers a sufficient dose of an ultrashort-acting agent to make the patient unconscious, yet able to

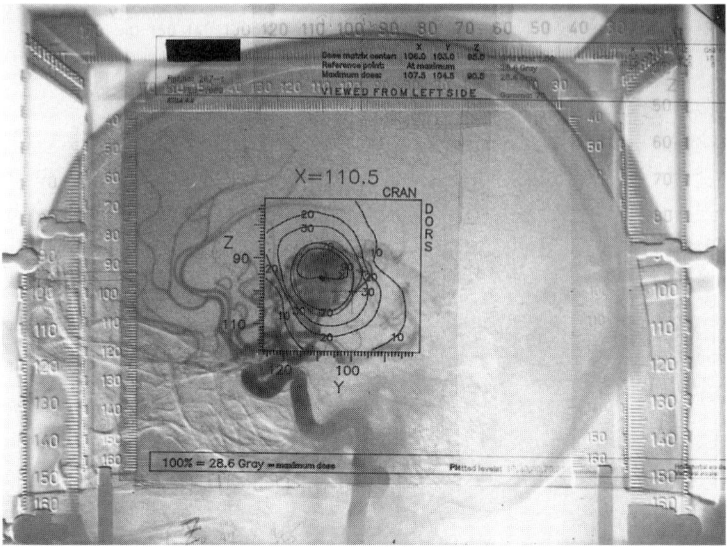

(a)

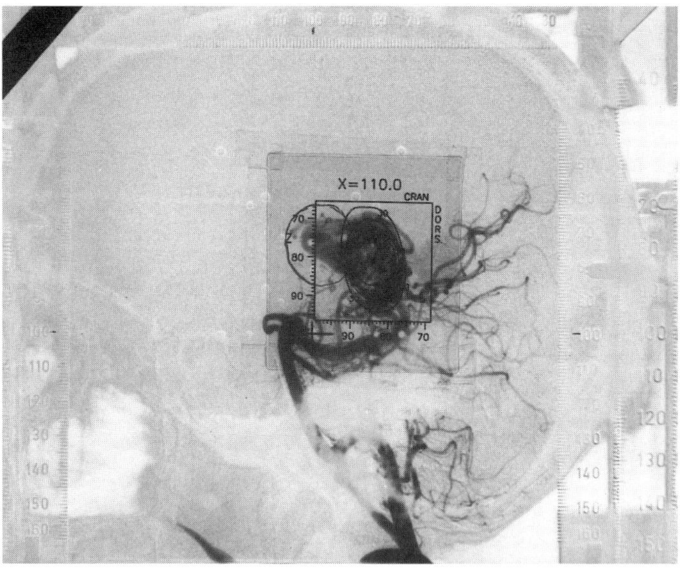

(b)

Figure 2 (a) Stereotactic left internal carotid angiogram with superimposed isodose distributions performed during initial radiosurgical treatment of a thalamic AVM that had bled repeatedly in years past. Vertebral angiography on the same date filled only the same nidus compartment. Radiosurgical dosimetry: 20 Gy at 70% isodose line using one 18-mm and one 8-mm isocenter. (b) Left vertebral stereotactic angiogram performed two years later during second radiosurgical procedure. The previously treated AVM com-

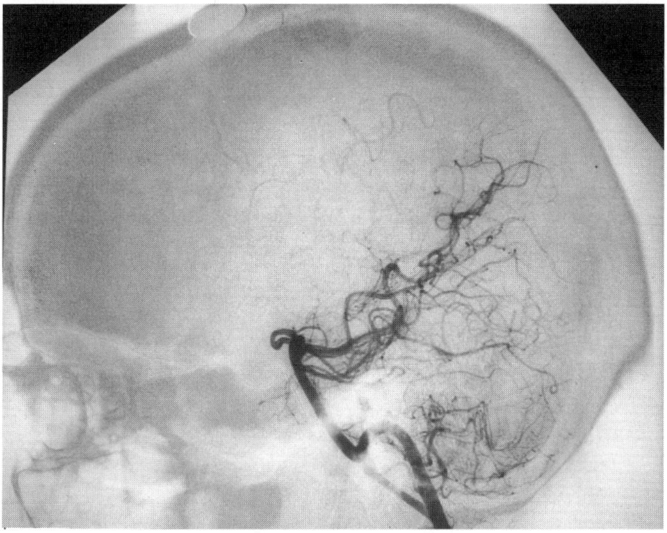

(c)

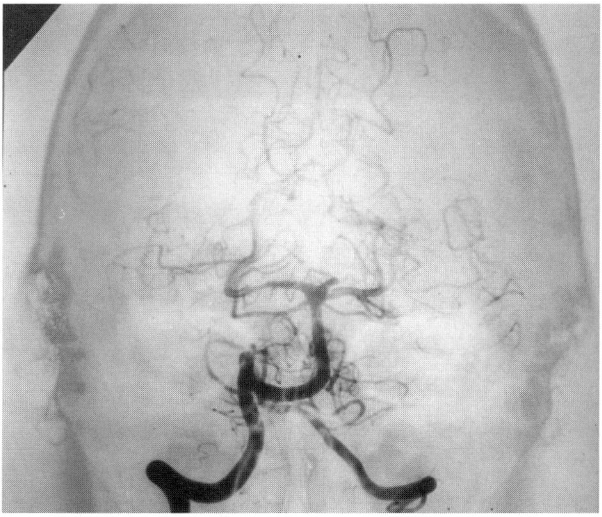

(d)

Figure 2 Continued.
partment (within the more anterior, dotted outline) had obliterated allowing a second, posteriorly located portion of the nidus to become more apparent. Radiosurgical dosimetry at second treatment: 18 Gy at 50% isodose line using a single 18-mm isocenter. (c) and (d) Follow-up lateral and AP vertebral angiogram films, respectively, two years after second radiosurgical procedure (four years after first treatment) showed complete obliteration of the AVM. The patient remained neurologically stable throughout this time period.

Table 2 Location of 121 AVMs Treated Using Radiosurgery

Location of AVM	Total series		AVM volume ≤10 cm^3		AVM volume >10 cm^3	
	Number	Percent	Number	Percent	Number	Percent
Lobar	78	64	53	59	25	81
Basal ganglia/thalamus	20	17	16	18	4	13
Corpus callosum	4	3	3	3	1	3
Ventricular	3	2	3	3	0	0
Brainstem/cerebellar	16	13	15	17	1	3
Total	121		90		31	

breathe spontaneously for the two to three minutes that it takes to apply the headframe. Once the patient awakens, mild sedation is given intermittently until the treatment is concluded and the headframe is removed.

Because each patient's head is shaped differently, because AVMs can be located anywhere in the cranial cavity, and because the range of coordinates attainable within the confines of the secondary collimator helmets of the gamma unit is limited, considerable ingenuity sometimes is required during headframe application to avoid the problem of an "unreachable" coordinate later in the case. In general, within the limits of the patient's physiognomy, the headframe is applied so as to shift the relative location of the target towards the center of the frame. After headframe placement, we record a series of skull radius measurements for input into the dose-planning computer. These measurements allow the construction of a wire frame diagram of the head in stereotactic space and form the basis for computer calculations of depth/dose to target for each of the 201 ^{60}Co sources.

Neuroimaging for radiosurgery requires the close cooperation of the radiology staff in order to generate useful data for stereotactic localization and dose

Table 3 Size (volume) of 121 AVMS Treated Using Radiosurgery

AVM Volume, cm^3	Cases Number	Percent
<1	8	6
1–4	42	35
4–10	40	33
>10	31	26

planning. Since each patient already has a known diagnosis, only an abbreviated imaging study is required. For AVMs, we employ conventional cut film angiography using photographic subtraction and a fixed magnification factor (approximately 1.35×, Figure 3A,B). An additional digital angiographic localizer is attached to the headframe over the standard one. This allows selected film images to be digitized for multimodality dose planning using the Leksell Gamma Plan system (Elekta Instruments, Atlanta, Georgia).

As part of our routine and especially for large, complex, unusually shaped, or critically situated AVMs, stereotactic MRI is utilized as an adjunct for treatment planning (Figure 3 C,D). We employ T_1 axial and coronal images, without contrast, spaced 1.5 or 3 mm apart, depending upon the size of the nidus. Direct coronal magnetic resonance images (MRI) are most useful for parasellar lesions close to the optic apparatus and for high-convexity lesions close to the calvarium. Direct network and/or magnetic tape transfer of the imaging data into the Gamma Plan computer is performed for high-speed interactive dose planning.

B. Radiosurgical Dosimetry

Treatment planning for AVMs involves definition of the lesion volume and coverage of the lesion using the optimal number and configuration of irradiation isocenters or "shots." Dose-planning computers of increasing speed and image resolution streamline the process considerably by permitting rapid review of minor dose-plan revisions almost instantaneously. However, in nearly all of our initial cases, we constructed the first dose plan manually (regardless of whether one or a dozen or more shots were involved) using scaled isodose overlays on hard copy angiogram and/or MRI films. Now, as dose planning proceeds, rapid correlation between angiography and MRI optimizes coverage of the nidus while drawing attention to sensitive structures nearby.

Selection of radiation dose to the margin of the lesion (at the 50% or greater isodose line) is based upon volume, with smaller lesions receiving the highest dose. Our current dose–volume schema is based upon a combination of predictive models, our own empirical observations, and the experience at other centers. Recently, on the basis of growing experience, we raised the dose applied to small, previously ruptured AVMs. Our current dose–volume schema is shown in Table 4. The entire dose-planning and dose-selection process, as well as the performance of actual treatment, is a cooperative effort of the neurosurgical, radiation oncology, and radiation physics team. Treatment begins once all members of the team have formally signed the computer printout of the dose plan. This document becomes a permanent part of the medical record, subject to review by the United States Nuclear Regulatory Commission. The formal dose plan lists the coordinates of each isocenter, collimator size, treat-

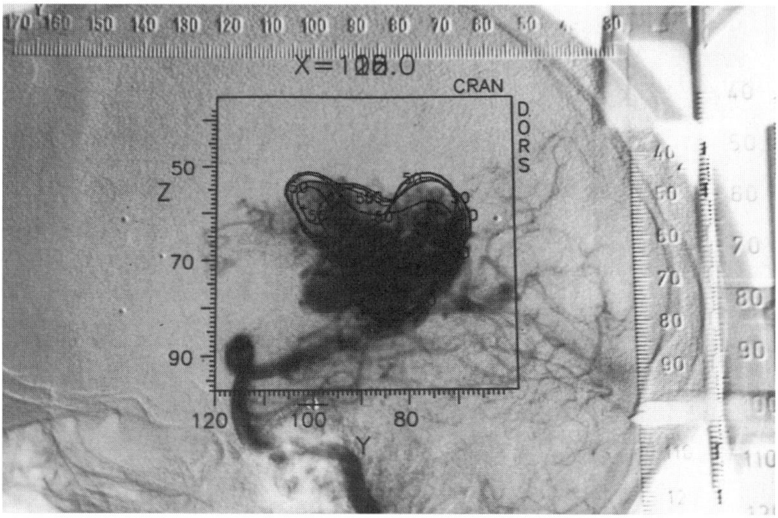

(a)

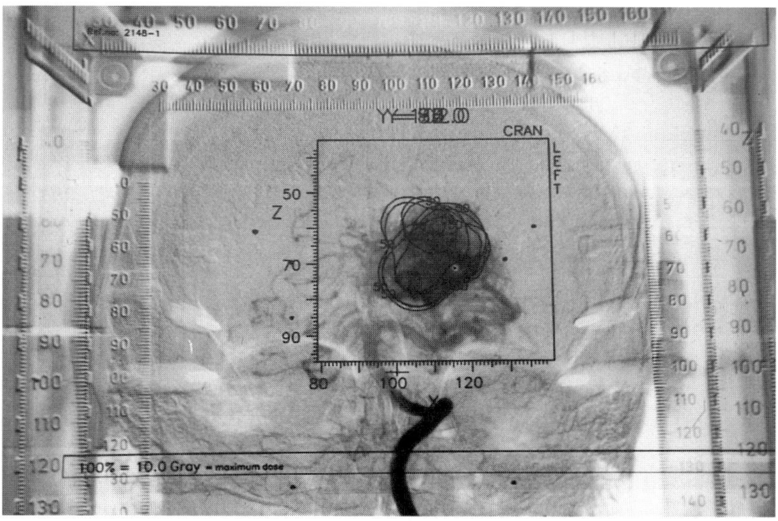

(b)

Figure 3 (a) and (b) Stereotactic angiogram films showing composite 50% isodose lines at coordinates corresponding to every irradiation isocenter used to treat a complex AVM involving the thalamus and choroidal fissure. (c) and (d) Stereotactic axial MRI series in the same patient showing coverage of the nidus and sparing of the surrounding normal brain by the dose plan. Instantaneous intercomparison between MR and angiographic images using an interactive video screen display promotes rapid optimization of the dose plan.

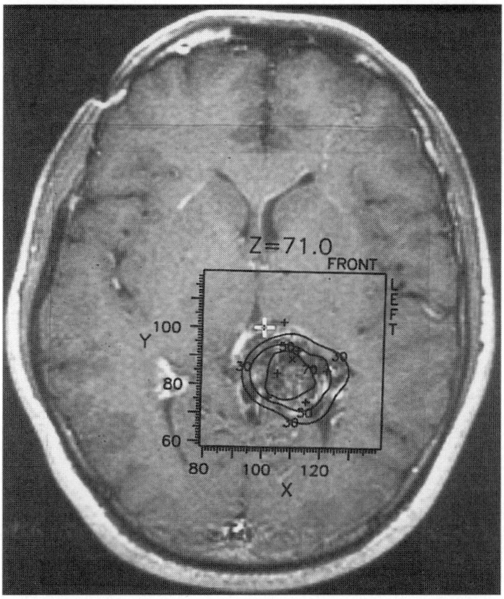

(c)

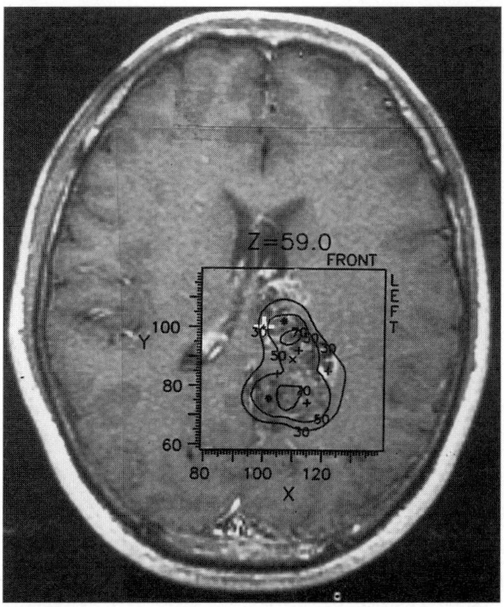

(d)

Figure 3 Continued.

Table 4 Dose–Volume Schema for AVM Radiosurgery

AVM size		
Average diameter (cm)	Volume (cm^3)	Margin dose (Gy)[a]
≤2.0	≤4.2	20
2.1–3.0	4.2–14.1	18
>3.0	>14.1	16

[a]At 50% or higher prescription isodose. Maximum prescription dose in brainstem AVMs is 18 Gy.

ment time for each shot, maximum dose, coordinate point of Dmax (maximum dose), and gamma angle (angle of the frame relative to the central beam) for each shot. During target irradiation the patient is monitored by closed-circuit television and audio monitors, pulse oximetry, and EKG. Once the final isocenter has been irradiated, the patient is removed from the treatment couch, the headframe is removed, and a turban-type head dressing is applied. Patients remain in the hospital overnight and are discharged the morning after treatment.

C. Followup Schedule and Plan

Because the therapeutic effects of radiosurgery as well as the potential neurologic complications occur in a delayed fashion in months to years, meticulous clinical and imaging followup is essential over an extended period. For patients with AVMs, MRI scans and clinical examinations are performed at six, 12, 24, and 36 months after treatment. Then, unless an obvious AVM nidus remains on MRI, cerebral angiography is performed. If the AVM is obliterated, the patient is discharged from further neurosurgical followup. In general, if any AVM nidus is still identified on the three-year study, even if it is much smaller than it was originally, repeat radiosurgical treatment is carried out, and followup continued. To date, radiosurgical retreatment of small nidus residue has been at least as effective as primary treatment. Patients are monitored carefully for potential management complications that include rebleeding during the latency period before obliteration and treatment-related neurologic deficits due to radiosurgery. Considering the size, location, arterial input, and venous drainage pattern of AVMs treated, our management outcome has been comparable to, if not better than, those of surgical series for similar lesions.

IV. CLINICAL AND IMAGING OUTCOME AFTER RADIOSURGERY

A. Clinical Followup

During clinical followup of all patients between 39 and 77 months after radiosurgery, 81 patients (67%) remained neurologically stable (Table 5). An additional 22 patients (18%) experienced neurologic improvement after treatment. For the most part, this consisted of a reduction or elimination of AVM-related seizures and/or amelioration of incapacitating vascular headaches. Overall, 85 percent of patients were stable or improved at last followup. Only five patients (4 percent) were clinically worse as a direct result of treatment. One such patient had a large AVM (30.1 cm^3) that involved the left basal ganglia and thalamus and was fed by anterior and posterior circulation vessels (Figure 4). Complete obliteration of the nidus occurred 34 months after treatment and was accompanied by the appearance of a left homonymous visual-field deficit. This was not disabling to the patient and, given the size and location of the lesion, was felt to be an acceptable clinical result.

Six patients with previously unruptured AVMs experienced nonfatal hemorrhages. In one such case, the patient had an AVM in the left temporal lobe and sylvian fissure with deep venous drainage. A routine MRI scan 18 months after treatment showed near-total obliteration of the nidus. The AVM ruptured 21 months after treatment, causing intraventricular hemorrhage but no permanent neurologic deficit. Complete cerebral angiography performed on the day of hemorrhage and repeated six weeks later showed no evidence of the nidus that, presumably, had bled during the final stages of obliteration. This case illustrates that some finite risk of hemorrhage persists until complete obliteration occurs.

Two patients with small, deep, previously ruptured AVMs died of rebleeding and one patient with a deep, previously unruptured AVM died between three and nine months after radiosurgery. In retrospect, radiosurgery still was

Table 5 Clinical Condition of 121 Patients with Cerebral AVMs Treated Using Radiosurgery

	Number	Percent
Improved	22	18.2
Stable	81	67
Permanent deficit	5	4
Fatal hemorrhage	3	2.5
Nonfatal hemorrhage	6	5
Death, other cause	4	3.3

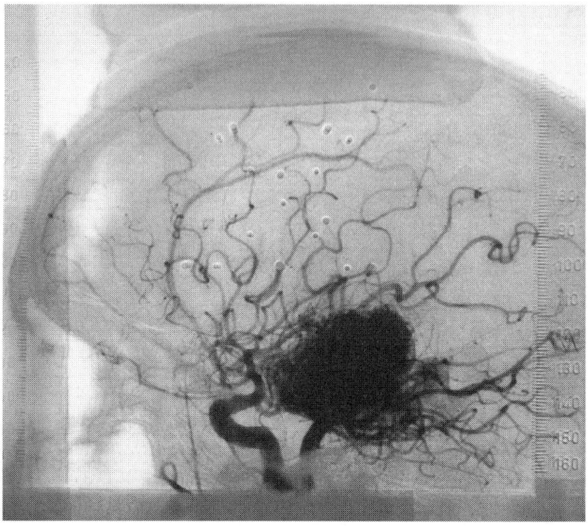

(a)

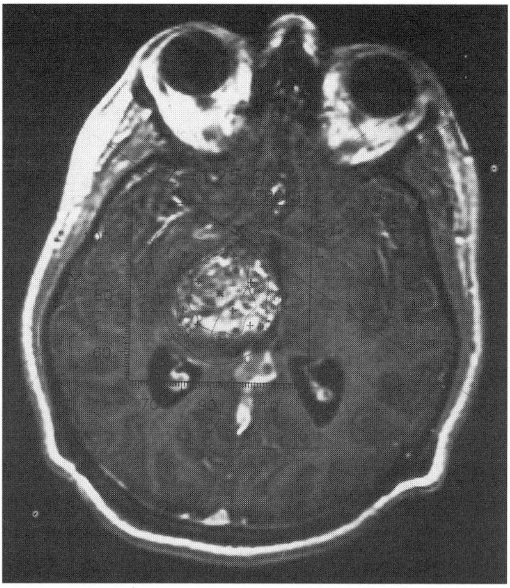

(b)

Figure 4 (a) Composite stereotactic angiogram showing superimposed carotid and vertebral artery injections. (b) Stereotactic axial MR image during radiosurgical treatment of a large right thalamic and brainstem AVM (volume, 30.1 cm^3). Although the patient had not experienced a clinical hemorrhagic ictus, other MRI sequences showed evidence

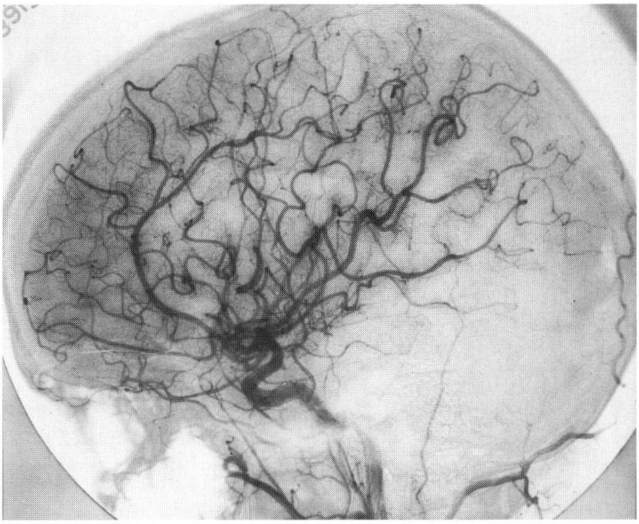

(c)

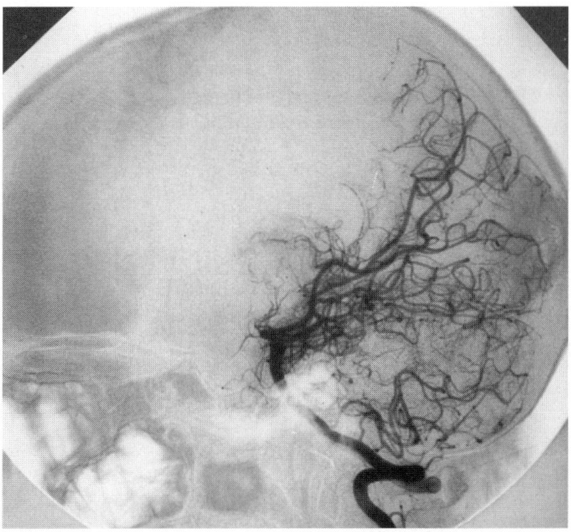

(d)

Figure 4 Continued.
of previous bleeding. Radiosurgical dosimetry: 16 Gy at 50% isodose line using ten 18-mm isocenters. (c) and (d) Follow-up carotid and vertebral angiogram films, respectively, 34 months after radiosurgical treatment showed complete obliteration of the AVM. The patient had a new, partial left-homonymous visual field defect that was not disabling to her.

the most reasonable treatment option for these small AVMs fed by lenticulostriate or thalamoperforating arteries and/or drained by the deep venous system. Four additional patients died of causes unrelated to their AVMs.

B. Imaging Followup and Angiographic Obliteration

Magnetic resonance imaging changes after radiosurgery characteristically involved the appearance of increased T_2 signal intensity around the nidus by 12 months after treatment. This sometimes was accompanied by decreased size of the nidus itself, or evidence of decreased flow within the nidus or draining veins. Even when T_2 signal changes were widespread, the patients most often were asymptomatic. Whether the signal changes represented interstitial edema or gliosis remains to be determined with certainty. However, the resolution of such changes over time favor the former. Coincident with the changes around the nidus, at 12–18 months after treatment (and occasionally longer) the target volume, including the nidus, began to show gadolinium contrast enhancement. The formerly prominent flow voids of the nidus diminished at this time, followed by regression of both the T_2 signal changes and contrast enhancement over the subsequent 6–12 months.

In our experience, even expert interpretation of both MRI and MR angiography have, at times, either overestimated or underestimated the degree of AVM obliteration compared to conventional angiography. So while MR is extremely useful in following the course of AVM obliteration, and is invaluable in demonstrating the condition of the brain in the vicinity of an AVM, conventional cerebral angiography remains the "gold standard" to confirm whether or not an AVM has been obliterated completely.

Table 6 summarizes the results of followup angiography. The obliteration rate is given as a function of AVM volume to allow for comparison with other radiosurgical series. To more precisely communicate the angiographic status and appearance of radiosurgically treated AVMs, the author no longer uses the confusing term "subtotal obliteration." Treated AVMs now are classified as having undergone total obliteration, near-total obliteration, partial obliteration, or no change. Near-total obliteration means that the AVM nidus is gone, only a subtle early vein is observed, no further treatment is warranted, and the patient is considered cured from the clinical standpoint. Partial obliteration means that a visible, shunting nidus remains and requires retreatment even if the nidus is tiny compared to the original AVM. To date we have observed an 81% complete or near-total obliteration rate, with only a single large AVM having been unchanged at three years after treatment. Partially obliterated AVMs were restudied three years after radiosurgery, and retreated if any nidus remained. Outside of the group of smallest AVMs (volume < 1 cm^3) that demonstrated a 100% oblit-

Table 6 Long-Term Angiographic Obliteration of AVMs After Radiosurgery (Volume $\leq$ 10 cm^3 versus $>$ 10 cm^3)

	All patients with 3-year or final postop angiography (80 cases)		AVMs $\leq$ 10 cm^3 (60 cases)		AVMs $>$ 10 cm^3 (20 cases)	
AVM status	Number	Percent	Number	Percent	Number	Percent
Total or near-total obliteration[a]	65	(81.25)	51[b]	(85)	14[c]	(70)
Partial obliteration	14	(17.5)	9	(15)	5	(25)
Unchanged	1	(1.25)	0	—	1	(5)

[a]clinical cure, no further treatment planned.
[b]includes 11 patients treated twice (4 elsewhere).
[c]includes 3 patients treated twice (1 elsewhere).

eration rate in this series, AVM volume and hence, radiation dose between 16–20 Gy, did not appear to correlate with obliteration rate (Figure 5).

Despite exhaustive efforts to obtain follow-up angiograms in all patients, a variety of psychological, social, and economic factors thwarted our plans. For example, 12 patients who have refused or postponed follow-up angiography have had good quality MRI studies that suggest total AVM obliteration. Inclusion of these individuals into final imaging statistics would increase the overall obliteration rate in this series to 84 percent. More complete followup of another 16 patients who have not even undergone adequate postoperative MRI might raise the obliteration rate even higher.

V. INDICATIONS FOR RADIOSURGERY VERSUS CONVENTIONAL SURGERY

Barely a decade ago AVM radiosurgery was an exotic, poorly understood treatment utilized as a last resort by a handful of neurosurgeons and radiation therapists to treat a small group of desperate patients with inoperable lesions [9,18–26]. More recently, our experience with radiosurgery has grown and matured, the natural history of intracranial AVMs has become more clear, realistic data regarding the risks of the various treatment options for AVMs have become available, and the financial and social costs of various AVM treatment strategies have been analyzed. Surprisingly, some individuals have opposed the practice

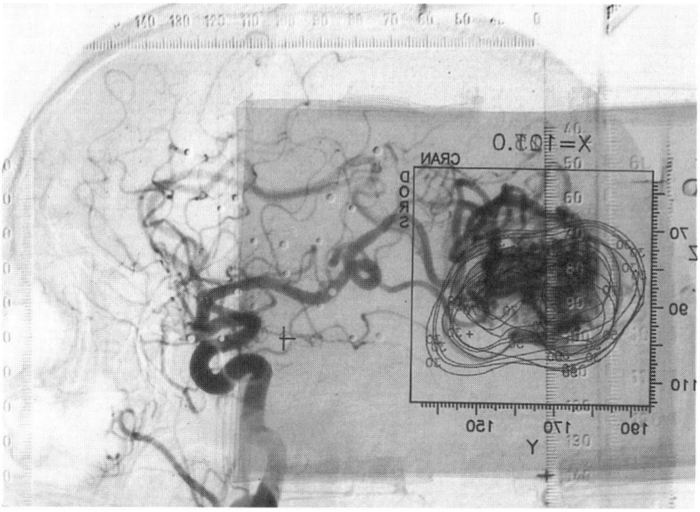

(a)

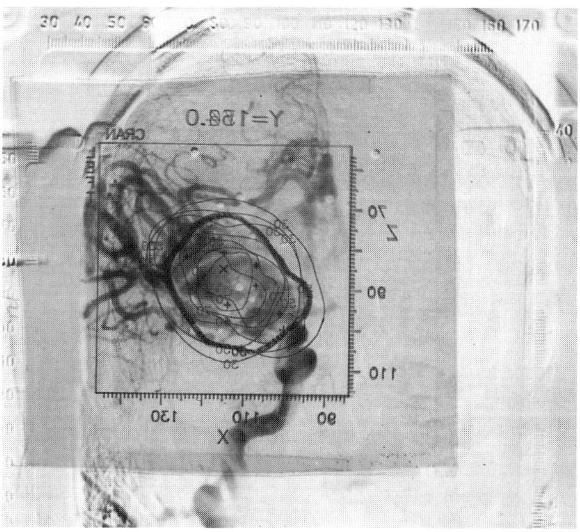

(b)

Figure 5 (a) and (b) Stereotactic right carotid angiogram films during radiosurgical treatment of a large mesial parietal lobe AVM (volume, 23.7 cm^3). The patient had focal sensory and visual seizures and frequent, severe migraine headaches. Radiosurgical dosimetry: 16 Gy at 50% isodose line using eight 18-mm isocenters. (c) and (d) Follow-

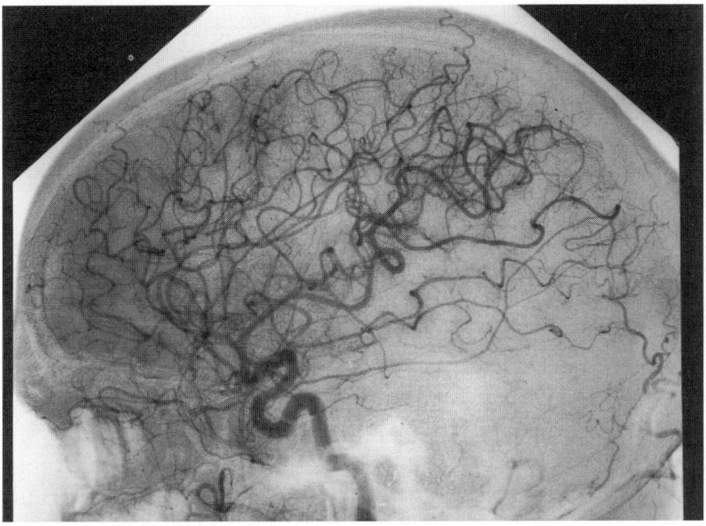

(c)

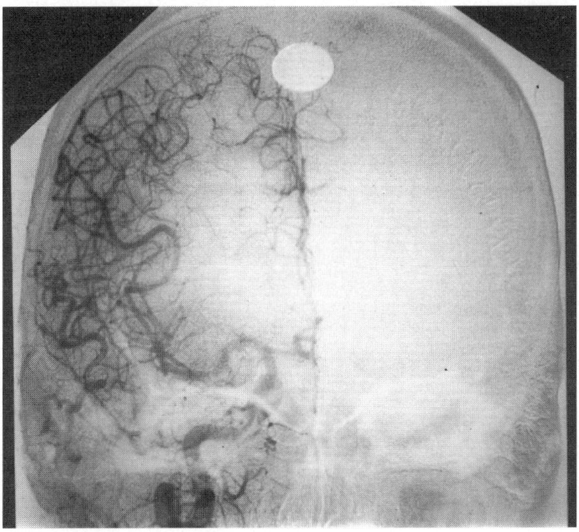

(d)

Figure 5 Continued.
up angiography two years after radiosurgery showed complete obliteration of the AVM. The patient remained neurologically normal and had no further seizures or severe migraine headaches.

of AVM radiosurgery categorically [27]. They have based their case against radiosurgery on mistaken notions regarding the natural history of AVMs, unrealistically low estimates of the morbidity and mortality associated with open AVM surgery, a fundamental misunderstanding of the obliteration or "cure" rate after radiosurgery, and lack of knowledge regarding the relatively low risk (compared to conventional surgery or no treatment) of properly performed radiosurgery, even for sizable AVMs.

Careful analyses of well-defined patient populations have shown that, in general, the presence of an intracranial AVM is a relatively benign condition over the short term of a few years. Rates of rebleeding for ruptured AVMs in patients who have not undergone definitive treatment are substantially the same after 12 to 24 months as the hemorrhage rate for unruptured AVMs: approximately two to four percent per year. A young or middle-aged patient's lifetime risk of AVM hemorrhage (or rebleeding) is on the order of 25 to 40% [28]. The risk of AVM hemorrhage must be calculated using actuarial methods rather than simply multiplying the "4 percent" figure by some number of years of projected life expectancy. So, the risk of an AVM bleeding is *not* 8% after two years, nor is it 100% after 25 years. In the majority of AVM patients, especially those with a newly discovered unruptured lesion, treatment is not an "emergency" to remove a "time-bomb that could go off any second." Rather, analysis of natural history data reveals that an effective, low-risk treatment for AVMs yields a clinical outcome superior to the natural history of the disorder *even if it takes three or more years for the AVM to obliterate*. While an analysis of the most optimistic surgical series also yields a predicted clinical outcome superior to the natural history of untreated AVMs, the results of radiosurgery may be even better.

Virtually all surgical series, even those from centers that handle complex cases routinely, suffer from an inescapable selection bias; surgeons only operate cases in which an acceptable outcome can be predicted with a fair degree of confidence. So any grading system based on surgical outcome becomes a tautology—the highest risk cases are never treated to begin with. In a similar fashion, reports of surgical series based upon measurements of AVM size also can be misleading. Unless stereotactic angiography and/or MRI are utilized, the chaotic magnification factors present on conventional angiographic films and the distortion present on digital images makes *accurate* determinations of the size of an AVM nidus nearly impossible, and *overestimation* of the AVM size quite likely. Surgical reports also tend to state only the single largest dimension of an AVM rather than the average of all three diameters or, better yet, the nidus volume.

A realistic appraisal of the results of modern AVM surgical series shows a mean mortality rate of 4.5% (range 2.4–11.6%), a mean neurologic morbidity rate of 8.5% (range 4.8–10%) and an additional nonneurologic surgical complication rate of up to 8% [7,29–34]. In the large series of Yasargil and Drake, 5%

and 6% of AVMs, respectively, could not be excised completely (with acceptable results in the judgement of the surgeon) upon exploration [7,33]. The morbidity and mortality of open resection of AVMs in the thalamus, basal ganglia and brainstem fall within the upper end of the range of figures quoted above [7,29,33].

In the present series, and in most other radiosurgical series, two- and three-year angiographic AVM obliteration rates are in the range of 70 to 92% [3,5,6,9,10,12,14,15]. In accordance with our experience, other investigators also have reported that progressive AVM obliteration begins after a 6 to 12 month latency period. Although some of the observed radiation-induced effect occurs by two years after treatment, the early selection of that interval for standard final followup was arbitrary and erroneous. We have observed considerable further reduction in angiographic AVM filling, in several cases to the point of complete obliteration, between two and three years after radiosurgery. So authors who criticize AVM radiosurgery on the grounds that 20 or 30% of patients are "not cured" are, at best, misinformed. Such a critique confuses the gradual, continuous, radiation-induced biological effect of radiosurgery with the immediate results of conventional surgery [35]. By taking the above line of reasoning to its absurd conclusion, one could compare the results of radiosurgery to conventional open surgery one day postoperatively. In that case, 100 percent of the radiosurgically-treated patients would remain "not cured," and open surgery would appear to be a much more successful form of therapy. In practice, when an AVM has not obliterated after three years, retreatment is performed even if the remaining portion of the nidus was irradiated previously. In our experience, and at other centers, repeat treatment carries as high a success rate as primary treatment, yielding gratifying results, albeit over an extended period of years.

In a hypothetical cohort of 100 AVM patients treated with radiosurgery, regardless of lesion location or grade, at least 70 patients (70%) will be cured by the first treatment over a two to three year period; 4 of the "cured" patients (4%) may have a new neurologic deficit, and 4 patients (4%) may rebleed fatally. Of the 26 remaining patients with a persistent AVM remnant retreated at the three-year point, another 18 AVMs (70%) will be obliterated after another two to three years. In summary, 88 patients will have been cured (4 of whom will have sustained a new deficit), 4 patients will have died of a hemorrhage during the latency interval, and only 8 patients will have a persistent AVM nidus remnant, most likely of little or no clinical significance or danger. This realistic appraisal of current practice leaves fewer than 8 percent of patients (not 20 percent of patients) "not cured" by radiosurgery and is superior to the results of any comprehensive surgical AVM series ever published.

Before the current generation of Gamma Knife instruments and a few advanced LINAC-based devices and treatment planning systems were developed, an arbitrary size limit for radiosurgical treatment of 2.5 to 3 cm was thought to exist. Using our current dose-volume schema and advanced treatment planning system, we now feel fairly confident in treating volumes over 33 cm^3 (equivalent to a sphere larger than 4 cm in diameter) safely and effectively without any greater risk of radiation-induced brain injury than in smaller lesions. Another safety issue, that of radiation-induced neoplasia after radiosurgery, has not been borne out in followup of thousands of patients subjected to the equivalent of tens of thousands of patient-years of observation.

In summary, radiosurgery is now a mainstay of treatment for patients with intracranial AVMs in the industrialized world. Radiosurgery yields clinical results that are far superior to the natural history of untreated AVMs and, in some instances, superior to the results of the best open surgical series presented to date.

ACKNOWLEDGMENTS

The author thanks members of the Department of Neurosurgery and the Division of Radiation Oncology for contributing patients to this series. Lorna N. Stevens, R.N. and Debb Gorman, R.N. assisted in the data analysis and Mrs. Mary Sawyer and Ms. Angela Kollasch prepared the manuscript.

REFERENCES

1. Lunsford LD. Stereotactic radiosurgery: at the threshold or at the crossroads? *Neurosurgery* 1993; 32:799–804.
2. Steiner L. Radiosurgery in cerebral arteriovenous malformations. In: Fein JM, Flamm ES, (eds). Vol IV. Cerebrovascular Surgery. New York: Springer-Verlag, 1985; 1161–1215.
3. Steiner L. Treatment of arteriovenous malformations by radiosurgery. In: Wilson CB, Stein BM, (eds). Intracranial arteriovenous malformations. Baltimore: Williams and Wilkins, 1984:295–313.
4. Steiner L, Lindquist C, Adler JR, Torner JC, Alves W, Steiner M. Clinical outcome of radiosurgery for cerebral arteriovenous malformations. *J Neurosurg* 1992; 77:1–8.
5. Betti O, Munari C, Rosler R. Stereotactic radiosurgery with the linear accelerator: treatment of arteriovenous malformations. *Neurosurgery* 1989; 24:311–321.
6. Colombo F, Benedetti A, Pozza F, Marchetti C, Chierego G. Linear accelerator radiosurgery of cerebral arteriovenous malformations. *Neurosurgery* 1989; 24:833–840.
7. Drake CG. Cerebral arteriovenous malformations: considerations for and experience with surgical treatment in 166 cases. *Clin Neurosurg* 1979; 26:145–208.

8. Fabrikant JI, Lyman JT, Frankel KA. Heavy charged–particle Bragg peak radiosurgery for intracranial vascular disorders. *Radiation Research* 1985; 104:5244–5258.
9. Fabrikant JI, Lyman JT, Hosobuchi Y. Stereotactic heavy–ion Bragg peak radiosurgery for intra–cranial vascular disorders: method for treatment of deep arteriovenous malformations. *Brit J Radiology* 1984; 57:479–490.
10. Friedman WA, Bova FJ. Linear accelerator radiosurgery for arteriovenous malformations. *J Neurosurg* 1992; 77:832–841.
11. Hosobuchi Y, Fabrikant J, Lyman J. Stereotactic heavy–particle irradiation of intracranial arteriovenous malformations. *Appl Neurophysiol* 1987; 50:248–252.
12. Kemeny AA, Dias PS, Forster DMC. Results of stereotactic radiosurgery of arteriovenous malformations: an analysis of 52 cases. *J Neurol Neurosurg Psychiat* 1989; 52:554–558.
13. Kjellberg RN, Hanamura T, Davis KR, Lyons SL, Adams RD. Bragg–peak proton–beam therapy for arteriovenous malformations of the brain. *N Engl J Med* 1983; 309:269–274.
14. Lunsford LD, Kondziolka D, Flickinger JC, Bissonette DJ, Jungreis CA, Maitz AH, Horton JA, Coffey RJ. Stereotactic radiosurgery for arteriovenous malformations of the brain. *J Neurosurg* 1991; 75:512–524.
15. Steinberg GK, Fabrikant JI, Marks MP, Levy RP, Frankel KA, Phillips MH, Shuer LM, Silverberg DG. Stereotactic heavy–charged–particle Bragg–peak radiation for intracranial arteriovenous malformations. *N Engl J Med* 1990; 323:96–101.
16. Coffey RJ, Nichols DA, Shaw EG. Stereotactic radiosurgical treatment of cerebral arteriovenous malformations. *Mayo Clinic Proceedings* 1995; 70:214–222.
17. Yamamoto Y, Coffey RJ, Nichols DA, Shaw EG. Interim report on the radiosurgical treatment of cerebral arteriovenous malformations. *J Neurosurg* 1995; 83:832–837.
18. Cushing H, Bailey P. Tumors Arising from the Blood Vessels of the Brain. Angiomatous Malformations and Hemangioblastomas. Springfield: Charles C Thomas, 1928.
19. French LA, Chou SN. Conventional methods of treating intracranial arteriovenous malformations. *Prog Neurol Surg* 1969; 3:274–319.
20. Johnson RT. Radiotherapy of cerebral angiomas, with a note on some problems in diagnosis. In: Pia HW, Gleave JRW, Grote F, Zierski J, (eds). Cerebral Angiomas. Advances in Diagnosis and Therapy. Berlin/Heidelberg/New York: Springer-Verlag, 1975:256–266.
21. Krayenbühl HA. Discussion des rapports sur "les angiomes supratentoriels." Premier Congrès International de Neurochirurgie, Rapports et discussions. Bruxelles, 1957.
22. Magnus V. Bidrag till Hjernchirurgiens Klinik og Resuhater. Merkur: Kristiana, 1921.
23. McKissock W, Hankinson J. The surgical treatment of supratentorial angiomas. Premier Congrès International de Neurochirurgie, Rapports et discussions. Bruxelles, 1957.
24. Pool JL. Aneurysms and arteriovenous anomalies of the brain. Diagnosis and treatment. New York: Harper and Row, 1965.
25. Potter JM. Angiomatous malformations of the brain; their nature and prognosis. *Ann Royal Coll Surg Engl* 1955; 16:227–243.

26. Tognetti F, Andaoli A, Cuscini A, Testa C. Successful management of an intracranial arteriovenous malformation by conventional irradiation. *J Neurosurg* 1985; 63:193–195.
27. Stein BM, Mohr JP, Sisti MB. Is radiosurgery all that it appears to be? [letter] *Arch Neurol* 1991; 48:19–20.
28. Auger RG, Wiebers DO. Management of unruptured intracranial arteriovenous malformations: a decision analysis. *Neurosurgery* 1992; 30:561–569.
29. Lee J-P. Surgical treatment of thalamic arteriovenous malformations. *Neurosurgery* 1993; 32:498–504.
30. Morgan MK, Johnston IA, Hallinan JM, Weber NC. Complications of surgery for arteriovenous malformations of the brain. *J Neurosurg* 1993; 78:176–182.
31. Parkinson D, Bachers G. Arteriovenous malformations. Summary of 100 consecutive supratentorial cases. *J Neurosurg* 1980; 53:285–299.
32. Piepgras DG, Sundt TM Jr., Ragoowansi AT, Stevens L. Seizure outcome in patients with surgically treated cerebral arteriovenous malformations. *J Neurosurg* 1993; 78:5–11.
33. Yasargil MG. Microneurosurgery. Vol 3B. New York: Thieme, 1988:369–392.
34. Yeh H-S, Tew JM, Gartner M. Seizure control after surgery of cerebral arteriovenous malformations. *J Neurosurg* 1993; 78:12–18.
35. Flickinger JC, Pollock BE, Kondziolka D, Lunsford LD. A dose–response analysis of arteriovenous malformation obliteration after radiosurgery. *Int J Radiation Oncology Biol Phys* 1996; 36(4):873–879.

17

Interventional Neuroradiology for the Treatment of Aneurysms, Vasospasm, and Arteriovenous Malformation

Douglas A. Nichols
Mayo Clinic, Rochester, Minnesota

I. ENDOVASCULAR TREATMENT OF INTRACRANIAL ANEURYSMS

The current therapy of choice for intracranial aneurysms is neurosurgical clipping. However, in a subset of patients with aneurysms, surgical clipping poses a high risk because of the location or size of the aneurysm, the presence of a wide or calcified aneurysm neck, a history of a recent severe subarachnoid hemorrhage, or the poor medical condition of the patient. Endovascular therapy of aneurysms has been directed at this subset of patients.

Endovascular therapy of intracranial aneurysms can be divided into two broad categories: 1. preservation of the parent artery by selective occlusion of the aneurysm with detachable balloons or metallic coils and 2. occlusion of the parent artery when selective occlusion of the aneurysm is not technically possible. The method of treatment depends on the location, size, and morphology of the aneurysm.

Fusiform aneurysms or aneurysms with wide necks are usually not amenable to selective aneurysm occlusion and are treated with detachable balloon occlusion of the parent artery. Before the parent vessel giving origin to an aneurysm is permanently occluded, it is temporarily occluded with a balloon catheter to test the patient's tolerance to occlusion.

Protocols for testing tolerance prior to permanent occlusion of the parent artery vary from institution to institution. In general, after systemic heparinization, the artery is occluded with a double lumen balloon catheter for thirty minutes during which time the patient's neurologic function is closely monitored. During the period of balloon occlusion, the collateral circulation through the circle of Willis to the vascular territory to be occluded is assessed by obtaining digital subtraction angiograms of the contralateral carotid artery and the dominant vertebral artery (when the internal carotid artery is occluded) or the contralateral vertebral artery and both internal carotid arteries (when the vertebral artery is occluded). Most institutions incorporate a form of functional imaging (either single photon emission computed tomography [SPECT] cerebral perfusion scanning or stable xenon-CT [computed tomography]) into their protocol for temporary balloon occlusion [1–3] (Figure 1).

Despite the functional testing just described, the temporary balloon occlusion test is not 100% predictive of tolerance to permanent occlusion of the parent artery [4]. Among 68 patients, Higashida et al. [5] reported that 7 (10.3%) had transient cerebral ischemia that responded to volume expansion or antiplatelet therapy and 3 (4.4%) had stroke after permanent balloon occlusion of the internal carotid artery.

If the patient tolerates temporary balloon occlusion of the parent artery, then the artery can be permanently occluded by detaching a balloon just proximal to the aneurysm. Detachable balloons come in various sizes and configurations and are made of either latex or silicone. Several delivery catheter and detachable balloon configurations are available [6,7]. In general, balloons are mounted on delivery catheters 1 to 2 French in diameter and are detached by either simple traction or "pushed" off the delivery catheter with a coaxial catheter. The balloons are inflated with a mixture of sterile water and iodinated contrast material iso-osmotic to blood. In most instances, after the first balloon is detached, a second "safety" balloon is detached just proximal to the initial balloon to protect against distal migration and embolization of the initially detached balloon if it should deflate prematurely (Figure 2).

Most aneurysms treated by permanent balloon occlusion of the parent artery are fusiform or wide-necked aneurysms involving the cavernous and paraclinoid segments of the internal carotid artery and present with symptoms secondary to mass effect. After permanent balloon occlusion of the carotid artery, the aneurysm thromboses and decreases in size over time and the symptoms secondary to mass effect resolve (Figure 3).

The two largest North American series [5,8] of cavernous and paraclinoid aneurysms treated by permanent balloon occlusion of the internal carotid artery reported 100% complete thrombosis of the aneurysms and a combined permanent morbidty rate of 2.8%.

When technically possible, it is desirable to selectively occlude the aneurysm with embolic materials while preserving the patency of the parent artery. Detachable balloons were the first embolic agent to be used on a widespread basis to selectively occlude aneurysms (Figure 4).

The available balloons come in a limited variety of sizes and shapes (spherical or cylindrical). Therefore, it is difficult to find a particular balloon or combination of balloons that will fill 100% of the volume of the aneurysm. There are multiple reports of delayed aneurysm enlargement or rupture after subtotal balloon occlusion of aneurysms [9–11]. A "water-hammer effect" from pulsating arterial blood on the balloon, which is transmitted to the aneurysm wall, is postulated to be the cause of delayed aneurysm enlargement or rupture after subtotal occlusion [11]. Balloons may also migrate into the thrombus of partially thrombosed aneurysms and cause subtotal occlusion.

Because the balloon exerts pressure on the aneurysm wall during the inflation process, most interventionalists were reluctant to treat aneurysms during the acute phase (first 72 hours) after subarachnoid hemorrhage. Therefore, selective balloon occlusion does not play a major role in the treatment of most intracranial aneurysms (that is, those that present with subarachnoid hemorrhage).

Because of the difficulties associated with detachable balloon therapy of intracranial aneurysms, investigative work was directed at finding other occlusive materials that could be placed inside an aneurysm. Early results from animal experiments and human trials demonstrate that selective occlusion with metallic coils could play a major role in the treatment of intracranial aneurysms [12–26].

A major technological advancement in the endovascular treatment of aneurysms was realized with the development of a "detachable" coil system. Guglielmi et al. [15] developed the Guglielmi detachable coil (Target Therapeutics, Inc., Fremont California), which has allowed for the controlled delivery of soft platinum coils within aneurysms.

The Guglielmi detachable coil system works on the principles of electrolysis and electrothrombosis (Figure 5). The platinum coils, which are available in various helical diameters and lengths, are attached to stainless steel guidewires with a microsolder. The tip of a microcatheter is navigated into the lumen of the aneurysm under fluoroscopic road-mapping and digital subtraction angiographic guidance. The platinum coil is pushed through the microcatheter with the stainless steel guidewire and as it exits the microcatheter it adopts a circular configuration, folds on itself, and conforms to the shape of the aneurysm. If the coil assumes an unsatisfactory position as it exits the microcatheter, it can be withdrawn back into the microcatheter by retracting the proximal end of the guidewire. Changing the position of the tip of the microcatheter within the aneurysm and advancement and withdrawal of the coil can be repeated until the coil assumes a satisfactory position within the aneurysm. Once satisfactory positioning of the coil within the aneurysm has been achieved, the coil is detached from the guidewire by the process of electrolysis. A 2.5-volt, 1.0-mA, direct electric current is applied to the proximal end of the guidewire. The current dissolves the microsolder junction between the guidewire and the coil

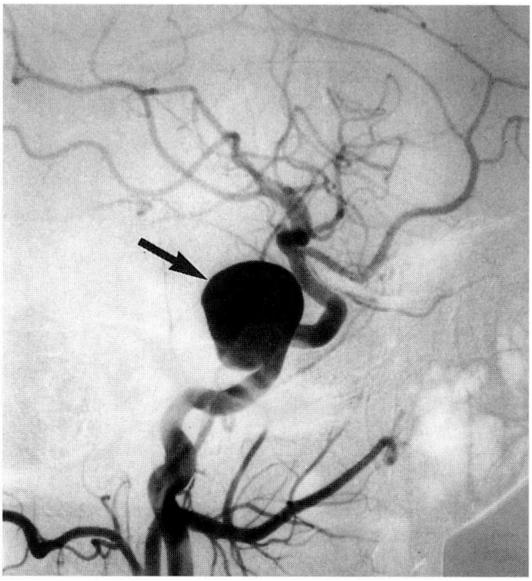

(a)

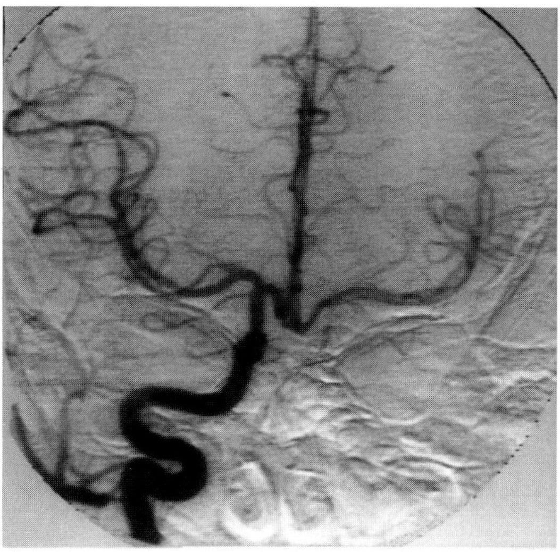

(b)

Figure 1 16-year-old male with several months history of diplopia on lateral gaze. Physical examination revealed a left VIth nerve palsy. (a) Lateral view of a left carotid angiogram demonstrates a giant fusiform aneurysm (arrow) of the cavernous internal carotid artery. (b) AP view of a right carotid angiogram obtained during temporary bal-

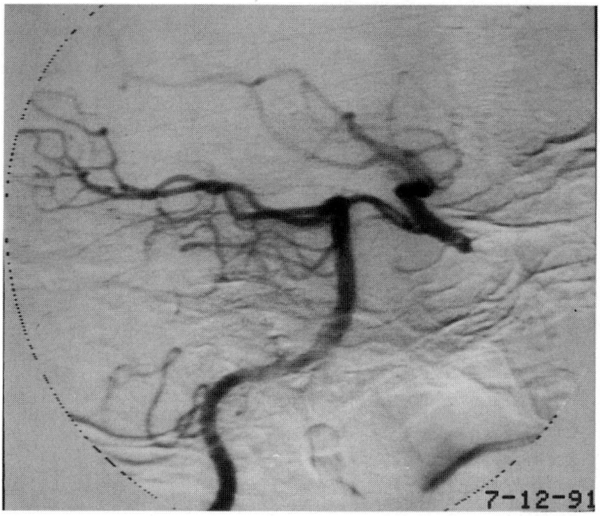

(c)

Figure 1 Continued.
loon occlusion of the left internal carotid artery demonstrates good collateral circulation to the left cerebral hemisphere via the anterior communicating artery. (c) Lateral view of a left vertebral angiogram obtained during temporary balloon occlusion of the left internal carotid artery also demonstrates good collateral circulation to the left cerebral hemisphere via the left posterior communicating artery.

over several minutes, which detaches the coil from the guidewire. During the process of coil detachment, the platinum coil assumes a positive charge, attracting negatively charged blood products such as platelets, fibrinogen, leukocytes, and erythrocytes. A thrombus forms around the coil within the aneurysm; this process is termed electrothrombosis. The platinum coil acts as a mesh, keeping the thrombus from embolizing out of the aneurysm. The aneurysm is occluded by a combination of the thrombus and the intertwined detached platinum coils (Figure 6). The best results immediately after the procedure and at delayed clinical and angiographic followup have been observed with small- and medium-sized aneurysms with small necks [20,25–27].

Because of the relatively atraumatic nature of the soft platinum coils, it has been possible to successfully treat aneurysms that present with subarachnoid hemorrhage within the first few hours after rupture. Treatment of recently ruptured aneurysms in the acute phase with an endovascular approach is theoretically attractive since it would markedly reduce or eliminate the possibility of rehemorrhage, allow for the aggressive medical or endovascular management

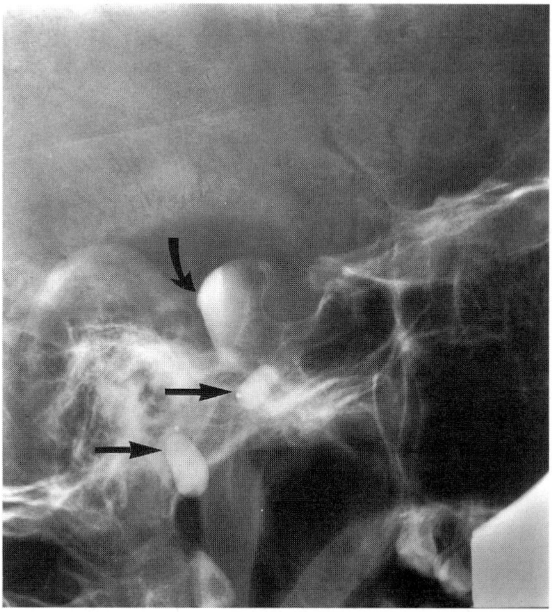

Figure 2 Same patient as in Figure 1. Lateral x-ray demonstrates two latex balloons (straight arrows) filled with an iso-osmotic mixture of sterile water and contrast detached in the cavernous and petrous segments of the left internal carotid artery. There is stagnant contrast present within the cavernous carotid aneurysm (curved arrow).

Figure 3 Same patient as in Figures 1 and 2. (a) Intermediate-weighted axial MRI obtained 6 weeks after balloon occlusion demonstrates thrombosis of the left cavernous carotid artery aneurysm (arrow). (b) Intermediate-weighted axial MRI obtained 18 months after balloon occlusion of the left internal carotid artery demonstrates nonvisualization of the left cavernous carotid aneurysm. The patient's left VIth nerve palsy had resolved on examination. Note absence of black "flow void" signal of the left internal carotid artery consistent with vessel occlusion. (Compare with the contralateral carotid artery [arrow]).

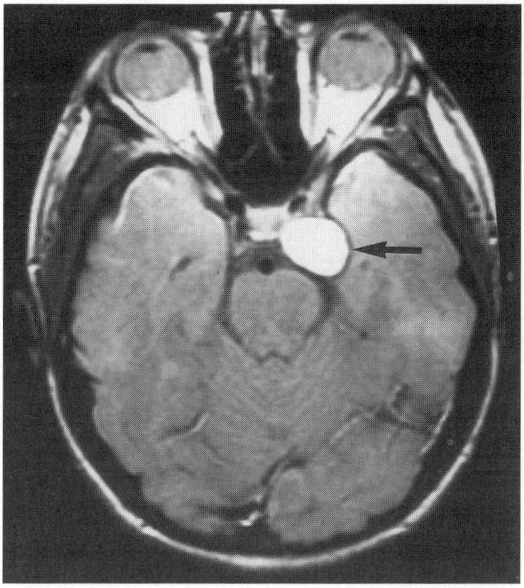

(a)

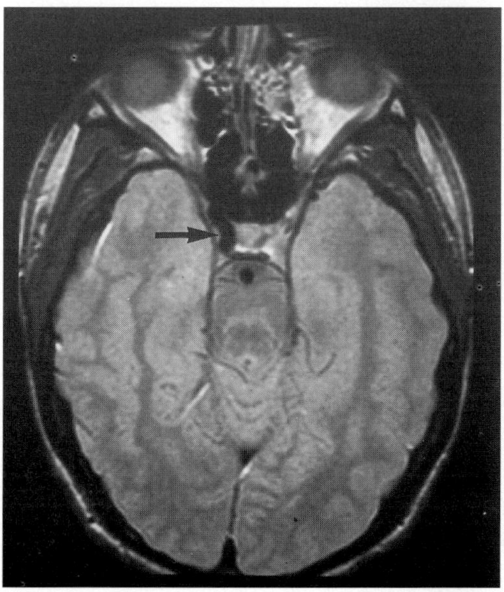

(b)

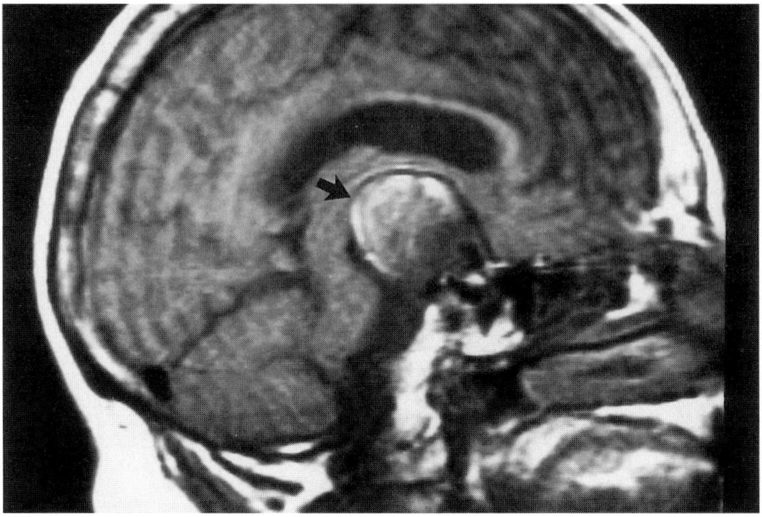

(a)

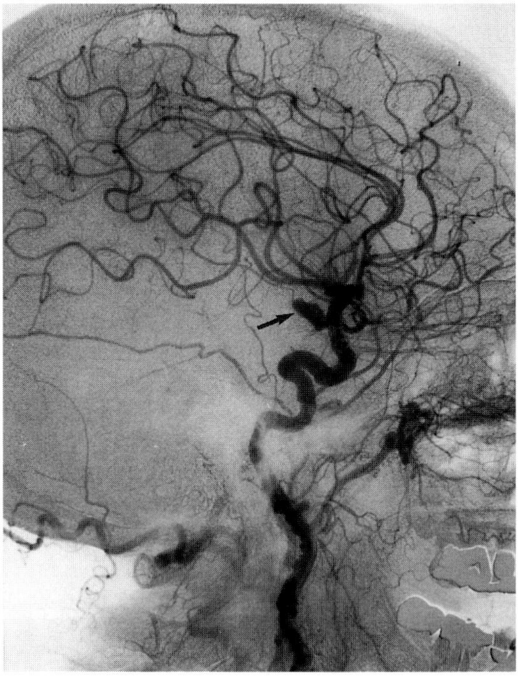

(b)

Figure 4 68-year-old female with a several month history of increasing confusion, left hemiparesis, and ataxia. (a) Sagittal T1-weighted MRI demonstrates a giant partially thrombosed aneurysm (arrow). (b) Lateral view of right carotid angiogram demonstrates

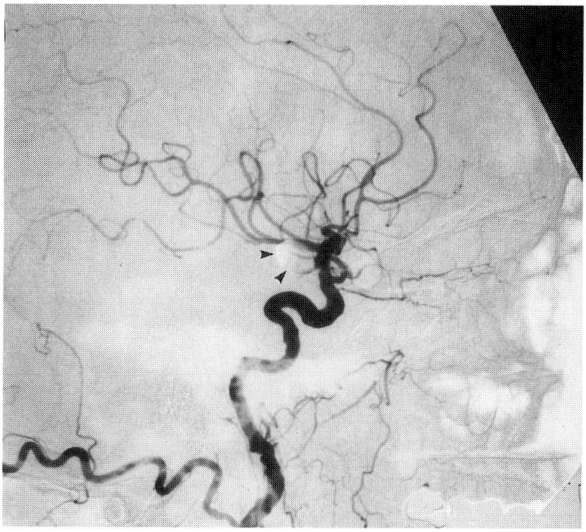

(c)

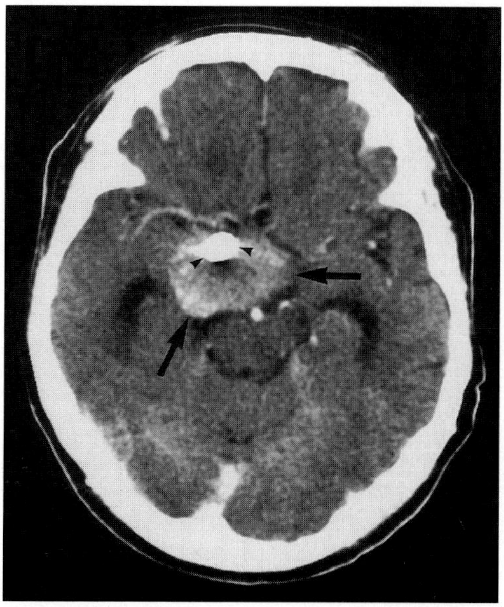

(d)

Figure 4 Continued.
a posterior communicating artery aneurysm (arrow). Note the small size of the patent lumen of the aneurysm compared to the thrombosed component of the aneurysm demonstrated on the MRI. (c) Lateral right carotid angiogram obtained after detachment of a latex balloon (arrowheads) within the patent lumen of the aneurysm. (d) CT obtained after balloon detachment demonstrates the balloon (arrowheads) within the thrombosed aneurysm (arrows).

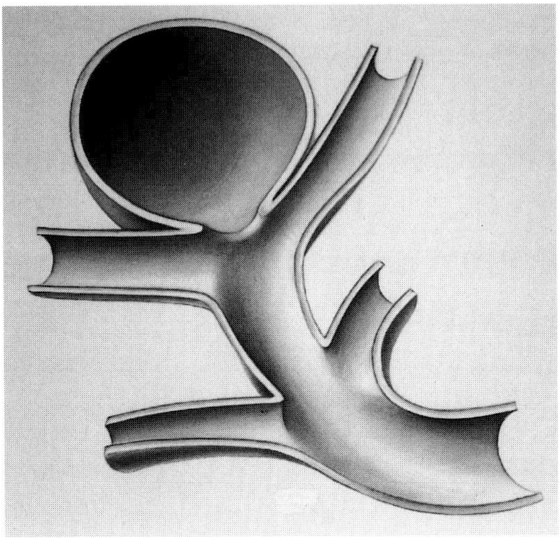

(a)

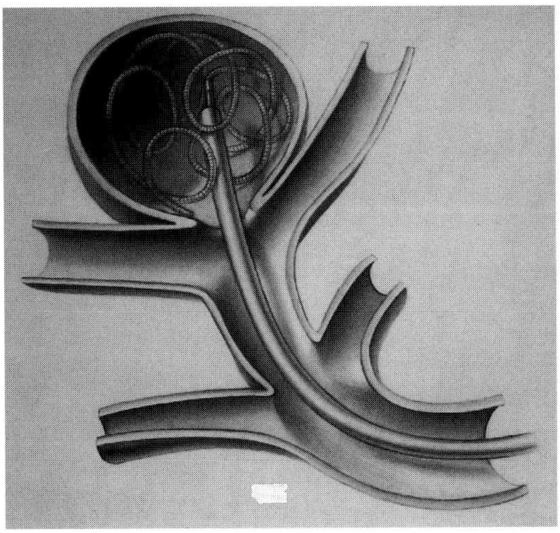

(b)

Figure 5 Schematic diagram of occlusion of an aneurysm with the Gugliemli detachable coil system. (a) Basilar caput aneurysm before treatment. (b) The tip of the microcatheter has been placed within the aneurysm and the first coil has been advanced

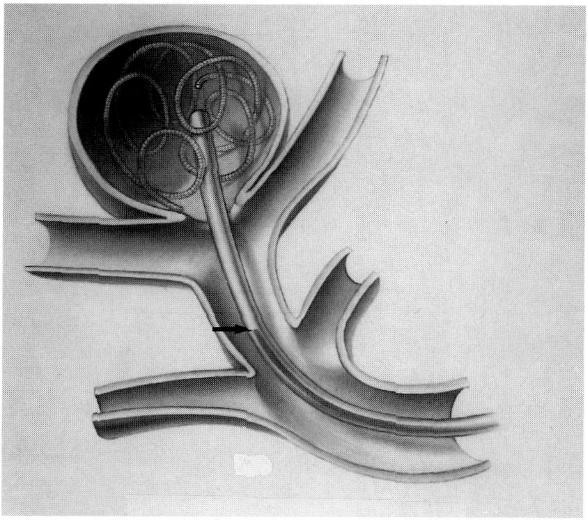

(c)

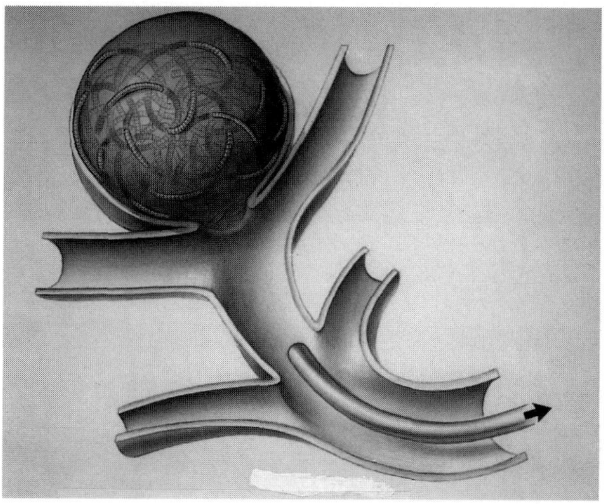

(d)

Figure 5 Continued.
through the catheter into the aneurysm. (c) The coil has been detached and the guidewire has been withdrawn into the microcatheter (arrow). (d) The process is repeated until the aneurysm is occluded with a combination of coils and thrombus.

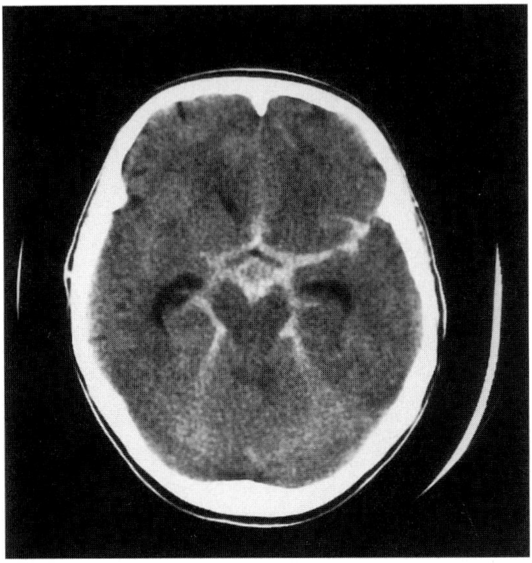

(a)

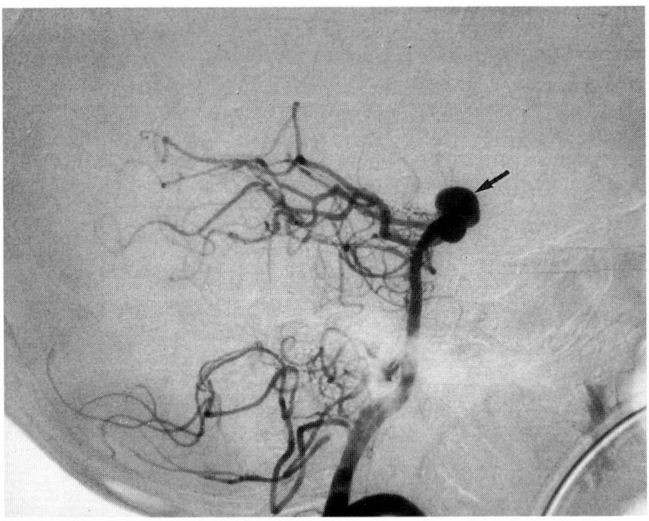

(b)

Figure 6 48-year-old woman with subarachnoid hemorrhage. Patient was treated with GDC coils three days after the subarachnoid hemorrhage (a) CT demonstrates dense subarachnoid blood in the basal cisterns. Lateral, (b), and submentovertex, (c), views of a left vertebral angiogram demonstrate an 11-mm diameter basilar caput aneurysm

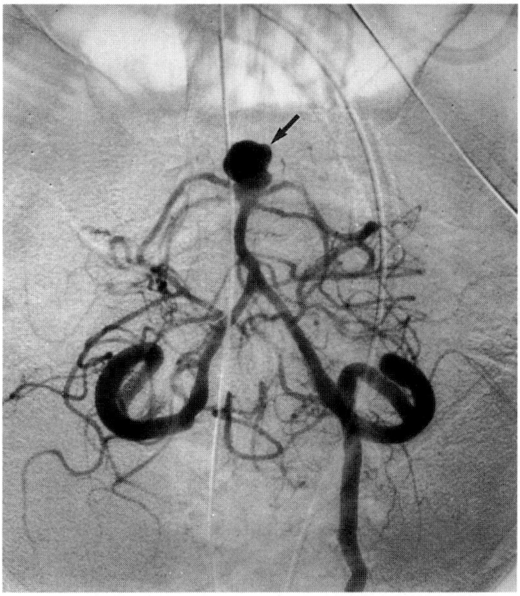

(c)

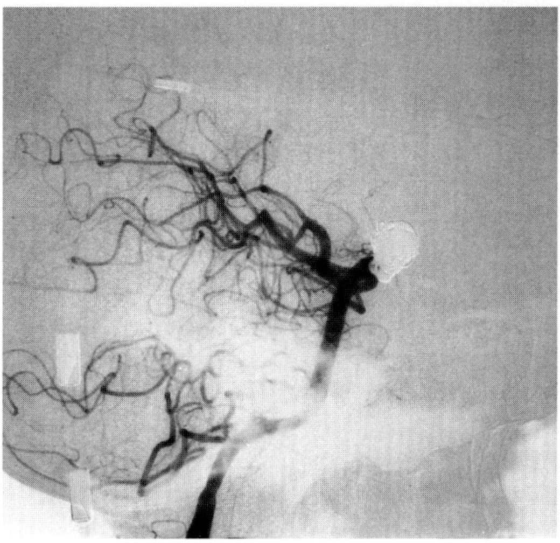

(d)

Figure 6 Continued.
(arrows). Lateral, (d), and submentovertex, (e), views of a left vertebral angiogram after the GDC coil occlusion procedure demonstrate 100% occlusion of the aneurysm. Lat-

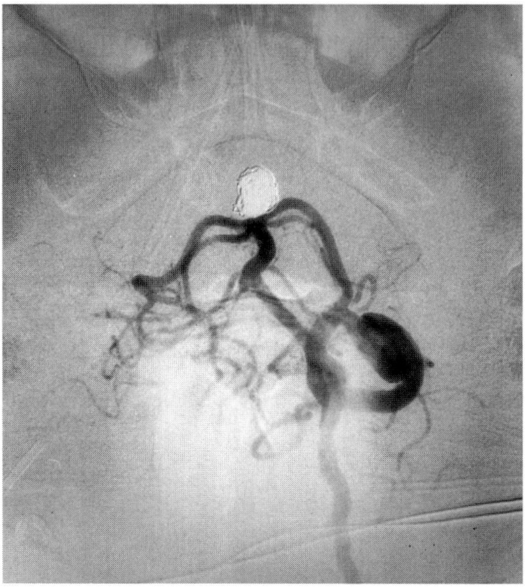

(e)

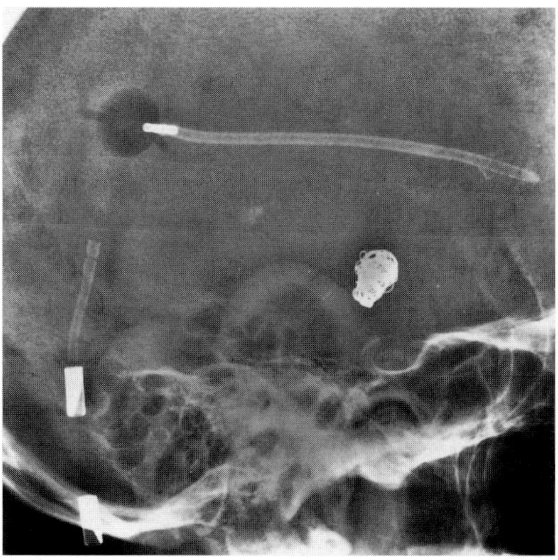

(f)

Figure 6 Continued.
eral, (f), and submentovertex, (g), x-rays demonstrate the detached coils. Eight coils measuring a total length of 108 cm were detached within the aneurysm.

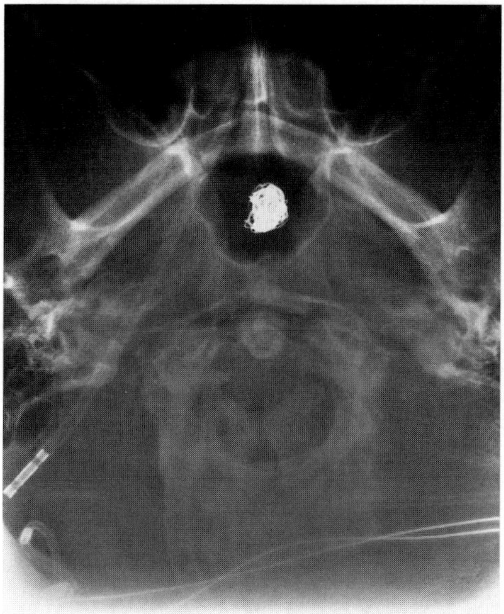

(g)

Figure 6 Continued.

of vasospasm, and avoid the difficulties of retracting an edematous and inflammed brain, thereby hopefully improving the long-term survival and outcome of patients with subarachnoid hemorrhage [28]. Additional technological advances are in various stages of development that will allow the interventional neuroradiologist to play an increasingly important role in the treatment of intracranial aneurysms.

II. ENDOVASCULAR TREATMENT OF VASOSPASM AFTER SUBARACHNOID HEMORRHAGE

Symptomatic vasospasm is initially treated medically by pharmacologically inducing hypertension and/or hypervolemia and by administering neuronal protection drugs. If medical treatment fails, then endovascular techniques may play a role in the treatment of vasospasm.

Balloon angioplasty of symptomatic vasospasm has the greatest chance of being successful and reversing the neurologic deficit if performed as soon as possible after the onset of symptoms that are unresponsive to maximal medical therapy [29]. Optimally, patients should be treated within the first six to twelve hours after the onset of symptoms. Other criteria for the selection of patients include angiographically demonstrating vasospasm in a location that can account for the neurologic findings and exclusion of other potential causes of a new neurologic deficit such as hydrocephalus or a hematoma. It is preferable that the aneurysm that was the source of the subarachnoid hemorrhage have been surgically clipped or treated by endovascular methods before balloon angioplasty because the increase in cerebral perfusion that occurs after angioplasty can lead to a rerupture of an untreated aneurysm.

A silicone balloon with physical properties that allow it to maintain a soft, low-tension shell after expansion (Target Therapeutics, Inc., Fremont, California) is the device most commonly used for vasospasm angioplasty procedures [30]. A transfemoral approach is used. The microcatheter with the attached angioplasty balloon is navigated into the vascular territory to be treated. Digital subtraction angiography and fluoroscopic road-mapping guidance are mandatory in order to avoid inflating the balloon in small branch arteries that may rupture. Vessel dilation is usually performed in a proximal to distal fashion. The balloon is inflated for 1 to 2 seconds and then deflated (Figure 7). Once a vessel has been dilated to its normal luminal diameter, it is rare to observe recurrent vasospasm on followup angiography.

Improvement in neurologic function after balloon angioplasty of symptomatic cerebral vasospasm occurs in approximately 70% of patients [29,31]. Vessel rupture and occlusion have been reported [29,32,33]. As stated above, morbidity also increases when the aneurysm that was the source of the hemorrhage has not been treated.

When the silicone balloon is maximally inflated, it is 4 mm in diameter and 12 mm in length. Although it is usually possible to achieve more distal catheterization, the angioplasty procedure is limited to the intracranial carotid artery, the M-1 segment of the middle cerebral artery, the A-1 segment of the anterior cerebral artery, the intracranial vertebral artery, the basilar artery, and the P-1 segment of the posterior cerebral artery. Balloon angioplasty of more distal vessels with the currently available angioplasty balloons carries a high risk of overdistention and rupture.

If, after balloon angioplasty of the accessible vessels, severe vasospasm is found to persist in the distal untreated vessels, the remaining vasospasm can be treated by infusing papaverine intraarterially either through a catheter placed in the high cervical segments of the internal carotid artery or vertebral artery or through a microcatheter placed in the intracranial circulation just proximal to the angiographically demonstrated vasospasm [34,35]. Dosages and rates of administration are still empirical but we have consistently observed angiographic improvement of distally located vasospasm after infusing 150 mg of papaverine diluted in 100 cc of normal saline over one-half hour via an intracranial microcatheter placed just proximal to the angiographically observed vasospasm. Corresponding improvement in neurologic function occurs in about 50% of patients in our experience. Unlike the results with balloon angioplasty, recurrent vasospasm of the treated vessels has been observed several days after the papaverine infusion necessitating retreatment in some instances.

III. ENDOVASCULAR TREATMENT OF BRAIN ARTERIOVENOUS MALFORMATIONS

Technological advances in catheter technology, embolic materials, and angiographic equipment have allowed the interventional neuroradiologist to play an important and active role in the management of brain arteriovenous malformations (AVMs). In experienced hands, the advances in technology have reduced complication rates. In a series of 482 adult patients with brain AVMs embolized between 1983 and 1990, Berenstein and Lasjaunias [36] reported a 1.6% mortality rate and 1.4% serious morbidity rate.

Endovascular therapy plays several different roles in the treatment of brain AVMs. First, some AVMs may present with "steal" symptoms and because of their size or a location involving eloquent brain structures may not be amenable to surgical resection or radiosurgery. The patients' "steal" symptoms may improve after partial embolization of the AVM [37] (Figure 8). Second, embolization of a brain AVM can reduce the size and volume of an AVM so that it may be amenable to treatment by radiosurgery with a higher probability of cure than if not reduced in size prior to treatment [38] (Figure 9). Third, approximately 10% of brain AVMs are amenable to cure by embolization alone without subsequent surgical resection or radiosurgery. Fourth, preoperative devascularization of brain AVMs has been proven to be of benefit in several series [39–41]. This is the most common indication for embolizing a brain AVM. Preoperative embolization of brain AVMs can be used for large AVMs in an attempt to decrease operating time, blood loss, and the possibility of perfusion pressure breakthrough postoperatively (Figure 10). It can also be employed in those AVMs with deep feeders that are difficult for the surgeon to control but which can be occluded preoperatively by embolization (Figure 11).

Embolization procedures are performed in the neuroangiography suite with the patient usually awake and under neuroleptic analgesia. Vascular access is obtained via the transfemoral route. Superselective catheterization of the arterial feeders to the AVM is performed under fluoroscopic road-mapping guidance with either a flow-directed microcatheter or a microcatheter-steerable microguidewire system. A superselective digital subtraction angiogram is performed of each catheterized arterial pedicle. This provides information about the AVM nidus such as

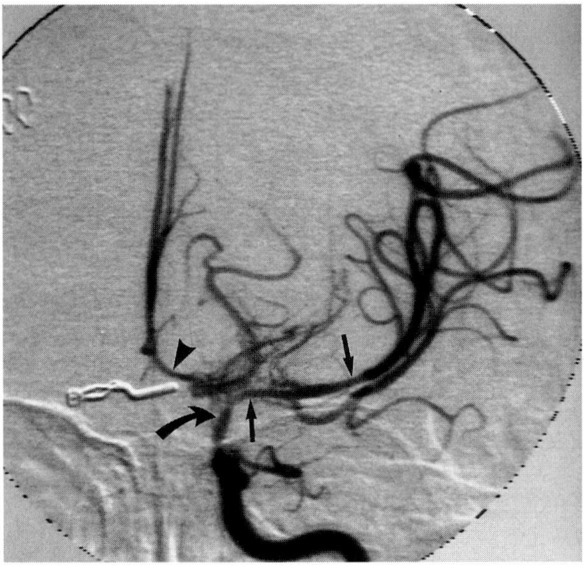

(a)

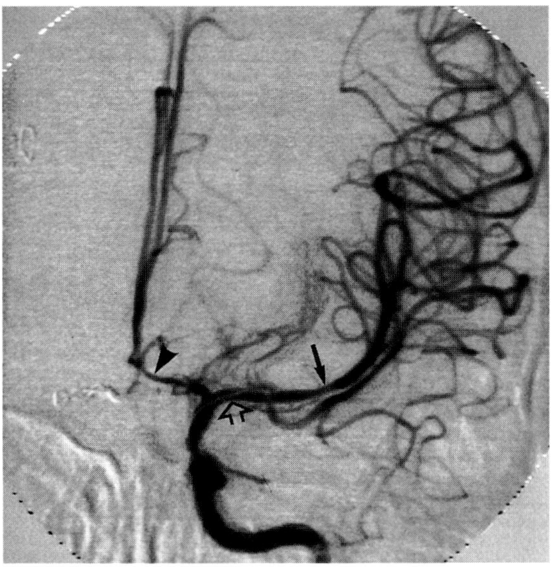

(b)

Figure 7 39-year-old female status/post clipping of a ruptured anterior communicating artery aneurysm. Ten days after the hemorrhage the patient developed aphasia and a

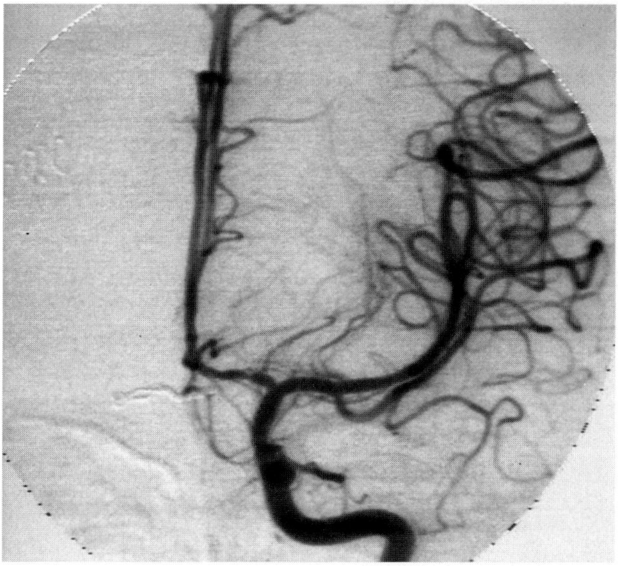

(c)

Figure 7 Continued.
decreased level of consciousness unresponsive to maximal medical therapy. (a) Towne view of the left internal carotid artery demonstrates severe vasospasm involving the supraclinoid internal carotid artery (curved arrow), the M-1 and M-2 segments of the left middle cerebral artery (straight arrows), and the A-1 segment of the left anterior cerebral artery (arrowhead). (b) Towne view of the left internal carotid artery after balloon angioplasty of the supraclinoid internal carotid artery, the M-1 segment of the middle cerebral artery, and the proximal A-1 segment of the anterior cerebral artery. Balloon angioplasty catheter is in the M-1 segment (open arrow). Note the improvement in the diameter of the vessels treated with balloon angioplasty compared to (a) Vasospasm involving the superior M-2 branch of the middle cerebral artery (arrow) and the distal A-1 segment of the anterior cerebral artery (arrowhead) persists. These vessel segments were not amenable to balloon angioplasty. (c) Towne view of the left internal carotid artery after infusion of 150 mg of papaverine over one-half hour into the supraclinoid internal carotid artery via a microcatheter. Note the improvement in diameter of the majority of the left carotid intracranial circulation vessels and in particular the vessels not amenable to balloon angioplasty compared to (b).

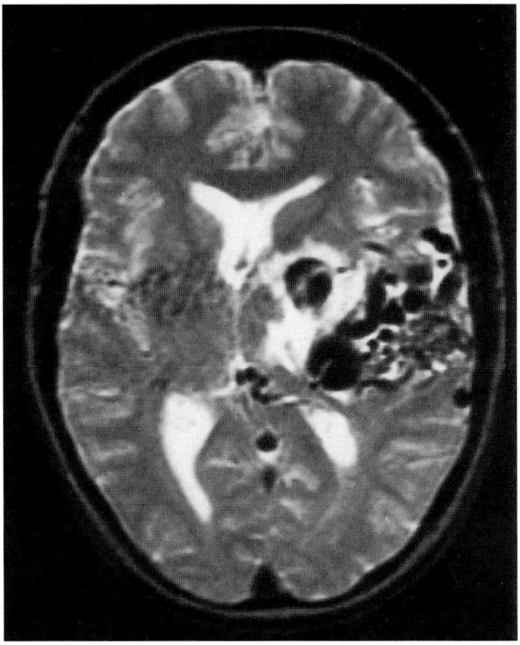

(a)

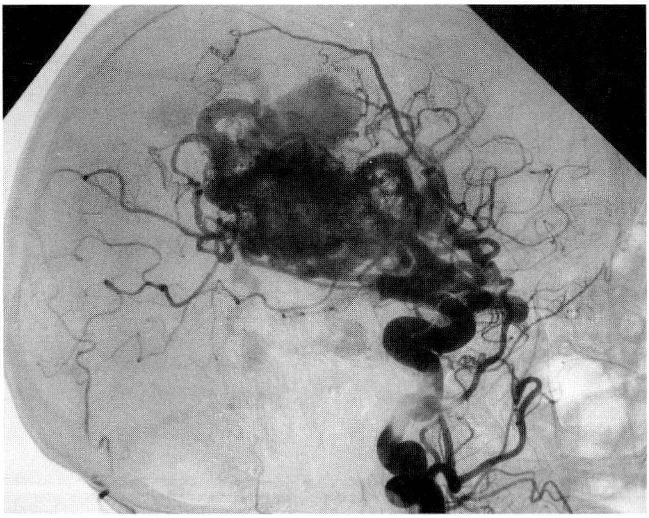

(b)

Figure 8 62-year-old woman with a several month history of worsening right hemiparesis, aphasia, and cognitive difficulties thought to be secondary to "steal" related to the patient's known left cerebral hemisphere AVM. (a) T2-weighted axial MRI demonstrates

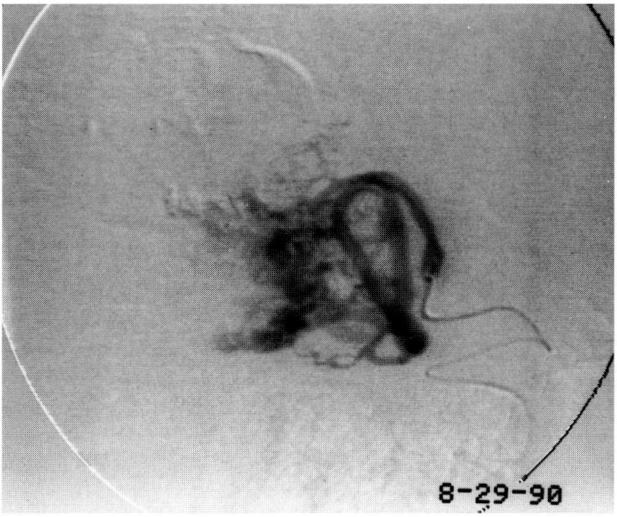

(c)

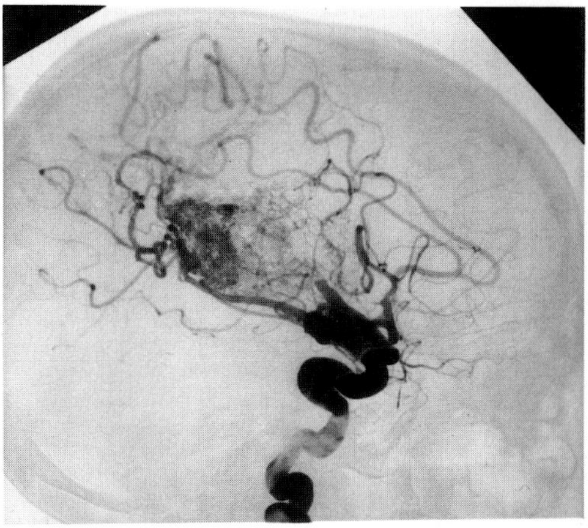

(d)

Figure 8 Continued.
a large left perisylvian AVM. (b) Lateral view of a left carotid angiogram demonstrates the high flow AVM. (c) Superselective lateral digital subtraction angiogram (DSA) obtained after selective catheterization of a frontal opercular branch of the left middle cerebral artery demonstrates opacification of the AVM nidus and no opacification of adjacent normal vasculature. Multiple arterial pedicles to the AVM were embolized with n-BCA. (d) Lateral view of a left carotid angiogram obtained after two embolization procedures demonstrates a decrease in the size of the AVM [compare to (b)]. The patient's "steal" symptoms improved after embolization.

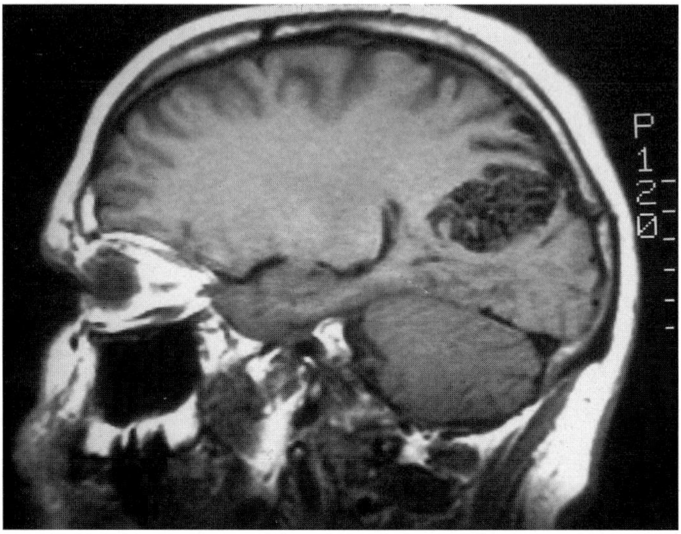

(a)

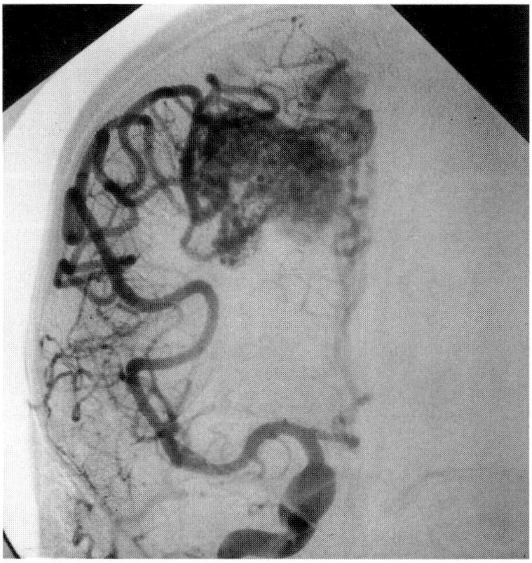

(b)

Figure 9 45-year-old male with history of severe headaches. (a) Sagittal T1-weighted MRI demonstrates a right parietal–occipital AVM. Towne views of the right carotid artery, (b) and left vertebral artery, (c) demonstrate the AVM. (d) AP superselective DSA obtained after catheterization of the parietal–occipital branch of the right posterior cerebral artery prior to embolization with n-BCA. (e) Towne view of the left vertebral artery obtained after

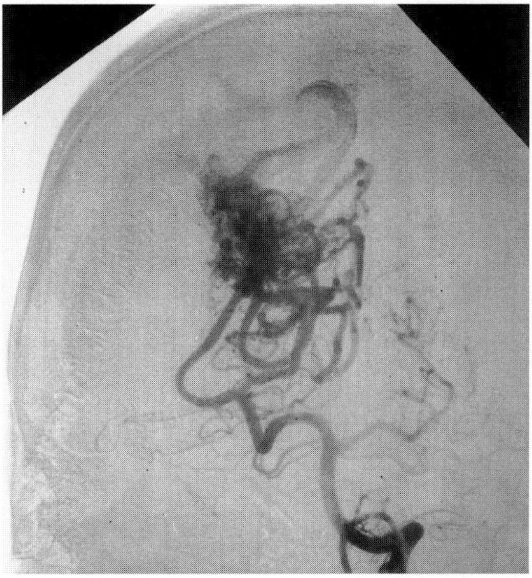

(c)

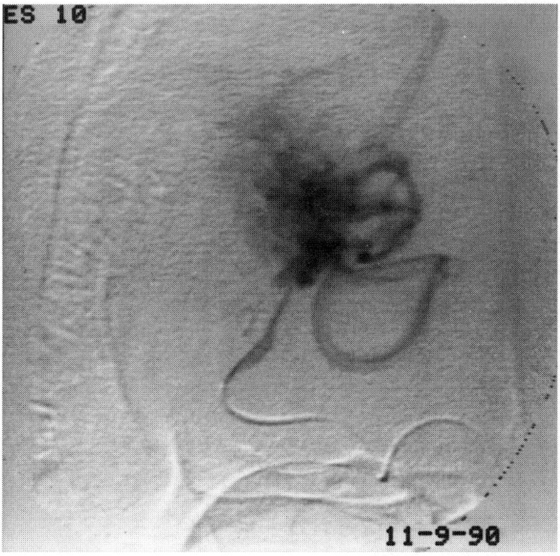

(d)

Figure 9 Continued.
embolization demonstrates significant reduction in size of the AVM nidus [compare to (c)]. Patient was treated with stereotactic radiosurgery. Sagittal T1-weighted MRI, (f) Towne view of the right carotid artery, (g) and Towne view of the left vertebral artery, (h) eighteen months after radiosurgery treatment demonstrate complete obliteration of the AVM.

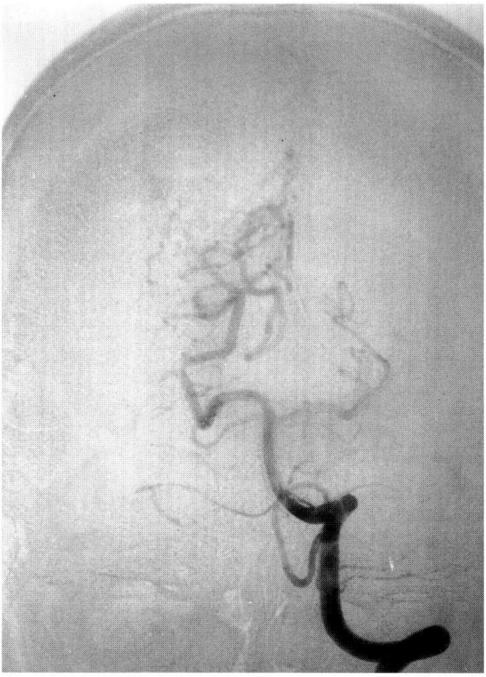

(e)

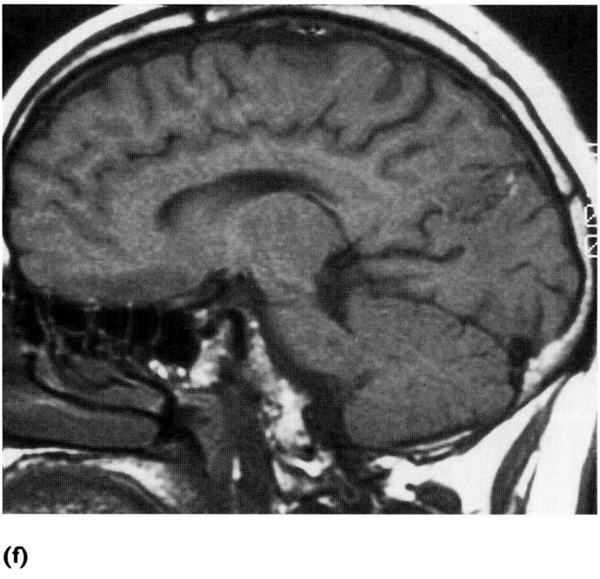

(f)

Figure 9 Continued.

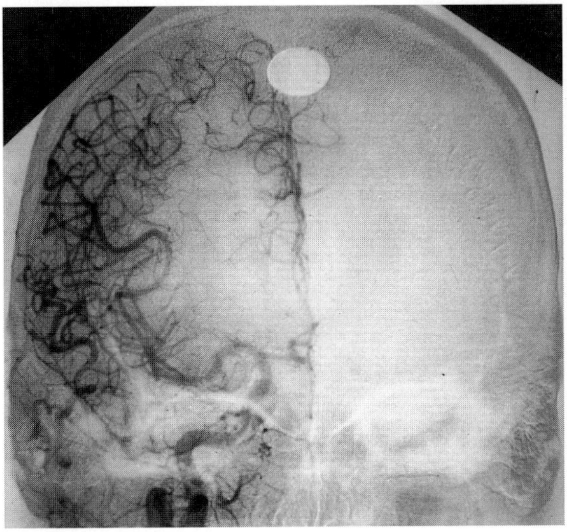

(g)

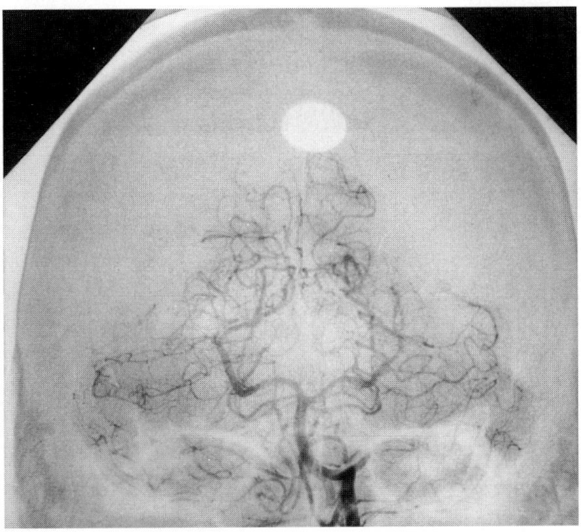

(h)

Figure 9 Continued.

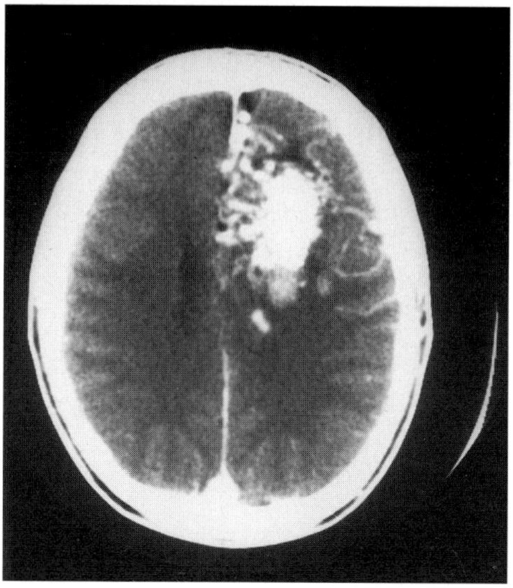

(a)

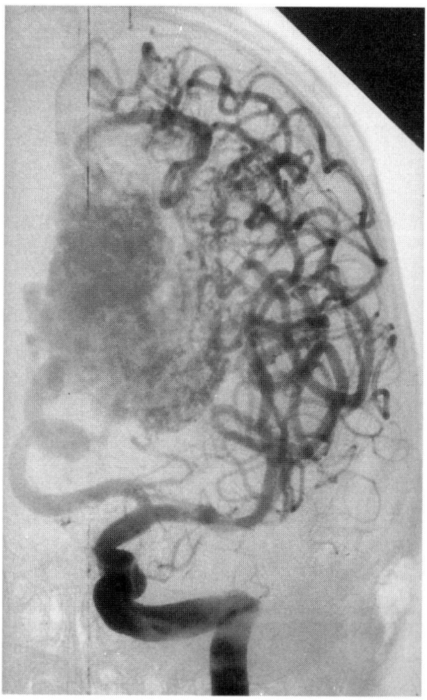

(b)

Figure 10 24-year-old male with seizures secondary to a left mid-frontal AVM. (a) Head CT with contrast demonstrates an approximately 5 cm in diameter left frontal

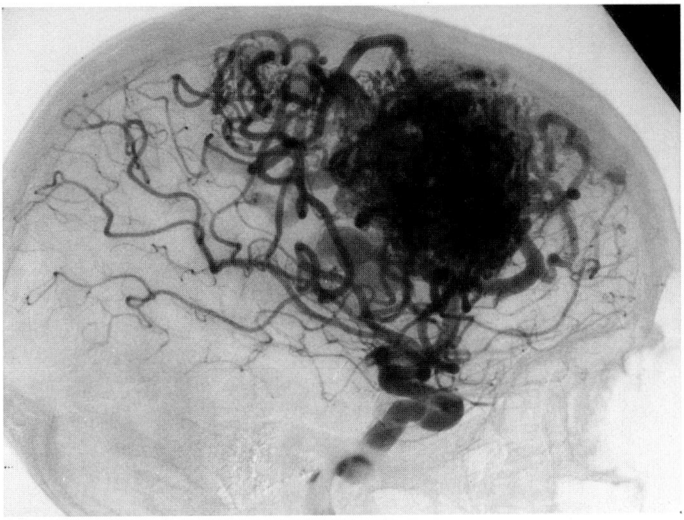

(c)

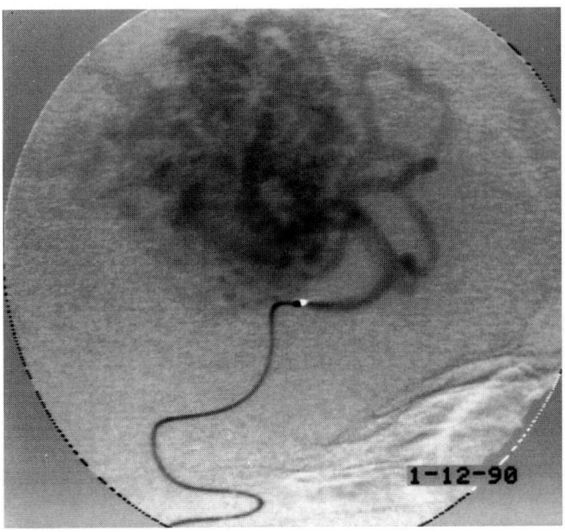

(d)

Figure 10 Continued.
AVM. Towne, (b) and lateral, (c) views of a left internal carotid angiogram demonstrates arterial supply to the AVM to be predominantly from the anterior cerebral circulation. (d). Superselective lateral DSA of the callosal marginal branch of the left anterior cerebral artery obtained before embolization. The AVM was embolized with *n*-BCA and particulate material. (e) Lateral view of the left internal carotid artery obtained after embolization of the anterior cerebral arterial supply to the AVM demonstrates reduction of flow to the AVM. The AVM was subsequently surgically resected without complications.

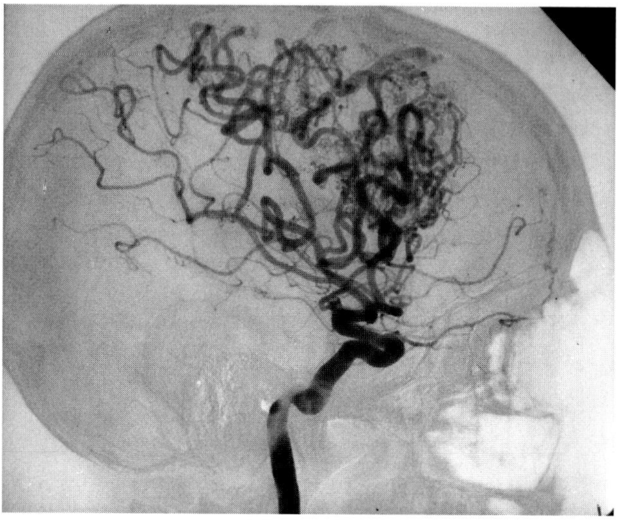

(e)

Figure 10 Continued.

the presence or absence of intranidal aneurysms or arteriovenous fisutlae that are not apparent on the conventional angiogram. This information may influence the choice of an embolic agent. Prior to embolizing the arterial pedicle, 30 mg of amytal is usually injected through the microcatheter in an attempt to predict neurologic dysfunction prior to embolization [42,43]. Superselective intravascular pressure monitoring is performed during the embolization procedure, which gives information regarding whether the embolic material is blocking the AVM nidus or passing through into the venous circulation [44,45].

There is considerable controversy regarding the choice of embolic agents used to embolize brain AVMs [46,47]. Multiple embolic agents are available and can be divided into those that occlude the nidus of the AVM and those that occlude the feeding arterial pedicles to the AVM.

The most commonly used embolic agent to achieve occlusion of the AVM nidus is *n*-butyl cyanoacrylate (n-BCA), a liquid acrylic which polymerizes to a solid when it comes in contact with an ionic solution such as blood. The n-BCA acrylic has the advantage of being able to permanently occlude the nidus of all or a portion of the AVM. Therefore n-BCA is considered by many therapists to be the agent of choice when embolizing an AVM for palliation of steal symptoms, prior to radiosurgery, or when attempting to cure an AVM. The main

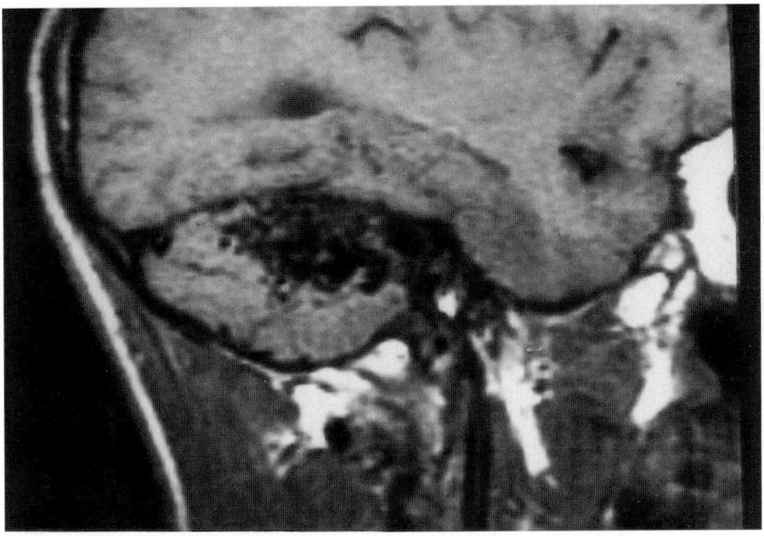

(a)

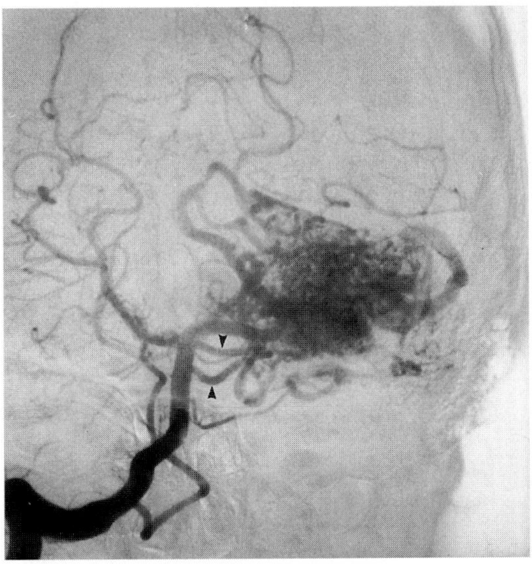

(b)

Figure 11 18-year-old male with a several-year history of severe headaches. (a) Sagittal T1-weighted MRI demonstrates a superior left cerebellar AVM. (b) Towne view of a right vertebral angiogram demonstrates arterial supply to the AVM from two left superior cerebellar arteries (arrowheads). (c) Superselective Towne DSA of one of the left superior

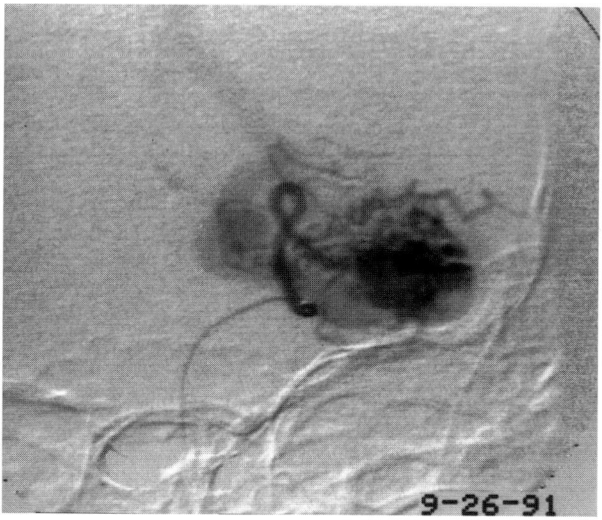

(c)

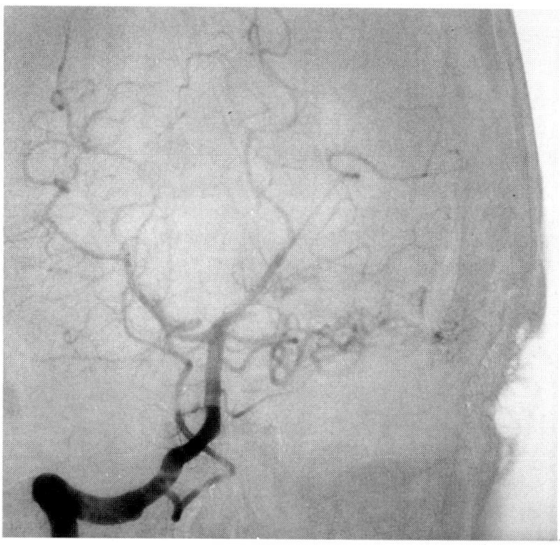

(d)

Figure 11 Continued.
cerebellar arteries prior to embolization. Both superior cerebellar arteries were embolized with particulate material. (d) Towne view of a right vertebral angiogram obtained after embolization demonstrates reduction of flow to the AVM. The AVM was surgically resected without complications.

disadvantage of n-BCA is that it is technically more difficult to use than agents that provide for proximal occlusion of the arterial pedicles to an AVM.

Many embolic agents are available for proximal occlusion of the arterial pedicles to an AVM. The most commonly used materials are polyvinal alcohol particles, silk suture material, microcoils, and detachable microballoons. The main advantage of the agents used for proximal occlusion of arterial pedicles is their relative ease of use compared to n-BCA. Their main disadvantage is their inability to provide a permanent occlusion of the AVM nidus. Therefore, these agents are most commonly used for the preoperative devascularization of brain AVMs.

Complications of embolization of brain AVMs include 1. hemorrhage secondary to perforation of an arterial pedicle during the catheterization process, 2. hemorrhage secondary to blockage of the venous outflow by embolic material while shunting through the AVM persists, and 3. ischemic stroke secondary to distal embolization of clots that form on the catheter or inadvertent embolization of normal arteries. Clinical severity of the complications ranges from mild and transient with complete recovery to severe with profound permanent neurologic deficits, coma, or death.

REFERENCES

1. Peterman SB, Taylor A Jr, Hoffman JC Jr. Improved detection of cerebral hypoperfusion with internal carotid balloon test occlusion and 99m Tc–HMPAO cerebral perfusion SPECT imaging. *AJNR* 1991; 12:1035–1041.
2. Eckard DA, Purdy PD, Bonte FJ. Temporary balloon occlusion of the carotid artery combined with brain blood flow imaging as a test to predict tolerance prior to permanent carotid sacrifice. *AJNR* 1992; 13:1565–1569.
3. Yonas H, Linskey M, Johnson DW, Horton JA, Janeck IP, Witt, JP, et al. Internal carotid balloon test occlusion does require quantitative CBF. (Letter to the editor). *AJNR* 1992; 13:1147–1148.
4. Eskridge JM. The challenge of carotid occlusion. *AJNR* 1991; 12:1053–1054.
5. Higashida RT, Halbach VV, Dowd C, Barnwell SL, Dormandy B, Bell J, et al. Endovascular detachable balloon embolization therapy for cavernous carotid artery aneurysms: results in 87 cases. *J Neurosurg* 1990; 72:857–863.
6. Higashida RT, Halback VV, Dormandy B, Bell JD, Hieshima GB. Endovascular treatment of intracranial aneurysms with a new silicone microballoon device: technical considerations and indications for therapy. *Radiology* 1990; 174:687–691.
7. Rufenacht DA, Nichols DA. A 1.1 F/2.7 F coaxial catheter system for intracranial balloon detachment. Presented at the American Society of Neuroradiology. Washington, D.C., June 9–14, 1991.
8. Fox AJ, Vinuela F, Pelz DM, Peerless Sj, Ferguson GG, Drake CH, et al. Use of detachable balloons for proximal artery occlusion in the treatment of unclippable cerebral aneurysms. *J Neurosurg* 1987; 66:40–46.

9. Strother CM, Lunde S, Graves V, Toutant S, Hieshima GB. Late paraophthalmic aneurysm rupture following endovascular treatment: case report. *J Neurosurg* 1989; 71:777–780.
10. Hodes JE, Fox AJ, Pelz DM, Peerless SJ. Rupture of aneurysms following balloon embolization. *J Neurosurg* 1990; 72:567–571.
11. Kwan ESK, Heilman CB, Shucart WA, Klucznik RP. Enlargement of basilar artery aneurysms following balloon occlusion—"water–hammer effect": report of two cases. *J Neurosurg* 1991; 75:963–968.
12. Graves VB, Partington CR, Rufenacht DA, Rappe AH, Strother CM. Treatment of carotid artery aneurysms with platinum coils: an experimental study in dogs. *AJNR* 1990; 11:249–252.
13. Hilal SK, Chi LT, Khandji A, Friedman D, Cross D, Solomon R. Preshaped thrombogenic coils for the treatment of intracranial aneurysms. Presented at the 28th meeting of the American Society of Neuroradiology. Los Angeles, California, March 19–23, 1990.
14. Graves VB, Strother CM, Rappe AH. Treatment of experimental canine carotid aneurysms with platinum coils. *AJNR* 1993; 14:787–793.
15. Guglielmi G, Vinuela F, Sepetka I, Macellari V. Electrothombosis of saccular aneurysms via endovascular approach: Part 1: Electrochemical basis, technique, and experimental results. *J Neurosurg* 1991; 75:1–7.
16. Guglielmi G, Vinuela F, Dion J. Duckwiler G. Electrothrombosis of saccular aneurysms via endovascular approach: Part 2: Preliminary clinical experience. *J Neurosurg* 1991; 75:8–14.
17. Gugliemli G, Vinuela F, Duckwiler G, Dion J, Lylyk P, Berenstein A., et al. Endovascular treatment of posterior circulation aneurysms by electrothrombosis using electrically detachable coils. *J Neurosurg* 1992; 77:515–524.
18. Casasco AE, Aymard A, Gobin YP, Houdart E, Rogopoulos A, Hodes J, et al. Selective endovascular treatment of 71 intracranial aneurysm with platinum coils. *J Neurosurg* 1993; 79:3–10.
19. Graves VB, Strother CM, Duff TA, et al. Early treatment of ruptured aneurysms with Gugliemli detachable coils: effect on subsequent bleeding. *Neurosurgery* 1995; 37:640–648.
20. McDougall CG, Halbach VV, Dowd CF, et al. Endovascular treatment of basilar tip aneurysms using electrolytically detachable coils. *J Neurosurg* 1996; 84:393–399.
21. Nichols DA, Meyer FB, Piepgras DG. Endovascular treatment of basilar artery aneurysms using Gugliemli deteachable coils. (Abstract). *J Neurosurg* 1994; 80:384A.
22. Nichols DA, Meyer FB, Piepgras DG, Smith PL. Endovascular treatment of intracranial aneurysms. *Mayo Clin Proc* 1994; 69: 272–285.
23. Pierot L, Boulin A, Castaings L, et al. Selective occlusion of basilar aneurysms using controlled deteachable coils: report of 35 cases. *Neurosurgery* 1996; 38: 948–954.
24. Raymond J, Roy D, Bojanowski M, et al. Endovascular treatment of acutely ruptured and unruptured aneurysms of the basilar bifurcation. *J Neurosurg* 1997; 86:211–219.
25. Viñuela F, Duckwiler G, Mawad M. Gugliemli detachable coil embolization of acute

intracranial aneurysm: perioperative anatomical and clinical outcome in 403 patients. *J Neurosurg* 1997; 86:475–482.

26. Nichols DA, Brown RD, Thielen KR, et al. Endovascular treatment of ruptured posterior circulation aneurysms using electrolytically detachable coils. *J Neurosurg*; In press.
27. Zubillage, Gugliemli G, Viñuela F, et al. Endovascular occlusion of intracranial aneurysms with electrically detachable coils: correlation of aneurysm neck size and treatment results. *AJNR* 1994; 15: 815–820.
28. Nichols DA. Guest Editorial: Endovascular treatment of the acutely ruptured intracranial aneurysm. *J Neurosurg* 1993; 79:1–2.
29. Eskridge JM, Newell DW, Pendleton GA. Transluminal angioplasty for treatment of vasospasm. *Neurosurg Clin North Am* April, 1990; 1:387–399.
30. Higashida RT, Halbach VV, Dormandy B, Bell J, Brant-Zawadzki M, Hieshima GB. New microballoon device for transluminal angioplasty of intracranial arterial vasospasm. *AJNR* 1990; 11:233–238.
31. Higashida RT, Halbach VV, Cahan LD, Brant-Zawadzki M, Barnwell S, Dowd C, Hieshima GB. Transluminal angioplasty for treatment of intracranial arterial vasospasm. *J Neurosurg* 1989; 71:648–653.
32. Linskey ME, Horton JA, Rao GR, Yonas H. Fatal rupture of the intracranial carotid artery during transluminal angioplasty for vasospasm induced by subarachnoid hemorrhage: case report. *J Neurosurg* 1991; 74:985–990.
33. Brothers MF, Hedlund LW, Friedman AH. Arterial rupture during "distal" vasospasm angioplasty (abstract). *Neuroradiology* 1991; 33 (Suppl):S155.
34. Kassell NF, Helm G, Simmons N, Phillips CD, Cail WS. Treatment of cerebral vasospasm with intra–arterial papaverine. *J Neurosurg* 1992; 77:848–852.
35. Kaku Y, Yonekawa Y, Tsukahara T, Kasakawa K. Superselective intraarterial infusion of papaverine for treatment of cerebral vasospasm after subarachnoid hemorrhage. *J Neurosurg* 1992; 77:842–847.
36. Berenstein A, Lasjaunias P. Endovascular treatment of cerebral lesions In: Surgical Neurangiography. Vol. 4. Berlin: Springer-Verlag, 1992:186–188.
37. Fox AJ, Girvin JP, Vinuela F, Drake CG. Rolandic arteriovenous malformations: Improvement in limb function by IBC embolization. *AJNR* 1985; 6:575–582.
38. Lunsford LD, Kondziolka D, Flickinger JC, Bissonette DJ, Jungreis CA, Maitz AH. Stereotactic radiosurgery for arteriovenous malformations of the brain. *J Neurosurg* 1991; 75:512–524.
39. Pelz DM, Fox AJ, Vinuela F, Drake CC, Ferguson GG. Preoperative embolization of brain AVMs with Isobutyl–2 cyanoacrylate. *AJNR* 1988; 9:757–764.
40. Viñuela F, Dion JE, Duckwiler G, Martin NA, Lylyk P, Fox A, et al. Combined endovascular embolization and surgery in the management of cerebral arteriovenous malformations: experience with 101 cases. *J Neurosurg* 1991; 75:856–864.
41. Jafar JJ, Davis AJ, Berenstein A, Choi IS, Kupersmith MJ. The effect of embolization with N–butyl cyanoacrylate prior to surgical resection of cerebral arteriovenous malformations. *J Neurosurg* 1993; 78:60–69.
42. Rauch RA, Viñuela F, Dion J, Duckwiler G, Amos EC, Jordan SE, et al. Preemboliza-

tion functional evaluation in brain arteriovenous malformations: the superselective amytal test. *AJNR* 1992; 13:303–308.

43. Rauch RA, Vinuela F, Dion J, Duckwiler G, Amos EC, Jordan SE, et al. Preembolization functional evaluation in brain arteriovenous malformations: the ability to superselective amytal test to predict neurologic dysfunction before embolization. *AJNR* 1992; 13:309–314.
44. Jungreis CA, Horton JA, Hecht ST. Hemodynamic changes in feeders to cerebral arteriovenous malformations during therapeutic embolization. *AJNR* 1989; 10: 1057–60.
45. Duckwiler G, Dion J, Vinuela F, Jabour B, Martin N, Bentson J. Intravascular microcatheter pressure monitoring: experimental results and early clinical evaluation. *AJNR* 1990; 11:169–175.
46. Purdy PD, Batjer HH, Risser RC, Samson D. Arteriovenous malformations of the brain: choosing embolic materials to enhance safety and ease of excision. *J Neurosurg* 1992; 77:217–222.
47. Editors Berenstein A, Lasjaunias P. Endovascular treatment of cerebral lesions In: Surgical Neurangiography. Vol. 4. Berlin: Springer-Verlag, 1992:186–188.

18

Rehabilitation After Subarachnoid Hemorrhage

Jeffrey R. Basford
Mayo Clinic and Mayo Foundation, Rochester, Minnesota

I. INTRODUCTION

Subarachnoid hemorrhage (SAH) produces cognitive and neurological deficits that range from the devastating to the minimal. The most devastating effects—coma, death and massive neurological injury—are well known. Less dramatic motor and cognitive effects are also well recognized and frequent. Nevertheless, 60–75% of SAH survivors may be "functionally" independent and have little or no significant motor or sensory deficits a year after the event [1,2]. However many of these survivors may suffer from unrecognized subtle cognitive and emotional effects [3–6]. This chapter reviews SAH rehabilitation and outlines rehabilitation approaches that may be helpful for the seriously impaired survivors as well as for those with milder sequelae.

Rehabilitation is a pragmatic science and the etiology of a central nervous system (CNS) injury is far less important than the impairment it produces. Despite this, two aspects of SAH, hemorrhage and vasospasm, are particularly relevant to rehabilitation. Hemorrhage is important due to the lethargy, confusion, and altered mental status that accompany its toxic effects in the subarachnoid space. Vasospasm is significant due to its association with ischemia and deficits beyond those resulting from hemorrhage alone [7–10]. Surprisingly, the site of hemorrhage, perhaps because of the diffuse location of blood in the cerebral spinal fluid (CSF), seems to have little association with outcome [8,11–15]. In any event cognitive deficits such as confusion, amnesia, and agitation [16,17] are often issues during early recovery with mood, judgment, and emotional lability having more importance in the later stages.

Subarachnoid hemorrhage accounts for only about 5% [1] of all strokes and as few as 7–20% of those with SAH may have clear physical impairments a year after the event [3]. This is a far different picture than that produced by the more common ischemic and intraparenchymal hemorrhagic strokes. As a result, SAH rehabilitation is often not addressed in discussions of stroke rehabilitation. In fact, SAH rehabilitation with its emphasis of diffuse cognitive issues in many ways more nearly approaches that of traumatic brain injury. This chapter follows this latter pattern, and gross motor rehabilitation, while important for some individuals, is not stressed here. The interested reader is referred to easily available texts and rehabilitation handbooks [18,19].

This chapter begins with a review of SAH rehabilitation in general. Next, it discusses specific aspects of the rehabilitation process for those with both severe and less major consequences. It then concludes with the suggestion that even SAH survivors with seemingly excellent outcomes be followed for cognitive and emotional problems that may interfere with family life and work.

II. ACUTE REHABILITATION

SAH rehabilitation, as is true for rehabilitation in general, should begin with early assessment, prevention of medical and musculoskeletal complications, and as rapid a progression of therapy as possible. The approach to each patient is individualized and will depend on that patient's presentation and rate of recovery. In some cases deficits will appear so minor that rehabilitation and therapy seem unnecessary. Regardless, since emotional and cognitive sequelae are possible in all patients, warnings about potential difficulties with concentration, emotional control, and anxiety, coupled with careful followup, are necessary.

Rehabilitation is clearly necessary for those with major deficits. In the most severe situations, initial efforts may be restricted to avoiding complications with a program of positioning; range of motion (ROM); bowel, bladder and skin care; family (and at times, staff) education; and cognitive stimulation.

The latter aspect, orientation and stimulation, takes place to some extent during any therapy session because even the simplest program involves verbal, tactile, and proprioceptive interaction between the patient and the therapist. Formalized and more intense programs involving the therapist, family, and staff are necessary for those with the most severe injuries. These programs are outlined in more detail below.

A. Specific Issues of Acute Rehabilitation

Controversy over the timing, intensity, benefits, and cost effectiveness exists in all areas of rehabilitation. Even for ischemic stroke with its high incidence and where outcomes have been studied for years, quantitative results have been elusive due to stroke variability, individualized treatment, and the lack of well-accepted quantitative outcome measures [20–23]. For SAH, with an incidence a small percentage of that of ischemic stroke [1], the difficulties are only more pronounced. Despite, this, there is evidence that early rehabilitation speeds recovery, reduces costs and lessens lengths of hospital stay for CNS injury in general [24–27]. As these findings agree with clinical experience, most involved in rehabilitation feel that comprehensive therapy programs are necessary for appropriate patients.

B. Therapy in the Acute Setting

Although the general approaches of early SAH rehabilitation, cognitive stimulation, rapid mobilization, and the limitation of complications have been outlined above, there are a number of issues that deserve fuller discussion.

1. Orientation and Stimulation

The extent, duration, and optimal approach to orientation and cognitive stimulation programs is debatable. Despite this, the approach is based on a number of reasonable premises. One of these is the concept that since a healthy mind grows best in a rich environment [28], a confused mind should also benefit from stimulation and orientating cues. In addition there is experimental evidence that stimulation improves cognition and counteracts neuro-anatomic changes seen in sensory deprived animals [29,30]. The jump to applying these concepts to humans does not seem excessive and controlled studies have shown that coma duration is shorter in those patients given an intensive, comprehensive stimulation program [31].

Stimulation programs for the comatose, or near comatose patient, ideally utilize all the senses—touch, sound, sight, smell, taste, and temperature sensing—in an attempt to speed orientation and cognitive recovery. Initially these programs are administered by a trained therapist, usually an occupational therapist (OT) on a twice a day schedule. Family involvement is encouraged from the outset as multiple brief episodes are thought to be the most effective, and family members should have the best rapport with the patient. In theory, the family and nursing staff can provide as complete and intense a program as the therapist. In practice, family reticence is often quite strong and nurses are subject to conflicting, and often more acute, care needs of other patients. Thus, while family members often assist with auditory input and bringing items (e.g., photographs, audio tapes) from home that are significant for the patient, they are frequently hesitant to work with more abstract modalities such as smell, light, and touch. In any event, the family and staff are instructed in the benefits of frequent short visits with a limited number of visitors, maintenance of a day–

night cycle, limiting stimulation intensity, orientation techniques, and alterations of the background environment (e.g., television and radio).

The therapist will frequently have a preassembled stimulation kit of items that are purposefully kept simple and easily duplicated by the patient's family. (For example terry cloth and sandpaper may be used for tactile sensation, voices and television for auditory input, photographs and flashlights for visual stimulation, sugar for taste, vanilla and citrus peels for smell, and a moist washcloth for warmth or cold.)

2. Physical Therapy

If the patient's consciousness remains severely depressed, the physical therapist's (PT's) role may be limited to preventing contractures and reducing tone with ROM, assistance with cognitive stimulation, and assisting nursing with mobilization. As the patient's condition improves, therapy will advance to "dangling" (sitting) on the side of the bed, transfers, standing balance, and ambulation. With further improvement, the patient may be taken to the therapy department to begin more focused efforts on ambulation, endurance, stair climbing, and addressing any focal motor deficits that might exist.

3. Occupational Therapy

The occupational therapist's (OT's) role in cognitive stimulation was outlined above. In addition, OTs are important in SAH rehabilitation because of their role in ADL (activities of daily living) training, swallowing assessment (often in conjunction with a speech therapist), safety and judgement evaluation, upper extremity function, and, particularly when the patient is too confused or aphasic to permit psychometric testing, cognitive assessment. For the SAH patient, where physical deficits may be relatively mild, the OT's role in safety assessment, home evaluation, and a "predriving" assessment may be invaluable.

Social services, speech therapy, and psychology all have varying and important roles during rehabilitation. At times they are essential for assessment and therapy during the initial period of hospitalization. However, the full impact of their benefits is often delayed until later in the hospitalization when the patient's alertness and improved level of cooperation permit fuller utilization of their resources.

III. REHABILITATION UNIT

Transfer to a rehabilitation unit is reserved for patients with deficits that are severe enough to require continuation of rehabilitation following the initial period of hospitalization, but which are not severe enough to preclude significant gains in function and independence with a further program of more intensive and comprehensive therapy. Lethargy may make assessment difficult, but transfer will typically require that the patient is actively participating in therapy and remembering new skills (if not the sessions) from day to day. Speed of improvement, safety, comorbidities, living situation, social support, as well as patient and family desires are also important considerations in any transfer considerations.

In short, the patient who will benefit the most from transfer to a rehabilitation unit is one who continues to have significant deficits but who has the capacity to regain independence, is working hard and acquiring new skills in therapy, has good social support, and has no insurmountable comorbidity or home accessibility issues. Frequently, decisions are relatively easy to make—the patient, family, team, and physician are all in agreement. In other cases the patient's goals may seem possible but extremely optimistic. In these situations an honest discussion with either a two week "trial" or temporary deferral of a rehabilitation unit stay may be the best approach.

The initial roles of the physical therapist and occupational therapist were described above. The responsibilities of the other members of the rehabilitation team are also important but were not well detailed. These are sketched below.

A. Physician

Rehabilitation physicians are typically board certified in Physical Medicine and Rehabilitation, but at times may be a neurologist or other physician with rehabilitation knowledge and skills. The physician's responsibilities are to medically assess and care for the patient, prevent complications and, with assistance from the team, coordinate the rehabilitation program.

B. Medical Issues

Medical issues can be important. The young individual with no medical problems other than the SAH itself has far fewer needs than an ill, debilitated elderly person with a history of poor medical care. Despite this, even the young, healthy patient has a number of issues that deserve consideration.

1. Deep Venous Thrombosis

Deep venous thrombosis (DVT) and pulmonary embolism are relatively common in patients with brain injury and stroke. Much, although not all, of the increased probability is due to the immobilization that accompanies the early stages of these processes. Whatever the cause, lower extremity vascular screening, (e.g., impedance plethysmography (IPG) or ultrasound) is reasonable for patients with SAH who have been immobile or have had paresis of a lower extremity. If evidence of a DVT is found, the evaluation is expanded and treatment begun with anticoagulation or filters as appropriate. In the absence of findings, routine protective measures such as rapid mobilization, follow-up scans, pneumatic leg compression, compressive stocking, and, in some cases, low-dose heparin are used.

2. Hydrocephalus

Hydrocephalus can occur after SAH and in some series 12–25% of SAH patients require shunting [32,33]. Classically, gait deterioration, urinary incontinence, and confusion are associated with hydrocephalus. In practice this seldom occurs in a rehabilitation unit because even subtle deterioration of performance is detected in therapy before a full complex manifests itself. Electrolyte disturbances and seizures associated with CNS are also relatively common and need to be monitored.

3. General Medical Care

Hypertension, diabetes mellitus, renal insufficiency and basic health-care maintenance may not be well evaluated during the initial hospitalization. These issues, as well as mammograms, pelvic examinations, and immunizations (influenza, pneumonia, and tetanus) should be considered and can usually be completed in the rehabilitation unit without interfering with a patient's progress.

C. Requirement for a Rehabilitation Unit

1. What Does Rehabilitation after Subarachnoid Hemorrhage Require?

Inpatient SAH rehabilitation requires a comprehensive therapy program and specialized facilities. Accreditation by organizations such as CARF (Committee for the Accreditation of Rehabilitation Facilities) or JCAHO (Joint Committee on the Accreditation of Healthcare Organizations), while helpful in evaluating rehabilitation programs, is not essential. At times the location of a program in the vicinity of a patient's home and family may be as important a criteria as nuances of therapy and quality of care. At other times, unique resources and a particular program may be required. At the very least, what is essential is an able staff with experience in neurological and cognitive rehabilitation.

2. What Are the "Bricks and Mortar" of a Rehabilitation Unit?

Rehabilitation units may be either free standing or attached to a hospital or skilled nursing facility. For a patient with an acute SAH, a hospital-attached unit seems necessary until medical and surgical stability is established. Ideally the unit will have the therapy areas (physical, occupational, speech, and recreational) as well as psychology, social service and examination, dining, and meeting areas contiguous with the nursing area.

Units should be self-contained and located out of the main flow of hospital traffic. In addition, many units will use magnetized clothing tags, door alarms, and closed circuit television (CCTV) as well as a few specific rooms for the most disoriented and agitated patients to enhance surveillance. These approaches are not infallible and more than one "confused" patient has left a rehabilitation unit despite the best efforts of the staff.

Physical therapy requires large open areas with contiguous "quiet" rooms to permit therapy of easily distractable, agitated, or disruptive patients. Equipment essentials are quite basic and include, in addition to the open areas, parallel bars, exercise platforms ("mats"), wall railings, short flights of stairs, gait aides, orthoses, and simple exercise equipment. Automobile mock-ups are helpful for training in car transfers but complex equipment such as ergonometers, biofeedback devices, and electrical stimulators has remained a surprisingly marginal need for most patients.

Occupational therapy also requires open areas and quiet rooms. Equipment needs are more prominent than in physical therapy but remain straightforward: adjustable tables, adapted equipment (e.g., dressing aides, eating, and hygiene utensils), cognitive assessment tools, fine motor training aides, computers and learning software, and orthotic fabrication supplies. Also important is a small workshop and an "apartment" with a kitchen and bathroom to permit realistic ADL training, home safety evaluation and overnight stays (if a stay at home is not feasible) prior to returning home.

Recreational therapy, despite its misnomer, is often an extremely important component of rehabilitation due to its emphasis on "community reentry" and the adaption of skills learned in the other therapies to more lifelike situations (e.g., working on a wood project to assist in task sequencing and improve fine motor skills). Space requirements include a large open area with easily accessible tables, craft supplies, game, and computer learning software. The recreational therapist often directs the first trip out of the hospital for the SAH patient and accessible transportation must be available.

Speech pathology, psychology, and social services as well as specialized therapies such as bowel and bladder training, all require accessible, quiet rooms for testing, treatment, and counseling. Conference rooms and classrooms for family education are also essential, although, with careful scheduling, multipurpose rooms can serve several functions and reduce space requirements.

Staffing and floor space requirements for a comprehensive unit are obviously considerable. For example, a 60-bed unit with the capabilities outlined above, might require 1400 m^2 (15,000 ft^2) of floor space and a full-time staff of 170: 23 PTs, 20 OTs, 65 nurses, five speech pathologists, five RTs, two psychologists, three social workers, four physicians as well as desk clerks, orderlies, secretaries and administrative personnel.

D. Length of Stay

The goal of rehabilitation is the return of a patient to the maximal level of independence possible. Despite this, rehabilitation in the rehabilitation unit may be involved in only a portion of this task: helping patients return to their home environment in a way that will maximize their current independence and facilitate further improvement over the longer term. As a result, complete restoration of baseline function, or maximal independence, is seldom a goal of a rehabilitation-unit stay.

Patients with relatively mild deficits may be in a rehabilitation unit for only a few days. For those with more severe impairments, rehabilitation may last two to three or even four weeks and display an overall rhythm: initial bedside therapy, increased endurance, more intensive therapy, conferences with the team and family, passes home, and discharge to outpatient therapy. "Full" recovery may require the efforts of a large number of additional vocational and rehabilitation agencies for a prolonged period over and above the rehabilitation unit stay.

E. Medication Used at the Rehabilitation Unit

Anticonvulsants, steroids, and calcium channel blockers are widely used during the initial course of SAH. As the steroids and calcium channel blockers are routinely discontinued early in the recovery period, their use is not discussed here. Anticonvulsant use, however, which is more persistent and controversial, does require discussion.

1. Anticonvulsants

The duration, frequency, and aggressiveness of seizure prophylaxis following CNS injury is declining rapidly. In the past, prophylactic treatment for a year or two was common. Now, with more awareness of the low incidence of seizures and more attention to potential cognitive impairment as a result of their use, prophylaxis of a seizure-free patient may last only a few weeks or months. Much of the treatment in this area is subjective and based on statistics: risks and benefits of any course should be carefully discussed with the patient and their family.

Phenytoin can be administered intravenously and as a result will probably remain the most common prophylactic anticonvulsants during the acute SAH period. If prolonged anticonvulsant therapy is necessary, a case can be made for switching to alternative agents such as carbamazepine in the hopes of improved alertness and cognition. Practice varies, however, and any alternative should be discussed in detail with the family.

2. "Rehabilitation" Medication

There is no uniform approach to the use of drugs to speed progress or improve cognition during rehabilitation. Nonetheless, theory and clinical experience support a trial of medication in a number of situations. The most common of these are discussed below.

a. *Lethargy, inattention, and distractibility*

Stimulants are often used to treat lethargy, inattention, and distractibility. Initial use was probably simple minded and pragmatic. Either as an attempt to "wake up" a poorly responsive patient, or in analogy with attentional deficit children, to improve attention and lessen distractibility. In any event, usage for these indications is bolstered by animal studies [34–36] and a few human investigations [37–39] that show that skill learning is enhanced following stroke if amphetamines are given in conjunction with instruction.

Day-to-day variations in patient behavior and the normal pattern of recovery makes quantitative evaluation of effectiveness difficult. Despite this, low doses of amphetamines or 5 to 10 mg of methylphenidate two or three times a day are well tolerated and often seem to produce quite dramatic results for lethargic, inattentive, or distractable patients. As disturbed sleep patterns are common in this patient population, treatment at 8:00 A.M. and noon might first be tried with the addition of doses later in the day as necessary. Seizure induction is not a concern with methylphenidate as this drug does not seem to lower seizure thresholds [40]. Who will benefit from stimulant therapy is difficult to establish prior to treatment and a trial with patients whose progress seems limited by lethargy, distractibility, or difficulty in initiating tasks seems reasonable. Both seriously and mildly impaired patients should be evaluated as stimulants may be the most beneficial for the severely impaired patient [40]. Benefits, if any, should be apparent within a few doses. If benefits are definite the drug should be maintained for a week or so followed by a trial of tapering. If benefits are equivocal, the drug should be discontinued or the dosage adjusted.

b. *Agitation, restlessness, and aggression*

Agitation, restlessness, and aggression are common following SAH with their presence ranging from the combative patient to the restless, sleepless individual incapable of completing a task and requiring constant reassurance. Initial treatment should involve reassurance, a calm environment, patience, and unobtrusive supervision. Often a few days of (grueling) "one-on-one" supervision during which the patient roams with nonconfrontational direction will produce a quieting of behavior. When it does not, the performance and safety of the patient, the staff and the other patients is jeopardized. At this point medication trials are reasonable.

Controlled medical trials are difficult to perform and limited in number. Not surprisingly, a wide variety of drugs (β-blockers, neuroleptics, carbamazepine, lithium, calcium channel blockers, and minor tranquilizers) are used on theoretical or pragmatic grounds with variable benefit. The most common of these are discussed below.

β–Blockers. Propranolol gained widespread use as a treatment of agitation following a report in 1977 of benefits in seven patients with anoxic and traumatic brain injury [41]. Subsequent studies, many of them controlled [42], have found several adrenergic blockers effective for agitation in a variety of organic brain dysfunctions [43]. In view of the relative safety of these medications, and the unclear benefits of alternatives, these drugs, particularly propranolol, are frequently used to treat disabling but nonemergent agitation.

Propranolol is usually begun at 20 mg one to three times a day and is increased by about 60 mg/day at three-day intervals. Patient selection is subject to the same restrictions as for any use, i.e., avoidance of asthma, diabetes mellitis, and cardiac failure. Our experience is similar to that of others: high dosages (e.g., 500+ mg/day) are well tolerated and may be needed. Effects may take several weeks to become apparent [40,42]. As a result it is often unclear whether improvement is due to medication or neurological improvement. For this reason, frequent attempts at a tapered reduction of use are necessary.

Neuroleptics. An experienced and trained staff is more tolerant [24,44] and more adept at avoiding disruptive behavior than is an untrained staff. In practice agitated and combative patients are rarer than might be expected. Nevertheless, abrupt aggressive outbursts occur. While forbearance is often the best treatment, the patient's behavior, staff training, and staffing levels do not always permit this. The allure of a medical solution increases as risk, stress, and behavior escalate.

Neuroleptics, particularly haloperidol, are the most commonly used medications when rapid control is necessary. Unfortunately, in addition to their well-known side effects, these drugs can lower seizure thresholds and should be tapered following long-term use [40]. Reports that neurological recovery is slowed in brain-injured animals given neuroleptics are also of concern [34].

Carbamazepine, lithium, and calcium channel blockers may also be effective treatments of agitation associated with organic brain dysfunction. Unfortunately, the evaluation of these and other drugs in this role is limited [40,42,45–47]. Sedatives, antihistamines, and minor tranquilizers are usually avoided due to concerns about sedation and impaired learning.

c. Dystonia and movement disorders

Although uncommon in SAH, movement disorders and dystonia can occur and be disabling. Treatment with ROM and prolonged terminal stretching, along with supplementary approaches such as air splints, is often effective. If these approaches do not provide significant relief, a trial of carbidopa-levadopa (beginning with low dosages and advancing to parkinsonian levels) is usually well tolerated and occasionally remarkably effective. Duration of need may be limited and periodic tapers are necessary. Baclofen, diazepam, and dantrolene are used upon occasion, but are avoided by many physicians due to their side effects and frequently limited benefits. If simple measures fail, review by a specialist in movement disorders may be beneficial.

d. Mood disturbance

Dysphoria associated with SAH is common and probably normal as the patients adjust to a new and different situation. Support by the family and rehabilitation staff, counseling by the psychologist, and watchful waiting seem to be the best initial approaches. If the patient performs fully in therapy, eats well, sleeps well, and seems to be adjusting well, there is little else that can or should be done. However, if progress stalls, sleep and appetite deteriorate, or the patient voices feelings of despair, worthlessness, or suicide, antidepressants and psychiatric evaluation are necessary. Mania and euphoria seem far less common and are usually less severe.

e. Insomnia

Patients with SAH may have profoundly altered sleep patterns and stay awake for phenomenal periods. While this may or may not be distressing for the patient, it can exacerbate confusion, is difficult for the staff to deal with and is impossible for the family to surmount if it doesn't resolve. Treatment depends first on establishing the patient's premorbid sleep habits (more than one nightworker has resisted all efforts at a nighttime sleep schedule), keeping a good sleep log and preventing (as much as possible) daytime napping. If these efforts are ineffective, a trial with nighttime sedation is reasonable. Preferences vary, but many will try low doses of sedating antidepressants with low anticholinergic effects such as trazedone in hopes that it will improve sleep patterns as well as ameliorate any underlying depression.

f. Disposition

Discharge of an individual from the hospital with SAH-associated deficits severe enough to require inpatient rehabilitation requires careful planning. Options depend on social support, recovery, comorbidities, and premorbid living situation. A healthy spouse, limited physical and cognitive deficits, an accessible home (e.g., single floor, one step entrance) foretell a good chance at a successful return to home. An isolated individual barely coping with life before a SAH will have a much more difficult time.

Severely impaired memory, poor judgement, speech and language limitations, and inability to perform most ADLs without assistance preclude a return to independent living in the absence of a committed family. Aphasia may present less of a problem than mildly impaired judgement and visual–spatial skills due to the supervision that these latter deficits may require. For all but the least involved, the social worker is invaluable in planning and coordinating passes; scheduling care conferences; obtaining welfare benefits and home services, and initiating vocational rehabilitation.

IV. REHABILITATION AFTER HOSPITALIZATION

As was noted above, even though 60–75% or more of those who have survived a ruptured intracranial aneurysm are left with minimal or no physical deficits [2,14], many will have cognitive and emotional problems that prevent full return to family life and work. In fact, while SAH survivors often demonstrate minimal deficiencies on psychometric testing six months to a year following injury [11,48], significant psychological residuals may be present in about half of those who have returned to "premorbid function" [48].

The relative impact of an SAH itself and the effect of an acute, terrifying, life-threatening event are impossible to fully separate [6]. Whatever the cause, many studies find that SAH patients with "good" clinical outcomes report excessive problems with fatigue, anxiety, aggression, concentration, emotional lability, social interaction, and mood that interfere with life and work [4,14,49–51]. Prediction of who will have such trouble is difficult and it should be remembered that while vasospasm may produce specific deficits [9], and that outcome may correlate with the amount of subarachnoid blood [52], the presence or absence of objective findings on imaging may not correlate with morbidity [53].

As a result, careful followup is essential. For those with severe sequelae, continued therapy, cognitive training, and intensive, prolonged vocational rehabilitation efforts may be necessary. For those with less severe impairment, empathetic questioning and concern about social adjustment, work, family life, and depression may be all that is needed. Medication changes, vocational rehabilitation, psychological counseling, and social support needs should be assessed at each visit. For all patients, attentive listening, open discussion, and help with problem solving is essential.

REFERENCES

1. Bamford J, Sandercock P, Dennis M, Burn J, Warlow C. A prospective study of acute cerebrovascular disease in the community: the Oxfordshire Community Stroke Project—1981–86. 2. Incidents, case fatality rates and overall outcome at 1 year of cerebro infarction, primary intracerebral and subarachnoid hemorrhage. *J Neurol Neuro Surg Psych* 1990; 53:16–22.
2. Saveland H, Hillman J, Brandt L, Edner G, Jakobsson KE, Algers G. Overall outcome in aneurysmal subarachnoid hemorrhage. *J Neurosurg* 1992; 76:729–734.
3. Lindeberg M, Anggquist KA, Fodstad H, Fugl-Meyer K, and Fugl-Meyer AR. Self–reported prevalence of disability after subarachnoid haemorrhage, with special emphasis on return to leisure and work. *Brit J of Neurosurg* 1992; 6:297–304.
4. Saveland H, Sonesson B, Ljunggren B, Brandt L, Uski T, Zygmunt S, Hindfelt B. Outcome evaluation following subarachnoid hemorrhage. *J Neurosurg* 1986; 64: 191–196.
5. Deruty R, Patet JD, Mottolese C, Portilla F. Long–term outcome of the management of ruptured intracranial aneurysm. *Neurological Research* 1988; 10:217–220.
6. McKenna P, Willison JR, Phil B, Lowe D, Neil-Dwyer G. Cognitive outcome and quality of life one year after subarachnoid haemorrhage. *Neurosurgery* 1989; 24: 361–367.
7. Adams CBT, Loach AB, O"laoire S. Intracranial aneurysms: analysis of results of microneursurgery. *Br Med J* 1976; 2:607–609.
8. Loach AB, DeAzevedo HRC. Some observations on the microneurosurgical treatment of intracranial aneurysms. Acta Neurochir 1976; 35:97–103.
9. Vilkki J, Holst P, Ohman J, Servo A, Heiskanen O. Cognitive deficits related to computed tomographic findings after surgery for a ruptured intracranial aneurysm. *Neurosurgery* 1989; 25:166–172.
10. Hijdra A, Van Gijn J, Stefanko S, Van Dongen KJ, Vermeulen M, Van Crevel H. Delayed cerebral ischemia after aneurysmal subarachnoid hemorrhage: clinicoanatomic correlations. *Neurology* 1986; 36:329–333.
11. Richardson JTE. Cognitive performance following rupture and repair of intracranial aneurysm. *Acta Neurol Scand* 1991; 83:110–122.
12. Artiola I, Fortuny L, Prieto-Valiente L. Long–term prognosis in surgically treated intracranial aneurysms. Part 2: Morbidity. *J Neurosurg* 1981; 54:35–43.
13. Hutter BO, Gilsbach JM. Cognitive deficits after rupture and early repair of anterior communicating artery aneurysms. *Acta Neurochir (Wien)* 1992; 116:6–13.
14. Desantis A, Laiacona M, Barbarotto R, et al. Neuropsychological outcome of patients operated upon for an intracranial aneurysm: analysis of general prognostic factors and of the effects of the location of the aneurysm. *Journal of Neurology, Neurosurgery, and Psychiatry* 1989; 52:1135–1140.

15. Smith B. Cerebral Pathology in Subarachnoid Haemorrhage. *J Neurol Neurosurg Psychiat* 1963; 26:535–539.
16. Vilkki J. Amensic syndromes after surgery of anterior communicating artery aneurysms. *Cortex* 1985; 21:431–444.
17. Alexander MP, Freedman M. Amnesia after anterior communicating artery aneurysm rupture. *Neurology* 1984; 34:752–757.
18. Garrison SJ, Rolak LA. Rehabilitation of the stroke patient. In: DeLisa JA, Currie DM, Gans BM, Cet al., (Eds.). Rehabilitation Medicine. 2nd Ed. Philadelphia: J. B. Lippincott Company, 1988.
19. Anderson TP. Rehabilitation of patients with completed stroke. In: Kottke FJ, Lehmann JF, (Eds.). Krusen's Handbook of Physical Medicine and Rehabilitation. 4th ed. Philadelphia: W. B. Saunders, 1990:656.
20. Keith RA M.D. Status of measurement in stroke rehabilitation outcomes. (Supplement to *Stroke*. A journal of cerebral circulation). September, 1990; 21:II–30.
21. Jongbloed L PhD. Problems of methodological heterogeneity in studies predicting disability after stroke. (Supplement to *Stroke*. A journal of cerebral circulation). September, 1990; 21:II–32.
22. Reding MJ M.D. A model stroke classification scheme and its use in outcome research. (Supplement to *Stroke*. A journal of cerebral circulation). September, 1990; 21:II–35.
23. Gresham GE M.D. Past achievements and new directions to stroke outcome research. (Supplement to *Stroke*. A journal of cerebral circulation). September, 1990; 21:II–1.
24. Cope DN, Hall K. Head injury rehabilitation: benefit of early intervention. *Arch Phys Med Rehabil* 1982; 63:433–437.
25. Mackay LE, Bernstein BA, Chapman PE, Morgan AS. Early intervention in severe head injury: long–term benefits of a formalized program. *Arch Phys Med Rehabil* 1992; 73:635–641.
26. Sivenius J, Pyorala K, Heinonen OP, Salonen JT. The significance of intensity of rehabilitation of stroke—A controlled study. *Stroke* 1985; 16:928–931.
27. Lehmann JF, DeLaeur BJ, Fowler RS, et al. Stroke: does rehabilitation affect outcome. *Arch Phys Med Rehabil* 1975; 56:375–382.
28. Piaget J. The Grains of Intelligence in Children New York: Norton, 1978.
29. Boddy J. Brain Systems and Psychological Concepts New York: John Wiley, 1978.
30. Will BE, Rosenzweig MR. Effets de l'environment sur la recuperation functionelle apres lesions cerebrates chez les rats adultes. *Biological Behaviour* 1976; 1:5–16.
31. Mitchell S, Bradley VA, Welch JL, Britton PG. Coma arousal procedure: a therapeutic intervention in the treatment of head injury. *Brain Injury* 1990; 4:273–279.
32. Larsson A, Wikkelso C, Bilting M, Stephensen H. Clinical parameters in 74 consecutive patients shunt operated for normal pressure hydrocephalus. *Acta Neurologica Scandinavica* 1991; 84:475–482.
33. Voldy B. Ruptured intracranial aneurysm. A clinical and pathophysiological study. *Dan Med Bull* 1986; 33:53–64.
34. Feeney DM, Gonzalez A, Law WA. Amphetamine, Haloperidol, and experience

interact to affect rate of recovery after motor cortex injury. *Science* 1982; 217:855–857.

35. Hovda DA, Fenney DM. Amphetamine with experience promotes recovery of locomotor function after unilateral frontal cortex injury in the cat. *Brain Research* 1984; 298:358–361.
36. Hurwitz BE PhD, Dietrich WD PhD, McCabe PM PhD, et al. Amphetamine promotes recovery from sensory–motor integration deficit after thrombotic infarction of the primary somatosensory rat cortex. *Stroke* 1991; 22:648–654.
37. Crisostomo EA, Duncan PW, Propst M, et al. Evidence that amphetamine with physical therapy promotes recovery of motor function in stroke patients. *Ann Neurol* 1988; 23:94–97.
38. Walker-Batson D, Unwin H, Curtis S, et al. Use of amphetamine in the treatment of aphasia. *Restorative Neurology and Neuroscience* 1992; 4:47–50.
39. Davis JN, Crisostomo EA, Duncan P, et al. Amphetamine and physical therapy facilitate recovery of function from stroke: correlative animal and human studies. In: Raichle ME, Powers WJ, (Eds.). Cerebrovascular Diseases. New York: Raven Press, 1987: 307.
40. Gualtieri CT. Review: pharmacotherapy and the neurobehavioural sequelae of traumatic brain injury. *Brain Injury* 1988; 2:101–129.
41. Elliott FA. Propranolol for the contro of belligerent behavior following acute brain damage. *Ann Neurol* 1977; 5:489–491.
42. Yudofsky SC, Silver JM, Schneider SE. Pharmacologic treatment of aggression. *Psychiatric Annals* 1987; 17:397–407.
43. Ratey JJ, Sorgi P, O'Driscoll GA et al. Nadolol to treat aggression and psychiatric symptomatology in chronic psychiatric inpatients: a double–blind, placebo–controlled study. *J Clin Psychiatry* 1992; 53:41–46.
44. Dunn ME, Umlauf RL, Mermis BJ. The rehabilitation situations inventory: staff perception of difficult behavioral situations in rehabilitation. *Arch Phys Med Rehabil* 1992; 73:316–319.
45. Foster HG, Hillbrand M, Chi CC. Efficacy of carbamazepine in assaultive patients with frontal lobe dysfunction. *Prog Neuro–Psychopharmacol and Biol Psychiat* 1989; 13:865–874.
46. Glenn MB M.D., Wroblewski B M.S., Parziale J M.D., et al. Lithium carbonate for aggressive behavior or affective instability in ten brain–injured patients. *Am J Phys Med Rehabil* 1989; 68:221–226.
47. Jackson RD M.D., Corrigan JD PhD, Arnett JA M.A. Amitriptyline for agitation in head injury. *Arch Phys Med Rehabil* 1985; 66:180–181.
48. Maurice-Williams RS, Willison JR, Hatfield R. The cognitive and psychological sequelae of uncomplicated aneurysm surgery. *Journal of Neurology, Neurosurgery and Psychiatry* 1991; 54:335–340.
49. Ljunggren B, Sonesson B, Saveland H, Brandt L. Cognitive impairment and adjustment in patients without neurological deficits after aneurysmal SAH and early operation. *J Neurosurg* 1985; 62:673–679.
50. Ropper AH, Zervas NT. Outcome 1 year after SAH from cerebral aneurysm. *J Neurosurg* 1984; 60:909–915.

51. Stegen G, Freckmann N. Outcome and rehabilitation after aneurymal subarachnoid haemorrhage. *Zentralblatt fur Neurochirurgie* 1991; 52:37–39.
52. Bell BA, Kendall BE, Symon L. Computed tomography in aneurysmal subarachnoid haemorrhage. *J Neurol Neurosurg Psychiatry* 1980; 43:522–524.
53. Rommer B, Sonesson B, Ljunggren B, Brandt L, Svaeland H, Holtas S. Late magnetic resonance imaging related to neurobehaviaoral functioning after aneurysmal subarachnoid hemorrhage. *Neurosurgery* 1989; 25:390–397.

Index